PEDIATRIC CARDIOLOGY BOARD REVIEW

Second Edition

PEDIATRIC CARDIOLOGY BOARD REVIEW

Second Edition

Benjamin W. Eidem, MD, FACC, FASE

Professor of Pediatrics & Medicine
Divisions of Pediatric Cardiology & Cardiovascular Diseases
Mayo Clinic
Rochester, Minnesota

Bryan C. Cannon, MD, FHRS

Associate Professor of Pediatrics
Divisions of Pediatric Cardiology & Cardiovascular Diseases
Mayo Clinic
Rochester, Minnesota

Jonathan N. Johnson, MD, FACC, FASE, FAAP

Associate Professor of Pediatrics
Divisions of Pediatric Cardiology & Cardiovascular Diseases
Mayo Clinic
Rochester, Minnesota

Anthony C. Chang, MD, MBA, MPH

Chief Intelligence and Innovation Officer
Medical Director
The Sharon Disney Lund Medical Intelligence and Innovation Institute
Medical Director
Heart Failure Program, Children's Hospital of Orange County
Orange, California

Frank Cetta, MD, FACC, FASE

Professor of Pediatrics & Medicine
Divisions of Pediatric Cardiology & Cardiovascular Diseases
Mayo Clinic
Rochester, Minnesota

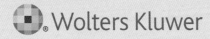
. Wolters Kluwer

Philadelphia • Baltimore • New York • London
Buenos Aires • Hong Kong • Sydney • Tokyo

Acquisitions Editor: Julie Goolsby
Development Editor: Andrea Vosburgh
Senior Production Project Manager: Alicia Jackson
Design Coordinator: Holly McLaughlin
Senior Manufacturing Coordinator: Beth Welsh
Prepress Vendor: Aptara, Inc.

© 2017 by Mayo Foundation for Medical Education and Research
200 First Street SW
Rochester, MN 55905 USA

9 8 7 6 5 4 3 2 1

Printed in China

Library of Congress Cataloging-in-Publication Data
Names: Eidem, Benjamin W., editor. | Cannon, Bryan C., editor. | Johnson,
    Jonathan N., editor. | Chang, Anthony C., editor. | Cetta, Frank, editor.
Title: Pediatric cardiology board review / [edited by] Benjamin W. Eidem,
    Bryan C. Cannon, Jonathan N. Johnson, Anthony C. Chang, Frank Cetta.
Description: Second edition. | Philadelphia : Wolters Kluwer, [2017] |
    Includes bibliographical references and index.
Identifiers: LCCN 2016015280 | ISBN 9781496351234 (paperback)
Subjects: | MESH: Heart Defects, Congenital | Heart Diseases | Child |
    Adolescent | Infant | Examination Questions
Classification: LCC RJ421 | NLM WS 18.2 | DDC 618.92/120076–dc23
LC record available at https://lccn.loc.gov/2016015280

LWW.com

Contributors

Heather N. Anderson, MD
Chief Resident Physician
Department of Pediatric and Adolescent Medicine
Mayo Clinic
Rochester, Minnesota

Jason H. Anderson, MD, FAAP
Pediatric Cardiology Fellow
Mayo Clinic
Rochester, Minnesota

Bryan C. Cannon, MD, FHRS
Associate Professor of Pediatrics
Divisions of Pediatric Cardiology & Cardiovascular Diseases
Mayo Clinic
Rochester, Minnesota

Frank Cetta, MD, FACC, FASE
Professor of Pediatrics & Medicine
Divisions of Pediatric Cardiology & Cardiovascular Diseases
Mayo Clinic
Rochester, Minnesota

Anthony C. Chang, MD, MBA, MPH
Chief Intelligence and Innovation Officer
Medical Director
The Sharon Disney Lund Medical Intelligence and
    Innovation Institute
Medical Director
Heart Failure Program, Children's Hospital of Orange
    County
Orange, California

Sheri S. Crow, MD, MSc
Assistant Professor of Pediatric and Adolescent Medicine and
    Health Services Research
Pediatric Critical Care Medicine
Mayo Clinic
Rochester, Minnesota

Sonja Dahl, APRN, CNP, DNP
Instructor in Pediatrics
Department of Pediatric & Adolescent Medicine
Mayo Clinic
Rochester, Minnesota

David J. Driscoll, MD
Professor of Pediatrics
Department of Pediatrics, Division of Pediatric Cardiology
Mayo Clinic
Rochester, Minnesota

Benjamin W. Eidem, MD, FACC, FASE
Professor of Pediatrics & Medicine
Divisions of Pediatric Cardiology & Cardiovascular Diseases
Mayo Clinic
Rochester, Minnesota

M. Eric Ferguson, MD
Assistant Professor of Pediatrics
Sibley Heart Center Cardiology
Emory University
Atlanta, Georgia

Jonathan N. Johnson, MD, FACC, FASE, FAAP
Associate Professor of Pediatrics
Divisions of Pediatric Cardiology & Cardiovascular Diseases
Mayo Clinic
Rochester, Minnesota

Angela M. Kelle, MD, FAAP
Assistant Professor of Pediatrics
Pediatric Cardiology Fellow
Mayo Clinic
Rochester, Minnesota

Brandon D. Morrical, MD
Pediatric Cardiology Fellow
Mayo Clinic
Rochester, Minnesota

Sabrina Phillips, MD, FACC, FASE
Associate Professor of Medicine
Department of Medicine, Cardiovascular Section
The University of Oklahoma Health Sciences Center
Oklahoma City, Oklahoma

Joseph T. Poterucha, DO
Assistant Professor of Medicine and Pediatrics
Pediatric Cardiology Fellow
Mayo Clinic
Rochester, Minnesota

Adam M. Putschoegl, DO, FAAP
Pediatric Cardiology Fellow
Mayo Clinic
Rochester, Minnesota

Muhammad Yasir Qureshi, MBBS
Assistant Professor of Pediatrics
Senior Associate Consultant
Division of Pediatric Cardiology
Mayo Clinic
Rochester, Minnesota

Andrew E. Schneider, MD, FAAP
Pediatric Cardiology Fellow
Mayo Clinic
Rochester, Minnesota

Nathaniel Taggart, MD
Assistant Professor of Pediatrics
Division of Pediatric Cardiology
Mayo Clinic
Rochester, Minnesota

Alex J. Thompson, MD
Pediatric Cardiology Fellow
Mayo Clinic
Rochester, Minnesota

Philip L. Wackel, MD
Assistant Professor of Pediatrics
Division of Pediatric Cardiology
Mayo Clinic
Rochester, Minnesota

Preface

Kudos to Drs. Chang and Eidem for beginning a decade of successful Pediatric Cardiology Review courses (2006–2016). Over the years, hundreds of seasoned practicing pediatric cardiologists and new graduates of fellowship training programs have provided the lifeblood to this educational venture. The 2nd edition of this text provides a comprehensive take home study guide for those agonizing about their upcoming board examination or for those who simply want to refresh their knowledge in the fundamentals of our field.

This 2nd edition provides expanded detailed answers in each chapter while also placing an added emphasis on adult congenital heart disease. This text recognizes the ever growing number of adults with CHD that will be encountered in daily practice. In addition, in the fall of 2015 the ABIM administered the first ACHD board examination. We aim to provide material in this edition which is directly applicable to that examination.

Not all questions in this book, nor on the official board examinations, are perfect. But the editors and authors feel that the concepts tested in each question will enhance the read-er's educational experience. Contrary to board examinations, many of the questions within this book have relatively short stems. Again this is designed to test as many concepts as possible while being cognizant of space and page limitations. Two messages are important with respect to test taking strategy: (1) When encountering a stem that is more than a few sentences long…read the answers first! In that way one has insight to find the pertinent clues in the stem, rather than feeling overwhelmed, fatigued, and lost at the end of a long question; and (2), most importantly, answer all of the questions—there are no points for unanswered questions!

For those who can make it to Dana Point, California for the upcoming Congenital Cardiology review courses in 2016 and 2018, we hope that this book serves as a handy resource. Feedback from readers of the 1st edition and prior course participants has been very positive and we hope that you feel the same with this 2nd edition!

THE EDITORS

Acknowledgments

I would like to thank my wife Jori for all of her love and support. I also would like to recognize the outstanding mentors and fellows at Mayo Clinic who have dedicated their careers to the advancement of our field—BWE

Thanks to my wife and children (Aaron, Ashleigh, and Avery) for their patience, love, and support—BCC

I would like to dedicate this book to all of my outstanding mentors and colleagues as well as the wonderful children and adults with congenital and acquired heart disease who have taught me throughout these years—ACC

I would like to thank my wife, Alissa, and daughter, Elliana, for their love, their support, and for always making me smile. I also want to express my appreciation to my mentors (including my coeditors) for their dedication to the education of decades of pediatric cardiology fellows—JNJ

I would like to thank Donald Hagler, MD, and David Driscoll, MD for all they taught me in fellowship and all they continue to teach me. They have made numerous contributions to grow the knowledge base and develop the careers of Mayo Clinic fellows for decades—FC

Abbreviations

ABG	arterial blood gas
ACE	angiotensin-converting enzyme
ADH	antidiuretic hormone
AH	atrium-His
AICD	automatic implantable cardioverter defibrillator
ALCAPA	anomalous left coronary artery arising from the pulmonary artery
ALTE	apparent life-threatening event
AP	aortopulmonary
APV	absent pulmonary valve
ARB	angiotensin receptor blocker
ARF	acute rheumatic fever
ARVC	arrhythmogenic right ventricular cardiomyopathy
ASD	atrial septal defect
AV	atrioventricular
AVM	arteriovenous malformation
AVSD	atrioventricular septal defect
BAS	balloon atrial septostomy
BMI	body mass index
BP	blood pressure
bpm	beats per minute
BT	Blalock–Taussig
CBC	complete blood count
CHD	congenital heart disease
CHF	congestive heart failure
CMR	cardiac magnetic resonance
CNS	central nervous system
CP	constrictive pericarditis
CPAP	continuous positive airway pressure
CPVT	catecholamine-sensitive polymorphic ventricular tachycardia
CRP	C-reactive protein
CS	coronary sinus
CT	computed tomography
CVP	central venous pressure
CW	continuous wave
CXR	chest x-ray
DBP	diastolic blood pressure
DCM	dilated cardiomyopathy
DCRV	double-chambered RV
df	degree of freedom
DKS	Damus–Kaye–Stansel
DORV	double-outlet right ventricle
ECG	electrocardiogram
ECMO	extracorporeal membrane oxygenation
EF	ejection fraction
EFE	endomyocardial fibroelastosis
ERP	effective refractory period
ESR	erythrocyte sedimentation rate
FEV	forced expiratory volume
FiO$_2$	fraction of inspired oxygen
FISH	fluorescence in situ hybridization
FRC	functional residual capacity
HCM	hypertrophic cardiomyopathy
HDL	high-density lipoprotein
HLHS	hypoplastic left heart syndrome
HR	heart rate
HV	His-ventricle
IAA	interrupted aortic arch
ICD	implantable cardioverter defibrillator
ICU	intensive care unit
IE	infectious endocarditis
INR	international normalized ratio
IPAH	idiopathic pulmonary arterial hypertension
IRT	isovolumic relaxation time
IV	intravenous
IVC	inferior vena cava
IVS	interventricular septum
JET	junctional ectopic tachycardia
LA	left atrium
LAD	left anterior descending
LAO	left anterior oblique
LBBB	left bundle branch block
LCA	left coronary artery
LDL	low-density lipoprotein
LIV	left innominate vein
LLSB	left lower sternal border
LMCA	left main coronary artery
LMWH	low–molecular-weight heparin
LPA	left pulmonary artery
LQTS	long QT syndrome
LSVC	left superior vena cava
LUSB	left upper sternal border
LV	left ventricular
LVEDP	left ventricular end diastolic pressure
LVEDV	left ventricular end diastolic volume
LVEF	left ventricular ejection fraction
LVH	left ventricular hypertrophy

LVOT	left ventricular outflow tract		**RHD**	rheumatic heart disease
LVOTO	left ventricular outflow tract obstruction		**RLSB**	right lower sternal border
MAPCA	major aortopulmonary collateral arteries		**ROC**	receiver operating characteristic
MDE	myocardial delayed enhancement		**RPA**	right pulmonary artery
MPA	main pulmonary artery		**RPCW**	right pulmonary capillary wedge
MRI	magnetic resonance imaging		**RUPV**	right upper pulmonary vein
MVP	mitral valve prolapse		**RV**	right ventricle
MVV	maximum voluntary ventilation		**RVED**	right ventricle end diastolic
NICU	neonatal intensive care unit		**RVEDP**	right ventricular end diastolic pressure
NPV	negative predictive value		**RVH**	right ventricular hypertrophy
PA	pulmonary valve atresia or pulmonary artery		**RVOT**	right ventricular outflow tract
PAC	premature atrial contraction		**RVSP**	right ventricular systolic pressure
PAH	pulmonary arterial hypertension		**SA**	sinoatrial
PAPVC	partial anomalous pulmonary venous connection		**SBP**	systolic blood pressure
pCO$_2$	partial pressure of CO_2		**SCD**	sudden cardiac death
PCWP	pulmonary capillary wedge pressure		**SD**	standard deviation
PDA	patent ductus arteriosus		**SEM**	standard error of the mean
PEP	positive expiratory pressure		**SLE**	systemic lupus erythematosus
PFO	patent foramen ovale		**SPAMM**	spatial modulation of magnetization
PGE	prostaglandin E		**SVASD**	sinus venosus atrial septal defect
PICU	pediatric intensive care unit		**SVC**	superior vena cava
PIG	peak instantaneous gradient		**SVR**	systemic vascular resistance
PJRT	permanent junctional reciprocating tachycardia		**SVT**	supraventricular tachycardia
PO	per os (by mouth)		**TAPVC**	total anomalous pulmonary venous connection
PPS	peripheral pulmonary stenosis		**TDI**	tissue Doppler imaging
PPV	positive predictive value		**TEE**	transesophageal echocardiography
PR	pulmonary regurgitation		**TOF**	tetralogy of Fallot
PRF	pulse repetition frequency		**tPA**	tissue plasminogen activator
PVC	premature ventricular contraction		**TSH**	thyroid-stimulating hormone
PVR	pulmonary vascular resistance		**TTE**	transthoracic echocardiography
PW	pulsed-wave		**TVI**	time velocity integral
PWP	pulmonary wedge pressure		**UVC**	umbilical venous catheter
RA	right atrium		**VAT**	ventilatory anaerobic threshold
RAP	right atrial pressure		**VEC**	velocity-encoded cine
RBBB	right bundle branch block		**VF**	ventricular fibrillation
RBC	red blood cell		**VQ**	ventilatory:perfusion
RCA	right coronary artery		**VSD**	ventricular septal defect
RCM	restrictive cardiomyopathy		**VT**	ventricular tachycardia
RF	rheumatic fever		**WPW**	Wolff–Parkinson–White

Contents

CHAPTER 1

Cardiac Anatomy and Physiology

Alex J. Thompson and Jonathan N. Johnson

QUESTIONS

1. Left ventricular isovolumic contraction continues until what cardiac event occurs?

   A. Mitral valve opens
   B. Passive atrial filling
   C. Increased ventricular volume
   D. Aortic valve opens
   E. Aortic pressure greater than left ventricular

2. A 12-year-old girl with newly diagnosed systemic lupus erythematosus is referred for an echocardiogram. During the echo, a verrucous Libman–Sacks lesion was noted. On which valve is this lesion most commonly found?

   A. Aortic valve
   B. Tricuspid valve
   C. Mitral valve
   D. Pulmonary valve
   E. Eustachian valve

3. Many metabolic factors are responsible for regulating coronary arterial blood flow. Which of the following metabolic factors is derived from the breakdown of high energy phosphates?

   A. Prostaglandin
   B. Nitric oxide
   C. Endothelin-1
   D. Adenosine
   E. Vascular endothelial growth factor

4. You diagnose a neonate with polysplenia. Which of the following is most likely to be true regarding this patient?

   A. Limb-length abnormalities are present
   B. There are multiple spleens on both the left and right sides
   C. Multiple gallbladders are common
   D. The SVC is interrupted
   E. The IVC is interrupted, with azygous continuation to SVC

5. In the mature cardiac myocyte, the majority of calcium involved in the binding of troponin C and thus the initiation of myocyte contraction is stored in which cellular space?

   A. Extracellular space
   B. T-tubule
   C. Mitochondria
   D. Lysosomes
   E. Sarcoplasmic reticulum

6. A 12-year-old boy is diagnosed with mild aortic stenosis. You suspect that he has an abnormal aortic valve. Echocardiographic imaging demonstrates that his valve is similar to the following pathology image (Fig. 1.1). Which of the following is the aortic leaflet pattern in this patient?

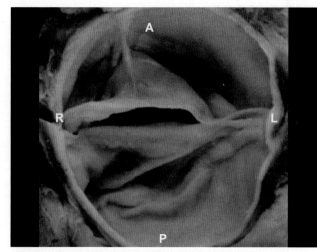

FIGURE 1.1 A, anterior; P, posterior; R, right; L, left. Image courtesy of Dr. William Edwards, Mayo Clinic.

  A. Bicuspid valve with fusion of the right and non-coronary cusps
  B. Quadricuspid valve with a cleft of the left coronary cusp
  C. Unicuspid valve with fusion of more than one cusp
  D. Bicuspid valve with fusion of the right and left cusps
  E. Bicuspid valve with fusion of the left and noncoronary cusps

7. A 5-day-old male infant is in the intensive care unit after a Norwood procedure and is hypotensive. In response to the decreased renal arterial pressure, which of the following hormones is released and subsequently induces cleaving angiotensinogen to angiotensin I?

  A. Angiotensin II
  B. Renin
  C. Vasopressin
  D. Norepinephrine
  E. Prostaglandin

8. Which of the following factors has the greatest impact on the pressure change across two points in a vessel?

  A. Vessel radius
  B. Blood viscosity
  C. Vessel length
  D. Maximum velocity of blood flow
  E. Hemoglobin concentration

9. The normal left aortic arch is primarily derived from which embryologic aortic arch?

  A. Fourth (IV) arch
  B. First (I) arch
  C. Second (II) arch
  D. Third (III) arch
  E. Sixth (VI) arch

10. Embryologically, the ductus arteriosus and the left pulmonary artery arise from the:

  A. Left fourth aortic arch
  B. Left sixth and fourth aortic arches, respectively
  C. Left fourth and sixth aortic arches, respectively
  D. Left sixth aortic arch
  E. Right fifth arch

11. You diagnose a 5-day-old female infant with tetralogy of Fallot. Of the following defects, which is most likely to be seen concurrently on echocardiogram?

  A. Right aortic arch
  B. Aortic stenosis
  C. Atrial septal defect or patent foramen ovale
  D. Coarctation of the aorta
  E. Mitral valve prolapse

12. A newborn female infant presents with cyanosis. The following echocardiogram is obtained (Fig. 1.2). In patients with this anatomy, which of the following is the most common coronary arterial abnormality?

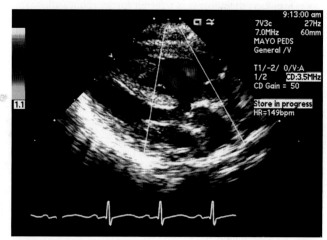

FIGURE 1.2

  A. Intramural left coronary
  B. Left anterior descending from the RCA
  C. Single right coronary
  D. Single left coronary
  E. Left circumflex from the RCA

13. A sonographer points out an echo-dark space around the aortic sinus in a parasternal short-axis echocardiographic image in a neonate. You note that this space extends anterior to the superior vena cava and posterior to the ascending aorta and pulmonary trunk. This echo-dark space is the:

- **A.** Oblique sinus
- **B.** Coronal sinus
- **C.** Transverse sinus
- **D.** Pericardial recess
- **E.** Longitudinal sinus

14. How does atrial natriuretic peptide (ANP) work on the kidney?

- **A.** Decreases tubular resorption of sodium
- **B.** Activates vasopressin receptors
- **C.** Inhibits ion exchange in the ascending loop of Henle
- **D.** Inhibition of sodium resorption in the proximal tubule
- **E.** Dilation of the efferent arteriole

15. In a normal adolescent heart, the average ratio of ventricular septal thickness to left free-wall thickness is:

- **A.** 1.1
- **B.** 2.9
- **C.** 1.9
- **D.** 0.6
- **E.** 2.4

16. A 3-year-old boy with a history of a ventricular septal defect presents to your office for follow-up. On examination, you hear a diastolic murmur at the apex. Echocardiography is performed (Fig. 1.3). Prolapse of which aortic cusp is most likely causing the diastolic murmur?

- **A.** Left
- **B.** Anterior
- **C.** Septal
- **D.** Right
- **E.** Noncoronary

17. An overriding atrioventricular valve:

- **A.** Has chordal attachments into both ventricles
- **B.** Must have chordal attachments to the ventricular septal crest
- **C.** Cannot coexist with straddling
- **D.** Is never associated with malalignment type of VSD
- **E.** Empties into two ventricles

18. A 17-year-old boy is involved in a head-on motor vehicle accident. In the emergency department, the physicians suspect he has pericardial tamponade secondary to myocardial rupture. Which of the following is the most likely chamber for the rupture to occur?

- **A.** Left ventricle
- **B.** Right atrium
- **C.** Right ventricle
- **D.** Left atrium
- **E.** Atrial appendage

19. You diagnose a neonate with asplenia. Which of the following is most likely to be present in this patient?

- **A.** The liver is midline with two mirror-image left lobes
- **B.** Descending aorta and IVC on the same side of vertebral column
- **C.** The biliary tree is patent with associated multiple gall bladders
- **D.** Stomach position is fixed to the right side
- **E.** Normal rotation of the bowels

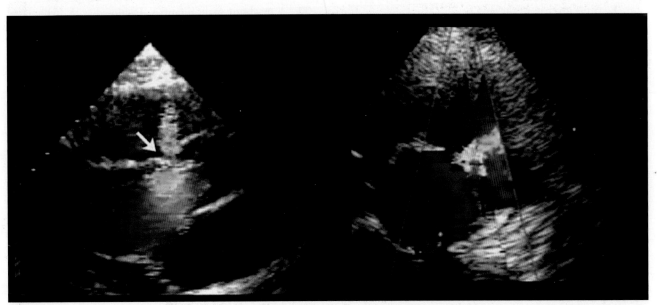

FIGURE 1.3

20. A 16-year-old boy is a long-distance runner in track for his high school. He has been training all year preparing for the state track meet. Compared to prior to training, which change in his resting hemodynamics will be seen in his currently trained state?

    A. Increased stroke volume
    B. Increased heart rate
    C. Decreased blood volume
    D. Increased myocardial oxygen demand
    E. Increased resting arterial blood pressure

21. The most reliable feature of the normal atrioventricular valve that distinguishes the mitral valve from the tricuspid valve is the:

    A. Level of attachment of AV valve at cardiac crux
    B. Shape of the orifice
    C. AV valve–semilunar valve continuity
    D. Presence of septal chordal attachments
    E. Number of leaflets

22. Which of the following factors would shift the O_2 dissociation curve to the left?

    A. Increased temperature
    B. Increased pCO_2
    C. Increased 2,3-DPG
    D. Increased pH
    E. Increased fetal hemoglobin concentration

23. A single sinoatrial node in a normal position is typically found in which of the following?

    A. Left juxtaposition of the atrial appendages
    B. Right atrial isomerism
    C. Right juxtaposition of the atrial appendages
    D. Left atrial isomerism
    E. Situs inversus of the atria

24. Systemic arteriolar vasodilation occurs in response to:

    A. Decreased pCO_2
    B. Decreased H^+
    C. Decreased pO_2
    D. Decreased K^+
    E. Decreased Mg^+

25. Which of the following is a valvular remnant located at the junction of the inferior vena cava and the right atrium?

    A. Thebesian valve
    B. Eustachian valve
    C. Valve of the fossa ovalis
    D. Chiari networks
    E. Valve of the SVC

26. Which term best describes the type of defect that is characterized by large atrial septal and ventricular septal defects as well as a common atrioventricular valve, but with separate left and right orifices?

    A. Partial AVSD
    B. Intermediate AVSD
    C. Complete AVSD
    D. Transitional AVSD
    E. Membranous VSD

27. Which fetal venous structure has the lowest oxygen saturation?

    A. Ductus venosus
    B. IVC
    C. Left hepatic vein
    D. Coronary sinus
    E. Right pulmonary vein

28. The most reliable anatomic feature that distinguishes the normal right ventricle from the left ventricle is:

    A. Course apical trabeculations
    B. Level of insertion of AV valve at cardiac crux
    C. Continuity between semilunar and AV valve
    D. Shape of the ventricle
    E. Presence of moderator band

29. The direction in which blood flows through an ASD primarily is related to the:

    A. Pulmonary vascular resistance
    B. Systemic vascular resistance
    C. Relative compliances of the left and right ventricles
    D. Morphology of eustachian valve
    E. Redundancy of atrial septum

30. A newborn male infant is diagnosed with hypoplastic left heart syndrome (HLHS). Of the following, which anatomic form of HLHS will most likely be seen in this patient?

    A. Aortic valve atresia with patent mitral valve
    B. Aortic valve stenosis with patent mitral valve
    C. Aortic valve stenosis with mitral valve stenosis
    D. Aortic valve atresia with mitral valve atresia
    E. Aortic valve atresia with mitral valve regurgitation

31. In the cardiac sarcomere, which of the following named features includes the entirety of the myosin contractile elements?

    A. E-line
    B. A-band
    C. I-band
    D. H-zone
    E. Z-disk

32. Truncus arteriosus is diagnosed in a newborn male infant. Of the following, which truncal valve morphology are you most likely to find?

   A. Unicuspid
   B. Bicuspid
   C. Quadricuspid
   D. Pentacuspid
   E. Sextacuspid

 33. The resting potential of which ion is primarily responsible for the baseline (phase 4) resting conductance of cardiac myocytes?

   A. Calcium
   B. Sodium
   C. Potassium
   D. Chloride
   E. Magnesium

34. The rapid depolarization of cardiac myocytes (phase 0) is driven by the rapid influx of which ion into the myocytes?

   A. Sodium
   B. Potassium
   C. Chloride
   D. Magnesium
   E. Calcium

35. You are called to see a cyanotic neonate in the neonatal intensive care unit. You note that the patient has an oxygen saturation of 69%. His chest x-ray shows decreased vascular markings in the lung fields. Which of the following is the most likely anatomy you will find on examination and echocardiography?

   A. Truncus arteriosus
   B. Total anomalous venous return
   C. Critical pulmonary stenosis
   D. Hypoplastic left heart syndrome
   E. Tricuspid atresia with transposed great arteries

36. A 9-year-old girl is diagnosed with a sinus venosus ASD on echocardiography. Relative to the fossa ovalis, where would you expect to find a sinus venosus ASD?

   A. Anterior and superior
   B. Anterior and inferior
   C. Posterior and superior
   D. Posterior and inferior
   E. Anterior and apical

37. What is the most abundant nonmyocyte cardiac cell in the mature heart?

   A. Fibroblasts
   B. Pericytes
   C. Vascular smooth muscle cells
   D. Macrophages
   E. Endothelial cells

38. A 4-year-old boy is referred for cardiomegaly on a chest x-ray. His four-chamber view is seen in Figure 1.4. Of the following, which additional cardiac diagnosis is most likely to be found in this patient?

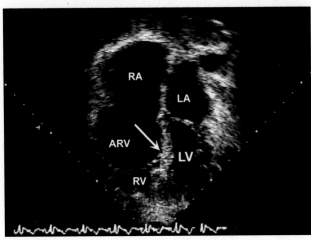

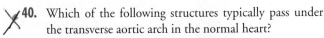

FIGURE 1.4 RA, right atrium; RV, right ventricle; LA, left atrium; LV, left ventricle; ARV, atrialized right ventricle.

   A. Ventricular septal defect
   B. Pulmonary valve stenosis
   C. Patent ductus arteriosus
   D. Mitral valve prolapse
   E. Atrial septal defect

39. Of the following, which structure in the fetus has the least saturated blood?

   A. Superior vena cava
   B. Inferior vena cava
   C. Patent ductus arteriosus
   D. Ductus venous
   E. Ascending aortic arch

40. Which of the following structures typically pass under the transverse aortic arch in the normal heart?

   A. Right pulmonary artery and left bronchus
   B. Right pulmonary artery and right bronchus
   C. Left pulmonary artery and left bronchus
   D. Left pulmonary artery and right bronchus
   E. Left pulmonary artery and thoracic duct

41. Which arterial vessel is partially formed by the remnants of the third aortic arch?

   A. Common carotid artery
   B. Left subclavian artery
   C. Brachiocephalic artery
   D. Maxillary artery
   E. Aortic arch three completely regresses

42. Which structures connect cardiac myocytes end to end and are responsible for structural integrity and synchronized contraction of cardiac tissue?

    A. Dystrophin
    B. T-tubules
    C. Costameres
    D. Intercalated discs
    E. Myosin

43. A 2-year-old boy undergoes repair of coarctation of the aorta. Postoperatively, he is able to be extubated, but develops intermittent stridor. Chest radiography is unremarkable. Which of the following is the most likely structure that was injured during the operation?

    A. Left vagus nerve
    B. Right recurrent laryngeal nerve
    C. Thoracic duct
    D. Right vagus nerve
    E. Left recurrent laryngeal nerve

44. A fetal echocardiogram is performed and demonstrates double outlet right ventricle. Which of the following positions of the aorta, relative to the pulmonary artery, are you most likely to find on further imaging?

    A. Right anterior
    B. Left anterior
    C. Side by side
    D. Left posterior
    E. Right posterior

45. A 4-year-old boy is seen because his pediatrician heard a murmur. An atrial septal defect (ASD) is found on echocardiography (Fig. 1.5). Which of the following types of defects is present?

    A. Coronary sinus ASD
    B. Primum ASD
    C. Sinus venosus ASD
    D. Secundum ASD
    E. Atrioventricular septal defect

46. The normal right superior vena cava is derived from which of the following embryologic structures?

    A. Left anterior cardinal vein
    B. Right vitelline vein
    C. Right anterior cardinal vein
    D. Ductus venosus
    E. Left umbilical vein

47. A term neonate presents with tachycardia, poor perfusion, and respiratory failure. The liver is enlarged on examination. Echocardiography reveals dilation of all four heart chambers. You note that the echo-calculated cardiac output is markedly elevated. Which of the following is the most likely source of the high-output cardiac failure?

    A. Lower extremity AVM
    B. Upper extremity AVM
    C. Hepatic AVM
    D. Vein of Galen malformation
    E. Pulmonary AVM

48. Which of the following is a characteristic of the morphologic tricuspid valve?

    A. Two leaflets are present
    B. Septal chordal attachments
    C. Elliptical-shaped orifice
    D. Two commissures are present
    E. Empties into the morphologic left ventricle

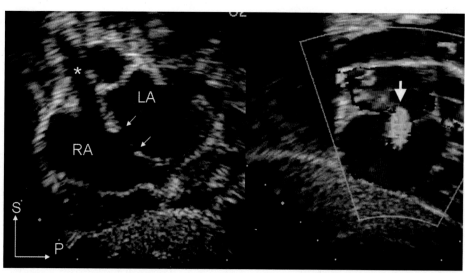

FIGURE 1.5

49. Which fetal remnant delivers blood from the right and left hepatic veins to the right atrium?

    A. Ductus arteriosus
    B. Ductus venosus
    C. Foramen ovale
    D. Aortic isthmus
    E. Umbilical arteries

50. A 5-day-old female infant has an echocardiogram performed (Fig. 1.6). Of the following abnormal coronary patterns, which are you most likely to find on this echocardiogram?

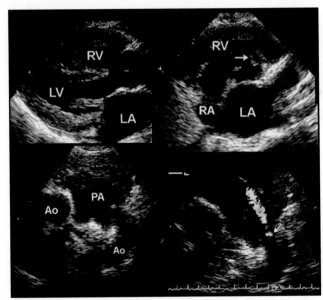

FIGURE 1.6 RV, right ventricle; LV, left ventricle; LA, left atrium; RA, right atrium; Ao, aorta; PA, pulmonary artery.

    A. Intramural left coronary artery
    B. Left anterior descending from the RCA
    C. Left circumflex from the RCA
    D. Single left coronary
    E. Single right coronary

51. Which of the following is an anatomic hallmark of the morphologic right atrium?

    A. Ostium of IVC
    B. Finger-like atrial appendage
    C. Smooth-surfaced free wall
    D. Ostium of the pulmonary veins
    E. More posterior location than the left atrium

52. A 4-day-old male infant has the following echo performed (Fig. 1.7). Which of the following great artery relationships are you most likely to find on echocardiography?

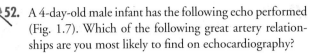
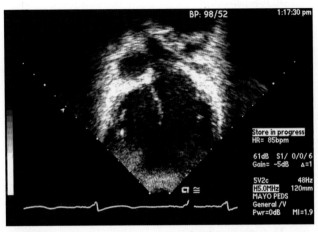

FIGURE 1.7

    A. D-transposition of the great arteries
    B. L-transposition of the great arteries
    C. Left anterior aorta
    D. Right anterior aorta
    E. Normally related great arteries

53. During the relaxation phase of the cardiac muscle contraction, the majority of Ca^{2+} is removed from the sarcoplasm by:

    A. Passive exchange through L-type Ca^{2+} channels
    B. Efflux via Na^+–Ca^{2+} passive exchange
    C. Ca^{2+}-ATPase pumps located on the sarcolemma
    D. Reuptake in the sarcoplasmic reticulum via SERCA pumps
    E. Efflux via K^+–Ca^{2+} passive exchange

54. You are evaluating a 3-week-old male infant with tricuspid atresia, transposition of the great arteries, moderate pulmonary stenosis, and a mildly restrictive ventricular septal defect. In this patient, where is the AV node most likely to be positioned?

    A. Posteriorly behind the ostium of the coronary sinus
    B. Anteriorly along the atrial septum in the right atrium
    C. Floor of the blind right atrium
    D. In the left atrium just medial to the left atrioventricular valve annulus
    E. Lateral to the ostium of the IVC in the right atrium

55. Which of the following is true regarding the right ventricle in the normal heart?

    A. Is typically a bipartite chamber
    B. Has small apical trabeculations
    C. Has a prominent crista terminalis
    D. Has a coarse septal surface
    E. There is tricuspid–pulmonary continuity

56. A neonate is diagnosed with d-transposition of the great arteries. In addition to the transposed great vessels, the most common concurrent finding on echocardiography in this patient is:

  A. Ventricular septal defect
  B. Mitral valve abnormalities
  C. Coarctation of the aorta
  D. Leftward juxtaposition of the atrial appendages
  E. Left ventricular outflow obstruction

57. A 12-year-old girl presents with cyanosis. An echocardiogram reveals severe Ebstein anomaly with severe tricuspid valve regurgitation. Which of the following is the most likely cause of her cyanosis?

  A. Left-to-right shunt at the atrial level
  B. Right-to-left shunt at the atrial level ✓
  C. Right-to-left shunt at the ventricular level
  D. Coronary fistula
  E. Stenotic outflow to the pulmonary arteries

58. Which of the following is an anatomic hallmark of the morphologic left atrium?

  A. Valve of fossa ovalis (septum primum)
  B. Limbus of the fossa ovalis
  C. More anterior location compared to the right atrium
  D. Entrance of the inferior vena cava
  E. Connection to tricuspid valve

59. Which of the following is true regarding fetal hemoglobin?

  A. Is composed of alpha and gamma subunits
  B. Is present in normal children until the age of 6 years
  C. Is replaced by adult hemoglobin by the 38th week of gestation
  D. Has a lower affinity for oxygen than adult hemoglobin
  E. Interacts more efficiently with 2,3-DPG than adult hemoglobin

60. Through which pathway does norepinephrine activate $\beta 1$ adrenergic receptors?

  A. Direct activation of Ca^{2+}-ATPase
  B. G_q-dependent activation of phospholipase C
  C. G_s-dependent activation of adenylate cyclase, increasing cAMP
  D. G_i-dependent inhibition of adenylate cyclase, decreasing cAMP
  E. Activation of guanylate cyclase, increasing cGMP

61. Which of the following changes occurs with inspiration in the normal heart and lungs?

  A. Increase in pleural pressure by 3 to 5 cm H_2O
  B. Decrease in intra-abdominal pressure
  C. Increased E′ velocity of the tricuspid valve
  D. Increased E′ velocity of the mitral valve
  E. Decrease in right ventricular stroke volume

62. A 3-month-old infant presents with a systolic murmur heard best at the apex. An echocardiogram is diagnostic of a mitral arcade. Which of the following would best describe a mitral arcade?

  A. Thickened mitral valve leaflets
  B. Fused papillary muscles
  C. Absent papillary muscle
  D. Absent/abnormal chordal insertions
  E. Decreased interpapillary muscle distance

63. The formation of an ostium primum ASD results from:

  A. Excessive resorption of the septum primum
  B. Insufficient growth of the septum secundum
  C. Abnormal endocardial cushion development
  D. Failure of the common pulmonary vein to connect to the left atrium
  E. Abnormal rotation of the dextrodorsal conal swelling

64. A vessel is noted running lateral and leftward to the pulmonary artery on high parasternal short-axis views, with flow heading inferiorly. The structure is seen again on a transesophageal echocardiogram running between the left pulmonary veins and the left atrial appendage, just posterior and superior to the mitral valve. What does this structure most likely represent?

  A. Membrane of cor triatriatum
  B. Persistent levoatrial cardinal vein
  C. Total anomalous venous return
  D. Descending aorta
  E. Persistence of the left horn of the sinus venosus

65. A 2-month-old female infant presents with cyanosis. Which of the following is true regarding the diagnosis of cyanosis in this patient?

  A. To visualize cyanosis, the patient has to have at least 5 g/dL of deoxygenated hemoglobin
  B. This patient most likely has an atrial septal defect
  C. The best indicator of cyanosis in this patient is examination of the nail beds
  D. The patient most likely has rib notching on chest radiography
  E. This patient most likely has a patent ductus arteriosus

66. Mutations in which protein may cause disassociation of the intracellular cytoskeleton and the extracellular matrix in cardiac myocytes, in addition to causing muscular dystrophy?

  A. Alpha-dystroglycan
  B. Syntrophin
  C. Cytoplasmic actin
  D. Dystrophin
  E. Caveolin

67. The sarcomere is the fundamental contractile unit of striated muscle. Which contractile protein binds to calcium, allowing cross-bridges to form and permitting contraction?
  A. Actin
  B. Troponin C
  C. Myosin
  D. Tropomyosin
  E. Troponin I

68. A 3-year-old girl is referred to you for a murmur. You uncover that the patient is a recent immigrant from Bolivia, having arrived in the last week. She had lived at an altitude of 10,000 feet since her birth. Which of the following are you most likely to find on a hemodynamic evaluation of this patient, compared to a patient living at sea level?
  A. Left atrial enlargement
  B. Decreased LV systolic function (EF ~40%)
  C. Elevated pulmonary artery pressure
  D. Decreased tricuspid regurgitant velocity
  E. Elevated systemic blood pressure

69. Baroreceptors are stretch receptors located in the carotid sinus and aortic arch. What is the outcome of increased arterial pressure on these receptors?
  A. Decrease in afferent impulses to CNS
  B. Decrease in parasympathetic efferent output
  C. Increased sinus atrial stimulus
  D. Increased cardiac output
  E. Decreased heart rate

70. What is the primary mechanism by which the myocardium compensates for increased oxygen demand?
  A. Increased oxygen extraction
  B. Increase parasympathetic stimulus
  C. Decrease adenosine release
  D. Increase coronary blood flow
  E. Decrease cardiac output

71. Relative to the fossa ovalis, where would you expect to find a coronary sinus ASD?
  A. Anterior and superior
  B. Posterior and superior
  C. Posterior and inferior
  D. Anterior and inferior
  E. Posterior and medial

72. A neonate is diagnosed with d-transposition of the great arteries. You hear a loud, single second heart sound. What is the explanation behind this examination finding?
  A. Ventricular septal defect
  B. Anterior position of aorta

  C. Pulmonary atresia
  D. Severe aortic stenosis
  E. Pulmonary vascular obstructive disease

73. A newborn baby is diagnosed with double outlet right ventricle. Which of the following is most likely to also be found?
  A. Secundum atrial septal defect
  B. Right aortic arch
  C. Primum atrial septal defect
  D. Pulmonary stenosis
  E. Subaortic stenosis

74. A 2-week-old male infant has an echocardiogram performed for a murmur. On echo, you note that the patient has moderate mitral valve stenosis and a single papillary muscle. Which of the following is the correct anatomical description of this patient's left AV valve?
  A. Supravalvar mitral web
  B. Congenitally stenotic mitral valve
  C. Parachute mitral valve
  D. Mitral arcade
  E. Mitral valve prolapse

75. Which of these sites contains contractile cardiac myocytes?
  A. Proximal aorta
  B. Epicardium
  C. Proximal main pulmonary artery
  D. Proximal pulmonary veins
  E. Distal inferior vena cava

76. What is the most common location of the pulmonary artery in patients with truncus arteriosus?
  A. Branch pulmonary arteries arise from posterior sides of the truncus
  B. Branch pulmonary arteries arise from lateral sides of the truncus
  C. Main pulmonary artery arises from the truncus
  D. Branch pulmonary arteries arise from descending aorta
  E. Main pulmonary artery arises from innominate artery

77. You diagnose a neonate with truncus arteriosus. It appears that this patient has a single pulmonary artery. Which artery is most likely to be absent in this patient?
  A. Left pulmonary artery
  B. Right pulmonary artery
  C. The pulmonary artery on the opposite side of the aortic arch
  D. Both left and right pulmonary arteries
  E. The pulmonary artery on the side of the aortic arch

78. Which of the following embryologic aortic arches regresses and typically does not contribute to any structure in the normal neonate?

    A. Left fourth arch
    B. Left fifth arch
    C. Right fourth arch
    D. Left third arch
    E. Left sixth arch

79. A 9-year-old boy is diagnosed with coarctation of the aorta. Which of the following is most likely to also be found in this patient?

    A. Ventricular septal defect
    B. Bicuspid aortic valve
    C. Parachute mitral valve
    D. Subaortic stenosis
    E. Tricuspid valve stenosis

80. Left ventricular isovolumic *relaxation* continues until what cardiac event occurs?

    A. Aortic valve opens
    B. Passive atrial filling
    C. Mitral valve opens
    D. Increased ventricular volume
    E. Aortic pressure greater than left ventricular

81. The atrioventricular node and proximal portion of the His bundle are located within the triangle of Koch. Which of the following is a border of the triangle of Koch?

    A. Eustachian valve
    B. Anterior leaflet of tricuspid valve
    C. Ostium of the coronary sinus
    D. Limbus of the fossa ovalis
    E. Crista terminalis

82. You are called by the neonatal intensive care unit regarding a new admission. The neonate's mother had a prior fetal echo which showed concern for total anomalous pulmonary venous return. Which of the following is the most likely type of total anomalous pulmonary venous return to be found?

    A. Infracardiac
    B. Supracardiac
    C. Infradiaphragmatic
    D. Mixed
    E. Cardiac

83. A 16-month-old toddler's status post repair of a partial AV canal defect has the following results of a blood gas:

    pCO_2: 37 mm Hg
    HCO_3: 33 mm/L
    pH: 7.54

Which of the following is the acid–base abnormality present in this patient?

    A. Acute respiratory alkalosis
    B. Acute respiratory acidosis
    C. Acute metabolic acidosis
    D. Acute metabolic alkalosis
    E. Chronic respiratory acidosis

84. A 15-year-old girl is admitted with chest pain. There is a concern for left ventricular inferior wall motion abnormalities on echocardiography. She admits to using cocaine in the past 24 hours. Which coronary artery typically supplies the inferior left ventricular wall and the posteromedial papillary muscle of the mitral valve?

    A. Right coronary
    B. Left circumflex
    C. Left anterior descending
    D. Obtuse marginal
    E. Conal branch

85. In the fetal circulation, which vascular structure has the highest oxygen content?

    A. Aorta
    B. Superior vena cava
    C. Umbilical artery
    D. Umbilical vein
    E. Ductus arteriosus

86. The great cardiac vein drains deoxygenated blood into the coronary sinus. What is the name of the valve at the ostium of the cardiac vein?

    A. Vieussens valve
    B. Eustachian valve
    C. Valve of the fossa ovalis
    D. Tricuspid valve
    E. Thebesian valve

87. The AV nodal artery arises from which coronary artery?

    A. Right coronary
    B. Left anterior descending
    C. Left circumflex
    D. Posterior descending
    E. Marginal

88. The most common coronary artery abnormality seen in patients with otherwise normal hearts is:

    A. Anomalous origin of right coronary artery from the left sinus of Valsalva
    B. Anomalous origin of the right coronary artery from the posterior sinus of Valsalva
    C. Single coronary artery
    D. Anomalous origin of left circumflex coronary artery from the right main coronary artery
    E. Anomalous origin of left coronary artery from the posterior sinus of Valsalva

89. A 15-year-old boy undergoes a chest CT after direct chest trauma in a car accident. He has no significant past medical history or prior symptoms. The radiologist identifies a congenital abnormality of the aortic arch. Which of the following is the most likely aortic arch malformation in this patient?
    A. Right aortic arch with left ductus arteriosus
    B. Double aortic arch
    C. Left aortic arch with anomalous right subclavian artery
    D. Cervical arch
    E. Anomalous RPA from ascending aorta

90. A 5-day-old infant presents with cyanosis and lower extremity edema. Hepatomegaly is apparent on physical examination. Echocardiography reveals a normal tricuspid valve, but the right ventricle is thinned and akinetic. Which of the following defects is most likely present?
    A. Tricuspid atresia
    B. Ebstein anomaly
    C. Uhl anomaly
    D. Arrhythmogenic right ventricular dysplasia
    E. Pulmonary stenosis

91. A straddling cardiac valve:
    A. Cannot coexist with overriding
    B. Is not associated with malalignment type of VSD
    C. Most commonly involves the pulmonary valve
    D. Is a common component of tetralogy of Fallot
    E. Involves anomalous insertion of chordae tendineae

92. Which of the following is thought to be most responsible for high pulmonary vascular resistance in the fetus?
    A. Low blood and alveolar oxygen tension
    B. Fetal secretion of vasoconstrictors (e.g., thromboxane, leukotrienes)
    C. Systemic vascular resistance
    D. Right-to-left shunting of blood
    E. Maternal and placental hormones

93. Around 1 month of gestation in the human embryo, the pulmonary venous plexus establishes a single connection to the sinoatrial portion of the developing heart, called the common pulmonary vein. What is the fate of this structure in the normal heart?
    A. Disappears, with eventual independent appearance of the four pulmonary veins
    B. Is incorporated into the coronary sinus
    C. Is incorporated into the wall of the right atrium
    D. Is incorporated into the back wall of the left atrium
    E. Becomes the supero-posterior portion of the atrial septum

94. Which phase of the cardiac action potential is characterized by entrance of Ca^{2+} into the cell through L-type voltage-gated channels?
    A. Phase 0
    B. Phase 1
    C. Phase 2
    D. Phase 3
    E. Phase 4

95. A 6-month-old female infant is brought to the emergency room with cyanosis, tachypnea, and irritability. Her father reports that a murmur was heard at her first checkup, but that he missed her appointment that had been scheduled with cardiology. What is most likely causing this patient's cyanosis?
    A. Increased pulmonary blood flow
    B. Increased systemic vascular resistance
    C. Decreased pulmonary vasculature pressure
    D. Increased right-to-left shunting
    E. Increased left-to-right shunting

96. Which of the following is true regarding T-tubules?
    A. Do not participate in excitation–contraction coupling
    B. Are a component of intercalated disks
    C. Are a continuation of the sarcolemma
    D. Envelop myofibrils at the level of the A-band
    E. Does not contain calcium ion channels

97. Which of the following will decrease myocardial oxygen consumption?
    A. Decreasing end diastolic volume
    B. Increasing wall tension
    C. Increasing heart rate
    D. Increasing cardiac contractility
    E. Sympathetic activation

98. A 2-month-old infant's status post repair of a complete AV canal has the following results of a blood gas:

    pCO_2: 36 mm Hg
    HCO_3: 14 mm/L
    pH: 7.21

    Which of the following is the acid–base abnormality present in this patient?
    A. Acute respiratory alkalosis
    B. Acute respiratory acidosis
    C. Acute metabolic acidosis
    D. Acute metabolic alkalosis
    E. Chronic respiratory acidosis

99. A 5-month-old infant's status post surgical repair of an atrioventricular septal defect has the following results of a blood gas:

pCO_2: 73 mm Hg
HCO_3: 25 mm/L
pH: 7.15

Which of the following is the acid–base abnormality present in this patient?

A. Acute respiratory alkalosis
B. Acute metabolic acidosis
C. Acute metabolic alkalosis
D. Acute respiratory acidosis
E. Chronic respiratory acidosis

100. Which of the following is true regarding the branching patterns of the right (RPA) and left (LPA) branch pulmonary arteries in a normal patient?

A. The RPA travels anterior to the right upper lobe bronchus, while the LPA travels posterior to the left upper lobe bronchus

B. The RPA travels posterior to the right upper lobe bronchus, while the LPA travels anterior to the right upper lobe bronchus

C. Both the LPA and RPA travel inferior to the left and right mainstem bronchi

D. Both the LPA and RPA travel posterior to their respective upper lobe bronchi

E. Both the LPA and RPA travel anterior to their respective upper lobe bronchi

101. The "power stroke" in cardiac muscle contraction (the interaction of the myosin head and actin that allows myosin to pull the actin filament inward) is powered by what process?

A. Ca^{2+} binding to troponin C
B. Troponin I binding to troponin C
C. Troponin T binding to tropomyosin
D. ATP hydrolysis and conversion to ADP
E. Release of ADP

ANSWERS

1. (D) Flow-volume loops are highly likely to be tested on the board examination (see the ICU section of this book for further questions on flow-volume loops). At end diastole, the LV filling is complete, and the mitral valve closes. There is a period of isovolumic contraction, after which the aortic valve opens secondary to a lower pressure in the aorta compared to the LV.

2. (C) The classic valve abnormality of systemic lupus erythematosus is the Libman–Sacks endocarditis lesion, a verrucous, nonbacterial lesion. They are most commonly found on the left-sided valves, and predominantly on the mitral valve. They appear in ~10% of patients newly diagnosed with SLE. On echo, they are irregular vegetations, <0.5 cm in diameter, on the valve or chordal apparatus.

3. (D) Adenosine is produced from the breakdown of ATP, which cannot be regenerated at times of low oxygen tension. Therefore, at times of low oxygen tension, AMP is made and then further broken down into adenosine, which causes coronary artery vasodilation. Nitric oxide induces the cyclic guanosine monophosphate which causes muscle relaxation. Endothelin-1 causes tonic vasoconstriction. Prostaglandin induces smooth muscle relaxation.

4. (E) In polysplenia, the multiple spleens are typically located all on the same side of the vertebral column as the stomach. The gall bladder is typically single, but patients may have concurrent biliary atresia. The abdominal situs is variable and can be normal, mirror image, or indeterminate. The IVC commonly is interrupted with azygous continuation to the SVC.

5. (E) In mature myocytes, the sarcoplasmic reticulum stores the most important source of calcium involved in the initiation of myocyte contraction. Calcium enters the myocyte during the action potential through L-type voltage-gated calcium channels. This calcium then activates the calcium release channel (also called the ryanodine receptor), causing release of calcium from the sarcoplasmic reticulum. In immature cardiac myocytes, the function and organization of the sarcoplasmic reticulum is not yet to mature levels, and activation is more dependent on flow through the L-type calcium channels.

6. (D) Of patients with a bicuspid aortic valve, by far the most common form is fusion of the right and left cusps (75%). The next most common are patients with fusion of the right and noncoronary cusps, followed by those with left and noncoronary cusp fusion. Fusion of more than one cusp can result in a unicuspid valve.

7. (B) The juxtaglomerular apparatus of the kidney, in response to lower renal perfusion pressures, will secrete renin. Renin will go on to induce cleaving of angiotensinogen to angiotensin I. This is then converted to angiotensin II by angiotensin-converting enzyme (ACE) in the lungs and vasculature. Angiotensin II will induce vasoconstriction and stimulate ADH (vasopressin) secretion.

8. (A) This question refers to the Poiseuille–Hagen relationship, where the resistance R between two points is a function of pressure and flow. This is ultimately described by the equation $R = (8 \times L \times \eta)/(\pi \times r^4)$, where the radius is raised to the fourth power (L = length of the vessel, η = viscosity).

9. (A) The majority of the aortic arch arises from the left fourth aortic arch, while the right fourth aortic arch gives rise to the proximal portion of the right subclavian artery. The pulmonary arteries and ductus arteriosus arise from the left sixth aortic arch.

10. (D) The pulmonary arteries and ductus arteriosus arise from the left sixth aortic arch. The majority of the aortic arch arises from the left fourth aortic arch, while the right fourth aortic arch gives rise to the proximal portion of the right subclavian artery. The fifth aortic arch most typically involutes.

11. (C) An atrial septal defect or a patent foramen ovale is present in over 80% of patients with tetralogy of Fallot (occasionally termed the "pentalogy of Fallot.)" Abnormalities of the left side of the heart are rare in patients with tetralogy. A right aortic arch occurs in around 25% of patients.

12. (E) The echocardiographic image represents a patient with d-transposition of the great arteries. Note the immediate posterior course of the great vessel arising from the left ventricle, indicative of the vessel being a pulmonary artery. There is a ventricular septal defect also present in the image. Patients with transposition of the great arteries most commonly have normal coronary anatomy (67%), but around 16% of patients will have an anomalous circumflex coronary artery arising from the right coronary. The next most common abnormalities are a single right coronary artery and an inverted right coronary and left circumflex (inverted origins of the RCA and LCx but normal origin of the LAD from the anterior facing sinus).

13. (C) The transverse sinus includes the intrapericardial space between the great arteries anterosuperiorly and the atrial walls posteroinferiorly. It can be visualized in some postoperative patients as the echo dark space around the aortic sinus in the parasternal short-axis echocardiographic image, if fluid is present in the sinus. Often in neonates, a small amount of fluid in the transverse sinus may have a similar appearance to the take-off of the left main coronary artery. The oblique sinus refers to the sinus between the posterior left atrium and the reflections of the great veins (superior vena cava and pulmonary veins).

14. (A) Atrial natriuretic peptide is released in response to stretch from either atrium. ANP works on the kidney by dilating the afferent arteriole and constricting the efferent arteriole, effectively increasing GFR. It also works on the distal tubules to decrease sodium resorption. ANP also has vasodilator and cardioinhibitory effects.

15. (A) In normal hearts in the first two decades of life, the thickness of the ventricular septum and left free wall are similar (mean = 1.1, range: 0.8 to 1.4). This ratio increases slowly in adulthood and averages greater than 1.2 by age 70. It can also be affected in diseases of asymmetric hypertrophy such as hypertrophic cardiomyopathy. The average ratio between left and right ventricular thickness is 3 (range: 2 to 5). Due to high right-sided pressure in utero, this ratio is lower in fetuses and neonates.

16. (D) The subarterial type of VSD (also called supracristal or infundibular) comprises around 5% of VSDs at autopsy, but is significantly more common in Asian populations. Due to the location of the VSD, there is deficiency of the support structure below the aortic valve, with subsequent herniation of the right coronary leaflet through the defect. This may also occur in some patients with perimembranous defects.

17. (E) The categorical definition of an overriding AV valve is one that empties into two ventricles. It is always associated with a malalignment ventricular septal defect. If there are also anomalous insertions of the chordae tendineae into the contralateral ventricle, then the valve is considered to be overriding and straddling.

18. (C) The right ventricle, being thin walled and the most anterior structure, is more commonly ruptured than the left ventricle. Ventricular rupture overall is more common than atrial rupture. Multiple ruptures are not uncommon, such as a combination of ventricular and aortic rupture. Survival is poor in patients with myocardial rupture, and surgical exploration is required emergently. If there is atrial rupture, the most common site of rupture is the atrial appendage.

19. (B) In most asplenia patients, the descending aorta and IVC will travel on the same side of the vertebral column. There is a high incidence of bowel malrotation, and the stomach can be located on the left, right, or midline. There is typically only one gall bladder, but it can be variable in position, depending on the site of the liver. Biliary atresia is uncommon. The liver is most commonly midline with two mirror-image right lobes.

20. (A) Repetitive exercise for prolong periods of time results in benefits on one's cardiovascular health and increases an individual's work capacity. Changes include increased blood volume and stroke volume and decreased heart rate, resting arterial blood pressure, and myocardial oxygen demand.

21. (A) The level of attachment of the AV valve is crucial in determining both the specific type of AV valve and ventricular morphology. The mitral valve typically inserts into the cardiac crux between 0 and 8 mm/m² higher than the tricuspid valve. Exceptions to this include Ebstein anomaly, where >8 mm/m² difference exists, and partial AV canal defects or double-inlet ventricles, where no difference between the valvular insertions exists. The other options are helpful in determining valve type, but are not as reliable in patients with congenital heart disease. See Figure 1.8.

22. (D) The hemoglobin–oxygen dissociation curve helps to understand the relationship between pO_2 and oxygen

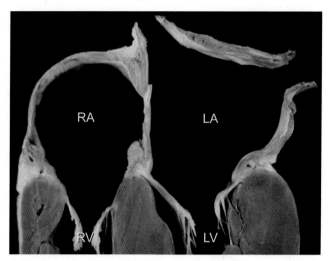

FIGURE 1.8 LA, left atrium; RA, right atrium; LV, left ventricle; RV, right ventricle. Image courtesy of Dr. William Edwards, Mayo Clinic.

saturations. Increasing the pH (alkalosis), decreasing temperature, and decreasing 2,3-DPG will shift the curve to the left; likewise, acidosis, increased temperature, and increasing 2,3-DPG shift the curve to the right.

23. (C) In patients with right atrial isomerism, bilateral sinus nodes can be encountered. In left atrial isomerism, the sinus node can be absent or malpositioned. In left-sided juxtaposition of the atrial appendages, the sinus node is often displaced anteriorly or inferiorly. Left juxtaposition is associated more with abnormal ventriculoarterial connections, while right-sided juxtaposition is more commonly associated with simpler lesions, like atrial septal defects.

24. (C) Specific tissues are able to regulate local blood flow in response to changing metabolic demands. A decrease in the pO_2 causes a systemic arteriolar vasodilation, as the local tissues attempt to get more oxygen delivery through increased volume of flow. Similarly, increasing pCO_2, increasing H^+ (acidosis), or increasing K^+ will cause local vasodilation. Some tissues will also release adenosine as a vasodilator in response to increased oxygen demand.

25. (B) The Eustachian valve is located at the entrance of the inferior vena cava. The crescent-shaped valvular remnant located at the os of the coronary sinus is the Thebesian valve. The Chiari network is a fine, filamentous structure that represents persistence of the valves of the sinus venosus, and typically extend from the crista terminalis to the Eustachian or Thebesian valves. It directs blood flow from the SVC and IVC through the foramen ovale to the left atrium. In normal patients, this regresses to form the crista terminalis, a ridge in the right atrium separating the sinus venosus portion of the right atrium from the muscular right atrium.

26. (B) An intermediate AVSD is a rare subtype of a complete defect where the common AV valve has separate left and right orifices. This is accompanied by a large primum ASD and inlet VSD, and the clinical picture is similar to complete AVSD. Partial AVSD consists of a septum primum ASD and cleft left AV valve anterior leaflet, but the left and right AV valves are separate.

AVSD Summary

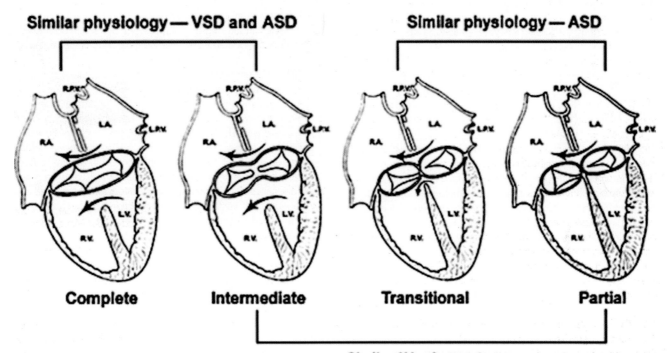

FIGURE 1.9 AVSD, atrioventricular septal defect; ASD, atrial septal defect; VSD, ventricular septal defect; LPV, left pulmonary vein; RPV, right pulmonary vein; RA, right atrium; LA, left atrium; RV, right ventricle; LV, left ventricle. Image courtesy of Dr. Frank Cetta, MD.

Transitional defects are a subtype of partial defects and include a small inlet VSD. See Figure 1.9.

27. (D) The least saturated blood in the fetus is in the coronary sinus and the superior vena cava, the oxygen having been used by the head and brain or the myocardium. The inferior vena cava, left hepatic vein, and ductus venosus will all receive some or all of their flow from the umbilical vein, and thus will not be at maximal desaturation.

28. (B) The most reliable feature that distinguishes the right ventricle from the left ventricle is the level of insertion of the respective AV valves at the cardiac crux. The pattern of trabeculations and the shape of the ventricle are not reliable in many forms of congenital heart disease. Continuity between AV and semilunar valves may be useful but is not as reliable as the level of AV valve insertion. Typically, the aortic and mitral valves are in fibrous continuity, while the tricuspid and pulmonary valves are not in fibrous continuity.

29. (C) The primary determinant of the direction of blood flow through an atrial septal defect is the relative compliances of the left and right ventricles. In the otherwise normal patient, the right ventricle will be more compliant than the left ventricle, with less resistance to filling from the right atrium, and thus left-to-right

shunting across the ASD. The vast majority of patients with ASDs have a relatively normal pulmonary resistance.

30. (D) Aortic atresia with mitral valve atresia occurs in 36% to 46% of patients with HLHS, compared to 13% to 26% of patients with aortic stenosis with mitral stenosis. About 20% to 29% of patients have aortic atresia with a patent mitral valve.

31. (B) The A-band, bisected by the M-line, contains all the myosin contractile elements of the sarcomere. The I-band, bisected by the Z-disk, contains purely actin elements of the sarcomere. The H-zone is a central subsection of the A-band that does not include the areas of myosin–actin overlap.

32. (C) The truncal valve in truncus arteriosus is most commonly *tricuspid* (~70%). The next most common form of truncal valve is quadricuspid (~20%), followed by bicuspid (~10%), pentacuspid (<1%), or unicommissural (<1%). The valve is in fibrous continuity with the mitral valve in all patients, but can also rarely be in fibrous continuity with the tricuspid valve.

33. (C) The I_{K1} potassium current is the dominant resting conductance of the myocyte. It keeps the myocyte negatively polarized around −85 mV, until an action potential arrives to activate the cell into phase 0. See Figure 1.10.

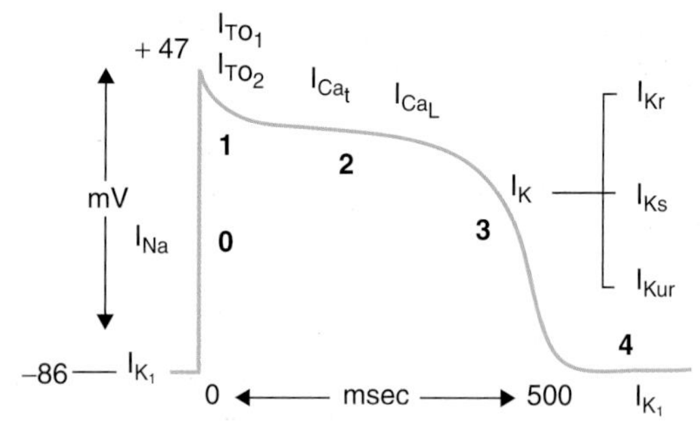

FIGURE 1.10

$+47$ I_{TO_1} I_{TO_2} I_{Ca_t} I_{Ca_L} I_{Kr}

mV 1 2 I_K I_{Ks}

I_{Na} 0 3 I_{Kur}

-86 — I_{K_1} 4

0 ← msec → 500 I_{K_1}

34. (A) When an action potential arrives to the cardiac myocyte, the cardiac sodium channels open, resulting in a rapid depolarization of the myocyte (phase 0). Once this primary depolarization has occurred, the sodium channels are inactivated in a time-dependant manner. Potassium and calcium conductance takes over at that point, providing the prolonged phase 1 and 2 depolarization required to achieve muscle contraction. Mutations in the sodium channel gene, *SCN5A*, may cause either type 3 long QT syndrome or Brugada syndrome.

35. (C) This patient is presenting with cyanosis and decreased pulmonary blood flow as evidenced by the lack of vascular markings in the lung fields. Critical pulmonary stenosis can present in this manner. All other options more commonly present with cyanosis and increased pulmonary vascularity.

36. (C) Relative to the fossa ovalis, a sinus venosus atrial septal defect will be posteriorly and superiorly placed. The defect is typically secondary to the absence of the usual rim of tissue between the right pulmonary veins and the right atrium. As such, it occurs commonly in the presence of anomalous right upper pulmonary venous return. See Figure 1.11.

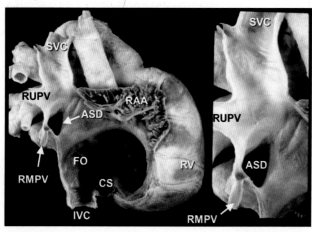

FIGURE 1.11 SVC, superior vena cava; FO, fossa ovalis; IVC, inferior vena cava; RAA, right atrial appendage; RUPV, right upper pulmonary vein; RMPV, right middle pulmonary vein; ASD, atrial septal defect; RV, right ventricle; CS, coronary sinus. Image courtesy of Dr. William Edwards, Mayo Clinic.

37. (A) Cardiac fibroblasts are vital for the structural integrity of the heart. They play a large role in remodeling and development. They are responsible for the deposition of the extracellular matrix

and also contribute to remodeling through secretion of metalloproteinases. They are also involved in the secretion of cytokines and growth factors which influence neighboring cells. Pericytes are contractile cells that help regulate blood flow in capillaries. Vascular smooth muscle cells are mostly found in medium caliber blood vessels in the heart. Macrophages are scattered throughout the heart. Endothelial cells line the inner wall of the ventricles.

38. (E) The four-chamber view demonstrates Ebstein anomaly, with marked apical displacement of the septal leaflet of the tricuspid valve. The most common additional abnormality seen in patients with Ebstein anomaly is an atrial septal defect, seen in >80% of patients. The next most common associated abnormality is pulmonary stenosis, followed by a ventricular septal defect. The degree of RV outflow obstruction is critical to determine prior to designing treatment plans in the neonate with severe Ebstein anomaly. Functional or true pulmonary atresia may be present in the neonate. Left ventricular noncompaction has been reported in some genetic association studies, but other left-sided lesions are uncommon.

39. (A) The superior vena cava drains unoxygenated blood from the upper body to the right atrium. The inferior vena cava carries blood from the lower body and the placenta. The patent ductus arteriosus carries mixed oxygenated blood from the pulmonary artery to the descending aorta. The ductus venous carries mixed blood from the hepatic veins to the inferior vena cava. The ascending aortic arch supplies the most oxygen-rich blood to heart and brain. The superior vena cava and coronary sinus have the lowest oxygen saturations of all vascular pathways in the fetus.

40. (A) The trachea divides into left and right bronchi just after passing the aortic arch, with the left bronchus heading under the arch. The pulmonary artery at its bifurcation is leftward of the ascending aorta. The right pulmonary artery heads under the arch to get to the right lung. The left pulmonary artery heads more posteriorly over the left bronchus.

41. (A) The first aortic arch forms part of the maxillary axillary, and the second aortic arch forms portions of the stapedial arteries. Aortic arch three forms the common carotid artery and the proximal portion of the internal carotid artery.

42. (D) Intercalated discs connect cardiac myocytes and are responsible for maintaining structural integrity and transmission of electric impulses. They are made up of adherens junctions, desmosomes, and gap junctions. Dystrophin and costameres are proteins which connect the myocytes to the extracellular matrix. T-tubules are invaginations of the sarcolemma which allows transmission of the action potential to the inner part of the cell. Myosin is involved in muscle contraction.

43. (E) The left recurrent laryngeal nerve is a branch of the vagus nerve that travels inferiorly around the aortic arch before traveling superiorly to innervate muscles in the larynx. The right recurrent laryngeal nerve takes a similar course but loops around the right subclavian artery. Injury to the left recurrent laryngeal nerve is possible during surgical manipulation of the aortic arch and often results in postoperative hoarseness and stridor.

44. (C) The most common aortic-pulmonary positions in patients with double outlet right ventricle (DORV) are the side-by-side configurations (aorta to the right of the pulmonary artery), accounting for around two-thirds of DORV patients. The aorta may arise more anteriorly (right anterior aorta) or posteriorly (right posterior aorta) in some patients or may be leftward and anterior to the pulmonary artery.

45. (D) Secundum ASDs are by far the most common (75%) and are located at the region of the fossa ovalis. Multiple factors can contribute to the formation of these ASDs, including deficient growth of the septum secundum, excessive resorption of the septum primum, or deficient valve tissue. Septum primum ASDs are the second most common (20%). Sinus venosus (5%) and coronary sinus (<1%) ASDs are less common, with the latter often associated with heterotaxy syndromes.

46. (C) The right anterior cardinal vein and right common cardinal vein give rise to the right superior vena cava. The left anterior cardinal vein typically regresses but may be persistent as a left superior vena cava. The ductus venosus remnant is termed the ligamentum venosum, and the umbilical vein remnants include the round ligament of the liver.

47. (D) The vein of Galen malformation is the most common hemodynamically significant extracardiac arteriovenous malformation in neonates. It affects male infants three times more than female infants. The infants commonly present with high-output cardiac failure soon after birth. A bruit can often be heard through the fontanelles. Other types of cerebral AVMs may also present similarly, but the vein of Galen malformation is the most common.

48. (B) Common features of the morphologic tricuspid valve include septal chordal attachments, a triangular-shaped orifice at the midleaflet level, the presence of three leaflets and commissures, and emptying into a morphologic right ventricle. All other answers listed in this question relate to a morphologic mitral valve.

49. (B) The ductus venosus receives blood flow from the hepatic veins and umbilical vein and delivers it to the right atrium. After birth the ductus venosus becomes the ligamentum venosum. The ductus arteriosus shunts blood from the main pulmonary artery to the descending aorta. The foramen ovale is an interatrial connection that allows oxygenated blood to flow across to the left atrium. The aortic isthmus is the segment of the aorta between the origin of the left subclavian artery and the ligamentum of arteriosum. Umbilical arteries bring deoxygenated blood from the internal iliac arteries to the placenta.

50. (B) This patient has tetralogy of Fallot; the echo images demonstrate aortic override, the presence of an RV outflow tract with a prominent conus, and a small left-to-right shunting ductus arteriosus. About 5% of patients with tetralogy have an origin of the left anterior descending artery arising from the right coronary artery. This coronary then takes a course anterior to the right ventricular outflow tract. This is an important anomaly to rule out, as the coronary's course can prevent the surgeon from using a transannular patch to open the right ventricular outflow tract. Around 10% to 15% of patients will have an accessory LAD (large conal

branch). Other coronary patterns are rare, occurring in less than 5% of patients.

51. (A) Since some patients with congenital heart disease may have absence of the typical left atrial (valve of the fossa ovalis) and right atrial (limbus of the fossa ovalis) characteristics, the next best marker for the right atrium is the ostium of the IVC. The suprahepatic IVC nearly always connects directly to the right atrium. This rule is particularly useful in the evaluation of complex heterotaxy patients. The finger-like atrial appendage and the smooth-surfaced free wall are more common characteristics of the left atrium. Pulmonary vein ostia are a poor predictor of atrial morphology due to the high frequency of anomalous pulmonary venous return in patients with heterotaxy.

52. (E) The infant has tricuspid atresia noted in this four-chamber image. The most common form of tricuspid atresia is type 1, or tricuspid atresia with normally related great arteries. The pulmonary outflow can vary from pulmonary atresia to widely patent pulmonary outflow without stenosis. The associated ventricular septal defect is expectedly larger in the presence of a widely patent pulmonary outflow and smaller in patients with pulmonary stenosis. Approximately 70% to 80% of patients with tricuspid atresia have normally related great arteries.

53. (D) About 80% of the calcium that is sequestered during the relaxation phase of the cardiac muscle contraction is done so via Ca^{2+}-ATPase SERCA pumps located on the sarcoplasmic reticulum. The remaining 20% is removed from the cell through $Na^+–Ca^{2+}$ and Ca^{2+}-ATPase pumps located on the sarcolemma.

54. (C) The AV node in tricuspid atresia is on the floor of the blind right atrium. The bundle of His then courses onto the crest of the intraventricular septum (muscular) and runs posterior to the VSD rim. This is important in the eventual repair or palliation of tricuspid atresia, in that care needs to be taken with any surgical procedure involving the VSD for fear of inducing heart block.

55. (D) The right ventricle is typically composed of the inlet, trabecular, and outlet regions (tripartite). There is typically a coarse septal surface, unlike the smooth-walled left ventricular septal wall. There are prominent apical trabeculations. The tricuspid and pulmonary valves are not in continuity in the normal patient, but can be in continuity in patients with tetralogy of Fallot with membranous VSD extension.

56. (A) A ventricular septal defect occurs in 40% to 45% of patients with d-TGA. The majority of VSDs are of the perimembranous, muscular, or malalignment type. Isolated LV outflow obstruction occurs in ~5% of patients. Coarctation, arch hypoplasia, or interrupted arch occurs in ~5% of patients. Leftward juxtaposition of the atrial appendages occurs in 2% to 5% of d-TGA patients. Around 20% of patients have been shown to have mitral valve abnormalities at autopsy; however, they are rarely functionally significant. Of these, cleft mitral valve is likely the most common.

57. (B) Most patients (80%) with Ebstein anomaly will also present with an atrial septal defect or patent foramen ovale. Patients with

Ebstein and cyanosis often have right-to-left shunting at the atrial level. This cyanosis often will worsen with exercise in older patients.

58. (A) The best and most specific hallmark of the morphologic left atrium is the valve of the fossa ovalis. In contrast, hallmarks of the right atrium include the limbus of the fossa ovalis and the entrance of the inferior vena cava. The left atrium is typically more posterior compared to the right atrium. The left atrial appendage is finger-like and trabeculated, compared to the broad-based appendage of the right atrium.

59. (A) Fetal hemoglobin has a higher affinity for oxygen as compared to adult hemoglobin and is composed of alpha and gamma subunits. Adult hemoglobin meanwhile is composed of alpha and beta subunits. The fetal hemoglobin has to have a higher affinity for oxygen in order for transport of oxygen across the placenta to be achieved. In the normal newborn, fetal hemoglobin has been replaced by adult hemoglobin by the age of 3 months.

60. (C) Norepinephrine activates β1 adrenergic receptors by activating the Gs subunit of the G-protein complex which activates adenylate cyclase. This enzyme converts ATP into cAMP, which activates protein kinase A. PKA phosphorylates multiple proteins involved in muscle contraction and action potentials of the heart, resulting in increased chronotropy and inotropy.

61. (C) With inspiration, there is a fall in pleural pressure and a rise in intra-abdominal pressure. These changes lead to increased right-sided venous return and increased RV stroke volume. E′ velocity across the tricuspid valve is increased (~5% to 10%), while E′ velocity across the mitral valve is slightly decreased (~5% to 10%).

62. (D) The mitral arcade, or hammock mitral valve, is characterized by absent or abnormal chordal insertions, and the leaflet edges may connect directly to the papillary muscles. The papillary muscles themselves are often small and abnormal. The leaflet edges are often thickened and rolled. Due to this direct insertion of the leaflets, the leaflets are relatively tethered and display poor coaptation. Mitral regurgitation is most common, although a functional mitral stenosis can also occur.

63. (C) A primum ASD is located anteriorly to the fossa ovalis in the inlet portion of the septum. Failure of the endocardial cushions to develop is the embryologic basis behind atrioventricular canal defects, including primum ASDs. Anomalous pulmonary venous return occurs when there is failure of the common pulmonary vein to connect to the left atrium. Excessive cell death and resorption of the septum primum, or insufficient growth of the septum secundum, are common etiologies behind secundum atrial septal defects.

64. (E) The circular structure seen in this location most commonly represents a dilated coronary sinus, due to a persistent left superior vena cava, which is the remnant of the left horn of the sinus venosus. This can be mistaken for the descending aorta, which should be seen more posteriorly outside the pericardium. The left SVC runs posteriorly along the left atrium before joining the coronary sinus in the left AV groove.

65. (A) In order for the examiner to be able to visualize true cyanosis, there must be at least 5 g/dL of deoxygenated hemoglobin. Thus, in a patient with anemia, a relatively low oxygen saturation may not result in the expected clinical cyanosis. The best indicator of cyanosis is the tongue due to the rich vascular supply and lack of pigmented cells. Rib notching is rare in a 2 year old even in the presence of a significant coarctation of the aorta. Atrial septal defect will rarely cause significant enough right-to-left shunt to produce cyanosis in a 2-year-old patient.

66. (D) Dystrophin is a protein that links the extracellular matrix and cytoplasmic actin, providing a vital link between extracellular and intracellular structures of the myocyte. Mutations in the gene encoding for this protein cause muscular dystrophy and are a known cause of dilated cardiomyopathy. Caveolin and syntrophin are proteins also involved in the linking of intracellular and extracellular structures and cause long QT syndrome and SIDS when mutated. Cytoplasmic actin and the dystroglycan complex are mutated in some patients with dilated cardiomyopathy.

67. (B) Calcium binds to troponin C, changing the tertiary structure of troponin C and other troponin subunits. This allows tropomyosin to shift positions and allows myosin and actin binding, leading to muscle cell contraction.

68. (C) Children living at elevation have been shown to have higher mean pulmonary artery pressures as compared to those living at sea level. This increase in pulmonary pressure is even more exacerbated with exercise. This may have a role in explaining the relatively increased risk of persistence of the patent ductus arteriosus in children living at altitude.

69. (E) Baroreceptors are found in each carotid sinus and aortic arch. These receptors respond to stretch of the arterial walls and send impulses to the brain. This stimulation results in a decreased blood pressure, by a decrease in heart rate and vasodilation.

70. (D) Due to high baseline oxygen extraction levels by the myocardium, the coronary oxygen tension is low (about 20 to 25 mm Hg). Increase in oxygen demand is fulfilled by increasing coronary blood flow, and not necessarily by changes in oxygen extraction.

71. (D) Relative to the fossa ovalis, which lays in a relatively midline position in the atrial septum, a coronary sinus atrial septal defect will be inferior and anteriorly placed, at the typical site of the coronary sinus ostium. It is typically seen in association with unroofing of the coronary sinus and a persistent left SVC. See Figure 1.12.

72. (B) The aorta and pulmonary artery are often located in an anterior–posterior position to each other, causing the narrow mediastinum and "egg-on-a-string" image seen on some chest x-rays. Due to the anterior aorta, the second heart sound is often single and loud.

73. (D) Pulmonic stenosis is the most commonly associated cardiac lesion and is seen in roughly 50% of patients with double

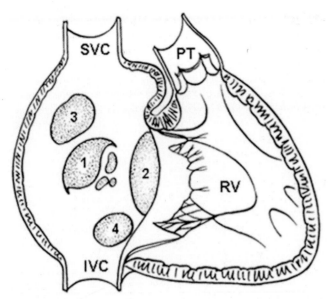

FIGURE 1.12 Types and locations of ASDs: 1, secundum; 2, inlet; 3, sinus venosus; 4, coronary sinus; RV, right ventricle; IVC, inferior vena cava; PT, pulmonary trunk; SVC, superior vena cava. Image courtesy of Dr. William Edwards, Mayo Clinic.

outlet right ventricle. Atrial septal defects are the next most common; 25% of patients have a secundum defect, while up to 8% may have a primum defect. Subaortic stenosis and right aortic arch may also be seen in these patients, but they are much less common.

74. (C) A mitral valve in which all of the chordal attachments occur to a single papillary muscle is called a parachute mitral valve. There is also a variant with attachments to two distinct papillary muscles, but with most attachments occurring to one of the papillary muscles. The chordae may be shortened and thickened. If the valve leaflets insert directly onto the papillary muscle, it would then be called a mitral arcade.

75. (D) The pulmonary veins contain cardiac myocytes instead of smooth muscle cells in the last 1 to 3 cm before insertion to the left atrium. This allows them to minimize retrograde flow during atrial systole. This can also be a source of atrial fibrillation, which is why pulmonary vein isolation procedures are often used in adults.

76. (C) About 48% to 68% of patients with truncus have type I, with the main pulmonary artery arising from the left postero-lateral aspect of the truncus right above the valve. About 29% to 48% of patients have type II, with branch pulmonary arteries arising from the posterior surface of the truncus. About 6% to 10% of patients have type III truncus, with branch pulmonary arteries arising from the lateral sides of the truncus. In type IV truncus, the branch pulmonary arteries arise from descending aorta.

77. (E) In tetralogy of Fallot, when a pulmonary artery is absent, the one affected is most commonly on the opposite side of the aortic arch. In contrast, in patients with truncus arteriosus, the absent pulmonary artery is typically on the same side of the aortic arch. This is a key distinction between absent pulmonary arteries in these two entities.

78. (B) The fifth aortic arch is typically rudimentary and does not usually develop into any known vessels in the normal neonate. It is not even present in many embryo specimens. Rare cases have been reported of persistence of the fifth arch, which can either be asymptomatic or be associated with other cardiac findings. If the fifth arch persists but there is interruption of the normal fourth arch, the patient may present with a clinical picture of coarctation.

79. (B) A bicuspid aortic valve may be seen in around 80% of patients with a coarctation of the aorta. Many investigators consider the combined findings an indication of a true "aortopathy," now proven by genetic linkage studies. Around half of patients with coarctation have a "simple" coarctation, implying normal intracardiac anatomy (other than the bicuspid aortic valve), while the other half have associated anomalies (VSD being the most common).

80. (C) At end systole, LV ejection is complete, and the aortic valve closes. This begins the period of isovolumic relaxation, with a subsequent drop in LV pressure. At the end of this period, the mitral valve opens, allowing filling of the ventricle due to lower pressures in the ventricle.

81. (C) The tricuspid valve annulus attaches to the septum slightly lower than the mitral annulus, resulting in a portion of the septum known as the atrioventricular septum. This septum is the location of the triangle of Koch, where the AV node is located. This area is bordered by the tendon of Todaro, the attachment of the septal leaflet of the tricuspid valve, and the ostium of the coronary sinus.

82. (B) Supracardiac total anomalous pulmonary venous connection is the most common type (46%) of TAPVC. The pulmonary veins form a confluence posterior to the left atrium and blood is directed through a venous channel to the left cardinal system. The most common anatomical site is the left innominate vein. Other forms of TAPVC include infracardiac (23%), cardiac (20%), and mixed (11%).

83. (D) The patient has an acute metabolic alkalosis, as evidenced by the elevated pH, relatively normal pCO2, and high bicarbonate. Causes of metabolic alkalosis can include vomiting, hypokalemia, the use of alkalotic medicines such as bicarbonate, hyperaldosteronism, and rare causes such as Bartter syndrome.

84. (A) While the anterolateral papillary muscle typically has a dual blood supply from the left anterior descending and circumflex coronary arteries, the posteromedial papillary muscle is typically solely supplied by the right coronary artery. The inferior wall of the left ventricle is also typically supplied by the right coronary artery.

85. (D) The umbilical vein is the structure that brings blood from the placenta to the fetus and has the highest oxygen content within the fetal circulation. The blood then passes from the umbilical vein, through the ductus venosus and left hepatic vein into the atrium. The superior vena cava and the coronary sinus typically have the lowest oxygen concentrations in the fetus.

86. (A) The Vieussens valve is a bicuspid valve located at the site of the cardiac vein that merges with the coronary sinus. The eustachian valve is located at the entrance of the inferior vena cava. The valve of the fossa ovalis is located in the atrial septum. The Thebesian valve is located where the coronary sinus drains into the right atrium.

87. (A) In 90% of the general population, the AV nodal artery arises from the right coronary artery and supplies the AV node. In the 10% of the general population, the left circumflex artery is dominant, and it supplies the AV nodal artery.

88. (D) Anomalous origin of left circumflex coronary artery from the right main coronary artery is the most common anomaly in patients with no evidence of other congenital heart disease and makes up approximately one-third of major coronary artery anomalies. Anomalous origin of right coronary artery from the left sinus of Valsalva is a close second at just under 30%. Single coronary arteries make up somewhere between 5% and 20% of coronary anomalies. Anomalous origin of the left or right coronary artery from the posterior sinus of Valsalva is a rare finding.

89. (C) The most common abnormality of the aortic arch is an anomalous right subclavian artery from a left aortic arch. This occurs in approximately 0.5% of the general population and is usually asymptomatic. The diagnosis is often made at autopsy or during imaging for another condition. It is seen commonly in patients with Down syndrome who have congenital heart disease (>30%).

90. (C) Uhl anomaly is a rare disorder characterized by partial or complete absence of the right ventricular myocardium with epicardium and pericardium opposed to each other. Valvular morphology is often normal as opposed to Ebstein anomaly. The normal tricuspid valve on echocardiography rules out tricuspid atresia. Arrhythmogenic right ventricular dysplasia is characterized by fatty infiltration and replacement of the right ventricular myocardium and arrhythmias or even sudden cardiac death. Pulmonary stenosis would result in hypertrophy of the right ventricle.

91. (E) The definition of a straddling atrioventricular valve is one that involves anomalous insertion of the chordae tendineae. It is important to identify preoperatively as it may prevent the surgeon from attempting certain repairs. There has to be a VSD, but it may or may not be a malalignment-type VSD.

92. (A) The normally low blood and alveolar oxygen tension is most associated with the high pulmonary vascular resistance in the fetus. The fetus also produces vasoconstrictive substances such as thromboxane and leukotrienes, but these do not appear to have as significant of an effect.

93. (D) The common pulmonary vein is the initial connection between the pulmonary venous plexus and the heart. The vein typically has four (or more) primary feeding veins, which eventually become the left and right upper and lower pulmonary veins. The common pulmonary vein is eventually incorporated into the back wall of the left atrium, with the atrium eventually appearing that the individual pulmonary veins connect independently to the atrium.

94. (C) Phase 2 (the plateau phase) is characterized by influx of Ca^{2+} into the cell through L-type Ca^{2+} channels. Phase 0 is the rapid depolarization phase due to Na^+ entry. Phase 1 involves early repolarization with K^+ efflux from the cell. Phase 3 is the repolarization phase and is dominated by K^+ efflux from the cell. Phase 4 is the return of the resting membrane potential and is maintained by Na^+/K^+-ATPase channels. See Figure 1.13.

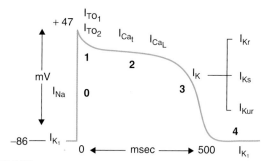

FIGURE 1.13

95. (D) Hypercyanotic ("tet") spells consists of abrupt onset of cyanosis, hypoxemia, dyspnea, and agitation. Events usually occur after the age of 2 months. Crying and agitation lead to increased pulmonary vascular resistance, with increased right-to-left shunting and decreased pulmonary blood flow. Infundibular spasm may also be involved in the limitation of RV outflow to the pulmonary arteries. In the modern era, the presence of hypercyanotic spells is widely considered an indication to proceed to surgical repair of the underlying tetralogy of Fallot.

96. (C) T-tubules are a continuation of the sarcolemma, enveloping myofibrils at the level of the Z-disks, and are important for rapid activation of the entire myocyte after the arrival of an action potential (excitation–contraction coupling). They are the site of numerous L-type calcium channels, which provide the initial calcium flow into the cell during excitation. Intercalated disks are junctions between adjacent myocytes. They link the myofibrils to costameres (which are intracellular protein complexes), transmitting force from the sarcomere to the extracellular matrix and adjacent myocytes. They also function to link the cytoplasmic actin filaments to the cytoskeleton and connect intermediate filaments between adjacent cells.

97. (A) Myocardial oxygen consumption is determined by wall tension which is related to intraventricular pressure and radius. Therefore, decreasing end diastolic volume decreases both the pressure and radius of the ventricle. Increased cardiac contractility increases the work that the ventricle is doing, thereby increasing the wall tension. Increased heart rate results in increased oxygen consumption over time due to an increase in the frequency of generating the pressure needed to overcome aortic pressure in left ventricular contraction. Sympathetic activation results in increased heart rate and contraction.

98. (C) The patient has an acute metabolic acidosis, as evidenced by the low pH, relatively normal pCO_2, and low bicarbonate.

99. (D) The patient has an acute respiratory acidosis, as evidenced by the low pH, elevated pCO_2, and normal bicarbonate. After the acute period of a respiratory acidosis, the bicarbonate will typically begin to increase to compensate and bring the pH closer to normal values.

100. (A) The right pulmonary artery travels anterior to the right upper lobe bronchus, while the left pulmonary artery travels posterior to the left upper lobe bronchus. Answer (B) may occur in patients with sinus inversus and mirror-image morphology. The branches may both travel anterior to their respective upper lobe bronchi in patients with bilateral morphologic right lungs, while they may both travel posterior to their respective upper lobe bronchi in patients with bilateral morphologic left lungs.

101. (D) Troponin is a complex made up of three proteins: troponin T, C, and I. During diastole, tropomyosin and troponin I prevent cross-bridging between actin and myosin. In systole, calcium ions bind to troponin C, which binds to troponin I and moves it from the ATP-reactive site on actin. Troponin T binds to tropomyosin which results in a conformational change, allowing the cross-bridging of actin and myosin. The myosin head has intrinsic ATPase activity, and when uninhibited, ATP becomes hydrolyzed which allows the myosin head to interact with actin and pull the filament inward, which is called the power stroke. After the power stroke, ADP is released which allows the myosin and actin to detach.

CHAPTER 2

Congenital Cardiac Malformations

M. Eric Ferguson /3

QUESTIONS

1. A 4-month-old girl is referred to you because of a cardiac murmur. She appears jaundiced. She has a grade 2–3/6 systolic ejection murmur along left upper sternal border that radiates to the back bilaterally. She has prominent facial features including a broad forehead and pointed chin. Her mother has similar features. A defect in which of the following genes would most likely explain her clinical findings?

    A. *NOTCH1*
    B. *PTPN11*
    C. *TBX1*
    D. *JAG1*
    E. *GATA*

2. A 28-year-old woman develops severe rubella infection late in the second month of pregnancy. The fetus is at increased risk for which congenital heart defect?

    A. Complex heterotaxy
    B. Ebstein anomaly
    C. Coarctation of the aorta
    D. d-Transposition of the great arteries (d-TGA)
    E. Valvar and supravalvar pulmonic stenosis

3. A 31-year-old primigravid woman drinks three cups of coffee daily. She is otherwise healthy. The fetus is at increased risk for which congenital heart defect?

    A. Tetralogy of Fallot (TOF)
    B. Tricuspid atresia
    C. Patent foramen ovale
    D. Secundum atrial septal defect
    E. No increased risk of cardiac defects

4. Which of the following defects is most likely to occur in a newborn whose mother had phenylketonuria?

    A. Ebstein anomaly
    B. Tricuspid atresia
    C. Coarctation of the aorta
    D. Anomalous pulmonary venous return
    E. Right aortic arch

5. You are asked to evaluate a 2-year-old boy for a cardiac murmur. You note that the child, for a 2-year old, is quite friendly, has stellate irises, a long philtrum, depressed nasal bridge, prominent lower lip, and enamel hypoplasia. There is a grade 3/6 systolic ejection murmur and no click. Which of the following chromosomal deletions is most likely in this patient?

    A. 18q
    B. 22p
    C. 8p23
    D. 7q11.23
    E. 22q11

6. A 4-month-old boy develops tachypnea and poor feeding. On examination, the blood pressure in the right arm is 110/60 mm Hg, in the left arm 105/60 mm Hg, and in the right leg 108/60 mm Hg. An echocardiogram demonstrates increased left ventricle (LV) wall thickness, moderate supravalvar aortic stenosis with estimated mean outflow gradient of 44 mm Hg, and mild supravalvar pulmonary stenosis. The aortic and pulmonary valves appear normal. The estimated LV ejection fraction (EF) is 20% with evidence of inferior wall hypokinesis. Which of the following is the most likely diagnosis in this patient?

    A. Velo-cardio-facial syndrome
    B. Down syndrome
    C. Williams syndrome
    D. Rheumatic heart disease
    E. Coarctation of the aorta

7. You are consulted to assess a small-for-gestational-age new-born with a heart murmur. Dysmorphic features include microcephaly, microphthalmia, short palpebral fissures, micrognathia, a prominent occiput, short sternum, and small nipples. The hands are clinched with overlapping fingers, and the feet have a convex shape. Which of the following statements is correct regarding this clinical scenario?

A. Trisomy 13 is the most likely clinical diagnosis

B. Associated congenital heart disease (CHD) occurs in ~50% of patients

C. Ventricular septal defect (VSD) and polyvalvular dysplasia are the most common CHD in this disorder

D. Most patients survive well into the second decade of life without surgery

E. If corrective cardiac surgery is performed successfully, the risk of death is decreased 10-fold

8. An infant presents in the newborn nursery with feeding difficulty and is noted to have a cleft palate, hypocalcemia, and lymphopenia. FISH testing is positive for a 22q11 deletion. Among the following, what is his echocardiogram most likely to demonstrate?

A. Ebstein anomaly of the tricuspid valve

B. Pulmonary atresia + intact ventricular septum (IVS)

C. Interruption of aortic arch between the left common carotid and left subclavian artery

D. Left ventricular diverticulum

E. Double outlet right atrium

9. You are seeing a female patient for a chief complaint of dyspnea with exertion. You note in her medical chart that she has a history of a large secundum atrial septal defect (ASD) that apparently went unrepaired. She last saw a physician at the age of 10 years, where the defect was noted to be 18 mm by echocardiography. The patient is now 31 years old. She has not had any cardiovascular interventions in the interim. You listen and fail to appreciate a widely split S2. In fact, you think the split is narrow and P2 is loud. There is a very short systolic murmur over the left upper sternal border (LUSB). There is no diastolic murmur. What is the most likely cause of the physical findings?

A. Spontaneous closure of the defect

B. Severe mitral valve regurgitation

C. Nonsustained ventricular tachycardia

D. Left ventricular diastolic dysfunction

E. Significant pulmonary hypertension

10. A 19-year-old male patient is found, by echocardiogram, to have a large sinus venosus defect with partial anomalous pulmonary venous connection with drainage of the right upper and middle pulmonary veins to the superior vena cava. The right ventricle appears severely dilated with moderately decreased function. The ventricular septum appears flattened throughout the cardiac cycle. The tricuspid valve does not leak. There is trace pulmonary insufficiency. What is your recommendation to the patient?

A. Dismiss from follow-up as there is nothing to be done

B. Begin propranolol immediately

C. Start IV epoprostenol

D. Cardiac catheterization with pulmonary vascular reactivity testing

E. Counsel that there is little to do at this point, as she is past the point of medical benefit

11. In a patient with typical auscultatory findings of an ASD and a P-wave axis of <30 degrees on the electrocardiogram, one should think immediately of which of the following type of atrial septal defect?

A. Unroofed coronary sinus

B. Sinus venosus

C. Secundum

D. Primum

E. Patent foramen ovale

12. Which of the following papillary muscle arrangements are seen most commonly with complete atrioventricular canal (septal) defect (AVCD or AVSD)?

A. The papillary muscles are closer together, the anterior muscle is closer to the septum than normal, and the posterior muscle is farther from the septum than normal

B. The papillary muscles are closer together, the anterior muscle is farther from the septum than normal, and the posterior muscle is closer to the septum than normal

C. The papillary muscles are closer together and positioned clockwise from their normal location

D. The papillary muscles are farther apart, the anterior muscle is closer to the septum than normal, and the posterior muscle is farther from the septum than normal

E. The papillary muscles are farther apart, the anterior muscle is farther from the septum than normal, and the posterior muscle is closer to the septum than normal

13. A 17-year-old man who underwent complete repair of a partial atrioventricular septal defect (AVSD) at 15 months of age presents with progressive shortness of breath. He has a grade 3/6 holosystolic murmur that is loudest over the apex and is less prominent with Valsalva maneuver. Chest x-ray reveals mild cardiomegaly and mildly increased pulmonary vascularity. Which of the following is the most likely cause of these symptoms?

A. Mitral regurgitation
B. Primary pulmonary hypertension
C. Left ventricular outflow tract obstruction
D. Mitral stenosis
E. Pulmonary valve stenosis

14. Which of the following is true regarding left ventricular outflow tract (LVOT) obstruction in patients with AVSD?

A. Obstruction may be due to displacement of the left atrioventricular (AV) valve annulus, resulting in shortening and narrowing of the LVOT
B. Nearly 30% of patients with AVSD will require reoperation for LVOT obstruction
C. Progressive LVOT obstruction is more common in patients with two atrioventricular (AV) valve orifices
D. Preoperative LVOT obstruction is often progressive, while postoperative obstruction is frequently static
E. LVOT obstruction is the most common indication for reoperation after partial AVSD repair

15. An 18-month-old boy undergoes operative repair of a moderate-sized ASD and moderate-sized mid-muscular ventricular septal defect (VSD). His preoperative chest x-ray revealed borderline cardiomegaly and an ECG at the same time was normal. He remains intubated on postoperative day 2, at which time you note a new finding of a widely split S_2 with no murmur. Which of the following is the most likely reason for your findings?

A. Residual ASD
B. Residual VSD
C. Postoperative decrease in pulmonary artery pressure
D. Right bundle branch block
E. Mechanical ventilation

16. Which of the following statements is true regarding VSD?

A. Flow across a large (unrestrictive) VSD is limited primarily by the size of the defect
B. Frequently, supracristal defects are partially or completely occluded by redundant tricuspid valve tissue
C. Prominent S_2 splitting is occasionally heard with a small VSD

D. After VSD repair, the LV mass decreases more prominently than left ventricular end-diastolic volume (LVEDV)
E. Patients who develop Eisenmenger physiology typically first manifest cyanosis between the ages 4 and 6 years.

17. You are seeing a 19-year-old woman who was diagnosed at the age of 6 months with a moderate-sized, isolated perimembranous VSD with outlet extension. The patient was then lost to cardiology follow-up. The patient presents for evaluation of a murmur that was noted during her required physical for her new job. She is asymptomatic and plays golf 2 to 3 times per week. On examination, she is acyanotic. There is a grade 2/6 systolic murmur over right upper sternal border and a grade 3/4 high-pitched decrescendo diastolic murmur at the left sternal border. What is the most likely explanation for the murmur?

A. Prolapse of left aortic cusp has closed the VSD, and the aortic valve is insufficient
B. Prolapse of the right aortic cusp has closed the VSD, and the aortic valve is insufficient
C. Prolapse of the septal leaflet of the tricuspid valve has closed the VSD, and the tricuspid valve is insufficient
D. Right and left ventricular pressures have equalized, and new pulmonary insufficiency has developed
E. Left atrial (LA) and LV volumes have increased secondary to unrestricted left-to-right shunting with secondary mitral valve insufficiency

18. What is the relationship of the bundle of His to an inlet VSD?

A. The bundle passes posterior-inferiorly to the defect
B. The bundle passes anterior-superiorly to the defect
C. The bundle courses caudally around the defect
D. The bundle courses through the right AV groove
E. The bundle passes laterally to the defect through the left ventricle

19. A 28-week preemie develops persistent abdominal distention, increasing residuals before feedings, blood in the stools, and decreasing bowel sounds. Abdominal x-ray reveals evidence of intramural air in the right lower quadrant. The patient has bounding pulses, and an echocardiogram confirms the presence of a hemodynamically significant patent ductus arteriosus (PDA). What is the best next step in management?

A. Referral to surgery for immediate surgical closure
B. Percutaneous closure of PDA with occluding coil
C. Trial of indomethacin
D. Trial of ibuprofen
E. Do nothing

20. You see an 8-year-old boy from Venezuela who presents for evaluation of a cardiac murmur. As an infant he had poor feeding, irritability, and tachypnea. Weight gain was slow. The symptoms gradually resolved after the age of 3 to 4 months, and he has grown steadily along the third percentile since then. He tires more easily than his peers. He has progressive myalgias, arthralgias, headache, and general malaise. Fever is relapsing and low grade, and his parents report marked diminution in appetite.

On examination, peripheral pulses are full and bounding. The precordium is hyperdynamic, and there is a thrusting apical impulse. A systolic thrill is palpable at the upper left sternal border. S_1 and S_2 are difficult to hear because they are masked by a loud continuous murmur. The murmur is intense and is heard throughout the precordium as well as posteriorly. It has a harsh quality with low-frequency components, and eddy sounds that vary from beat to beat give it a machinery quality. A third heart sound is heard at the apex. Blood cultures are positive for *Streptococcus viridans*. His CXR is shown in Figure 2.1:

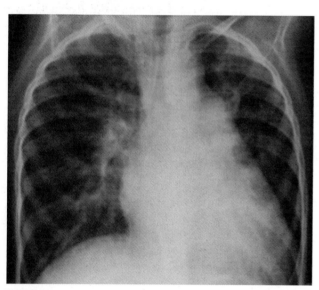

FIGURE 2.1

Which of the following statements is most likely to be true in this clinical setting?

A. Vegetation is likely, and it will be seen on the pulmonary arterial (PA) end of the ductus arteriosus

B. Vegetation is likely, and it will be seen on the aortic end of the ductus

C. *Streptococcus viridans* is very unlikely to cause endocarditis in this setting

D. Abscess is much more common than vegetation in this setting

E. Vegetation is unlikely, but if present would be seen on the aortic end of the ductus

21. Which of the following events is most responsible for early, functional closure of the ductus arteriosus?

A. Hemorrhage and necrosis in the subintimal region

B. Medial smooth muscle cell migration in the wall of the ductus

C. Equalization of pulmonary and systemic vascular resistance

D. Infolding of the endothelium

E. Thinning of the intimal layer

22. What is the theoretical benefit of ibuprofen over indomethacin for closure of PDA in premature infants?

A. Decreased risk of intraventricular hemorrhage

B. Decreased risk of pulmonary hypertension

C. Decreased risk of gastrointestinal bleeding

D. Greater rate of ductal closure

E. Less effect on cerebral blood flow

23. A 2-week-old infant is found to have anomalous left coronary artery from the pulmonary artery (ALCAPA). Surgical correction is planned. What preoperative comorbidity has been found to be a risk factor for mortality and for late reoperation?

A. Mitral insufficiency

B. Tricuspid insufficiency

C. Aortic valve insufficiency

D. Pulmonary valve insufficiency

E. Patent foramen ovale

24. You examine a 17-year-old boy with a 2-year history of progressive dyspnea on exertion and 2 months of orthopnea. Vital signs: pulse (P), 80 beats per minute; Blood pressure (BP), 118/44 mm Hg; and respiratory rate (RR), 24 breaths per minute. Physical examination reveals a lift along the left sternal border and a continuous murmur with maximal intensity in the third to fourth intercostal space near the right sternal edge. On the basis of the available information, of the following diagnoses, which is most likely?

A. Sinus of Valsalva fistula from the aorta to the right atrium

B. Sinus of Valsalva fistula from the aorta to the left atrium

C. Anomalous left coronary artery from the pulmonary artery

D. Patent ductus arteriosus

E. Severe isolated aortic regurgitation

25. A 3-week-old infant has had several episodes of acute onset of agitation and crying. During these episodes, the baby is inconsolable. On examination, there is a high-frequency systolic murmur audible at the apex with radiation to the left axilla. Which of the following coronary artery anomalies most likely would be responsible for these symptoms?

 A. Anomalous origin of right coronary artery from left sinus of Valsalva
 B. Anomalous origin of left main coronary artery from right sinus of Valsalva
 C. Anomalous origin of left coronary artery from the pulmonary artery
 D. Anomalous origin of left anterior descending artery from the right main coronary artery
 E. Origin of left circumflex coronary artery from right main coronary artery

26. Which of the following is true regarding aneurysms of the sinus of Valsalva?

 A. The most common location is the noncoronary sinus
 B. There is no gender predilection for aneurysm formation
 C. Concomitant VSD is seen up to 50% of the time
 D. The most common site of rupture is into the left atrium
 E. Most VSDs seen with coronary sinus aneurysms are paramembranous

27. A neonate presents at birth with high-output cardiac failure secondary to a cerebral arteriovenous malformation (AVM). If left untreated, what is the approximate risk of mortality during the first week of life?

 A. 3%
 B. 15%
 C. 30%
 D. 50%
 E. 90%

28. Which of the following is true regarding pulmonary AVM?

 A. Pulmonary AVM in the setting of hereditary hemorrhagic telangiectasia (HHT) tend to shrink as the patient grows older
 B. In patients with pulmonary AVM, cardiac output typically is twice that of normal
 C. If there are multiple pulmonary AVMs, there is a >80% chance of the patient having HHT
 D. Patients with pulmonary AVMs typically are hemodynamically unstable and require significant respiratory support in infancy
 E. Most pulmonary AVMs in children are acquired

29. Which of the following statements is correct regarding transcatheter embolization of pulmonary AVM?

 A. To avoid device embolization, liquid adhesive is more effective than coil device closure

 B. Embolization effectively prevents strokes and transient ischemic attacks, but not brain abscesses
 C. Embolization effectively prevents brain abscess but does not prevent strokes
 D. Greatest success if achieved by decreasing systemic arterial oxygen tension to <50 mm Hg
 E. Embolization provides persistent relief of desaturation but not of orthodeoxia

30. Which of the following measurements has the best potential to distinguish a large AVM from a large PDA in a young infant?

 A. Pulse pressure as determined by sphygmomanometry
 B. Cardiothoracic ratio on plain chest x-ray
 C. Systemic vein oxygen saturation measurements obtained during cardiac catheterization
 D. QRS axis on electrocardiogram
 E. Liver span by physical examination

31. An 11-year-old boy is evaluated for swallowing difficulty and moderate exercise intolerance. A barium esophagram shows evidence of anterior indentation, and pulmonary function testing shows evidence of obstruction. What is the most likely diagnosis?

 A. Retroesophageal left subclavian artery
 B. Pulmonary artery sling
 C. Tracheoesophageal fistula
 D. Innominate artery compression of the trachea
 E. Retroesophageal fistula of Phillips

32. A CT scan is done to assess a neck mass in a 3-year-old child with a history of murmur but no prior cardiac history. This patient has no trouble swallowing and has no history of respiratory problems. The scan incidentally showed a right aortic arch with mirror image branching. What additional action is warranted?

 A. Barium swallow
 B. Echocardiography
 C. Bronchoscopy
 D. Surgical referral
 E. No further action needed

33. Which of the following typically results in a vascular ring?

 A. Right aortic arch with retroesophageal innominate artery, left patent ductus arteriosus
 B. Right aortic arch with retroesophageal left subclavian artery, no patent ductus arteriosus
 C. Right aortic arch with mirror-image branching, right ligamentum arteriosus
 D. Left aortic arch with cervical origin of right subclavian artery
 E. Left aortic arch with retroesophageal right subclavian artery

34. A newborn infant presents in acute cardiovascular collapse on day 3 of life. Physical examination reveals absence of all limb pulses with strong carotid pulses bilaterally. Echocardiography is most likely to reveal which of the following?

A. Critical aortic stenosis

B. Interruption of the aortic arch, type A, with anomalous subclavian artery

C. Interruption of the aortic arch, type B

D. Interruption of the aortic arch type B with anomalous subclavian artery

E. Right aortic arch with retroesophageal diverticulum of Kommerell

35. A 5-month-old girl presents with stridor and wheezing since birth. She has been treated with albuterol and inhaled steroids without any improvement. Her parents have noticed that she has been coughing and gagging since starting baby foods 2 weeks prior. Which of the following diagnoses is most likely?

A. Right aortic arch with retroesophageal diverticulum of Kommerell

B. Left aortic arch with retroesophageal diverticulum of Kommerell

C. Right aortic arch with mirror image branching

D. Left aortic arch with retroesophageal right subclavian artery

E. Right aortic arch with retroesophageal innominate artery

36. Which of the following statements is true regarding anomalies of pulmonary venous return?

A. An untreated infant born with total anomalous pulmonary venous connection (TAPVC) has a 50% chance of surviving until the age of 1 year

B. The cardiothymic silhouette tends to be shifted leftward in Scimitar syndrome

C. Patients with cor triatriatum have enlargement of the right atrium and right ventricle

D. Normal p-wave size (<2.5 mm) on ECG effectively rules out cor triatriatum

E. Ventricular arrhythmias are common following TAPVC repair

37. A 3-year-old asymptomatic boy has a 2/6 systolic ejection murmur at the left upper sternal border and fixed splitting of S_2. An echocardiogram reveals a sinus venosus ASD. This defect results from which of the following?

A. Deficiency of septum primum

B. Deficiency of septum secundum

C. Excessive resorption of septum primum

D. Anomalous insertion of the superior pulmonary vein

E. Deficiency of the common wall of the superior vena cava and the pulmonary vein

38. What is the catheter course in Figure 2.2?

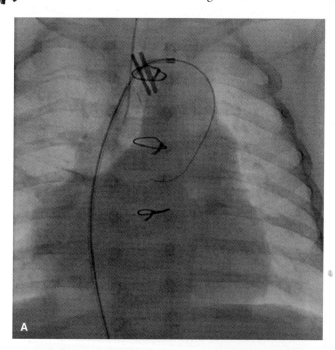

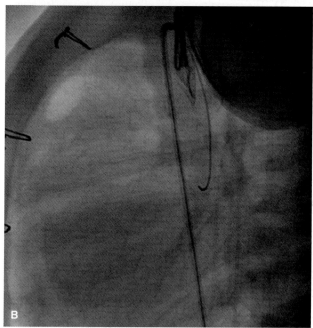

FIGURE 2.2

A. Aorta → right aortic arch → innominate artery → BT shunt → RPA

B. Aorta → right aortic arch → right sinus of Valsalva

C. Scimitar vein → right SVC → innominate vein → left SVC → coronary sinus

D. IVC → right atrium → SVC → innominate vein → left SVC → coronary sinus

E. IVC → right atrium → SVC → innominate vein → vertical vein → anomalous pulmonary venous confluence

39. A newborn is diagnosed with infradiaphragmatic total anomalous pulmonary venous connection (TAPVC) to the portal vein. Echocardiography demonstrates high-velocity, continuous, nonphasic venous flow in the anomalous vein. PGE_1 has been started. The cardiorespiratory and metabolic states have been optimized. What is the best immediate plan of action?

A. Supportive therapy for 24 to 48 hours to allow PA pressures to fall before operation

B. Bedside balloon atrial septostomy

C. Cardiac catheterization to determine pulmonary vascular resistance (PVR) and to perform blade atrial septostomy if needed

D. Balloon dilation +/− stent placement in anomalous pulmonary vein

E. Immediate corrective surgery

40. A 19-year-old woman presents with a several-month history of worsening breathlessness. Past medical history is significant for five episodes of pneumonia over her lifetime. Chronic medications include inhaled fluticasone, budesonide, and montelukast. She carries a rescue inhaler of albuterol. Physical examination reveals an RV heave, loud P2, and pulmonary systolic ejection click. There is a soft, blowing systolic murmur along the left sternal border. Echocardiography reveals the following (Figure 2.3):

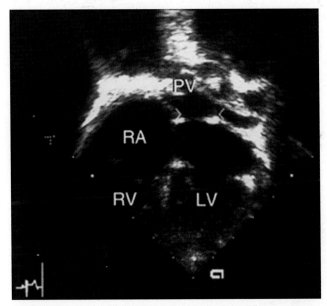

FIGURE 2.3

What is the most correct statement about this condition?

A. Surgical correction is universally futile

B. Medical management offers a better chance of 20-year survival than operative correction

C. Perioperative risk is low

D. In patients who survive operative correction, prognosis is excellent

E. Atrial fibrillation is common

41. Which of the following statements is correct regarding anomalous drainage of the left pulmonary veins to the left innominate vein (LIV)?

A. The left lung drains typically by a left SVC

B. A primum ASD is common

C. The vertical vein represents a persistent embryologic connection between the splanchnic plexus of the lung buds and the cardinal veins

D. This is a normal variant and found in 0.5% of the general population

E. This condition has never been described

42. A 3-year-old child has complex single ventricle, bilateral superior vena cavae, and interrupted IVC with azygous continuation to the right SVC. At operation, he has construction of bilateral bidirectional superior vena caval–pulmonary anastomoses. Two months postoperatively his systemic arterial blood oxygen saturation is 87%, and he is doing well. Six months postoperatively his saturation is 82%, and he is doing well. Two years postoperatively his saturation is 75%, and he is a bit more fatigued. Which of the following factors, unique to the operation he had, contribute the most to his progressive desaturation?

A. Increased coronary sinus drainage

B. Increased pulmonary arteriolar resistance

C. Erythrocytosis

D. Pulmonary arteriovenous fistulae

E. Decreased chest wall compliance

43. An 8-year-old girl with palpitations has an echocardiogram that demonstrates an outpouching originating in the coronary sinus that has a distinct neck and extends behind the LV. What is the most likely source of her palpitations?

A. RVOT-origin ventricular tachycardia

B. Accessory pathway-mediated SVT

C. AV nodal reentry tachycardia

D. Torsades de pointes

E. Brugada syndrome

44. A 14-day-old infant presents with irritability. He has been eating poorly due to tachypnea (RR = 80s) and is 15% below his birth weight of 3,216 g. Physical examination reveals tachypnea and a loud systolic murmur over his entire precordium. There is a soft low-pitched diastolic murmur at the apex. Distal pulses are slightly diminished. An ABG demonstrates pH = 7.27, pCO_2 = 31, and HCO_3 = 16 on room air. Echocardiogram reveals tricuspid atresia, d-TGA, and a moderately restrictive VSD. His aortic arch is moderately hypoplastic, although there is no evidence of a definite posterior shelf at the isthmus. Of the following procedures, what is the best initial surgical palliation option?

A. Modified Blalock–Taussig (BT) shunt only

B. PA banding only

C. Bidirectional cavopulmonary anastomosis

D. Anastomosis between main pulmonary artery (MPA) and ascending aorta (Damus–Kaye–Stansel [DKS]) with aortic arch augmentation and BT shunt

E. VSD closure + patch enlargement of LVOT (modified Konno)

45. Which of the following features are more specific for Uhl anomaly than Ebstein anomaly?

A. The presence of significant cyanosis on physical examination

B. Large P-waves and diminished right ventricular voltages on ECG

C. Thin appearing, dysfunctional RV myocardium on echocardiography

D. Similar pressure wave contours in the RA and RV during cardiac catheterization

E. Ventricular endocardial potentials recorded past the expected anatomic tricuspid valve annulus during electrophysiologic assessment

46. An 11-year-old boy with a history of pulmonary stenosis presents for evaluation. His blood pressure at rest is 100/70 mm Hg. Echocardiography reveals normal inspiratory collapse of his IVC. The following Doppler-derived velocities are obtained (at rest):

Tricuspid regurgitation (CW) = 3.5 m/s

Infundibulum (PW) = 2 m/s

RVOT (CW) = 4 m/s

Assume RA pressure is 6 mm Hg. Using traditionally accepted Doppler-derived criteria to determine severity, what degree of pulmonary stenosis is present in this patient?

A. Trivial

B. Mild

C. Moderate

D. Severe

E. Not enough information provided

The following clinical scenario pertains to Questions 47 and 48:

A 1-day-old term newborn is admitted to the NICU with cyanosis and a murmur. He is diagnosed with critical pulmonary stenosis and a moderate-sized PDA. Percutaneous pulmonary valvotomy is performed. Cardiac hemodynamics obtained during the catheterization are shown in Table 2.1.

TABLE 2.1 Cardiac Hemodynamics Obtained during Catheterization		
	Pre-Valvotomy	Post-Valvotomy
RA (mean)	10	9
RV (systolic/EDP)	100/11	72/10
MPA	35/18	37/20
RPCW (mean)	Not done	7
Systemic BP	51/21	53/25

RA, right atrial; RV, right ventricular; EDP, end-diastolic pressure; MPA, main pulmonary artery; RPCW, right pulmonary capillary wedge pressure.

That night, the baby continues to have low oxygen saturations in the mid-80s despite being mechanically ventilated and on PGE_1. On examination, there is a grade 4/6 late-peaking harsh systolic murmur at the left upper sternal border, which is increased in intensity from his admission examination, and a new, soft diastolic murmur. Blood pressure is 52/24 mm Hg. Blood gas reveals a base deficit of −2.

47. Which of the following would be the next best step?

A. Urgent repeat percutaneous valvotomy

B. Urgent open pulmonary valvotomy

C. STAT echocardiogram

D. Increase the PGE dosage

E. Continued close observation

48. Which of the following is the most likely underlying cause of his desaturation?

A. Pulmonary vein stenosis

B. Infundibular RVOT obstruction

C. Right-to-left shunting across the PDA

D. Undiagnosed VSD

E. Severe pulmonary regurgitation

49. You are performing an echocardiogram on an asymptomatic 4-month-old girl referred for a cardiac murmur. You note discrete stenosis of the proximal LPA, measuring 2 mm. The distal LPA is 6 mm. The RPA is 8 mm. The pulmonary valve and MPA are normal. There is no ASD or VSD. Peak Doppler velocity across the LPA stenosis is 2.0 m/s. Right ventricular systolic pressure (RVSP) is estimated to be 25 mm Hg. There is mild RV hypertrophy. Which of the following statements is true?

A. The degree of LPA stenosis is mild
B. RVSP is likely underestimated considering the degree of LPA narrowing
C. Invasive pressure measurements would be likely to show an MPA to LPA gradient that is much higher than that estimated by Doppler flow velocity.
D. If angioplasty is performed, a 6- to 8-mm balloon should be used
E. The risk of restenosis after angioplasty is approximately 3% to 5%

 50. A newborn infant is cyanotic, and echocardiography reveals pulmonary atresia with intact ventricular septum. The right ventricle is bipartite and quite small. The baby is receiving PGE-1. Which of the following is the next step in the management of this patient?

A. Balloon atrial septostomy
B. Surgical outflow tract reconstruction
C. Cardiac catheterization and angiography
D. Cardiac CT scan
E. Cardiac MRI

51. Which of the following anatomical substrates most likely predicts a successful decompression of the RV using radiofrequency ablation and balloon pulmonary valvotomy in patients with pulmonary atresia with intact ventricular septum?

A. Unipartite RV
B. Muscular pulmonary atresia
C. RV-dependent coronary circulation
D. Severe tricuspid stenosis
E. Tricuspid valve Z score = −2

52. The angiogram demonstrated in Figure 2.4 is performed in a 9-month-old boy with pulmonary atresia and intact ventricular septum.

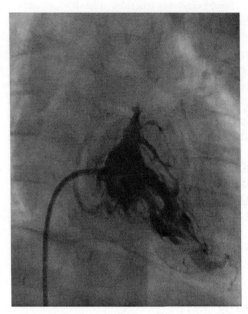

FIGURE 2.4

Which of the following operations is best for this patient?

A. Bidirectional Glenn alone
B. RV to PA conduit with a bidirectional Glenn
C. RV to PA conduit alone
D. Pulmonary valvotomy alone
E. Pulmonary valvotomy with a bidirectional Glenn

53. For the above patient, a takedown of his BT shunt is performed along with the placement of an RV to PA conduit. That evening he develops congestive heart failure (CHF). Which of the following ECG findings would you most likely see in this patient at this time?

A. Complete heart block
B. Left bundle branch block
C. ST segment elevation in I, aVL
D. ST segment elevation in II, III, aVF
E. Increased voltages in V1, V2, V3

54. You are seeing a 4-day-old infant with cyanosis. Echocardiography reveals pulmonary atresia with intact ventricular septum. There is significant subpulmonary (infundibular) obstruction. The RV appears tripartite but severely hypoplastic. By echocardiography, there is no evidence of RV-dependent coronary circulation. You are planning an eventual biventricular repair beginning with a surgical pulmonary valvuloplasty and RVOT patch enlargement. What is the best next step in surgical planning?

A. Go to surgery without further testing
B. Cardiac catheterization with hemodynamic study only
C. Catheterization with hemodynamic assessment and RV angiography
D. MRI with RV volume quantification
E. Biopsy of RV myocardium to evaluate for spongy myocardium and/or endocardial sclerosis

55. A newborn is found to have cyanosis shortly after birth. A holosystolic murmur is heard and PGE-1 is started. An echocardiogram is performed (Figure 2.5):

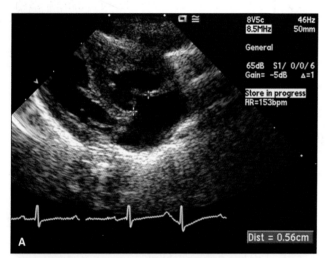

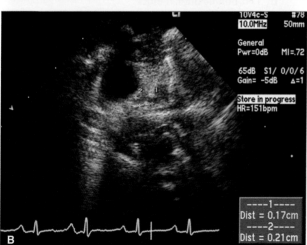

FIGURE 2.5

Color flow Doppler fails to show antegrade flow in the MPA. The ventricular septum is intact. Which of the following is true regarding neonates with this form of congenital heart disease?

A. Coronary artery perfusion is wholly RV dependent in about 45% of cases
B. Pulmonary blood flow most often is supplied by aortopulmonary collaterals
C. This form of congenital heart disease is more common in males
D. By definition, the right ventricle is always bipartite
E. A main pulmonary trunk almost always is present

56. A 3-year-old boy has pulmonary atresia with VSD. He has a history of hypoplastic central pulmonary arteries and multiple major aortopulmonary collateral arteries (MAPCA), with multiple surgeries including a central shunt as well as right and left unifocalization surgeries. He is admitted for complete repair. Following reconstruction of the central confluence, placement of an RV–PA conduit, takedown of two MAPCAs, and VSD closure, he does not tolerate coming off bypass. His blood pressure is 84/60 mm Hg on multiple pressors. His saturation is 87% on 100% oxygen. His RV pressure is 69/15 mm Hg. TEE demonstrates patency of the conduit. What is the best course of action?

A. Placement of ECMO until hemodynamics improve
B. Reinstitution of bypass, takedown of RV–PA conduit and placement of a central shunt
C. Replacement of the RV–PA conduit with a larger conduit
D. Treatment with nitric oxide to improve PVR
E. Reopening the VSD

57. An 11-year-old boy with history of pulmonary atresia with VSD is status post a BT shunt early in life and is also status post multiple unifocalization procedures. He is in the operating room for a complete repair. The surgeon has completed the operation. You are performing an echocardiogram. You note that the VSD is now closed and the RV–PA conduit has laminar flow by color Doppler. The estimated RV systolic pressure is 80 mm Hg. Biventricular function appears reasonable. You see that the radial arterial pressure tracing is 100/50 mm Hg. You advise the surgeon to:

A. Do nothing further
B. Replace the conduit with a smaller one
C. Replace the conduit with a larger one
D. Reopen the VSD
E. Place a BT shunt in addition to what has been done already

58. A 4-month-old infant with pulmonary atresia with VSD undergoes complete repair, including unifocalization, RV–PA conduit and closure of the VSD. Before sternal closure in the operating room she becomes hypotensive. Systemic arterial pressure is 65/45 mm Hg. She is edematous with hepatomegaly. TEE reveals RV hypertrophy and moderately decreased biventricular systolic function. She has moderate tricuspid regurgitation with a velocity of 3.5 m/s. Which of the following interventions is most urgent at this time?

 A. Milrinone
 B. Leave the chest open and return to the ICU
 C. Reopen the VSD
 D. Placement of a bidirectional Glenn
 E. ECMO

59. A neonate with pulmonary atresia with VSD undergoes heart catheterization. The angiogram in Figure 2.6 is obtained.

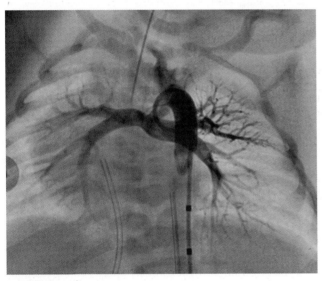

FIGURE 2.6

What is the primary source of pulmonary blood flow in this patient?

 A. Ascending aorta
 B. Descending aorta
 C. Patent ductus arteriosus
 D. BT shunt
 E. Right subclavian artery

 60. In a patient with pulmonary atresia with VSD, where is the proximal His bundle located relative to the VSD?

 A. Along the posteroinferior rim of the VSD on the left ventricular side
 B. Along the posterosuperior rim of the VSD on the right ventricular side
 C. Along the anterolateral rim of the VSD on the left ventricular side
 D. Along the anteromedial rim of the VSD on the right ventricular side
 E. Not enough information provided

61. A 12-year-old patient with unrepaired TOF presents to clinic for preoperative evaluation before a planned complete surgical repair. Physical examination reveals severe cyanosis with marked clubbing of the fingers. Cardiac examination reveals a normal S_1, single S_2, with a grade 2/6 systolic ejection murmur at the left upper sternal border. There is also a soft continuous murmur over interscapular area. Echocardiography demonstrates severe right ventricular hypertrophy, anterocephalad malalignment of the conal septum, and a large perimembranous VSD with an overriding aorta. Owing to difficult visualization of the pulmonary artery anatomy, a cardiac catheterization is planned for the next morning at 8:30 AM. Which of the following should be done to decrease the chance of a hypercyanotic spell in the morning?

 A. Make the patient NPO after midnight and start an IV at 7:00 AM
 B. Use a general anesthesia-inducing agent that decreases systemic vascular resistance more than PVR
 C. Make the patient NPO after midnight, perform phlebotomy to decrease Hgb to <14 before starting the IV
 D. Start an esmolol drip as soon as the procedure starts
 E. Make the patient NPO after midnight, start IV fluid when NPO starts, and use a topical anesthetic such as EMLA before attempting vascular access

62. A 17-year-old girl with a history of tetralogy of Fallot (TOF) with a left aortic arch presents with progressive dyspnea on exertion. She describes a history of multiple operations including an RV–PA conduit revision 2 years ago. As part of her evaluation, cardiac catheterization is performed, from which the data in Table 2.2 are obtained.

TABLE 2.2 Cardiac Catheterization Data		
	Pressure	**SpO$_2$**
SVC	Mean 9	74
RA	Mean 8	76
RV	76/6	73
MPA	65/15, mean 46	74
RPA	27/13, mean 22	74
LPA	63/14, mean 44	74
RPCW	Mean 12	100
LPCW	Mean 12	
LV	112/10	99
Asc AO	110/68, mean 80	
Desc AO	102/67, mean 80	

SVC, superior vena cava; RA, right atrial; RV, right ventricular; MPA, main pulmonary artery; RPA, right pulmonary artery; LPA, left pulmonary artery; RPCW, right pulmonary capillary wedge pressure; LV, left ventricular; AO, aortic.

On the basis of the information, which of the following is most likely to be true?

A. She would benefit from sildenafil
B. She would benefit from closure of her left-to-right shunt
C. She should have a conduit revision
D. Her symptoms are primarily related to diastolic dysfunction
E. She has a history of a Waterston shunt

63. A 6-day-old male infant presents with cyanosis and tachypnea. An echocardiogram confirms the diagnosis of Tetralogy of Fallot with absent pulmonary valve. He is in moderate respiratory distress. His heart rate (HR) is 190 beats per minute, RR is 55 breaths per minute, and his ABG shows PaO$_2$ = 67, PaCO$_2$ = 68, pH = 7.25, Bicarb = 17, and an oxygen saturation of 84%. What should be done next in an attempt to alleviate his respiratory distress?

A. Inhaled albuterol
B. Intubation and mechanical ventilation

C. IV solumedrol
D. Emergent surgical repair of his congenital heart disease
E. Placement in prone position

64. A 3-day-old male infant presents to the emergency department with cyanosis. He was diagnosed prenatally with tetralogy of Fallot. He was born at home at 35 and 4/7 weeks of gestation. Over the first 48 hours of life, his color was good and he was nursing effectively. However, over the past 2 to 4 hours, he appeared progressively blue. At the time of presentation, his oxygen saturations are 60% to 65%, and he appears dusky. He is becoming duskier. On examination, he has no appreciable murmur. A UVC has been placed. What is the best next step in management?

A. Echocardiogram to ascertain whether his prenatal echo had the correct diagnosis
B. Hyperoxia test to try to ascertain if he has a pulmonary component of his cyanosis
C. Emergent surgical repair
D. IV prostaglandin
E. IV morphine to encourage left-to-right shunting across his VSD

65. A 6-day-old male infant presents with a cardiac murmur and cyanosis. His saturation is 69% and his cuff blood pressure is 65/37 mm Hg. An echocardiogram reveals the following: TOF; severe infundibular obstruction (narrowest diameter 2 to 3 mm); a bicuspid pulmonary valve measuring <5 mm at the annulus; almost entirely right-to-left shunting at the VSD with a peak Doppler VSD velocity of 2.5 m/s; accessory tricuspid valve tissue prolapsing into the VSD during systole; and a tricuspid regurgitation velocity of 4.5 m/s. He has an enlarged coronary sinus draining a left SVC. He has a large conal branch from his right coronary artery. Among the findings below, which feature is the most unusual in patients with TOF?

A. Large conal branch
B. Left SVC
C. Restrictive VSD
D. Pulmonary valve stenosis
E. Predominant right-to-left shunting through the VSD

66. A 3-week-old infant presents with tachypnea and poor feeding. Her prenatal screening ultrasound was suggestive of a severe conotruncal defect, but she was lost to follow-up and was a home delivery. Today, vital signs are as follows: P, 140 beats per minute; BP, 80/35 mm Hg; RR, 60 breaths per minute, O_2 saturation 93% (room air). Cardiac examination reveals an active precordium, normal S_1, single S_2 with a grade 2/6 systolic murmur at left-mid sternal border. When the baby is quiet, a soft continuous murmur becomes apparent in the back. Which of the following statements is correct regarding this scenario?

- **A.** The continuous murmur strongly suggests a diagnosis of truncus arteriosus
- **B.** The continuous murmur is the result of truncal valve stenosis and regurgitation
- **C.** Physical examination findings suggest a diagnosis of pulmonary atresia with VSD more than truncus arteriosus
- **D.** Physical examination findings suggest a diagnosis of pulmonary atresia with intact ventricular septum more than truncus arteriosus
- **E.** The presence of an apical diastolic murmur in this patient suggests anatomical mitral valve stenosis

67. Which of the following statements is correct regarding coronary artery anatomy in truncus arteriosus?

- **A.** The posterior descending coronary artery arises from the left circumflex artery (left coronary dominance) in <3% of patients
- **B.** The left anterior descending artery is relatively large and displaced rightward
- **C.** The conus branch of the right coronary artery is usually small
- **D.** The left coronary artery arises from the pulmonary trunk in ~40% of patients
- **E.** Left coronary usually arises from the left posterolateral truncal surface

68. A 6-year-old girl from Mongolia presents for surgical consideration of her congenital heart disease. Echocardiogram reveals type I truncus arteriosus with a large VSD. The atrial septum is intact and there is trivial tricuspid regurgitation. Heart catheterization is performed, whereupon the data in Table 2.3 are obtained:

TABLE 2.3 Heart Catheterization Data

	Pressure	SpO₂
IVC		58
SVC	Mean 9	52
RA	Mean 8	54
RV	102/12	62
Truncus	92/60, mean 72	82
RPA	83/49, mean 62	79
LPA	85/50, mean 63	79
RPCW	Mean 12	99
LPCW	Mean 13	99
LV	93/11	87
FA	96/58, mean 71	79

IVC, inferior vena cava; SVC, superior vena cava; RA, right atrial; RV, right ventricular; RPA, right pulmonary artery; LPA, left pulmonary artery; RPCW, right pulmonary capillary wedge pressure; LV, left ventricular; FA, femoral arterial.

Her systemic cardiac index is 4.0 L/min/m². Which of the following is true regarding this patient?

- **A.** No corrective intervention is indicated (palliation only)
- **B.** She should undergo closure of her VSD and placement of an RV–PA conduit
- **C.** Decision about whether or not to repair her lesions should be deferred until her hemodynamics are reassessed while she receives 100% oxygen
- **D.** She should be listed for cardiac transplantation
- **E.** She may benefit from balloon angioplasty of her pulmonary arteries

69. A neonate presents with cyanosis and a murmur. He is found to have type I truncus arteriosus with a bicuspid truncal valve and right aortic arch. He has a large secundum ASD and a left SVC draining into the coronary sinus. There is moderate RVH with normal biventricular function. Among the anatomic findings in this patient, which is most common among patients with truncus arteriosus?

- **A.** Type I truncus
- **B.** Bicuspid truncal valve
- **C.** Interrupted aortic arch (IAA)
- **D.** ASD
- **E.** Left SVC

70. You are performing an echocardiogram on a cyanotic neonate. You note a large, thickened semilunar valve that is mildly incompetent and appears to originate from both RV and LV with a large outlet VSD. The pulmonary arteries originate separately from the ascending aorta. You also note interruption of the aortic arch. Which of the following is this baby most likely to have?

A. Bicuspid truncal valve
B. Right aortic arch
C. Absent ductus arteriosus
D. Absent left or right pulmonary artery
E. Chromosome 22q11 deletion

71. A cardiac catheterization is performed on an 18-month-old boy with unrepaired truncus arteriosus. He has a moderate-sized ASD with no ductus arteriosus. The data in Table 2.4 are obtained.

TABLE 2.4 Cardiac Catheterization Data

	Room Air		100% FiO₂	
	Pressure	SpO₂	Pressure	SpO₂
SVC	Mean 5	60	Mean 5	65
RA	Mean 4	68	Mean 4	70
RV	78/8	72	75/8	74
Truncus	85/52, mean 63	78	83/52, mean 62	89
RPA	83/49, mean 56	79	81/50, mean 58	87
LPA	82/50, mean 56	79	80/51, mean 58	87
RPCW	Mean 11	98	Mean 10	100
FA	90/51, mean 60	79	88/50, mean 60	87

SVC, superior vena cava; RA, right atrial; RV, right ventricular; RPA, right pulmonary artery; LPA, left pulmonary artery; RPCW, right pulmonary capillary wedge pressure; FA, femoral arterial.

If pulmonary blood flow is 5.0 L/min/m² on room air and 6.8 L/min/m² on 100% FiO₂, what course of treatment is recommended for this patient?

A. Home oxygen therapy with repair in 1 to 2 years
B. Pulmonary artery banding
C. Surgical repair now
D. Listing for heart–lung transplant
E. Home oxygen (palliation only)

72. You are seeing a new patient in clinic with a history of truncus arteriosus. On auscultation, you hear a split second heart sound at the left sternal border. What is the most likely cause of the splitting of S₂?

A. Referred tricuspid valve closure sound
B. Ejection click after truncal valve opening

C. Delayed closure of some of the cusps of the abnormal truncal valve
D. Increased flow across the mitral valve
E. Pulmonary artery ostial stenosis

73. Echocardiography of a newborn infant is performed. There is a large ventricular septal defect with an overriding semilunar valve. The pulmonary arteries are widely patent with laminar, increased flow and arise from a common trunk. The aortic arch is right-sided. There is a single semilunar valve that is large in diameter, quadricuspid, and has moderate-to-severe regurgitation. There are no other complicating factors. What is the best treatment plan for this newborn infant?

A. Perform bilateral BT shunts in the first week of life, then a bidirectional Glenn at 4 to 6 months, with Fontan completion at 2 years of life
B. Diuretics, digoxin, and afterload reduction for first 2 to 4 months if tolerated. Plan complete repair at 6 months (divide MPA from aorta, aortic valve repair, homograft conduit from RV to MPA)
C. Band the pulmonary arteries in the first 2 weeks of life, then manage medically until 4 to 6 months, when complete surgical repair can be more safely performed
D. Complete repair by 3 weeks of age consisting of VSD closure, division of main pulmonary trunk from the aorta, aortic valve repair, placement of homograft conduit from RV to main PA
E. Complete repair within the first 72 hours of life consisting of VSD closure, division of main pulmonary trunk from the aorta, place an aortic valve tissue prosthesis and homograft RV–MPA conduit

74. In the setting of asymmetric congenital mitral stenosis with unbalanced cord attachment, which of the following papillary muscle arrangements is the most common?

A. Absence of both papillary muscles
B. Absence of the anterolateral papillary muscle
C. Absence of the posteromedial papillary muscle
D. Presence of two separate papillary muscles
E. Presence of two fused papillary muscles

75. A 1-month-old infant presents with tachypnea and poor feeding. A cardiac murmur is heard and an echocardiogram is performed (Figure 2.7).

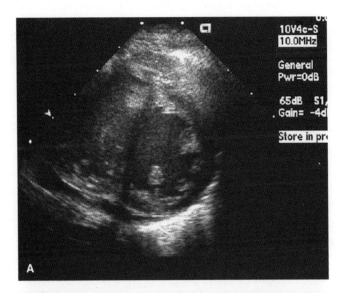

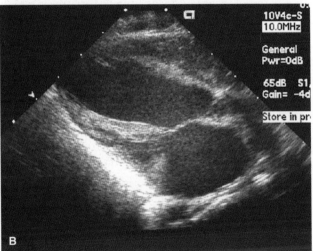

FIGURE 2.7

The echocardiogram also suggests moderate mitral inflow obstruction (mean gradient, 8 mm Hg), severe mitral regurgitation, and LA and LV enlargement. Which of the following is the most likely diagnosis?

A. Double orifice mitral valve
B. Mitral arcade
C. Supramitral ring
D. Parachute mitral valve
E. Cor triatriatum

76. A 4-year-old girl presents with tachypnea and heart failure and is found to have mitral stenosis. She undergoes a transatrial repair of her mitral valve. Attempts to extubate on postoperative day 2 are unsuccessful. Her examination is significant for a soft holosystolic murmur at the apex, a loud P2, and a liver edge palpable 3 cm below the costal

margin. An echocardiogram documents a mitral inflow mean gradient of 5 mm Hg and the pulmonary vein Doppler flow pattern in Figure 2.8.

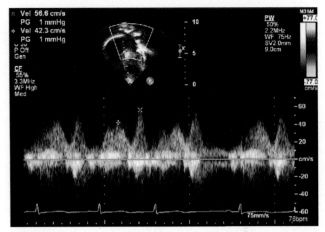

FIGURE 2.8

The RV is moderately dilated with moderately decreased systolic function, which is not significantly changed from her preoperative echocardiogram. Which of the following is the most likely cause for the patient's symptoms?

A. Pulmonary hypertension
B. Residual mitral stenosis
C. Unrecognized supramitral ring
D. Pulmonary vein stenosis
E. Right coronary infarction

77. Unlike the "cleft" in atrioventricular septal defects (AVSD), which of the following is true about the isolated cleft of the mitral valve?

A. It is more truly a commissure as there is typically a papillary muscle associated with it
B. It causes more significant mitral regurgitation
C. It is associated with both mitral stenosis and regurgitation
D. It is directed anteriorly towards the LVOT
E. It is not associated with ASD or VSD

78. A 4-month-old infant is found to have congenital mitral insufficiency without stenosis due to a cleft in the anterior leaflet. By echocardiography, the valve appears repairable. The left ventricular end-diastolic dimension (LVEDD) is at the upper limit of normal, and left ventricular function is normal. The left atrium has mild enlargement. CXR reveals a normal cardiac silhouette. ECG is normal for age. Vital signs are normal. What is the best next step in management?

A. Furosemide and captopril
B. Propranolol and verapamil
C. Propranolol and captopril
D. Surgical referral
E. No therapy at the present time

79. A 16-year-old girl presents for clearance to participate in competitive volleyball. She has a history of vasodepressor–vasovagal syncope following a stressful event at school 2 years prior. Evaluation at that time revealed a normal physical examination and normal ECG. Now, physical examination while supine reveals a systolic click shortly after S_1 at the apex. With sitting, you note that the click moves towards S_1 and is followed by a 1/6 systolic murmur at the apex that ends before systole concludes. These findings prompt an echocardiogram which reveals bileaflet mitral valve prolapse (MVP) with moderate mitral regurgitation, with a left ventricular EF of 53%. She then has a 24-hour ambulatory ECG monitor that shows frequent sustained SVT. Her resting blood pressure is 108/55 mm Hg. Along with her MVP, which of her findings would be an indication to restrict her from competitive volleyball?

   A. Degree of mitral regurgitation
   B. Left ventricular ejection fraction
   C. History of syncope
   D. Ambulatory ECG results
   E. Her blood pressure

80. An infant is diagnosed with critical aortic stenosis and resultant LV hypoplasia. According to the "Rhodes criteria" and other literature, which of the following echocardiographic criteria would indicate that the patient would benefit more from a Norwood-type palliation as opposed to a two-ventricle repair?

   A. LV long axis to heart long axis ratio of 0.9
   B. Aortic root diameter of 8 mm (4 cm/m²)
   C. Indexed mitral valve area of 8 mm (4 cm/m²)
   D. LV mass index of 10 g (50 g/m²)
   E. Antegrade flow in the ascending aorta

81. A 17-year-old girl immigrant presents with a 3-month history of progressive dyspnea on exertion. She had a childhood history of rheumatic fever, but she cannot remember the details of her underlying cardiac status except the painful IM antibiotic every month. On examination, she appears comfortable. Palpation reveals no thrill. Her S_1 and S_2 are normal. There is a grade 3/6 harsh systolic murmur audible along the mid-left sternal border radiating to the neck. There is no diastolic murmur or click. During auscultation, she has a few premature ventricular contractions. The systolic murmur becomes much louder in intensity following the extra beat. What is the most likely etiology of these physical examination findings?

   A. Tricuspid valve regurgitation
   B. Mitral regurgitation
   C. Pulmonary valve stenosis
   D. Subaortic stenosis
   E. Innocent murmur

82. Aortic balloon valvuloplasty is indicated in which of the following patients? All patients have bicuspid aortic valves, and all have undergone cardiac catheterization. "Peak-to-peak gradient" refers to the pressure gradient across the aortic valve.

   A. Asymptomatic 2-year-old boy with normal growth who has a peak-to-peak gradient of 45 mm Hg
   B. Asymptomatic 20-year-old woman who is planning to become pregnant and whose peak-to-peak gradient is 40 mm Hg
   C. Asymptomatic 18-year-old man who wants to play American football with a peak-to-peak gradient of 40 mm Hg
   D. A 1-day-old newborn who has an LV EF of 45% and a peak-to-peak gradient of 30 mm Hg
   E. Asymptomatic 20-year-old man with a normal ECG whose peak-to-peak gradient is 50 mm Hg

83. In assessing left ventricular myocardial function in patient with significant aortic valve stenosis, echocardiography with tissue Doppler imaging (TDI) is often used. Which of the following underlying assumptions is true in regards to the assessment of myocardial function by TDI?

   A. The echocardiographically derived ratio of early mitral inflow velocity (E) to early diastolic mitral annular velocity (E') correlates with catheter-derived LV end-diastolic pressure
   B. Measurement of mitral annular systolic velocity (S') by tissue Doppler imaging (TDI) demonstrates systolic short-axis dysfunction
   C. Longitudinally oriented fibers are present primarily in the subepicardial region
   D. The subendocardium is remarkably resilient to ischemia
   E. Transverse axis dysfunction typically precedes long-axis dysfunction

84. A 15-year-old boy with congenital aortic valve stenosis presents for interval follow-up. He underwent successful balloon dilatation at the age of 4 years with a reduction in Doppler peak instantaneous gradient from 87 mm Hg to 22 mm Hg. He has been followed up annually for the past 10 years without further intervention. Blood pressure is normal. By echocardiography, his peak gradient today is 42 mm Hg (mean 26 mm Hg). There is mild LV hypertrophy without mid-cavitary obstruction. He is interested in playing hockey for his high school team. Try-outs start in 8 weeks. He is asymptomatic. What is the best recommendation?

   A. Start low-dose lisinopril, then allow participation if blood pressure remains normal
   B. Balloon dilate the valve, then allow to play after 6 weeks
   C. Replace the valve with a homograft, then allow to play
   D. Replace the valve with a mechanical valve and prohibit participation
   E. Perform an exercise ECG and reassess

85. You are asked to consult on a term neonate with a cardiac murmur. He has a harsh grade 2–3/6 systolic ejection murmur consistent with left ventricular outflow tract (LVOT) obstruction. He has good distal pulses and perfusion with no increased work of breathing. Echocardiography reveals a thickened bicuspid aortic valve with a velocity across the valve of 3.0 m/s and a PDA. The left ventricle has good function with no endomyocardial fibroelastosis. Which of the following is true regarding LVOT obstruction?

A. Mild congenital subaortic stenosis, as a rule, rapidly progresses in the first few months of life

B. The amount of endomyocardial fibroelastosis (EFE) is independent of the degree of stenosis

C. Significant retrograde diastolic flow in the distal arch from the PDA is consistent with severe stenosis

D. Echo-derived pressure gradient is independent of other hemodynamic variables, such as preload and afterload

E. Relative to balloon valvuloplasty, open surgical valvotomy results in a greater degree of aortic regurgitation

The following stem applies to Questions 86 and 87.

A 10-day-old male infant presents to the emergency room with vomiting and respiratory distress. Pregnancy history was uncomplicated, and the infant was delivered at term. The patient was discharged from the hospital at day 2 of life. At day 4 of life, the patient began to have some difficulty with feeds. He was slow to feed due to fast breathing. No color changes were noted with feeds. His oral intake and urine output had been decreased over 24 hours before presentation.

Vital signs at the time of presentation are: HR, 169 beats per minute; RR, 70 breaths per minute; BP (right arm), 90/60 mm Hg; and BP (right leg), 70/30 mm Hg. On physical examination, there are no facial dysmorphic features. The skin is mottled and pale. There is a hyperactive RV impulse, normal S₁, single S₂ with S₃ gallop, and a soft systolic murmur at apex. Brachial pulses are normal, but femoral pulses are absent bilaterally. There are bilateral subcostal retractions. The liver is palpated 4 cm below the right costal margin. Extremities are cool.

ECG and CXR are obtained (Figure 2.9).

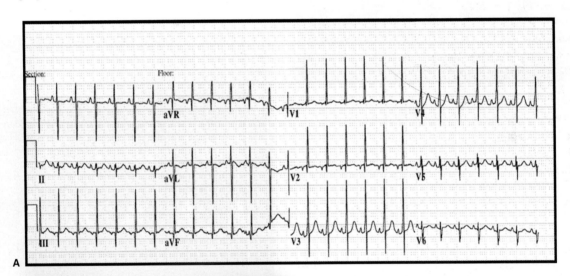

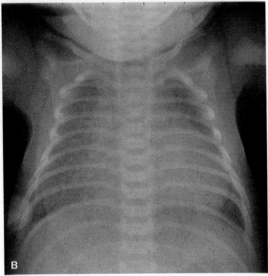

FIGURE 2.9

86. What would be the appropriate next step in management?

A. Perform an echocardiogram
B. IV access and give Lasix
C. IV access and start dobutamine
D. IV access and start PGE1
E. IV access and give sodium bicarbonate

87. While IV access is being obtained, emergent echocardiography is performed on the baby. Pulsed wave Doppler interrogation of the abdominal aorta is performed (Figure 2.10).

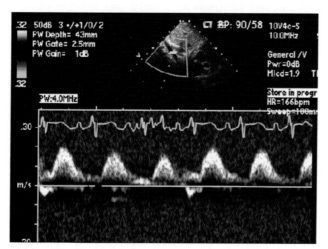

FIGURE 2.10

Which of the following statements is true?

A. The Doppler profile suggests that surgical correction is unlikely to be necessary before 12 months of age
B. A bicuspid aortic valve is unlikely to be associated with this defect
C. Severe aortic regurgitation is likely to be present
D. VSD is commonly associated with this defect
E. Secundum atrial septal defect is the defect responsible for this clinical presentation

88. A 1-year-old child is referred for a cardiac murmur. She is asymptomatic. Her blood pressure in the right arm is 104/56 mm Hg and in the left leg is 84/50 mm Hg. Echocardiogram confirms isolated coarctation of the aorta. When do you recommend the patient have surgical repair?

A. At Age 2 to 3 years
B. At Age 6 to 8 years
C. At Age 12 to 14 years
D. Only operate if systolic pressure gradient >50 mm Hg
E. Only operate if symptoms develop, such as lower-extremity claudication

The following clinical stem is used to answer Questions 89 to 91.

A 9-day-old female infant presents to the Emergency Department with respiratory distress. She is pale, irritable, and diaphoretic with RR, 80 breaths per minute; HR, 210 beats per minute; 4-extremity BP: right arm 48/32 mm Hg, left arm 68/34 mm Hg, right leg 47/31 mm Hg, left leg 48/31 mm Hg. Auscultation reveals a gallop rhythm. A grade 2–3/6 murmur is heard at the upper left sternal border, at the base, and in the left interscapular area posteriorly. The murmur is heard throughout systole and disappears in early diastole. Moderate hepatomegaly is noted. She has widely spaced nipples and a webbed neck. She undergoes an echocardiogram.

89. What is the echocardiogram most likely to reveal?

A. Mitral valve stenosis with moderate mitral regurgitation
B. Anomalous left coronary artery from the pulmonary artery
C. Isolated large outlet VSD with severe pulmonary valve stenosis
D. Isolated severe coarctation of the aorta
E. Coarctation of the aorta with anomalous aortic arch branching pattern

90. The above patient undergoes an echocardiogram following initiation of PGE₁. The pulsed wave Doppler profile in Figure 2.11 is obtained.

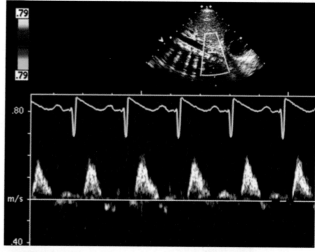

FIGURE 2.11

What is the most likely explanation for the tracing?

A. Aortic arch is normal
B. Ductus arteriosus is widely patent
C. Cardiac output is extremely low
D. Pulmonary hypertension is present
E. Thrombus is present in the descending aorta

91. The above patient undergoes genetic testing. What is the most likely result?

A. 45,XO genotype
B. *JAG1* gene mutation
C. *PTPN11* gene mutation
D. 46,XY/47,XYY mosaicism
E. *TBX5* gene mutation

92. A 12-year-old girl who is status post repair (end–end anastomosis) of coarctation of the aorta as a young child now complains of headaches with exercise. A neurologic work-up including an MRI/MRA of her neck and head are negative. She is noted to have exercise hypertension on a bicycle exercise test. Further cardiology evaluation with an echocardiogram reveals no significant anatomical obstruction of the aorta. Which intervention or next step in evaluation would be beneficial to help relieve her exercise hypertension?

A. Nothing, wait and watch
B. Heart catheterization with possible stent placement as needed
C. CT angiography to further evaluate aorta
D. β-Blocker pharmacotherapy
E. Nephrology consult

 93. A 5-day-old term infant is 2 days status post a Norwood procedure with an RV–PA shunt (Sano) for hypoplastic left heart syndrome. His chest is closed and he is mechanically ventilated. Over the past 6 hours, you have noticed worsening acidosis and increasing hepatic enzymes. Creatinine has increased from 0.4 to 0.8. Urine output has been adequate. His vital signs are: HR, 145 beats per minute; BP, 60/38 mm Hg; and RR, 24 breaths per minute (all ventilator-initiated). His saturation is 77% on 30% FiO$_2$; hemoglobin is 12 g/dL. Echocardiogram shows patent surgical connections with normal RV function. Which of the following interventions is most likely to improve this patient's clinical status?

A. Start milrinone
B. Increase inspired oxygen to 50%
C. Start nitric oxide
D. Transfuse 15 mL/kg packed RBCs
E. Increase ventilator rate to 30/min

94. A neonate is diagnosed with d-TGA with an anterior malalignment VSD and subaortic stenosis. Which of the following is most likely to be concurrently found in this patient?

A. Coarctation of the aorta
B. Peripheral pulmonary stenosis
C. Pulmonary atresia
D. Mitral arcade
E. Ebstein anomaly

95. Which of the following statements is correct regarding pathologic anatomy of complete d-TGA with an intact ventricular septum (IVS)?

A. There is complete resorption of subaortic conus
B. Ventricular septum is relatively sigmoid in shape rather than straight
C. Functional (dynamic) subpulmonic obstruction from bulging of ventricular septum into LVOT usually occurs immediately after birth

D. Sinus node and AV nodes are typically in their normal locations
E. LV mass usually regresses much faster in d-TGA with IVS compared with d-TGA with VSD

96. A neonate is found to have d-TGA with VSD and ASD. There is a small patent ductus arteriosus. The VSD is nonrestrictive, but there is severe LVOT obstruction. The patient's oxygen saturation is 68% on room air. What is the most appropriate initial surgery/procedure for this patient?

A. Jatene arterial switch with LeCompte maneuver
B. Mustard operation
C. BT shunt
D. LVOT balloon arterioplasty
E. PDA ligation

97. A 15-year-old boy presents with lightheadedness for the past 2 weeks. He has never fainted. On physical examination, he has a loud second heart sound, normal right parasternal impulse, and no cardiac murmurs. His ECG shows complete AV block, Q-waves in V1 and no Q waves in V6. What is the most likely explanation for his A-V dissociation?

A. Maternal systemic lupus erythematosus
B. Q-fever
C. Congenitally corrected transposition of the great arteries (l-TGA)
D. Recent tick bite
E. Myocarditis

98. Where is the AV node located in patients with congenitally corrected TGA?

A. Along the anterior aspect of the atrioventricular ring, near the atrial septum
B. Along the anterolateral aspect of the atrioventricular ring
C. Along the posterior aspect of the atrioventricular ring, near the coronary sinus
D. Along the posterior aspect of the atrioventricular ring, near the atrial septum
E. Along the posterior aspect of the atrioventricular ring, near the IVC

99. An echocardiogram is performed on a cyanotic newborn infant in the NICU. It reveals double-outlet right ventricle (DORV) with side-by-side great arteries, a large inlet VSD with mitral valve straddle, moderate subaortic stenosis, and severe coarctation of the aorta. What is the most appropriate initial surgery for this patient?

A. Patch VSD to aorta, repair coarctation
B. Repair coarctation, close VSD, and repair the mitral valve
C. Repair coarctation only
D. Norwood palliation with Sano shunt
E. Patch VSD to aorta, repair coarctation, resection of subaortic stenosis

100. What is the surgical procedure of choice for patients with DORV and a subpulmonary VSD without pulmonary stenosis?

A. Pulmonary artery banding
B. Arterial switch operation with patch closure of VSD
C. Systemic to pulmonary shunt
D. Patch closure of the VSD
E. VSD stenting

101. You are called to the emergency department to evaluate a 6-month-old infant with cyanosis. The infant is thin, frail, cyanotic, and breathing comfortably. You note oxygen saturations of 75% to 80% on room air, which do not change significantly with supplemental oxygen. His parents state that he has become gradually bluer over the past 4 months. On examination, you appreciate a gallop rhythm with a loud, harsh systolic ejection murmur. On the basis of this initial assessment, of the following diagnoses of double-outlet right ventricle (DORV), which is most likely?

A. DORV with subpulmonic VSD and no pulmonary stenosis
B. DORV with subpulmonic VSD and pulmonary stenosis
C. DORV with subaortic VSD and no pulmonary stenosis
D. DORV with subaortic VSD and pulmonary stenosis
E. DORV with subaortic VSD and suprasystemic pulmonary hypertension

The following clinical stem refers to Questions 102 and 103.

You are called to perform an echocardiogram on a 2-day-old neonate with cyanosis. The patient is mildly tachypneic with retractions. Pulse oximetry reveals oxygen saturation of 63% to 65%. Chest x-ray demonstrates normal heart size with increased pulmonary vascular markings. On examination, you appreciate a loud S$_2$ with no significant murmurs.

102. Which of the following is most likely?

A. DORV with subpulmonic VSD and no pulmonary stenosis
B. DORV with subpulmonic VSD and pulmonary stenosis
C. DORV with subaortic VSD and no pulmonary stenosis
D. DORV with subaortic VSD and pulmonary stenosis
E. DORV with subaortic VSD and suprasystemic pulmonary hypertension

103. An echocardiogram is performed and documents DORV Taussig–Bing type, with a nonrestrictive VSD, a large PDA with low-velocity bidirectional shunt, and a tiny PFO. The aortic arch appears mildly hypoplastic but

unobstructed. An IV is obtained and prostaglandin is started. The patient's clinical status does not improve. Which of the following interventions is likely to be of the most immediate benefit?

A. Increase the rate of PGE-1 infusion
B. Start nitric oxide
C. IV furosemide
D. Balloon atrial septostomy
E. Surgical repair in 2 to 3 weeks

104. A 3-year-old girl presents to your clinic with double-inlet left ventricle (DILV), left-sided hypoplastic subaortic right ventricle, V-A discordance, with a mildly restrictive bulboventricular-foramen-type VSD. She had a pulmonary band placed at 3 months of age and is now status post bidirectional Glenn anastomosis. She is being considered for Fontan palliation. Which of the following of her cardiac catheterization findings are associated with the highest mortality in patients with DILV undergoing Fontan?

A. PVR = 2.5 Wood units
B. Mild left AV-valve regurgitation
C. Patent left SVC
D. Resting subaortic gradient = 45 mm Hg
E. Mild right atrioventricular valve regurgitation

105. A 2-year-old child presents to your clinic for initial assessment after moving from another state. He was born with double-outlet right ventricle, multiple muscular VSDs, and normally related great arteries with no sub-aortic or sub-pulmonary stenosis. He had a prior intervention, but the parents do not recall the details. He is now found to have a resting peak subaortic gradient of 50 mm Hg by echocardiography. What prior intervention is most likely the cause of the subaortic gradient in the patient?

A. Pulmonary artery banding
B. Ligation of patent ductus arteriosus
C. Balloon atrial septostomy
D. Balloon dilation of left pulmonary artery stenosis
E. Device closure of atrial septal defect

106. A term neonate with a harsh systolic murmur at birth is found to have DILV with a hypoplastic subaortic RV, and a restrictive bulboventricular foramen and severe subaortic stenosis. A prostaglandin infusion is started. A subsequent echocardiogram documents a large PDA. Which of the following is the most appropriate initial operation for this child?

A. Enlargement of the VSD
B. Aortopulmonary anastomosis (DKS) with BT shunt
C. Pulmonary artery banding only
D. Bidirectional cavopulmonary anastomosis
E. Pulmonary artery banding with aortic arch augmentation

The following stem and angiograms apply to Questions 107 and 108.

You are performing a cardiac catheterization on a 2-year-old girl with heterotaxy syndrome with atrial and visceral situs ambiguus, asplenia, dextrocardia, complete AV septal defect, and DORV with left anterior aorta (Figure 2.12).

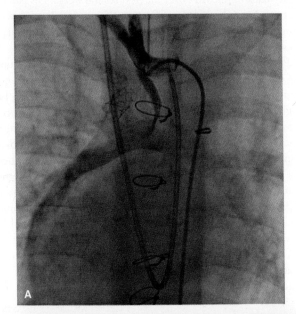

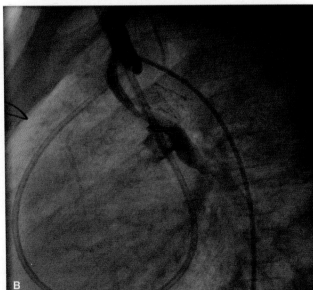

FIGURE 2.12

107. What is the course of the venous catheter?
  A. Right IJ → SVC → anomalous pulmonary vein → pleural space
  B. Right IJ → SVC → MPA → common ventricle → Aorta
  C. Right IJ → SVC → common atrium → common ventricle → MPA

D. Right IJ → SVC → common atrium → common ventricle → aorta
E. Right IJ → SVC → azygous vein → IVC → common atrium → left SVC

108. What is the course of the arterial catheter?
  A. Femoral artery → descending aorta → aortic arch → BT shunt
  B. Femoral artery → descending aorta → left SVC → MPA
  C. Femoral artery → descending aorta → Waterston shunt → MPA
  D. Femoral artery → descending aorta → Potts shunt → MPA
  E. Femoral artery → descending aorta → aortic arch → anomalous pulmonary vein

109. A 17-year-old boy has been experiencing chest pain for the past several months with exertion. One event occurred with syncope. His past medical history is negative. Physical examination revealed normal auscultation with a hyperactive impulse that is slightly displaced to the left. A chest radiograph revealed a slightly displaced cardiac silhouette to the left and prominent bulges of the aortic knob and pulmonary artery. Which diagnostic evaluation will most likely be helpful in confirming your clinical suspicion/etiology for his chest pain?

  A. Auscultation
  B. Chest x-ray
  C. Echocardiography
  D. Cardiac catheterization
  E. Magnetic resonance imaging

110. You are seeing a 14-year-old male patient for the first time. His mother died suddenly at the age of 39 and was found to have hypertrophic cardiomyopathy (HCM) on autopsy. Your patient had a negative echocardiogram performed at the age of 5 years due to a history of a murmur. His electrocardiogram is normal for his age. His current echocardiogram now reveals a maximal left ventricular wall thickness of 17 mm. When should the next echocardiogram and follow-up visit be performed?

  A. 6 months
  B. 1 year
  C. 3 years
  D. 5 years
  E. Only if symptoms arise

111. What is the known pattern of inheritance in HCM?
  A. Autosomal recessive
  B. X-linked recessive
  C. Autosomal dominant
  D. Sporadic
  E. X-linked dominant

112. A 17-year-old boy with a family history of sudden cardiac death collapsed while watching the finale of a singing competition on television. He stood up to get something from the refrigerator and fell without warning. His girlfriend performed successful CPR. He was brought to the Emergency Department and subsequently admitted to the PICU. A bedside echocardiogram revealed a 28-mm interventricular septal thickness with systolic anterior motion of the mitral valve. A maximal instantaneous Doppler gradient of 100 mm Hg was demonstrated across the left ventricular outflow tract. What is your recommendation regarding management?

A. Place ICD only
B. Surgical septal myectomy only
C. Perform surgical septal myectomy, then place ICD
D. Start nadolol only
E. Perform surgical septal myectomy, then start nadolol

113. Which of the following will increase the outflow murmur in a patient with obstructive HCM?

A. β-Blocker
B. Squatting
C. Isometric handgrip
D. Phenylephrine
E. Amyl nitrate inhalation

114. Regarding the risk of sudden death in individuals with HCM, which of the following statements is the most correct?

A. Most HCM-related sudden deaths occur during or just after vigorous exercise.
B. The strongest predictor of sudden death is degree of LVOT obstruction
C. A drop in blood pressure during exercise is associated with an increased risk of sudden death
D. Sudden death in patients with HCM is most often due to primary pulseless electrical activity
E. For patients at high risk of sudden death, septal myectomy is a valid alternative to ICD placement

115. A 14-year-old boy is found to have his family's genetic mutation for HCM. He has no symptoms attributable to his heart. His echocardiogram is normal. There is no family history of sudden death. According to the 36th Bethesda Conference, which of the following management strategies is most appropriate?

A. Prophylactic ICD placement
B. β-blocker therapy alone
C. β-blocker therapy and activity restriction
D. Activity restriction alone
E. No medical therapy or activity restriction

The following stem is used for the Questions 116 and 117.

A 4-year-old boy presents to the Emergency Department with fever, irritability, increased work of breathing, and poor feeding. Symptoms initially began 4 weeks before presentation while visiting family in southern Mexico, but they seemed to improve over the next several days. However, he never seemed to be "back to himself" over the next several weeks. His parents report a 2 to 3 day history of fever, vomiting, and diarrhea with progressive worsening of his condition in the hours prior to presentation.

Physical examination reveals an anxious, diaphoretic, grunting child. Vitals: Temperature (T), 39.2°C; RR, 64 breaths per minute and labored; P, 186 beats per minute; BP, 98/40 mm Hg (right arm); O$_2$ sat 93% on room air. Lung examination reveals accessory muscle use and wheezing. Cardiac examination reveals a downwards, laterally displaced apical impulse. S$_1$ is normal, S$_2$ is increased. An S$_3$ gallop rhythm is audible. There is a grade 2/6 holosystolic murmur over the left lower sternal border. His abdomen is distended. The liver edge is palpable 6 cm below the right costal margin. His extremities are somewhat cool. Capillary refill time is 4 to 5 seconds. Peripheral IV access is obtained. Laboratory results are pending.

Chest x-ray reveals cardiomegaly. Echocardiography demonstrates a severely dilated left atrium and a dilated, poorly functioning left ventricle.

116. What drug is most likely to be of initial benefit to this patient?

A. Nebulized albuterol
B. Epinephrine
C. High-dose dobutamine
D. Milrinone
E. Digoxin

117. A Spanish translator obtains further history. It turns out that the family saw a doctor in Mexico 3 weeks before presentation who started the boy on nadolol for suspected long QT syndrome. The patient took a dose 2 hours before arrival in the Emergency Department. Given this new information, what is the best therapy for the patient?

A. Nebulized albuterol
B. Dobutamine
C. Norepinephrine
D. Milrinone
E. Digoxin

118. A 10-month-old boy presents in severe respiratory distress with poor perfusion requiring admission to the pediatric ICU for mechanical ventilation and inotropic support. His history is remarkable for poor weight gain and hypotonia. He has been treated for the last 10 days with antibiotics and albuterol inhalers for a respiratory infection and reactive airway disease.

Oxygen saturation by pulse-oximetry is 88% on 60% FiO_2. His CXR shows severe cardiomegaly with diffuse pulmonary infiltrates consistent with pulmonary venous congestion. An arterial blood gas reveals the following: pH 7.28, $PaCO_2$ 48, PaO_2 55, HCO_3 15, base deficit −9. A complete blood count reveals the following: WBC 2.6 (4% neutrophils, 65% monocytes, 22% lymphocytes, 6% basophils, 3% eosinophils), Hgb 14, Hct 45, Platelets 220,000. This CBC is very similar to a CBC done 2 weeks ago when his illness started. His family history is significant for a maternal uncle and maternal great uncle who both died of heart disease in childhood. On general examination he is not dysmorphic. Which of the following laboratory test results would you expect to be present in this patient?

A. Decreased acid α-glucosidase activity in skin fibroblasts

B. Elevated mucopolysaccharides in urine

C. Elevated 3-methylglutaconic acid in urine

D. Mutation in fibrillin-1 (FBN-1)

E. SCN5A mutation

119. A cardiac catheterization is performed to differentiate between restrictive cardiomyopathy (RCM) and constrictive pericarditis (CP). Which hemodynamic parameters would be more consistent with RCM rather than CP?

A. Right atrial pressure (RAP) = pulmonary wedge pressure (PWP)

B. RV systolic pressure <50 mm Hg

C. Pulmonary wedge pressure 10 mm Hg higher than RV end-diastolic pressure

D. RVEDP = LVEDP

E. Normal PVR index

120. An 18-year-old previously healthy man presents with weight loss, intermittent fever, cough, and a systemic macular rash. He has progressively worsening shortness of breath. A chest x-ray reveals vascular congestion in the lung fields. Physical examination reveals a gallop rhythm, loud P2, and a palpable liver 5 cm below the costal margin. A CT scan shows evidence of prior splenic and hepatic infarcts. Serial blood work reveal normal Hgb, WBC, and platelet counts, but show a persistently elevated eosinophil count of >3,000 eosinophils/mm^3. Echocardiography is consistent with restrictive cardiomyopathy. Which of the following is the most appropriate initial outpatient treatment regimen for this patient?

A. Digoxin, Lasix, Coumadin, Aspirin

B. Digoxin, Enalapril, Aldactone

C. Digoxin, Lasix, Diuril, Enalapril, Coumadin

D. Digoxin, Lasix, Enalapril, Coumadin, Prednisone

E. Lasix, Enalapril, Coumadin, Methotrexate

121. According to the WHO classification of cardiomyopathies, which of the following findings precludes the diagnosis of restrictive cardiomyopathy?

A. Reduced RV diastolic volume

B. LV EF 50%

C. Normal LV wall thickness

D. Right atrial enlargement

E. Mildly increased LV end-diastolic volume

122. A 10-year-old boy with Duchenne muscular dystrophy is undergoing an orthopedic surgical procedure for which he will be placed under general anesthesia. Which medication should be avoided during the procedure?

A. Fentanyl

B. Succinylcholine

C. Midazolam

D. Milrinone

E. Vecuronium

123. A 4-year-old boy is noted, during a primary care evaluation, to have gross motor delay. He is suspected to have Duchenne muscular dystrophy and gene testing is pending. He was referred for cardiac evaluation. What characteristic ECG findings would you most likely expect?

A. Ventricular premature contractions

B. Q waves in leads II, V1, V2, and V3

C. Atrial premature contractions

D. First-degree AV block

E. Q waves in leads I, aVL, V5, and V6

124. You are seeing a 4-year-old boy with a waddling gait and calf pseudohypertrophy. What type of murmur do you expect to hear on cardiac examination?

A. Systolic ejection murmur with a click

B. No murmur

C. Continuous murmur

D. Diastolic murmur

E. High-pitched holosystolic murmur

125. Which of the following is the most commonly reported arrhythmia among children with restrictive cardiomyopathy?

A. Atrial fibrillation

B. Atrial flutter

C. Wolff–Parkinson–White syndrome

D. Second-degree AV block, type II

E. Symptomatic sinus bradycardia

ANSWERS

1. (D) This clinical scenario is most consistent with a diagnosis of Alagille syndrome. Alagille syndrome is an autosomal dominant disorder associated with liver disease secondary to bile duct paucity, cholestasis, congenital heart disease, skeletal or ocular abnormalities, or typical facial features. Mutations in the Notch ligand, *JAG1*, are responsible for the clinical phenotype. Alagille syndrome is characterized by right-sided heart disease including peripheral pulmonary stenosis (diffuse hypoplasia of the pulmonary arterial bed as well as discrete stenosis), pulmonary valve stenosis, and tetralogy of Fallot (TOF). Left-sided lesions and septal defects have also been reported.

NOTCH1 mutations result in aortic valve pathology but not the other findings given here. *PTPN11* mutations result in Noonan syndrome (characterized by hypertelorism, ptosis, short stature, and CHD, most commonly pulmonary valve stenosis and HCM). Additional cardiac manifestations include secundum-type atrial septal defect, VSD, TOF, pulmonary artery stenosis, coarctation of the aorta, partial AVSD (primum-type atrial septal defect), and polyvalvulopathy. Other noncardiac anomalies of Noonan syndrome include webbed neck, skeletal anomalies, bleeding diathesis, lymphatic disorders, mental retardation, and cryptorchidism. *TBX1* is a gene that resides in the area of chromosome 22q11; mutations of *TBX1* lead to features of DiGeorge syndrome (hypocalcemia, immunodeficiency, and severe CHD, most commonly interruption of the aortic arch [IAA] type B, truncus arteriosus, or Tetralogy of Fallot). *GATA4* mutations appear to be involved in septation defects but are not associated with a classic syndrome as described in the vignette.

2. (E) Heart defects in congenital rubella syndrome include pulmonic stenosis (valvar, supravalvar, or peripheral) and patent ductus arteriosus. Tetralogy of Fallot has also been reported.

3. (E) Caffeine intake during pregnancy has not been shown to result in an increased risk of congenital heart disease in the fetus.

4. (C) Women with maternal phenylketonuria who have high levels of phenylalanine when pregnant have a high likelihood of having children with microcephaly and mental retardation. There is an increased risk for left-sided defects, septal defects, and Tetralogy of Fallot.

5. (D) This vignette describes Williams syndrome, which is characterized in part by CHD, hypercalcemia in infancy, skeletal and renal anomalies, cognitive deficits, social personality, and so-called "elfin facies." Approximately 90% of patients with the clinical diagnosis of Williams syndrome have a deletion at chromosome 7q11.23, which is not generally apparent on a routine karyotype but can be detected by FISH. Approximately 55% to 80% of patients with Williams syndrome have CHD, which typically include supravalvar aortic stenosis and/or supravalvar pulmonary stenosis. Therefore, a click may not be present despite a murmur and significant gradient across the involved outflow tract.

18q deletion is associated with ASD, VSD, and pulmonary stenosis and is associated with cleft palate and GU anomalies. Tetrasomy 22p is known as "cat eye syndrome" and is associated with rectoanal anomalies, coloboma, genitourinary anomalies, and preauricular pits/tags. Deletion of 8p23 is associated with septal defects, GU anomalies, abnormally formed ears, and minor hand anomalies. Chromosome 22q11 deletion is known as DiGeorge syndrome or velocardiofacial syndrome and is characterized by hypocalcemia, immunodeficiency, and severe CHD, most commonly IAA type B, truncus arteriosus, or TOF.

6. (C) Approximately 55% to 80% of patients with Williams syndrome have congenital heart disease, which typically include supravalvar aortic stenosis and/or supravalvar pulmonary stenosis. The degree of cardiovascular involvement varies widely. Supravalvar pulmonary stenosis tends to improve with time, while supravalvar aortic stenosis usually progresses. Sudden death has been described in Williams syndrome. Suspected etiologic factors include coronary artery stenosis and severe biventricular outflow tract obstruction. Presumably, sudden cardiac death results from myocardial ischemia, decreased cardiac output, or arrhythmias. Patients with Williams syndrome are prone to develop hypertension because of renal artery stenosis.

7. (C) This scenario describes trisomy 18. The distinctive phenotype of trisomy 18 includes growth retardation, short palpebral fissures, small mouth, and micrognathia. Specific features include a prominent occiput, short sternum, small nipples, clenched hands, disorganized or hypoplastic palmar creases, hyperconvex nails, and "rocker bottom feet." Congenital heart disease is the rule (>90% incidence). Most common associated defects include perimembranous VSD, TOF, DORV, and polyvalvular dysplasia. Approximately 90% of affected individuals die in the first year of life and usually not of their heart disease.

8. (C) The most common CHD associated with a 22q11 deletion include Tetralogy of Fallot, Interrupted Aortic Arch type B, truncus arteriosus, perimembranous VSD, and aortic arch anomalies. A wide range of CHD has been reported in patients with a 22q11 deletion, including pulmonary valve stenosis, atrial septal defect, heterotaxy syndrome, and hypoplastic left heart syndrome.

9. (E) This clinical scenario describes pulmonary hypertension resulting from a large unrepaired atrial septal defect. Although rare, severe irreversible hypertensive pulmonary vascular disease can develop from unrepaired ASDs. There is a female preponderance for this association. Spontaneous closure is rare for defects >8 mm in size. Although severe mitral regurgitation, nonsustained VT, and LV diastolic dysfunction can contribute to dyspnea on exertion, they are not the primary cause as indicated by this scenario.

10. (D) In general, cardiac catheterization is unnecessary for the diagnosis of sinus venosus ASD. Occasionally, however, questions about pulmonary vascular obstructive disease or associated cardiac defects arise that require catheterization. In this case, it is important to assess the presence and degree of pulmonary vascular vasoreactivity to determine appropriate treatment. It would be premature to start therapy without a thorough understanding of the pulmonary artery pressures and reactivity.

11. (B) Sinus venosus ASD accounts for 5% to 10% of ASDs and is located posterior and superior to the fossa ovalis. The sinus venosus defect commonly is associated with anomalous connection of the right pulmonary veins to either the right atrium or the superior vena cava near the caval–atrial junction. Electrocardiogram shows that about half of patients have a frontal plane P-wave axis of <30 degrees. The other types of atrial septal defects are associated with normal P-wave axes.

12. (A) The complete form of AVSD is characterized by a large septal defect with interatrial and interventricular components and a common atrioventricular valve that spans the entire septal defect. The septal defect extends to the level of the membranous ventricular septum, which is usually deficient or absent.

The common atrioventricular valve has five leaflets. Beneath the five commissures are five papillary muscles. The two left-sided papillary muscles are oriented closer together than in a normal heart, and the lateral leaflet is smaller than usual. In addition, the two papillary muscles are often rotated counterclockwise, thus positioning the posterior muscle farther from the septum than normal and the anterior muscle closer to the septum. This papillary muscle arrangement, along with a large anterolateral muscle bundle, can contribute to progressive LVOT obstruction.

13. (A) In partial AVSD, the mitral and tricuspid annuli are separate. Partial AVSD consists of a primum ASD and a "cleft" anterior mitral valve leaflet. Although patients with partial AVSD may be asymptomatic until adulthood, symptoms of excess pulmonary blood flow typically occur in childhood. Tachypnea and poor weight gain occur most commonly when the defect is associated with moderate or severe mitral valve regurgitation or with other hemodynamically significant cardiac anomalies. Patients with a primum ASD usually have earlier and more severe symptoms, including growth failure, than patients with a secundum ASD. Repair of residual/recurrent mitral valve regurgitation or stenosis is the most common reason for reoperation.

In this clinical scenario, surgical correction was required early, suggesting a hemodynamically significant cleft mitral valve. This patient presents with progressive shortness of breath. Physical examination and chest x-ray findings suggest mitral valve regurgitation. Mitral stenosis may also be involved, but the murmur on examination suggests regurgitation is significant. The patient may indeed have pulmonary hypertension, but it would be secondary rather than primary in origin. LVOT obstruction is an important consideration for all forms of AVSD, and it is usually progressive. However, it would be characterized by a systolic ejection-type murmur. Pulmonic stenosis also would have an ejection murmur but would be heard best over the left upper sternal border.

14. (C) In the normal heart, the aortic valve is wedged between the mitral and the tricuspid annuli. In AVSD the aortic valve is displaced or "sprung" anteriorly. This anterior displacement creates an elongated, so-called gooseneck deformity of the LVOT. LVOT obstruction may occur in all forms of AVSD. It is more frequent when two atrioventricular valve orifices are present than when there is a common orifice. Ten percent of patients with AVSD may require reoperation to relieve LVOT obstruction (while the most common indication for reoperation is left AV valve regurgitation or stenosis). Progressive LVOT obstruction is more common in partial than in complete AVSD. Mechanisms of LVOT obstruction include attachments of superior bridging leaflet to ventricular septum, extension of the anterolateral papillary muscle into the LVOT, discrete fibrous subaortic stenosis, tissue from an aneurysm of the membranous septum bowing into the LVOT. Obstruction may develop *de novo* after initial repair of the AVSD and closure of the mitral valve cleft.

15. (D) Right bundle branch block is common and may be due to ventriculotomy or direct injury to the right bundle itself. However, right bundle branch block occurs after a transatrial repair as well. Of the other options, a residual ASD would likely not be the cause of a newly split S_2, a residual VSD would be accompanied by a murmur. Ventilation changes would not result in a newly split S_2.

16. (C) The valve closure sounds in patients with a small VSD are usually normal. Some patients, however, have wide splitting of the second sound. If there is associated pulmonary stenosis or mitral insufficiency in a patient with VSD, these lesions may be suspected when the systolic murmur is transmitted to the upper left sternal border or apex, respectively. Flow across a large (unrestrictive) VSD is limited primarily by relative resistances of the systemic and pulmonary circulations.

Minor anomalies of the tricuspid valve may be acquired secondary to left-to-right shunting across perimembranous defects. These anomalies include redundant septal leaflet tissue that can partially or completely occlude the defect. After VSD repair, the LV mass and volume decrease, but volume decreases at a much greater rate than mass. Finally, patients who develop Eisenmenger physiology typically begin manifesting cyanosis before 2 years of age.

17. (B) Prolapse of one of the aortic valve cusps may occur with outlet or perimembranous VSDs. Patients with outlet defects usually have deficiency of muscular or fibrous support below the aortic valve with herniation of the right coronary leaflet through the VSD. The aortic commissures themselves are usually normal. In contrast, patients with perimembranous VSDs and aortic insufficiency have herniation of the right or much less commonly the noncoronary cusp, have frequent abnormalities of aortic commissures (usually the right/noncoronary), and may have associated infundibular pulmonary stenosis. Echocardiography and angiography can show that the prolapsed aortic leaflet partially closes a moderate to large VSD and limits the left-to-right shunt. The associated aortic valve insufficiency is progressive.

The murmur of an incompetent tricuspid valve or mitral valve would be systolic. The patient is asymptomatic and acyanotic; hence, Eisenmenger physiology is not present. Therefore, RV and LV pressures have not equalized.

18. (B) The relationship of the atrioventricular conduction pathways to VSDs is important to surgical repair. In perimembranous defects, the bundle of His lies in a subendocardial position as it courses along the posterior-inferior margin of the defect. In inlet defects, the bundle of His passes anterosuperiorly to the defect. In muscular VSDs and outlet defects, there is little danger of heart block because the conduction tissue generally is far removed unless these defects extend into the perimembranous area.

19. (A) When signs of necrotizing enterocolitis develop in an infant with significant left-to-right shunting through a PDA, early surgical closure of the ductus arteriosus has significantly reduced mortality. Therefore, if abdominal distention is persistent, increasing residuals before feedings, blood in the stools or gastric aspirate, decreasing bowel sounds, and, particularly, intramural air occur in association with a significant left-to-right shunt through a PDA, immediate surgical closure is recommended.

20. (A) This vignette describes a child with a hemodynamically significant PDA that has gone unrepaired and is now infected. Bacterial endarteritis or endocarditis is uncommon in developed countries, although it remains a serious complication of PDA in undeveloped countries. In such countries, PDA accounts for up to 15% of all endocarditis cases. *Streptococcus viridans* and *Staphylococcus aureus* are the most common organisms. Vegetations are almost always seen on the pulmonary artery end of the duct.

21. (B) Postnatal closure of the ductus arteriosus occurs in two phases. The first phase, "functional closure," occurs within 12 hours after birth. There is contraction and cellular migration of the medial smooth muscle in the wall of the ductus arteriosus that causes the vessel walls to become thick and protrude into the vessel lumen. The second stage is usually completed by 2 to 3 weeks and results from infolding of the endothelium, disruption, and fragmentation of the internal elastic lamina, proliferation of the subintimal layers, and hemorrhage and necrosis in the subintimal region. There is connective tissue formation and replacement of muscle fibers with fibrosis with subsequent permanent sealing of the lumen, thus forming the *ligamentum arteriosum.*

22. (E) Ibuprofen has been evaluated as a possible alternative to indomethacin in preterm infants. Studies have shown a similar rate of ductal closure after ibuprofen treatment with fewer negative effects on renal function, cerebral vasculature, and cerebral blood flow than indomethacin. The risk of intraventricular hemorrhage is equivocal. Of note, using ibuprofen for prophylaxis is associated with increased risk of pulmonary hypertension.

23. (A) Surgical correction of ALCAPA involves direct reimplantation of the origin of the left coronary artery into the aorta and is considered the standard corrective surgical approach in many centers. An alternative approach is the Takeuchi procedure, in which an aortopulmonary window is created and then a tunnel fashioned that directs blood from the aorta to the left coronary ostium.

Because of papillary muscle infarction and dysfunction, significant preoperative mitral insufficiency has been found to be a risk factor for both mortality and need for late mitral valve surgery.

24. (A) A localized weakness of the wall of a sinus of Valsalva leads to aneurysmal bulging. If the aneurysm ruptures, the size of the fistula determines how large the shunt will be, and its site of entry into the heart often determines the specific features. Thus, aneurysmal rupture into the left heart does not produce signs of a left-to-right shunt, whereas rupture into the right heart produces a left-to-right shunt. With a small fistula, there may be only a continuous murmur with its maximal intensity in the third or fourth intercostal space near the sternal edge. If the fistula enters the right atrium, the murmur may be maximal to the right of the sternum. With larger fistulas, there will be a wide pulse pressure, a collapsing pulse, and left ventricular hyperactivity. If the fistula enters

the right side, there will be right ventricular hyperactivity as well. A large fistulae entering the left ventricle may display a to-and-fro murmur and simulate aortic incompetence. Occasionally, there is only a diastolic murmur in fistulae entering the left ventricle or the high-pressure right ventricle in a neonate.

25. (C) In this anomaly, the left coronary artery arises from the pulmonary artery, usually from the left posterior facing sinus. In fetal life, pressures and oxygen saturations are similar in the aorta and pulmonary artery, so myocardial perfusion is normal. After birth, the pulmonary arteries have low pressures and desaturated blood, which does not bode well for myocardial perfusion. Myocardial ischemia subsequently occurs. Ischemia is worsened with exertion such as feeding or crying. As time passes, infarction of the anterolateral LV free wall occurs. The mitral valve papillary muscles are affected, and mitral regurgitation develops.

Anomalous coronary artery origins from the wrong sinus of Valsalva are generally asymptomatic in infancy. The most common anomaly (a third of all major coronary arterial anomalies) is origin of the left circumflex from the right main coronary artery. This anomaly has no general clinical significance in the absence of intracardiac surgery.

The origin of the left main coronary artery from the right sinus of Valsalva is less common but more important clinically. If the anomalous vessel passes between the aorta and the RVOT, the child is at risk for sudden death during or just after vigorous exercise. In many of these cases, the ostium of the left main coronary artery is slit-like, increasing the risk further.

26. (C) A localized weakness of the wall of a sinus of Valsalva leads to aneurysmal bulging. Localized aneurysms are usually congenital, with thinning just above the annulus at the leaflet hinge. However, aneurysms can follow infective endocarditis. Approximately 75% of patients are male. Approximately 65% of aneurysms are located in the right aortic sinus, 25% in the noncoronary sinus, and 10% in the left aortic sinus. Up to 50% of cases may be associated with VSDs, especially right sinus aneurysms associated with defects of the outlet septum. Aneurysms can rupture into any cardiac chamber. Rupture is most often of the right sinus aneurysm into the right ventricle in the setting of an outlet VSD. Rupture into the pericardium is rare.

27. (E) Central nervous system AVMs manifest symptoms according to their hemodynamic effects. Infants presenting with CHF typically have large AVMs. The most common cerebral AVMs presenting with CHF are located deep (vein of Galen), superficial (pial), or dural. Affected infants have high-output CHF with dilation of all cardiac chambers, feeding arteries, and draining veins. If there is venous obstruction, flow can be restricted through the AVM, so patients may present with venous hypertension or cerebral ischemia.

The prognosis for most patients with large cerebral arterial malformations is grave. If untreated, most newborns (90%) die during the first week of life from intractable CHF or neurologic complications (seizures, intracranial hemorrhage). Those who do survive the neonatal period often suffer profound neurologic morbidity (hydrocephalus, mental retardation, hemorrhage).

28. (C) Most pulmonary AVMs are congenital or associated with HHT. Pulmonary AVMs enlarge as the child grows older. A high proportion (>85%) of patients with multiple pulmonary AVMs have HHT. Overall, 30% to 50% of patients with pulmonary AVMs have HHT.

Patients with pulmonary AVMs generally are hemodynamically stable. In contrast to systemic AVMs, cardiac output is not increased, while pulmonary blood flow and pressures are unchanged. Of note, during cardiac catheterization, the total PVR is normal. That is, resistance within the AVM is low, whereas the resistance in the other lung segments may be elevated.

29. (B) Transcatheter embolization has become the treatment of choice for pulmonary AVMs. Embolization provides persistent relief of hypoxemia, resolution of orthodeoxia, and minimal growth of small remaining AVMs. The embolization procedure is effective for preventing stroke and transient ischemic attacks but does not appear to reduce the risk of brain abscess.

To avoid device embolization (through the AVM to the systemic circulation), transcatheter occlusion of the afferent artery or fistula is usually accomplished using a coil or umbrella rather than liquid adhesive or beads. The goal is to raise the systemic arterial oxygen tension (some authors suggest to 60 mm Hg) by occluding the most significant afferent arteries (generally considered those to be >3 mm in diameter).

30. (C) Large AVMs and large patent ductus arteriosus have similar hemodynamic effects (large extracardiac left-to-right shunts) and thus are indistinguishable in terms of pulse pressure, liver span, cardiothoracic ratio on chest x-ray, and QRS axis on ECG. Diagnostic cardiac catheterization is usually unnecessary, as the diagnosis is suspected by clinical examination and confirmed by noninvasive imaging. When performed, catheterization demonstrates high cardiac output, elevated atrial and ventricular end-diastolic pressures, a widened systemic arterial pulse pressure, and a large difference in the oxygen saturation between the superior and inferior vena cava (higher saturation from the involved area).

31. (B) A barium esophagram which shows an anterior indentation is virtually pathognomonic for a pulmonary artery sling or a tumor. Origin of the left pulmonary artery from the right pulmonary artery, known as a pulmonary artery sling, is a rare anomaly in which the lower trachea is partially surrounded by vascular structures. The left pulmonary artery arises as a very proximal branch of the right and then loops around the trachea. It is the only situation in which a major vascular structure passes between the trachea and esophagus.

Pulmonary sling is frequently associated with complete cartilaginous rings in the distal trachea resulting in tracheal stenosis. It usually appears as an isolated abnormality but can be associated with other congenital cardiac defects, including tetralogy of Fallot.

32. (B) Right aortic arch with mirror image branching describes an aortic arch that traverses the right mainstem bronchus. The first branch is a left innominate artery that divides into left carotid and left subclavian arteries. The second branch is the right carotid, and the third is the right subclavian. The ductus arteriosus (or ligamentum arteriosum) is usually on the left side and arises from the base of the innominate artery. This lesion typically does not form a vascular ring. However, this arch anomaly is frequently associated with congenital intracardiac disease. The most common association is with TOF, but other conotruncal anomalies may also be seen, as well as DORV. Therefore, an echocardiogram

should be considered in this patient to evaluate the intracardiac anatomy.

The patient is asymptomatic at this time, so further work-up for a vascular ring (such as swallowing study or bronchoscopy) is not necessary.

33. (A) A vascular ring is an aortic arch anomaly in which the trachea and esophagus are completely surrounded by vascular structures. The clinical picture typically includes respiratory symptoms, especially stridor. Pneumonia, bronchitis, or cough may also be present. Infants may demonstrate a posture of hyperextension of the neck. A common history is that of a 1- to 3-month-old with "noisy breathing since birth" who develops more significant respiratory distress in association with an intercurrent upper respiratory infection. Less commonly (and usually in toddlers or older children), the presentation will be swallowing difficulty. Of the listed options, only a right aortic arch with retroesophageal innominate artery and a left PDA complete the ring.

34. (D) Interrupted aortic arch (IAA) is defined as a complete separation of ascending and descending aorta. Celoria and Patton classified IAA into three types: type A if the interruption was distal to the left subclavian artery, type B if between carotid and subclavian arteries, and type C if between carotid arteries. These patients typically present with acute cardiovascular collapse or heart failure after spontaneous closure of the ductus arteriosus in the first days of life.

Absence of all limb pulses suggests a type B interruption with an anomalous subclavian artery. In this situation, both carotid arteries are proximal to the interruption, while both subclavians are distal to the interruption. Strong carotid pulses help to differentiate interrupted arch from critical aortic stenosis in which all pulses are diminished.

35. (A) Right arch with diverticulum of Kommerell is the second most common vascular ring after double aortic arch.

In right aortic arch with mirror image branching, there usually is no left-sided ductus arteriosus or ligamentum arteriosum and thus no vascular ring. Left aortic arch with retroesophageal right subclavian artery is the most common aortic arch anomaly, but does not form a ring and is usually asymptomatic. Right aortic arch with retroesophageal innominate artery is a very rare abnormality of the aortic arch system. The ductus arteriosus (or ligamentum arteriosum) completes a vascular ring as it connects the left pulmonary artery with the base of the innominate artery. However, it is much less common than right arch with retroesophageal diverticulum of Kommerell.

36. (C) In classic cor triatriatum, a membrane separates the more proximal chamber, which receives the pulmonary veins, from the more distal left atrium, which communicates with the mitral valve. To allow for cardiac output, typically there is a hole in the membrane that ranges from <3 mm to about 1 cm. The distal, true left atrium is in continuity with the left atrial appendage. The fossa ovalis usually is located between the distal left atrial chamber and the right atrium; occasionally, a patent foramen ovale/ASD is present in this area. Right ventricular hypertrophy and dilation are almost invariably found. Right atrial hypertrophy and dilation are present in <25% of cases. Hypertrophy and dilation of the right atrium results in tall, broad, oftentimes peaked P waves on ECG.

The prognosis in TAPVC is influenced by the size of the interatrial communication and by the degree of obstruction in anomalous venous pathways. Overall mortality for unrepaired TAPVC is 80% or more at 1 year. Long-term prognosis depends on the state of the pulmonary vascular bed at the time of surgery as well as the patency of the pulmonary venous–left atrial anastomosis. Late arrhythmias may develop in a small number of these patients. Atrial arrhythmias are most common and include sinus bradycardia, atrial flutter, and supraventricular tachycardia. Ventricular rhythm problems are unusual.

Scimitar syndrome describes the chest x-ray findings present in anomalous connection of the right pulmonary veins to the IVC. There is a crescent-like shadow in the right lower lung field; the shape of the shadow resembles a Turkish sword, or scimitar. Frequent coexistent anomalies include hypoplasia of the right lung and chest, mesocardia or dextrocardia, and lung parenchymal abnormalities.

37. (E) A superior sinus venosus defect (also called SVC type) results from deficiency of the common wall between the SVC and the right upper pulmonary vein (RUPV). This defect "unroofs" the RUPV. The unroofed pulmonary vein then drains into the SVC, while its left atrial orifice becomes the interatrial communication. This interatrial communication is not a defect of the atrial septum.

38. (E) The correct catheter course is IVC → right atrium → SVC → innominate vein → vertical vein → anomalous pulmonary venous confluence.

39. (E) In infradiaphragmatic TAPVC, the most common site of obstruction is at the anomalous vessels' connection with the portal vein or the hepatic veins. By 2D echo, there frequently is seen a dilated venous channel proximal to the site of stenosis. If unobstructed, the anomalous vessel is characterized by a low-velocity, phasic laminar flow pattern with brief flow reversal during atrial systole. Luminal narrowing is associated with flow acceleration and turbulence by color Doppler.

Corrective surgery for the infant or child with TAPVC should be performed as soon as possible. In the sickest infants, the patient's clinical condition should be optimized, including the cardiorespiratory and metabolic states. When possible, surgery should be done on the basis of echocardiography rather than cardiac catheterization in an effort to lessen the time to operation and therefore reduce mortality.

Balloon atrial septostomy and blade atrial septostomy have been used in the past as palliative procedures. Septostomy delays the definitive procedure and is of little value when an anomalous venous channel is obstructed. Balloon dilation of obstructed anomalous venous channels is usually unsuccessful.

40. (D) The echocardiogram image demonstrates cor triatriatum. Most patients with classic cor triatriatum have onset of symptoms within the first few years of life. However, some patients present in the second or third decade of life. Frequently, these patients will present with a history of dyspnea, frequent respiratory issues including "asthma," and pneumonia. They often are considered to have primary pulmonary disease.

Untreated cor triatriatum results in pulmonary hypertension. Physical examination findings include a loud pulmonary component of the second heart sound, right ventricular heave, and pulmonary systolic ejection click. A murmur of tricuspid regurgitation

may be present. Less often, a diastolic murmur is detected at the mitral area, or a continuous murmur may be heard. Right-sided heart failure is common. Pulmonary rales are heard if pulmonary edema is present.

In the patient with pulmonary edema or right heart failure, the disease frequently is progressive despite maximal medical management. Surgical intervention should be planned as soon as possible. Surgical resection of the cor triatriatum membrane under cardiopulmonary bypass is the effective treatment of choice. When pulmonary edema and right heart failure occur, survival is usually only a matter of months. However, in patients who survive operative correction, the severe pulmonary arterial changes that result in pulmonary hypertension can regress. In these patients, the prognosis seems excellent.

41. (C) Other than partial anomalous pulmonary venous connection (PAPVC) to the right SVC and to the right atrium (sinus venosus defect and malposition of the septum primum, respectively), the most common type of PAPVC is of the left pulmonary veins to the left innominate vein (LIV). The left-sided pulmonary vein(s) connect(s) to the LIV through a persistent early embryonic pathway. The connecting vein (often called a "vertical vein") between the left pulmonary veins and the LIV may incorrectly be termed a persistent left superior vena cava (LSVC). This term is incorrect both embryologically and anatomically.

Embryologically, the vertical vein represents a persistent early embryonic connection between the splanchnic plexus of the lung buds and the cardinal veins. Anatomically, it is positioned more posteriorly than the LSVC, which is located immediately behind the left atrial appendage. An LSVC usually connects with the coronary sinus, although it may connect with the left atrium when the coronary sinus is unroofed. When a left pulmonary vein drains into the LSVC, the LSVC should still connect with the coronary sinus or with the left atrium.

A secundum atrial septal defect is commonly associated with PAPVC to the LIV. A primum atrial septal defect is very uncommon. Rarely, the atrial septum is intact.

42. (D) Absence of the hepatic segment of the IVC with azygous continuation into the right or left SVC is referred to as an interrupted IVC. Pulmonary AVMs have been known to develop after a classic or bidirectional Glenn anastomosis owing to the exclusion of hepatic venous blood or "hepatic factor" to the lungs. This malformation can develop in one or both lungs if preferential blood flow is present. In the case described in this vignette, there is likely inadequate hepatic venous blood flow to the pulmonary arteries.

43. (B) Congenital malformations of the coronary sinus are frequently associated with arrhythmias. SVT and sudden cardiac death have been reported in a significant percentage of patients with diverticula of the coronary sinus. Patients with diverticula of the coronary sinus usually present with SVT associated with accessory pathways that transverse the diverticulum to form an atrioventricular connection.

44. (D) This patient is a set-up for inadequate systemic blood flow, given his tricuspid valve atresia and transposition of the great arteries with a restrictive VSD. He has evidence of systemic underperfusion with acidosis. He requires a stable source of systemic blood flow. Of the given options, only a DKS procedure results in a stable systemic circulation.

45. (E) Uhl anomaly is a congenital cardiac malformation consisting of an almost total absence of the RV myocardium. Cyanosis and hepatomegaly are often present, as is jugular venous distension. The precordium usually is quiet, and peripheral pulses are diminished. The heart tones are decreased. A pansystolic murmur of tricuspid insufficiency may be present, but patients may have no murmurs or other nonspecific murmurs present.

ECG usually shows prominent P waves and diminished QRS amplitude, especially in the right precordial leads. The chest x-ray demonstrates cardiomegaly with normal to diminished pulmonary vascularity (which can appear similar to Ebstein anomaly of the tricuspid valve).

Echocardiography demonstrates marked dilation of the right-sided cardiac chambers. An important finding is the presence of the tricuspid valve leaflets arising appropriately from the annulus, differentiating this lesion from Ebstein anomaly.

At cardiac catheterization, similar pressure wave contours are obtained from the pulmonary artery, right ventricle, and right atrium. The right atrial *a wave* is dominant. Endocardial potentials, if recorded during catheterization, show normal transition between the ventricular and atrial complexes, helping to rule out Ebstein anomaly.

Most patients die in infancy or childhood. The typical pathologic finding is the markedly dilated, "parchment-like" right ventricle. Histologically, the endocardium is thickened, and there are few if any true myocardial cells in the right ventricular free wall. The tricuspid valve arises normally from a dilated valve annulus and may be dysplastic, but is not displaced into the right ventricular cavity.

46. (C) In patients with relatively normal cardiac output, classification of severity of pulmonary stenosis routinely is based on measurements of RV pressure and valve gradient. Mild stenosis is characterized by an RV pressure less than half the LV pressure or a peak valve gradient <35 mm Hg to 40 mm Hg. In moderate stenosis, the RV pressure is <50% to 75% of the LV pressure, or the peak gradient is <40 mm Hg to 60 mm Hg. Severe stenosis is defined as a RV pressure ≥75% of the LV pressure or a peak gradient >60 mm Hg to 70 mm Hg.

In this case, TR velocity predicts an RV-to-RA pressure gradient of 49 mm Hg, or an RV systolic pressure of 55 mm Hg. Using the modified Bernoulli equation $4(V_2^2 - V_1^2)$, the peak gradient across the pulmonary valve is $4(16 - 4)$ or 48 mm Hg. Both of these measurements indicate moderate pulmonary valve stenosis.

47. (E) If discontinuation of prostaglandin E1 and subsequent ductal constriction are not tolerated immediately after valvuloplasty, these infants can be maintained on prostaglandin for 2 to 3 weeks while intermittently assessing whether constriction of the ductus is tolerated with O_2 saturations remaining ≥70%. Neonates who immediately remain cyanotic following valvuloplasty often demonstrate improvement over weeks to months as RV compliance improves and the atrial right-to-left shunt decreases. Ultimately, those in whom a shunt was created can undergo shunt closure either surgically or by transcatheter techniques.

48. (B) As a result of pulmonary valve stenosis, secondary changes in the RV and pulmonary arteries can occur. The infundibular region of the RV becomes hypertrophied with resultant dynamic subvalvular obstruction. This hypertrophy can persist in the immediate postvalvuloplasty period, resulting in limited pulmonary outflow. Over time, once the fixed pulmonary obstruction is removed, this hypertrophy resolves.

49. (D) In the setting of unilateral branch pulmonary artery stenosis without a significant left-to-right shunt, resting RV systolic pressure remains normal. The contralateral pulmonary artery accommodates the cardiac output without an increase in pressure. Because flow to the stenotic side is lower than normal, the severity of obstruction may be underestimated by systolic pressure difference estimations (though the diastolic pressure difference is proportional to the severity of obstruction).

The protocol for angioplasty consists of positioning a balloon dilation catheter across the stenotic segment of the pulmonary artery. In contrast to pulmonary valve dilation, the balloon diameter should be three to four times the narrowest pulmonary artery segment.

Percutaneous balloon angioplasty of peripheral pulmonary artery stenosis has a lower success rate than pulmonary valvuloplasty. The overall acute success rate for branch PA angioplasty is <50% to 60%. The rate of recurrent stenosis has been 15% to 20% in short-term to mid-term follow-up.

50. (C) It is important to confirm the coronary circulation in patients with pulmonary atresia with intact ventricular septum before proceeding with an intervention. "Right ventricular–dependent coronary artery circulation" describes the situation whereby the myocardium is supplied by blood that originates in the RV at systemic or supersystemic systolic pressure and supplies the myocardium in a retrograde fashion. Myocardial ischemia, infarction, and death may result if significant ventriculocoronary connections are present and the right ventricular pressure is reduced secondary to an intervention.

In the normal circulation, the aortic diastolic pressure primarily drives coronary blood flow. Factors that reduce aortic diastolic pressure (or shorten diastole) will compromise coronary blood flow. The presence of ventriculocoronary artery connections may result in coronary artery stenosis and/or interruption. In this case, aortic diastolic pressure may not be sufficient to drive coronary blood flow; elevated RV pressures are necessary. Interference with blood flow into the RV or other reduction of RV systolic pressure has deleterious effects.

51. (E) Transcatheter perforation of the atretic pulmonary valve with subsequent balloon dilation is an alternative to surgical valvotomy. The ideal patient (lowest risk) would have a tripartite right ventricle of near normal size with valvar pulmonary atresia and a well-developed pulmonary arterial circulation. There would not be RV-depending coronary circulation.

In general, the smallest RVs are associated with the most ventriculocoronary connections. Unipartite or bipartite ventricles are much more likely to have ventriculocoronary communications. Using the convention of the tricuspid Z value, data from the CHSS demonstrated a positive correlation with ventriculocoronary connections: a more negative tricuspid Z value correlates with the presence of ventriculocoronary connections.

52. (A) This patient demonstrates evidence of RV-dependent coronary circulation. Therefore, decompression of the RV is not warranted, eliminating an RV-to-PA conduit or pulmonary valvotomy.

53. (D) The angiogram demonstrates evidence of RV-dependent coronary circulation in the inferior distribution. Therefore, he would exhibit evidence of myocardial ischemia in an inferior distribution, including ST elevation in leads II, III, and aVF.

54. (C) Despite the lack of evidence of RV-dependent coronary circulation by echocardiography, cardiac catheterization is still necessary to rule out such circulation. MRI does not have a role in the preoperative management of a 4-day-old infant. Biopsy is not indicated.

55. (E) These images demonstrate pulmonary atresia with intact ventricular septum. Ventriculocoronary connections are observed in <45%, but <10% of patients are considered to have wholly RV-dependent coronary circulation (CHSS database). Confluent pulmonary arteries usually are supplied by a left-sided ductus arteriosus. A main pulmonary artery is almost always present. Rarely, nonconfluent pulmonary arteries are supported by bilateral ductus arteriosus or aortopulmonary collaterals. Some patients with this disease have all three RV components present; in others, the RV is extremely underdeveloped and may have an inlet only. There is no known gender predilection.

56. (E) For patients whose pulmonary artery anatomy appears amenable to reconstruction, procedures leading to complete repair are indicated. Connecting the RV to the central pulmonary artery using a conduit is performed; this may promote growth of the central pulmonary arteries. Unifocalization procedures are performed to incorporate the maximum number of pulmonary artery segments into the eventual RV outflow reconstruction. The ultimate goal is complete repair (closure of all septal defects, interruption of all extracardiac sources of pulmonary arterial blood flow, and incorporation of at least 14 pulmonary arterial segments in a connection to the right ventricle).

At the end of a full repair, the central pulmonary artery size should be at least 50% of normal size. At the end of the operation, the RV pressure should be ≤70% than that measured in the LV. If higher, the VSD should be reopened.

57. (D) At the end of the operation, the right ventricular pressure should be ≤70% of the left ventricle. If higher, the VSD should be reopened.

58. (C) This patient has an estimated RVSP of >50 mm Hg, based on the modified Bernoulli equation. Given that her systemic BP is 65 mm Hg, her VSD should be reopened. RV systolic pressure at the conclusion of the operation should be <70% of LV systolic pressure.

59. (C) In PA–VSD, the blood supply to the lungs is entirely from the systemic arterial circulation. These include the ductus arteriosus, multiple systemic-to-pulmonary collateral arteries, occasionally a coronary artery, and plexuses of bronchial or pleural arteries. Ductal and collateral sources may be present in the same patient but rarely in the same lung.

The caliber of the central pulmonary arteries appears to be directly related to the amount of blood flow present through that segment. When the ductus or collateral arteries connect proximally to the central pulmonary arteries (as in this patient), the pulmonary arteries may be mildly hypoplastic or even normal in size. When multiple collateral arteries are present more distally, the central pulmonary arteries are usually hypoplastic.

60. (A) In pulmonary atresia with VSD, the sinus node is normal. The AV node occupies its normal position within the triangle of Koch. The nonbranching proximal portion of the His bundle penetrates the central fibrous body and lies along the left ventricular aspect of the posteroinferior rim of the VSD.

61. (E) Hypercyanotic spells constitute a medical, and possibly surgical, emergency. Treatment is directed towards lowering impedance to pulmonary flow and further increasing systemic vascular resistance. Typical treatment includes administration of supplemental oxygen, volume expansion, β-blockade, and sedation with morphine or ketamine. If needed, vasopressors (such as phenylephrine) can be used to increase systemic vascular resistance and decrease the relative ratio between pulmonary and systemic resistance. Occasionally, emergent surgical palliation or repair is required.

To prevent such spells, dehydration should be avoided; hence, making the patient NPO after midnight and starting an IV at 7:00 AM or performing phlebotomy to decrease Hgb to <14 before starting the IV are incorrect. Using a general anesthesia-inducing agent that decreases systemic vascular resistance more than PVR is the inverse of what is advisable. Starting an esmolol drip as soon as the procedure starts is not a bad choice, per se, because β-blockade is used to treat a hypercyanotic spell. However, making the patient NPO after midnight, starting IV fluid when NPO starts, and using a topical anesthetic such as EMLA before attempting vascular access is better because such measures can help prevent a spell, rather than treat a spell once it is started.

62. (E) Waterston shunts (anastomosis of the ascending to the right pulmonary artery) or Potts shunts (descending aorta to left pulmonary artery) may result in pulmonary artery distortion with consequent inconsistent transmission of flow and pressure to the pulmonary arterial bed. Pulmonary arterial stenosis and/or pulmonary vascular disease preclude routine use of these palliative procedures.

The catheterization data demonstrate a significant gradient between the MPA and the RPA. The patient may or may not benefit from sildenafil; further testing with inhaled NO would help make such a determination. She does not have evidence of a left-to-right shunt based upon her SpO$_2$ measurements. At this point, she does not have evidence of RV–PA conduit stenosis as the RV-to-MPA systolic gradient is <10 mm Hg. Her dyspnea on exertion more likely is due to her pulmonary vascular disease than her mild LV diastolic dysfunction (LVEDP = 10 mm Hg).

63. (E) Some newborns with TOF with absent pulmonary valve may be asymptomatic with only mild cyanosis and no findings of heart failure. As PVR drops in early infancy, a net left-to-right shunt can develop with pathophysiology of a VSD. These patients may require minimal medical intervention and undergo elective surgical correction at a later age. Other newborns can present with respiratory failure. In the most serious cases, central bronchial compression from massively dilated pulmonary arteries can result in respiratory failure despite conventional mechanical ventilation. In this case, respiratory distress may be improved by placing the patient prone to suspend the pulmonary arteries off the airways.

64. (D) This patient demonstrates evidence of critically restricted antegrade flow to the lungs. Given a prenatal diagnosis of TOF, it is reasonable at this point to start prostaglandin to reopen the ductus arteriosus. Once he is stabilized, he can be considered for either total repair or a systemic-to-pulmonary shunt. While most newborns with TOF do not have ductal-dependent pulmonary blood flow and may be followed without specific early intervention, this patient demonstrates that he is "ductal-dependent." PGE1 should be started without delay. Then other studies, such as echocardiogram, can be performed. He should not go to surgery before attempts at medical stabilization have been attempted.

65. (C) All patients with TOF demonstrate anterior and cephalad deviation of the outlet septum. The degree and nature of this deviation determines the severity of subpulmonic obstruction, the size of the VSD, and the degree of aortic override. In virtually all patients with severe infundibular obstruction, there is an associated large, nonrestrictive VSD and a prominent overriding aorta. In this case, it is very uncommon to have a restrictive VSD. Among other findings, a large conal branch, or accessory left anterior descending artery, is seen in ≤15% of hearts. A left SVC is found in <10% of patients.

66. (C) A truly continuous murmur is uncommon in truncus arteriosus. When present, it usually suggests pulmonary artery ostial stenosis. Continuous murmurs are common in patients with PA/VSD. Patients with PA/VSD can have either a patent ductus arteriosus or systemic collateral arteries to the pulmonary arteries. Because the differential diagnosis of truncus arteriosus includes this lesion, a continuous murmur is strongly suggestive of pulmonary atresia rather than of truncus arteriosus.

67. (E) In truncus arteriosus, the left coronary artery tends to arise from the left posterolateral truncal surface and the right coronary artery from the right anterolateral surface. The left anterior descending coronary artery is frequently relatively small and displaced leftward. The conal branch of the right coronary artery is usually prominent and supplies several large branches to the right ventricular outflow tract.

The posterior descending coronary artery arises from the left circumflex artery (left coronary dominance) in 25% to 30% of truncus arteriosus patients. Anomalies of coronary ostial origin are common, involving 37% to 49% of patients.

68. (A) Patients with truncus arteriosus are at risk of having pulmonary vascular obstructive disease developing at an early age, and this has provided the major impetus for early surgical correction. For patients presenting beyond infancy, PVR must be assessed to select the best treatment.

Patients with truncus arteriosus who have two pulmonary arteries and a pulmonary arteriolar resistance >8 units m^2 are at high operative risk. In most centers, corrective surgery is not offered to most of these patients. Some centers might offer repair to children who are <2 years of age and whose resistance decreases <8 units m^2 with vasoreactivity testing. In a child of 6 years, unfortunately, pulmonary artery changes are irreversible.

Cardiac transplantation is not a good option because this patient will have irreversible obstructive pulmonary vascular disease.

69. (A) The pulmonary arteries most commonly arise from the left posterolateral aspect of the truncus arteriosus, a small distance above the truncal valve. Type I truncus arteriosus is observed in <50% to 65% of patients, type II in 30% to 45%, and type III in 5% to 10%.

The truncal valve is tricuspid in <70%, quadricuspid in <20%, and bicuspid in <10%.

A right aortic arch with mirror-image brachiocephalic branching is associated fairly commonly with truncus arteriosus, occurring in up to 35% of patients.

IAA occurs relatively frequently (<10% to 20% of patients). It is frequently associated with DiGeorge syndrome.

Among other associated anomalies, a secundum atrial septal defect has been noted in <10% to 20% of patients, an aberrant subclavian artery in <5% to 10%, a persistent LSVC draining into the coronary sinus in <5% to 10%, and mild tricuspid stenosis in <6%.

70. (E) IAA in the setting of truncus arteriosus is frequently associated with DiGeorge syndrome (chromosome 22q11 deletion).

71. (C) This child is younger than 2 years of age. His PVR decreases to <8 units m^2 when 100% oxygen is breathed. In such young patients, surgery may still be offered if the parents are willing to accept a higher surgical risk because it is possible that the increased resistances may result from arteriolar or medial smooth muscle hypertrophy and vasoconstriction rather than advanced intimal occlusive disease. These changes may be reversible.

72. (C) The second heart sound usually is loud and single in truncus arteriosus. The occasionally heard split second sound in these patients may be caused by delayed closure of some of the cusps of the abnormal truncal valve.

73. (D) Corrective surgery for truncus arteriosus is preferred in the first weeks of life. Delay of operation runs the risk of ischemia of the hypertrophied ventricle secondary to desaturated blood at a low diastolic perfusion pressure (caused by runoff through the pulmonary arteries as well as "aortic" insufficiency, if present). Repair of truncus at 6 to 12 months of age carries a mortality rate twice that for repair between 6 weeks and 6 months. Pulmonary vascular obstructive disease also can develop early, which provides additional impetus for correction in the first few months of life.

The preferred operation is complete repair during the neonatal period. Although techniques of repair that do not include an extracardiac conduit have been described, most prefer a valved conduit when complete repair is performed because of the presence of pulmonary hypertension.

The presence of a regurgitant truncal valve is almost always amenable to various repair techniques, and replacement is rarely required in the neonatal period. If recurrent truncal valve incompetence occurs, repair or replacement of the truncal valve can be performed at the time of reoperation for conduit replacement.

74. (D) Asymmetric congenital mitral stenosis, with unbalanced cord attachment, is often termed parachute mitral valve. In the more common type, there are two papillary muscles. However, the valve is parachute-like with unbalanced chordae predominantly attached to one papillary muscle, mimicking the appearance of a classic parachute mitral valve. Less common are valves with hypoplastic, fused, or single papillary muscles and focalized cord attachments (the so-called classic parachute mitral valve).

75. (B) In this rare condition, also known as "hammock valve," the mitral valve leaflets are thickened and chordae are markedly shortened or absent. The leaflets insert directly to the papillary muscles or to the posterior ventricular wall, resulting in limited mitral valve excursion, stenosis, and insufficiency. An abnormal band of fibrous tissue often extends along the free margin of one or both valve leaflets, thus tethering the leaflets and papillary muscles.

76. (A) It is common, after surgical relief of mitral valve stenosis, for pulmonary hypertension to persist. In this vignette, physical examination findings are consistent with pulmonary hypertension and mitral valve regurgitation. The echocardiogram documents a mitral inflow gradient of 5 mm Hg, making residual mitral stenosis or an unrecognized supramitral ring unlikely. Also, the valve was repaired through an atrial approach, making an unrecognized ring very unlikely. The pulmonary vein Doppler is not suggestive of pulmonary vein stenosis.

77. (D) A cleft of the anterior mitral valve leaflet is rare and associated with significant mitral insufficiency presenting in infancy or young children. It may also occur as an isolated defect in asymptomatic individuals. In isolated cleft, the atrioventricular septum is intact, and the left ventricular outflow tract is not elongated. The valve is somewhat dysplastic, as the cleft edges usually are thickened and rolled. The cleft is directed anteriorly towards the outflow septum, as opposed to an atrioventricular canal defect where the cleft is more posteriorly directed towards the inlet septum.

In isolated cleft of the mitral valve, the papillary muscles are generally normal. In most cases, chordae attach to the papillary muscles. There may be accessory chords which attach to the membranous and muscular septum. In some cases of complete cleft, accessory chords are absent, and the anterior leaflet is usually flail and grossly insufficient. Associated left ventricular outflow tract obstruction may be caused by the accessory chords.

The mitral annulus is commonly dilated. The most commonly associated congenital heart anomalies include ASDs, VSDs, and transposition of the great arteries.

78. (A) Management of young infants and children with moderate mitral insufficiency remains primarily medical, including diuretics and afterload-reducing agents such as angiotensin-converting enzyme inhibitors. Some patients may require antiarrhythmic medication for atrial arrhythmias as well. Platelet antagonists or anticoagulation may be used in patients with atrial thrombosis (which develops secondary to severe left atrial enlargement and/or atrial fibrillation).

Patients with severe mitral insufficiency and heart failure unresponsive to medical management require surgical management.

79. (D) The physical examination findings are suggestive of MVP. While usually innocuous, there is a small subset of patients who may be at risk for sudden cardiac death. MVP patients with the following conditions are restricted to low-intensity competitive sports only (class 1A: arrhythmogenic-mediated syncope; repetitive nonsustained or sustained supraventricular tachycardia or frequent/complex ventricular tachyarrhythmias on ambulatory Holter monitoring; color Doppler evidence of severe mitral regurgitation; left ventricular ejection fraction <50%. Otherwise, MVP patients are permitted participation in all competitive sports.

80. (C) In neonates with critical aortic stenosis and a small left ventricle, therapeutic direction requires a decision regarding adequacy of the left heart to support a two-ventricle circulation. Several studies have addressed methods of quantitatively assessing adequacy of the left heart to handle the entire systemic circulation. Infants with nonapex-forming left ventricle, small aortic annulus (<5 mm), and small mitral valve annulus (<9 mm) may have improved survival with Norwood-type palliation or cardiac transplant than with treatment strategies to achieve a two-ventricle circulation.

Rhodes and colleagues developed a predictive equation for success of two-ventricle management plan in neonates with critical aortic stenosis. The parameters that were most predictive of success or failure included aortic root dimension indexed to body surface area, the ratio of the long axis of the left ventricle to the long axis of the heart, and the indexed mitral valve area. In a prospective multicenter analysis performed by the Congenital Heart Surgeons Society, a regression equation was used to predict 5-year survival probability with Norwood-type palliation versus two-ventricle approach. Discriminating parameters included age, aortic valve Z score, grade of EFE, diameter of ascending aorta, presence of significant tricuspid valve regurgitation, and left ventricular length Z score. Significant retrograde flow in the distal aortic arch through the patent ductus arteriosus is also associated with lower likelihood of success with a two-ventricle approach.

81. (D) The case describes aortic stenosis or subaortic stenosis. The systolic ejection murmur is loudest at the mid left sternal border and radiates to the upper sternal borders and into the suprasternal notch. A systolic click is rare, which helps to differentiate subvalvular aortic stenosis from valvular aortic stenosis. The left ventricular impulse may be hyperdynamic, and associated findings of aortic regurgitation and/or mitral valve regurgitation may be present.

82. (D) The American College of Cardiology/American Heart Association guidelines for management of aortic stenosis recommend the following:

- Asymptomatic children and young adults with Doppler mean gradient >40 mm Hg be considered for cardiac catheterization and possible balloon valvuloplasty.
- Patients who desire to participate in competitive sports or are contemplating pregnancy and have Doppler mean gradient >30 mm Hg should be considered for catheterization and possible valvuloplasty.
  - If the catheter measured peak-to-peak gradient is >60 mm Hg, balloon valvuloplasty is indicated.
  - If the patient desires to play competitive sports or become pregnant, balloon valvuloplasty is indicated if the peak-to-peak gradient is >50 mm Hg.
- Patients with symptoms (angina, syncope, dyspnea on exertion) or ischemic or repolarization changes on rest or exercise ECG should have valvuloplasty if the peak-to-peak gradient is >50 mm Hg.
- Valvuloplasty is not recommended for asymptomatic patients with peak-to-peak gradients <40 mm Hg unless cardiac output is impaired.

83. (A) Tissue Doppler Imaging (TDI) may be helpful in assessment of systolic and diastolic dysfunction in patients with aortic stenosis. Doppler parameters derived from mitral or pulmonary vein flow have been used for estimation of left ventricular filling pressure, but limitations to these measurements are dependent on loading conditions and heart rate. TDI directly measures myocardial velocities, typically the systolic and diastolic mitral annular velocities. This practice allows quantification of systolic long-axis function and diastolic function.

In patients with aortic stenosis, the ratio of early mitral inflow velocity (E) to early diastolic mitral annular velocity (E') correlates with the LV end-diastolic pressure, thereby providing a clinically useful noninvasive method of assessing diastolic dysfunction. In addition, measurement of the mitral annular systolic velocity (S') by TDI may demonstrate systolic long-axis dysfunction in patients with aortic stenosis who have otherwise normal ejection fractions.

Because longitudinally oriented fibers are present in the subendocardial region, and the subendocardium is most susceptible to ischemia in patients with aortic stenosis, these fibers are at greater risk than the circumferentially oriented fibers. Long-axis dysfunction therefore might precede transverse axis dysfunction.

84. (E) The 36th Bethesda Conference Task Force recommendations for competitive athletics defines aortic stenosis severity as follows (PIG):

- Mild: peak-to-peak gradient <30 mm Hg, mean Doppler gradient <25 mm Hg, or PIG <40 mm Hg
- Moderate: peak-to-peak gradient 30 mm Hg to 50 mm Hg, mean Doppler gradient 25 mm Hg to 40 mm Hg, or PIG 40 mm Hg to 70 mm Hg
- Severe: peak-to-peak gradient >50 mm Hg, mean Doppler gradient >40 mm Hg, or PIG >70 mm Hg

Patients with mild stenosis, if asymptomatic and possessing normal exercise tolerance, are permitted to participate in all competitive sports. Patients with severe aortic stenosis should not participate in any competitive sports.

Asymptomatic patients with moderate aortic stenosis, absent or mild left ventricular hypertrophy, absence of repolarization abnormality on ECG, and a normal exercise test may participate in sports with a low static component and low-to-moderate dynamic component (such as golf, bowling, baseball/softball, and volleyball).

If such patients have no history of supraventricular tachycardia or ventricular tachyarrhythmias at rest or with exercise, they may participate in sports with moderate static component and low dynamic component (such as diving, archery, equestrian, and motorcycling).

For aortic valve stenosis patients who also have aortic regurgitation, these recommendations must be considered in concert with the Task Force recommendations for aortic regurgitation.

For details regarding indications for balloon aortic valvuloplasty, please refer to **Answer 82**.

85. (C) Subaortic stenosis is a lesion that occasionally progresses rapidly. However, the rate of progression of mild subvalvular aortic stenosis is variable, and the obstruction may remain mild for many years. Factors associated with more rapid progression of obstruction include higher initial pressure gradient, short distance between the obstructive lesion and the aortic valve, and anterior mitral valve leaflet involvement.

Left ventricular hypertrophy and myocardial fibrosis are seen in patients with aortic stenosis. EFE and papillary muscle infarction can be seen in infants with severe aortic stenosis but typically are not present in mild forms of disease. Myocardial fibrosis may also be present in asymptomatic children with hemodynamically moderate congenital aortic stenosis.

Traditionally, Doppler estimates of pressure gradients across stenotic valves have been used for estimation of severity of obstruction. These measurements are dependent on loading conditions, heart rate, and other factors.

For infants with severe or critical aortic valve stenosis who are thought to be candidates for two-ventricle circulation, initial therapy usually entails balloon valvuloplasty or surgical valvotomy. For critical neonatal aortic stenosis, open surgical valvotomy or percutaneous balloon valvuloplasty procedures may be performed. Balloon valvuloplasty is the preferred procedure in most centers. Open surgical valvotomy may result in higher likelihood of residual or recurrent stenosis, whereas balloon valvuloplasty may be associated with a higher incidence of important aortic regurgitation.

86. (D) This patient has a history and physical examination concerning for a ductal-dependent lesion, most likely coarctation of the aorta. Prostaglandin E1 should be started immediately. Medical therapy and further imaging studies should not take priority until PGE1 has been started.

87. (D) This Doppler profile is suggestive of aortic arch obstruction, consistent with coarctation of the aorta. Children who present in infancy are much more likely than older children to have complex coarctation (associated lesions). Approximately 50% of patients who require surgical correction before 12 months of age have a simple coarctation. Among the remaining <50% with complex coarctation, a large VSD is the most common associated lesion. VSDs associated with coarctation include the perimembranous, muscular, or malalignment types. A malalignment VSD may occur with posterior deviation of the conal septum and left ventricular outflow tract obstruction. Such subvalvular aortic stenosis is particularly common in the critically ill infant who presents with coarctation and VSD.

A bicuspid aortic valve occurs in up to 85% of patients with coarctation, and the valve may be stenotic or the annulus hypoplastic. Mitral stenosis also occurs in patients with coarctation and may be caused by a supravalvar mitral ring, thickening and dysplasia of the mitral leaflets, short dysplastic chordae tendineae, or the presence of a single "parachute" papillary muscle. The association of multiple left-sided obstructive lesions with coarctation has been referred to as Shone syndrome.

88. (A) Coarctation more commonly presents in an asymptomatic child as upper-extremity hypertension or a heart murmur. Coarctation repair is generally recommended at 2 to 3 years of age in asymptomatic children without severe upper-extremity hypertension. The risk for late recurrence of coarctation appears to be increased when repair is performed on a patient younger than 1 year of age. Studies demonstrate that the normal descending aorta has attained <50% of its final adult diameter by 3 years of age. Because significant hemodynamic obstruction at rest occurs only if the aortic diameter is reduced by ≥50%, restenosis following coarctation repair after 3 years of age should be uncommon. Furthermore, because of an increased risk for residual hypertension and early atherosclerotic cardiovascular disease, elective repair should not be delayed into late childhood and adolescence.

89. (E) This patient has evidence of Turner syndrome and coarctation. An echocardiogram is warranted. Her left arm systolic blood pressure is 20 mm Hg higher than her right arm or lower extremities. This indicates that she likely has an anomalous right subclavian artery distal to the coarctation.

90. (B) A normal abdominal aortic Doppler profile does not rule out coarctation of the aorta. If the ductus arteriosus is patent, the pulsed wave Doppler profile can appear normal.

91. (A) Turner syndrome is associated with a 45, XO genotype.

92. (D) Exercise-induced upper-extremity hypertension is usually associated with an increase in the coarctation pressure gradient during exercise. This is believed to be secondary to an increase in aortic blood flow across a relatively nondistensible coarctation repair site. Patients with exercise hypertension, but without significant anatomic stenosis following coarctation repair, may benefit from β-blocker therapy with a decrease in exercise hypertension and coarctation gradient.

The long-term prognosis following repair of coarctation may be adversely affected by systemic arterial hypertension and an associated increase in premature atherosclerotic disease. Systolic and diastolic hypertension may occur at rest, most commonly in patients whose coarctation repair is delayed beyond late childhood. The risk for late hypertension may be as high as 10% to 20%, even when the coarctation is repaired in infancy. The cause of late postoperative hypertension in patients without a residual resting coarctation gradient may relate to anatomic and functional changes in the arterial vasculature proximal to the coarctation.

93. (D) This patient is suffering from inadequate tissue delivery to end organs, as evidenced by his acidosis, elevated liver function studies, and elevated creatinine. Matching of oxygen delivery to changes in oxygen consumption is more effective through interventions in total cardiac output or hemoglobin concentration than by precise manipulation of Qp/Qs balance. In this case, the patient is relatively anemic (Hgb 12 g/dL), and therefore, transfusion is warranted.

For those patients in whom Qp/Qs is elevated and systemic perfusion is compromised, therapy with milrinone might be warranted. Milrinone, however, has also been shown to reduce PVR and carries the undesired risk of increasing Qp/Qs. Furthermore, milrinone could result in significant hypotension in a patient already at risk for decreased perfusion.

Increasing the amount of inspired oxygen or starting nitric oxide both could increase the pulmonary blood flow at the expense of systemic perfusion. Increasing the ventilator rate from 24 to 30 could drive down pCO_2, which could increase pulmonary blood flow at the expense of systemic perfusion and would not be as helpful as increasing the hemoglobin concentration.

94. (A) Anterior malalignment VSDs are associated with varying degrees of overriding of the pulmonary annulus into the right ventricle. With increasing degrees of override, the anatomy becomes more and more similar to DORV with subpulmonary defect (Taussig–Bing anomaly). The subaortic stenosis caused by the anterior malalignment of the infundibular septum is frequently associated with aortic arch hypoplasia, coarctation, or even complete interruption of the aortic arch.

95. (D) Consistent with the normal atrial anatomy, the sinus and AV nodes are in their usual locations.

The normal conus is subpulmonary, left sided, and anterior, and it prevents fibrous continuity between the pulmonary and tricuspid valve rings. In d-TGA, the infundibulum is usually subaortic, right sided, and anterior, and it prevents fibrous continuity between the aortic and tricuspid valve rings. d-TGA is hypothesized to result from the abnormal growth and development of the subaortic infundibulum with concurrent absence of growth of the subpulmonary infundibulum.

With intact ventricular septum, the entire septum is usually a relatively straight structure and does not have the sigmoid curvature typical of the normal heart.

Dynamic obstruction is rare in the neonate with elevated pulmonary artery resistance or in the presence of a nonrestrictive ductus arteriosus, as the left ventricle pumps against systemic systolic pressure and retains "normal" geometry.

Following atrial level repair, frequently there is a small-to-moderate systolic pressure difference across the subpulmonary outflow tract.

96. (C) In the infant with d-TGA/large VSD and severe left ventricular outflow obstruction, there may be markedly restricted pulmonary blood flow and severe hypoxemia. In some neonates, a palliative systemic-to-pulmonary arterial shunt may be performed, with intracardiac correction carried out at a later age. Alternatively, corrective surgery can be performed in early infancy. However, none of the surgical corrections listed among the answer choices would be appropriate for this patient.

One appropriate corrective surgery in this case would be the Rastelli operation, a combination of intraventricular repair and placement of an extracardiac right ventricle-to-pulmonary artery conduit. The Rastelli repair has been considered the most appropriate operation for d-TGA with large VSD and extensive LVOTO because it achieves complete bypass of the LVOTO and an anatomic correction of the transposition pathology.

An alternative technique, termed REV (*Réparation à l'étage ventriculaire*), could potentially be used. The REV procedure appears to have some advantages over the Rastelli operation: application in younger patients, avoidance of prosthetic extracardiac conduit, and avoidance of intracardiac tunnel obstruction. This operation involves performing a high, anterior right ventricular incision and a radical excision of the outlet septum to create an unobstructed anterior right ventricular cavity; establishing a short and direct intraventricular tunnel from the LV to the aorta; closure of the pulmonary artery orifice; and reimplantation of the transected pulmonary artery directly onto the right ventricular outflow cavity without a prosthetic conduit.

Finally, posterior translocation of the aortic root and coronary arteries can be performed, with enlargement of the left ventricular outflow tract, with conduit placement from the right ventricle to the pulmonary arteries anteriorly, as originally described by Nikaidoh and advocated by others.

97. (C) In ccTGA, the interventricular septum has a sagittal position. With ventricular inversion, both its surfaces and ventricular bundle branches are inverted, and thus the sequence of initial activation is oriented from right to left and usually in a more superior and anterior direction. This results in a reversal of the normal Q-wave pattern in the precordial leads: Q waves are present in the right precordial leads but are absent in the left precordial leads. The electrocardiographic changes identified in patients with ccTGA include reversal of Q-wave distribution in the precordial leads with QS complexes in the right precordial leads, large Q waves in leads III and aVF, and left axis deviation.

98. (A) The AV node is located along the anterior aspect of the atrioventricular ring, near the atrial septum.

99. (D) Varying degrees of left ventricular outflow obstruction may be observed in patients with DORV. Subaortic stenosis appears to result from extensive hypertrophy of the aortic conus and conal septum. In addition, subaortic stenosis has resulted from marked malalignment of the conal septum. With compression of the aortic outflow tract and reduction of aortic flow, there may be secondary hypoplasia of the aortic annulus and the aorta. Thus, an association has been described with interruption of the aortic arch or coarctation of the aorta in patients with DORV and subpulmonary VSD. Coarctation of the aorta, however, has also been described in instances of subaortic, doubly committed, and remote VSD.

Complete correction of DORV depends on the complexity of the intracardiac anatomy. Because of the complexity of intracardiac repair of these anomalies, it may be necessary to palliate some infants and small children who become symptomatic in the first year of life.

In this case, mitral valve straddling indicates that complete two-ventricle repair will be impossible. To establish a stable source of systemic perfusion, aortic arch reconstruction will be necessary. Therefore, a Norwood-type palliation is indicated.

100. (B) For patients with DORV and subpulmonary VSD, physiology is that of complete transposition of the great arteries. Therefore, the arterial switch operation appears to be the procedure of choice and can be performed in the neonatal period. The VSD should be closed at the time of the arterial switch.

101. (D) Patients with subaortic VSDs and pulmonary stenosis display varying degrees of cyanosis. Their clinical presentations are similar to that in TOF. When the pulmonary stenosis is severe, early cyanosis, failure to thrive, exertional dyspnea, and polycythemia may be present. The precordium may show evidence of a right ventricular impulse at the left sternal border, and a prominent systolic thrill is often palpable over the upper left sternal border. This is associated with a grade 4–5/6 systolic ejection murmur, which radiates into the lung fields. The first heart sound is normal, and the second heart sound is usually single. A third heart sound may be noted at the cardiac apex. In older children, clubbing also may be evident.

102. (A) Patients with DORV with subpulmonic VSD and no pulmonary stenosis typically present clinically with features resembling those in d-TGA with VSD. Commonly, these patients present with cyanosis and heart failure in early infancy. Patients in this group who have associated coarctation of the aorta may present in infancy with heart failure, cyanosis, and diminished or absent femoral pulses.

Like patients with TGA, these patients exhibit severe failure to thrive and may have frequent respiratory tract infections. Typically there is severe cyanosis. A precordial bulge and right ventricular impulse are present at the left sternal border. A grade 2–3/6 high-pitched systolic murmur may be present at the upper left sternal border. When PS is present, a systolic thrill may be present, and the murmur is loud (grade 3–4/6). The second heart sound is loud and single because of the proximity of the aorta to the chest wall. With increased pulmonary flow, an apical diastolic rumble may be present.

103. (D) This patient has physiology similar to d-TGA and, as such, would benefit from increased mixing at the atrial level. Increasing the rate of PGE-1 would not help, as the ductus arteriosus is already patent. Nitric oxide would potentially decrease PVR and increase pulmonary blood flow, but would not have an effect on mixing such as would a septostomy. Diuresis with furosemide would not help mixing. The patient may require surgery, but it would be inappropriate to wait several weeks without first doing a septostomy.

104. (D) Systemic outflow tract obstruction in the heart with a functional single ventricle promotes myocardial hypertrophy, and this has been shown to be an unequivocal risk factor for poor outcome at the Fontan procedure.

105. (A) Pulmonary arterial banding will reduce pulmonary flow and protect the pulmonary arterioles from obstructive pulmonary arteriopathy, but may induce or aggravate subaortic stenosis due to hypertrophy of the subaortic conus. However, banding may be appropriate in the setting of DORV with multiple muscular VSDs or a remote VSD.

106. (B) DILV with a right-sided hypoplastic subaortic right ventricle is at risk for failing a two-ventricle-type surgical repair. In this case, the patient has a restrictive bulboventricular foramen and severe subaortic stenosis. Therefore, systemic perfusion is at risk and the infant needs a stable systemic blood supply. Of the choices, an aortopulmonary anastomosis (DKS) procedure is most likely to result in a stable, long-term systemic blood supply.

Pulmonary artery banding is not the best option because it can set the stage for progressive ventricular hypertrophy and obstruction in patients who have naturally occurring mild restriction at the VSD.

PA banding with arch augmentation does not address the problem of subaortic obstruction.

107. (D) The arterial catheter is injecting the BT shunt. The venous catheter takes the course Right IJ → SVC → common atrium → common ventricle → aorta.

108. (A) The arterial catheter takes the course femoral artery → descending aorta → arch → BT shunt.

109. (E) Clinical suspicion is high for a partial pericardial defect. The best way to demonstrate a defect of the pericardium is by magnetic resonance imaging.

Partial or total absence of the pericardium are rare congenital anomalies that may be associated with significant symptoms. Eighty percent of defects occur on the left side. They appear to be secondary to premature atrophy of the left duct of Cuvier during embryologic development. Most cases of pericardial defect are identified incidentally. Symptomatic cases are rare. Symptoms, if present, may include syncope, chest pain, arrhythmias, and death. Severe symptoms have been described secondary to herniation or incarceration of the left atrial appendage through the defect, torsion of the great arteries, or constriction of a coronary artery at the rim of the defect.

The techniques of magnetic resonance imaging and computer-assisted tomography are very useful in demonstrating the pericardial defect. By MRI, a tongue of pulmonary tissue between the aorta and the main pulmonary artery is a common finding. MRI is ideal for evaluating the pericardium and is the procedure of choice to identify this diagnosis.

Chest radiography in complete absence of the pericardium may demonstrate leftward displacement of the cardiac border with a posterior bulging of the heart. Herniation of the left atrial appendage may be apparent on the chest radiograph, where the herniated appendage resembles an enlarged main pulmonary artery.

Electrocardiography frequently may be normal, but may also show right bundle branch block or other abnormalities of conduction.

By echocardiography, the right ventricle may appear enlarged, excessive cardiac motion may be apparent, and the left atrial appendage may appear prominent. Importantly, the actual defect in the pericardium cannot be imaged by echocardiography.

Cardiac catheterization is of little diagnostic value other than to document coexisting heart disease. Thoracoscopy may be necessary to confirm the diagnosis.

110. (B) The greatest risk for sudden death in children with HCM appears to be associated with one or more of the following clinical risk markers: (a) prior cardiac arrest or sustained ventricular tachycardia; (b) family history of one or more premature HCM-related deaths, particularly if sudden and multiple; (c) syncope; and (d) massive degrees of LV hypertrophy (maximum wall thickness ≥30 mm).

In clinical practice, prospective screening of HCM family members to ascertain affected or unaffected genetic status usually takes place without access to DNA analysis and is performed primarily with 2D echocardiography and 12-lead ECG, as well as history-taking and physical examination.

The traditional recommended strategy for screening first-degree relatives calls for such evaluations on a 12- to 18-month basis, usually beginning at least by age 12. If these studies do not show evidence of LV hypertrophy by 21 years of age, echocardiographic screening can be every 5 years.

111. (C) HCM is an autosomal dominant trait.

112. (C) The greatest risk for sudden death in children with HCM appears to be associated with one or more of the following clinical risk markers: (a) prior cardiac arrest or sustained ventricular tachycardia; (b) family history of one or more premature HCM-related deaths, particularly if sudden and multiple; (c) syncope; and (d) massive degrees of LV hypertrophy (maximum wall thickness ≥30 mm). The risk of sudden death increases when septal thickness is >20 mm.

For any patient who has a history of aborted cardiac death, an ICD should be placed as primary prevention. Also, since the patient's septum is severely hypertrophied, and a significant gradient is present with associated symptoms, a myectomy should also be performed.

113. (E) The subaortic gradient and systolic ejection heart murmur in HCM are dynamic. They can be reduced or abolished by interventions that decrease myocardial contractility (e.g., β-blocking adrenergic drugs) or increase ventricular volume or arterial pressure (e.g., squatting, isometric handgrip, or phenylephrine administration). They can be augmented by interventions that decrease arterial pressure or ventricular volume (e.g., the Valsalva maneuver or administration of nitroglycerin) or that increase contractility, such as standing, amyl nitrite inhalation, administration of isoproterenol, or exercise.

114. (C) Sudden death due to HCM occurs most commonly during adolescence and young adulthood (12 to 35 years of age) and rarely before 10 years of age. These events are due to primary ventricular tachycardia and/or ventricular fibrillation. Most patients die while sedentary or during normal or modest physical exertion. Importantly, however, an important proportion die suddenly during or just after vigorous activity.

HCM is the most common cause of sudden cardiac death in the young, including competitive athletes. Therefore, standard recommendations are to disqualify young individuals with HCM from intense competitive sports (guidelines of the 36th Bethesda Conference).

At present, the greatest risk for sudden death in children with HCM appears to be associated with one or more of the following clinical risk markers: (a) prior cardiac arrest or sustained ventricular tachycardia; (b) family history of one or more premature HCM-related deaths, particularly if sudden and multiple; (c) syncope; and (d) massive degrees of LV hypertrophy (maximum wall thickness ≥30 mm).

Septal myectomy is performed to improve symptoms, but it is not used as a sudden death-preventative procedure. To prevent sudden death, an ICD is recommended.

115. (E) This patient is at low risk, as he is asymptomatic, has a negative family history, and a normal echocardiogram. There is at present no recommendation to limit activity or treat medically on the basis of a genetic test.

116. (D) This patient has CHF from dilated cardiomyopathy. The phosphodiesterase inhibitor milrinone increases stroke work and cardiac output. Both systemic and pulmonary vascular resistances are decreased, and the drug evokes unique lusitropic properties affecting relaxation and ventricular compliance. This drug is thought to promote increase in intracellular calcium concentration by inhibition of phosphodiesterase III.

117. (D) Nadolol is a long-acting β-blocker. Phosphodiesterase inhibitors are the treatment of choice for patients who are taking β-blocker drugs. Milrinone retains its full hemodynamic effects in the presence of β-blocker therapy. Therefore, there is no reason to change therapy.

118. (C) This vignette describes a classic presentation of Barth syndrome. Barth syndrome is an X-linked disorder characterized by skeletal myopathy, congenital dilated cardiomyopathy, short stature, and neutropenia. Affected individuals usually die early in childhood. It is diagnosed by urinalysis revealing elevated 3-methylglutaconic acid.

Typically, boys with Barth syndrome present with hypotonia and dilated cardiomyopathy, including labored breathing, poor appetite, and/or slow weight gain, typically within the first few months after birth. Another important feature of Barth syndrome is a history of bacterial infections because of neutropenia.

The gene for Barth syndrome, Tafazzin (*TAZ*), is located on chromosome Xq28. Mutations in the *TAZ* gene lead to decreased production of an enzyme required for the synthesis of cardiolipin. There is no specific treatment for Barth syndrome, but each of the individual problems can be successfully controlled, and short stature often resolves after puberty.

119. (C) Cardiac catheterization is an important part of the evaluation in patients with RCM and should be performed at the time of diagnosis. Catheterization can help differentiate between RCM and CP, although many hemodynamic features can overlap.

Both diseases typically have an early diastolic dip and subsequent plateau pattern, also called the square root sign. In classic RCM the left ventricular end-diastolic pressure, left atrial pressure, and pulmonary capillary wedge pressure are markedly elevated and ≥4 mm Hg to 5 mm Hg (preferably 10 mm Hg) greater than the RAP and right ventricular end-diastolic pressure. In cases in which the pressures are essentially equal, volume loading may bring out the differences in pressure between the right and left sides.

120. (D) This vignette describes a classic case of Löffler endocarditis (hypereosinophilic syndrome, or HES). HES is typically seen in temperate climates and is more common in adult males. Persistent hypereosinophilia is present. HES includes persistent eosinophilia with 1,500 eosinophils/mm³ for ≥6 months or until death with evidence of other organ involvement. Usually, in HES, various organs besides the heart are involved (lungs, bone marrow, and brain). The cause of the eosinophilia is unknown.

Cardiac histologic findings include eosinophilic myocarditis: inflammatory reaction in the small intramural coronary vessels with thrombosis and fibrinoid change, and endocardial mural thrombosis and fibrotic thickening.

The clinical picture may include weight loss, fever, cough, rash, and heart failure. Systemic embolism is frequent. Death is usually secondary to the cardiac manifestations of the disease. Therapy for the hypereosinophilia may include corticosteroids, hydroxyurea, or vincristine. Cardiac therapy has included digoxin, diuretics, afterload reduction, and anticoagulation. Surgical approaches have included mitral and/or tricuspid valve repair or replacement and excision of fibrotic endocardium.

121. (E) RCM, by definition, has small ventricular volumes with normal or near-normal systolic function. Ventricular wall thickness is usually normal. The atria are enlarged.

122. (B) It is important to realize that patients with Duchenne and Becker muscular dystrophies can have severe complications from anesthesia, including cardiac arrest. Most complications seem to be related to use of succinylcholine, a muscular relaxant that may trigger hyperkalemia. Others have been attributed to use of volatile anesthetic agents. Patients also can have a reaction similar to malignant hyperthermia, develop rhabdomyolysis, and have masseter muscle spasm.

123. (E) The characteristic electrocardiogram in Duchenne muscular dystrophy shows deep Q waves in leads I, aVL, V5, and V6, and occasionally in leads II, III, and aVF. There is often a tall right precordial R wave and an increased R/S ratio. The P–R interval is shortened in many patients. Some have reported QT prolongation and QT dispersion abnormalities. Holter analysis has shown that automaticity is also affected whereby there is a resting sinus tachycardia, loss of circadian rhythm, and reduced heart rate variability in many patients with Duchenne muscular dystrophy.

There are frequent arrhythmias in older patients including ectopic atrial tachycardia, atrial fibrillation, transient second- and third-degree AV block, and more ominous ventricular tachycardias. The presence of multiform premature ventricular contractions and ventricular tachycardia on Holter monitoring portends possible sudden death owing to ventricular fibrillation.

124. (B) This vignette describes Duchenne muscular dystrophy. The cardiac examination is seldom abnormal, even in the presence of cardiomyopathy. Occasionally, third or fourth heart sounds may be present. There may be neck vein distention or hepatomegaly. The examination is often distorted by chest wall deformities, especially in older patients with scoliosis.

125. (B) Of the pediatric studies reporting arrhythmias in RCM, <15% of the patients had arrhythmias and/or conduction disturbances. Atrial flutter was the most commonly reported arrhythmia. High-grade second-degree and third-degree heart block were the next most commonly reported rhythm disturbances. Atrial fibrillation and atrial tachycardias, Wolff–Parkinson–White syndrome with supraventricular tachycardia, symptomatic sinus bradycardia requiring pacing, and ventricular tachycardia and torsade were also reported.

CHAPTER 3

Diagnosis of Congenital Heart Disease

Jonathan N. Johnson

QUESTIONS

X **1.** A 4-year-old child presents with new-onset ventricular tachycardia. Echocardiography after treatment of the arrhythmia reveals a single large mass in the wall of the left ventricle (Fig. 3.1). Which of the following is the most likely diagnosis?

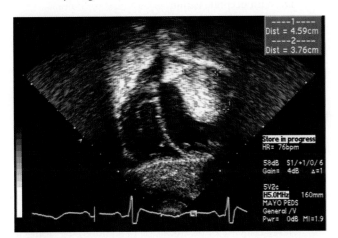

FIGURE 3.1

    A. Rhabdomyoma
    B. Fibroma
    C. Myxoma
    D. Pericardial teratoma
    E. Lymphoma

2. A 32-year-old pregnant woman undergoes fetal echocardiography due to an abnormal obstetrical scan. The echo reveals a diagnosis of tetralogy of Fallot with absent pulmonary valve. At the time of delivery, what is the most important initial step in management?

    A. Immediate sternotomy and VSD repair
    B. Initiation of prostaglandin drip

    C. Balloon atrial septostomy
    D. Respiratory support
    E. Initiation of epinephrine drip

3. You are seeing a 9-year-old patient in clinic who has hypertrophic cardiomyopathy. On examination, the patient has a crescendo–decrescendo systolic murmur along the left sternal border. Which of the following provocative maneuvers or medications would *decrease* the intensity of the patient's murmur?

    A. Phenylephrine
    B. Exercise
    C. Straining portion of Valsalva
    D. Nitroglycerine
    E. Isoproterenol

X **4.** A mother with phenylketonuria gives birth to a term male infant. The obstetricians note that she had not adhered well to her prescribed diet and likely had elevated blood phenylalanine levels during pregnancy. Which of the following defects are you most likely to see on echocardiography of the neonate?

    A. Ebstein anomaly
    B. Hypoplastic left heart syndrome
    C. Branch pulmonary stenosis
    D. Total anomalous pulmonary venous return
    E. Interrupted inferior vena cava

5. A 2-month-old male infant is referred for failure to thrive and is diagnosed with supravalvar pulmonary stenosis and supravalvar aortic stenosis on echocardiography. The child is described as having an "elfin" face, with flared eyebrows, bright stellate irides, and a wide mouth. On which of the following chromosomes is there most likely to be a deletion?

A. 11q
B. 22q
C. 7q
D. 1p
E. 8p

6. You are referred a 10-month-old male infant with a history of atrial septal defect. On examination, you note that the patient also has a missing thumb on his right hand. The patient's father has a similar missing thumb. Laboratory values including a CBC and electrolytes are normal. Genetic analysis reveals a mutation in the *TBX5* gene. Which of the following is the most likely diagnosis?

A. Thrombocytopenia-absent radii (TAR) syndrome
B. LEOPARD syndrome
C. Holt–Oram syndrome
D. CHARGE association
E. Rubenstein–Taybi syndrome

7. A 2-year-old girl is diagnosed with myocarditis. Her parents relate to you that she recently had a viral upper respiratory infection. Which of the following viruses are most likely implicated in this patient?

A. Epstein–Barr virus (EBV) and RSV
B. Parainfluenzae virus and coxsackie virus
C. HIV and parainfluenzae virus
D. Coxsackie virus and adenovirus
E. RSV and influenza A virus

8. A neonate is diagnosed with truncus arteriosus. Which of the following genetic syndromes is most likely in this patient?

A. Down syndrome
B. Turner syndrome
C. DiGeorge syndrome
D. Klinefelter syndrome
E. Holt–Oram syndrome

9. A 14-year-old girl is referred for an unusual sound heard on auscultation by her pediatrician. There is a high-frequency "click" audible immediately after S_1 and heard best at the apex. The most likely cause of this click is:

A. Mitral valve prolapse
B. Subvalvar pulmonary stenosis
C. Pulmonary valve stenosis
D. Pericardial rub
E. Bicuspid aortic valve

10. A 13-year-old girl is seen for a heart murmur. Her parents note that she has numerous dark-brown freckle-like spots throughout her body, which seem to have increased in number as she has gotten older. She has a prior diagnosis of sensorineural deafness, as well as short stature. Her parents report that a murmur was heard in many well-child visits, but was always thought to be benign. An ECG is performed and shows first-degree AV block. Which of the following is most likely to be seen on echocardiography?

A. Coarctation of the aorta and bicuspid aortic valve
B. Atrial and ventricular septal defects
C. Pulmonary stenosis and left ventricular hypertrophy
D. Double aortic arch
E. Rhabdomyoma

11. A 3-year-old healthy boy is referred for evaluation of a recently heard heart murmur. His peripheral pulses are normal. The first and second heart sounds are normal. There is a grade 2/6 low-to-mid frequency "vibratory" murmur along the left sternal border. One would expect this murmur to increase in intensity:

A. When going from sitting to standing position
B. When squatting
C. When going from sitting to supine position
D. With deep inhalation
E. During the third phase of the Valsalva maneuver

12. Which of the following is the most appropriate indication for performing a pericardiocentesis?

A. Pulsus paradoxus
B. Presumed viral pericarditis
C. Hypertension
D. Asymptomatic patient with hypothyroidism
E. Asymptomatic patient with renal failure

13. A 14-year-old boy is referred to your clinic. He has a history of recurrent sinusitis for which he has undergone numerous courses of antibiotics. A chest x-ray is performed which shows evidence of dextrocardia. In addition, the stomach bubble is located on the right side of the x-ray. A CT scan of the chest reveals bronchiectasis. Which of the following is the most likely diagnosis?

A. Carney complex
B. Kartagener syndrome
C. DiGeorge syndrome
D. Wiskott–Aldrich syndrome
E. Turner syndrome

14. You are seeing a neonate in the ICU who presented with cyanosis. The sonographer has started the echo and reports there is an aortopulmonary (AP) window with intact ventricular septum. There is also an interrupted aortic arch. Which type of interrupted arch is most likely for this patient?

  A. Type A (interruption distal to the left subclavian artery)
  B. Type B (interruption between the left carotid and left subclavian arteries)
  C. Type C (interruption between the carotid arteries)
  D. Type D (interruption proximal to the innominate artery)
  E. All types occur with equal frequency

15. A 3-day-old patient is referred to you for a murmur. On ECG, they have evidence of left axis deviation. Which of the following is the most likely diagnostic cause of the left axis deviation?

  A. Total anomalous pulmonary venous connection
  B. Concentric LVH
  C. Tricuspid atresia
  D. Secundum atrial septal defect
  E. Double outlet right ventricle

16. A 13-year-old girl presents to the clinic complaining of a rapid heart rate, which she has noticed for the past month. She denies any chest pain, syncope, or presyncope. Heart rate is 120 beats per minute while sitting on the examination table. Blood pressure is 115/72 mm Hg. BMI is 15. A faint systolic ejection murmur is heard. Of the following, the most appropriate laboratory test to order would be:

  A. Electrolyte panel
  B. Chromosome panel (karyotype)
  C. Hemoglobin A1C
  D. Thyroid-stimulating hormone (TSH)
  E. Serum cortisol

17. A 7-year-old girl is brought to the emergency department with new-onset pain in her knees and wrists. Her knees are swollen and red and are tender to the touch. You also note several erythematous, serpiginous, macular lesions with pale centers on her trunk that are not pruritic. She is febrile (temp = 39.5°C) and is found to have an elevated serum streptococcal antibody titer. Of the following, the most likely diagnosis is:

  A. Juvenile rheumatoid arthritis
  B. Systemic lupus erythematosus (SLE)
  C. Juvenile dermatomyositis
  D. Rheumatic fever
  E. Kawasaki disease

18. An outreach echocardiogram performed on a 2-day-old female infant reveals ventricular hypertrophy and an abnormal aortic arch. The baby is transported to your institution, and on arrival, the nurse performs four-extremity blood pressure measurements. The findings are as follows:

  Right leg: 40/25
  Left leg: 42/22
  Right arm: 73/36
  Left arm: 72/35

Which of the following is the most likely diagnosis?

  A. Coarctation of the aorta
  B. Complete AV canal defect
  C. Truncus arteriosus with pulmonary artery ostial stenosis
  D. Tetralogy of Fallot
  E. Coarctation of the aorta with aberrant right subclavian artery

19. A 38-week-old term infant with congenital heart disease is diagnosed with necrotizing enterocolitis (NEC). Which of the following diagnoses is associated with the highest risk of developing NEC in a term neonate?

  A. Tetralogy of Fallot
  B. Patent ductus arteriosus
  C. Tricuspid atresia
  D. Complete AV canal
  E. Hypoplastic left heart syndrome

20. A 5-year-old boy presents to the emergency department following a motor vehicle accident. The attending physician notes that his blood pressure is now 70/40 mm Hg and that his heart sounds are distant. Which of the following physical examination findings would be consistent with traumatic cardiac tamponade?

  A. A third heart sound
  B. A precordial rub
  C. A precordial knock
  D. Neck vein distention
  E. Bradycardia

21. You are seeing a 12-year-old girl in clinic, who was referred to you for cardiomegaly. On examination, you hear distant breath sounds as well as pulsus paradoxus. Her heart rate is 65 beats per minute. She has complained of progressively worsening fatigue over the last 2 months, which she attributes to her recent 20 lb weight gain. Which of the following is the most likely cause of her pericardial effusion?

  A. Rheumatic fever
  B. Hypothyroidism
  C. Recent isoniazid administration
  D. Renal failure
  E. Purulent pericarditis

22. A 5-year-old girl presents with fatigue and is found to have complete heart block. Echocardiography reveals a moderate-sized secundum atrial septal defect. A mutation in which gene is most likely to be found in this patient?

    A. NKX2.5
    B. TBX5
    C. MLL2
    D. JAG1
    E. PTNP11

23. A 5-year-old boy presents to your office with exercise intolerance. You note a 3/6 systolic ejection murmur at the left upper sternal border with a widely fixed split S_2 and a soft middiastolic rumble. Which of the following would you most likely find on further investigation?

    A. Right atrial enlargement on EKG
    B. Evidence of LVH on EKG
    C. Q_p:Q_s = 1.2
    D. Accessory left anterior descending coronary artery
    E. Spontaneous closure of the defect by age 10

24. You are consulted on a 1-day-old neonate in the NICU for a heart murmur. On examination, you note a loud systolic ejection murmur radiating throughout the precordium, with a prominent LV impulse. The neonate has poor peripheral perfusion and weak femoral pulses. On echocardiography, you obtain a right parasternal image with the following velocity in the ascending aorta (Fig. 3.2). Of the following, which is the most appropriate next intervention to perform?

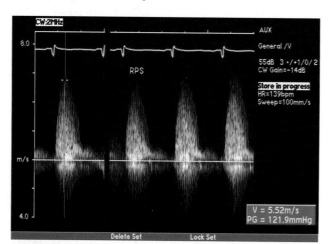

FIGURE 3.2

    A. Initiation of IV milrinone
    B. Pericardiocentesis
    C. Urgent aortic valvuloplasty
    D. Urgent atrial balloon septostomy
    E. Initiation of ECMO

25. A murmur is heard at a 1-week well-child examination. The infant is referred for an echocardiogram, which reveals several well-circumscribed masses in the left and right ventricular walls (Fig. 3.3). What is the most likely diagnosis?

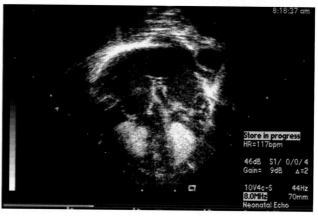

FIGURE 3.3

    A. Fibroma
    B. Myxoma
    C. Blood cyst
    D. Hemangioma
    E. Rhabdomyoma

26. You see a 5-year-old boy with aortic stenosis in follow-up. You note that he has a single S_2 heart sound. Which of the following is characteristic of the S_2 heart sound in patients with aortic stenosis?

    A. The S_2 becomes more widely split with inspiration in severe AS
    B. Paradoxical splitting of S_2 often occurs with mild AS
    C. The pulmonic component of S_2 is often decreased with severe AS
    D. The S_2 has normal physiologic splitting in patients with mild AS
    E. The S_2 is single in mild AS

27. A 14-year-old male patient is referred to you for a murmur. On history, the patient reports recurrent low-grade fevers, malaise, and a 20 lb weight loss in the last 2 months. On the echocardiogram, you find a pedunculated mass (2 cm × 2 cm) attached to the fossa ovalis in the left atrium. What is the most likely diagnosis?

    A. Rhabdomyoma
    B. Myxoma
    C. Teratoma
    D. Fibroma
    E. IVC extension of Wilms tumor

28. A 17-year-old male basketball player is referred to you for a murmur. On examination, you note that he has significant scoliosis, pectus carinatum, and pes planus (flat feet). His height is 190 cm, and his arm span is 210 cm. He has positive "thumb" and "finger" signs. His aortic sinus of Valsalva measures 45 mm in diameter (Z-score = 5.2). His carotid arteries, aortic arch, and descending aorta are normal. There is no significant family history. He admits to being admitted twice in the past with spontaneous pneumothoraces. Which of the following is true regarding this young man's diagnosis?

  A. He has Loeys–Dietz syndrome
  B. He should have a repeat echocardiogram in 5 years
  C. He does not need an eye examination
  D. He has Marfan syndrome
  E. He needs an ECG to assess for a prolonged QT interval

29. A 12-year-old boy with congenital heart disease is noted to have complete AV block. Which of the following is the most likely structural cardiac diagnosis for this patient?

  A. Ventricular septal defect
  B. d-Transposition of the great arteries
  C. Asplenia with tetralogy of Fallot
  D. Maternal lupus
  E. Congenitally corrected transposition of the great arteries

30. An echo performed on a 2-day-old male infant demonstrates severe tricuspid and mitral valve dysplasia with prolapse (Fig. 3.4). He is diagnosed with congenital polyvalvular dysplasia. Which of the following is the most likely genetic diagnosis in this patient?

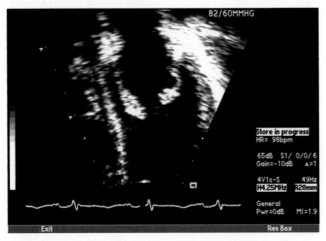

FIGURE 3.4

  A. Down syndrome
  B. Noonan syndrome
  C. Trisomy 18
  D. DiGeorge syndrome
  E. Alagille syndrome

31. Which of the following genetic syndromes are associated with an increased incidence of partial anomalous pulmonary venous return?

  A. Trisomy 18 and trisomy 21
  B. Holt–Oram and Marfan
  C. Turner and trisomy 21
  D. Turner and Noonan
  E. Noonan and Alagille

32. A 5-year-old boy is diagnosed with Wolff–Parkinson–White syndrome. He is found to have an abnormal echocardiogram. Which of the following forms of congenital heart disease is most commonly associated with WPW?

  A. Hypertrophic cardiomyopathy
  B. Ventricular septal defect
  C. Bicuspid aortic valve
  D. Tetralogy of Fallot
  E. Atrial septal defect

33. You have been following a 2-year-old boy with pulmonary stenosis. Which of the following would be a clinical clue that the degree of stenosis has worsened?

  A. The murmur peaks earlier
  B. The ejection click occurs later
  C. The "a" wave becomes less prominent
  D. S_1 becomes more prominent
  E. The split of S_2 becomes wider

34. A 9-year-old girl presents to you for evaluation of a murmur. The patient is asymptomatic, but does not participate in athletic activity. Her family history is significant for a paternal uncle, grandfather, and great grandfather who had "thick heart muscle." On examination, she has short stature, a triangular face, pectus excavatum, and a webbed neck. Her heart examination reveals an RV lift and a soft short systolic ejection murmur at the LUSB. What are you most likely to find on her echocardiogram?

  A. Bicuspid aortic valve with or without coarctation
  B. Thickened pulmonary valve with mild stenosis
  C. Discrete supravalvular pulmonary stenosis
  D. Bilateral pulmonary branch stenosis
  E. Right aortic arch

35. An 19-month-old female infant presents for evaluation due to a cardiac murmur. On examination, a high-frequency continuous murmur is present at the right upper sternal border. The murmur is maximal in the upright position and is softer when the neck is turned. This murmur is most likely:

  A. Aortic insufficiency murmur
  B. Patent ductus arteriosus
  C. Peripheral pulmonary branch stenosis
  D. Venous hum
  E. Carotid bruit

36. A 15-year-old boy is referred for dyspnea on exertion. On examination, his S_1 and S_2 sounds are normal, but there is a harsh 3/6 systolic murmur with a musical quality heard from the sternal border down to the apex. There are no clicks, thrills, or rubs, and diastole is quiet. Just after a PVC that you note on his cardiac monitor, the murmur increases in intensity. What is the most likely cause of the murmur?

   A. Aortic stenosis
   B. Ventricular septal defect
   C. Mitral regurgitation
   D. Pulmonary stenosis
   E. Innocent murmur

37. As part of an evaluation for short stature, a 12-year-old girl is noted to have streaked gonads on abdominal and pelvic ultrasound examination. A karyotype determines that she has Turner syndrome. Which of the following is most likely to be found on echocardiography?

   A. Bicuspid aortic valve
   B. Mitral valve stenosis
   C. Subaortic membrane
   D. Aortic root dilatation
   E. Atrial septal defect

38. A 17-year-old boy is referred to you for a murmur heard over the left scapula. Basic laboratory studies are normal. The patient is noted to be hypertensive, and an abdominal ultrasound with renal Doppler is normal. An echocardiogram is performed and thought to be normal, but images are difficult secondary to the patient's size (particularly subcostal images). The following chest x-ray is taken (Fig. 3.5). Which of the following is the next best diagnostic test to order?

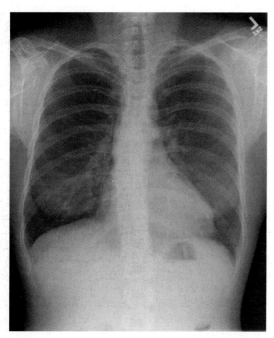

FIGURE 3.5

   A. Left and right heart catheterization
   B. Computed tomography scan of the chest
   C. Stress echocardiogram
   D. Exercise treadmill test using the Bruce protocol
   E. Urine metanephrines

39. You diagnose a 2-month-old male infant with congenitally corrected transposition of the great arteries (cc-TGA or L-TGA). What is this patient most likely to also have on echocardiography?

   A. Atrial septal defect
   B. LVOT obstruction
   C. Ventricular septal defect
   D. Tricuspid valve dysplasia
   E. Mitral valve dysplasia

40. A 14-year-old basketball player is referred to you after having an episode of syncope while running during a game. He has a known history of seizures for which he has been treated with antiepileptic medication. He relays to you that his uncle died suddenly while swimming on vacation at the age of 34 and that his anatomical autopsy was normal. Your patient's echocardiogram reveals normal ventricular size and function and normal coronary artery anatomy. An ECG has been performed but is pending. Which of the following is the most likely diagnosis?

   A. Brugada syndrome
   B. Coronary artery vasospasm
   C. Benign vasovagal syncope
   D. Long QT syndrome
   E. Idiopathic ventricular fibrillation

41. You are called to perform an echocardiogram on a 5-day-old female infant with cyanosis. The patient is mildly tachypneic with retractions. Pulse oximetry reveals an oxygen saturation of 70%. Chest x-ray shows a normal heart size with mildly increased pulmonary vascular markings. On examination, you appreciate a loud S_2 with no significant murmurs. Echocardiography shows side-by-side great arteries. Which of the following diagnoses is most likely?

   A. DORV with subpulmonic VSD and no pulmonary stenosis
   B. DORV with subpulmonic VSD and pulmonary stenosis
   C. DORV with subaortic VSD and no pulmonary stenosis
   D. DORV with subaortic VSD and pulmonary stenosis
   E. DORV with subaortic VSD and coarctation of the aorta

42. A 6-week-old female infant with biliary atresia is found to have a murmur on examination. When you see the patient, you note that she has a broad forehead, deep-set eyes, and a pointed chin, which give her face a triangular appearance. She is significantly jaundiced. Auscultation reveals a 2/6 systolic murmur heard best at the left upper sternal border and radiating to the axillae bilaterally. Which of the following is the most likely diagnosis?

A. CHARGE association
B. Alagille syndrome
C. Williams syndrome
D. Noonan syndrome
E. DiGeorge syndrome

43. A 15-year-old patient with hypertrophic cardiomyopathy is referred to your clinic. You hear a murmur consistent with LV outflow obstruction. Which of the following maneuvers will increase the outflow murmur in this patient?

A. Beta blocker
B. Squatting
C. Exercise
D. Isometric handgrip
E. Phenylephrine

44. A 17-year-old athlete is found to have thickened LV myocardium. Which of the following characteristics supports a diagnosis of hypertrophic cardiomyopathy over "athlete's heart"?

A. Increased LV end diastolic volume
B. Symmetric ventricular hypertrophy
C. Male gender
D. T-wave inversions in the lateral leads
E. Mitral inflow E/A = 1.5

45. A 3-year-old child presents with dilated cardiomyopathy. The child was adopted 2 weeks ago from Chile, but birth records report no family history of congenital heart disease, cardiomyopathy, or HIV. Which of the following is the most likely infectious cause of DCM in this patient?

A. Human papillomavirus
B. Human immunodeficiency virus
C. Chagas disease
D. Lymphocytic choriomeningitis
E. West Nile virus

46. A series of studies are undertaken to differentiate between restrictive cardiomyopathy and constrictive pericarditis in a 14-year-old boy. Which of the following findings would be more consistent with restrictive cardiomyopathy?

A. "Septal bounce" on echocardiography
B. RVSP <30 mm Hg on catheterization
C. Increased atrial size on echocardiography

D. RVEDP = LVEDP on catheterization
E. Normal pulmonary vascular resistance index on catheterization

47. You are seeing a 7-year-old boy in clinic with mitral valve regurgitation from a prior episode of rheumatic fever. How would you ask the patient to be positioned in order to best hear his murmur?

A. Sitting
B. Left lateral decubitus
C. Sitting-up and leaning forward
D. Standing
E. Right lateral decubitus

48. A 3-month-old male infant is referred to you for a murmur. The patient has already been referred to medical genetics for a history of low birth weight, hypotonia, and microcephaly. On examination, you note the patient has hypertelorism, epicanthal folds with down-slanting palpebral fissures, a flat nasal bridge, micrognathia, single palmar creases, and a high-pitched cry. Which of the following are you most likely to find on echocardiography?

A. Coarctation of the aorta
B. Transposition of the great arteries
C. Double outlet right ventricle
D. Ebstein anomaly
E. Ventricular septal defect

49. A 7-year-old boy presents with polyarthritis and is diagnosed with rheumatic fever. Which of the following major manifestation of rheumatic fever is also most likely to be seen in this same patient?

A. Carditis
B. PR prolongation on ECG
C. Chorea
D. Subcutaneous nodules
E. Erythema marginatum

50. A 3-year-old patient is referred to you with postaxial polydactyly, large atrial septal defect, dwarfism, and fingernail dysplasia. Which of the following is the most likely genetic syndrome in this patient?

A. Holt–Oram syndrome
B. DiGeorge syndrome
C. Alagille syndrome
D. Ellis–van Creveld syndrome
E. Down syndrome

51. A 16-year-old football player presents with an episode of syncope while singing in church. His pediatrician obtained an ECG and referred him to you for sports clearance. Which of the following findings on the ECG are most concerning for an underlying pathology (i.e., not related to training)?

A. Left bundle branch block
B. Incomplete right bundle branch block
C. First-degree AV block
D. Early repolarization
E. Isolated QRS voltage for LVH

52. A 2 month old with tuberous sclerosis is referred to your practice. On echocardiography, you find several moderate-sized cardiac tumors, all located within the walls of the LV and RV without obstruction of the LVOT or RVOT. The patient is asymptomatic. What is the most likely future course for this patient?

A. The patient will eventually have to undergo surgical resection
B. Around 50% chance of requiring surgical resection
C. Complete resolution of the tumors
D. The tumors will resolve after an interventional procedure
E. The tumors will not resolve, but the patient will remain asymptomatic

53. A male neonate is diagnosed with tetralogy of Fallot. What is the inheritance pattern of the most frequently identified genetic cause of tetralogy of Fallot?

A. X-linked dominant
B. Mitochondrial
C. Autosomal recessive
D. X-linked recessive
E. Autosomal dominant

54. A 6-month-old infant presents with recurrent respiratory infections and stridor. A vascular ring is found on echocardiography. Which type of vascular anomaly is most likely to be found in this patient?

A. Retroesophageal right subclavian artery with left aortic arch
B. Retroesophageal left subclavian artery with right aortic arch
C. Left pulmonary artery sling
D. Double aortic arch
E. Persistent fifth aortic arch

55. A 10-year-old girl presents with chest pain and diffuse ST-segment elevation. You diagnose her with acute pericarditis. On examination, you hear a typical friction rub.

Which of the following maneuvers will cause the rub to become louder on auscultation?

A. Have the patient blow out as much air as possible
B. Have the patient lie on their side
C. Have the patient stand up straight
D. Have the patient lean forward
E. Have the patient lie supine

56. An 8-year-old, developmentally delayed boy presents with shortness of breath. Echocardiography reveals a mitral valve arcade with severe stenosis (mean gradient = 14 mm Hg). On further questioning, his family reports a history of short stature and thrombocytopenia. Examination demonstrates wide-spaced eyes, mild ptosis, and small ears. A microarray is sent and reveals a deletion in chromosome 11q23. Which of the following is the diagnosis?

A. Williams syndrome
B. DiGeorge syndrome
C. Turner syndrome
D. Jacobsen syndrome
E. Noonan syndrome

57. A neonate is admitted with concerns for congenital rubella infection. Which of the following congenital heart defects is mostly likely to be found on echocardiography?

A. Pulmonary stenosis
B. Coarctation of the aorta
C. Transposition of the great arteries
D. Hypoplastic left heart syndrome
E. Ectopia cordis

58. A 12-year-old boy is referred for evaluation of a murmur by his pediatrician. On examination, there is a systolic click heard in early to midsystole with the patient standing; however, the click moves later in systole with the patient in the squatting and supine positions. There is also a late systolic murmur heard best at the apex. Which of the following is the most likely diagnosis?

A. Bicuspid aortic valve
B. Subvalvar pulmonary stenosis
C. Mitral valve prolapse
D. Pulmonary valve stenosis
E. Pericardial rub

59. Which of the following chromosomal abnormalities portends the highest incidence of congenital heart disease for affected patients?

A. Trisomy 21
B. Trisomy 18
C. Turner syndrome
D. DiGeorge syndrome
E. 5p– syndrome

60. Which of the following patients is most likely to harbor a 22q11.2 deletion?

A. 2-month-old male infant with tetralogy of Fallot

B. 4 year old with a small ventricular septal defect

C. 4 month old with double outlet right ventricle and subaortic VSD

D. 2-day-old infant with d-transposition of the great arteries and VSD

E. 2-week-old infant with interrupted aortic arch type B

61. You are caring for a 16-year-old boy who had a cardiac arrest during a football game. Which of the following is the most likely underlying diagnosis?

A. Short QT syndrome

B. Long QT syndrome

C. Hypertrophic cardiomyopathy

D. Mitral valve prolapse

E. Aortic dissection

62. An outreach echocardiogram performed on a critically ill 3-day-old male infant reveals ventricular hypertrophy and an abnormal aortic arch. The baby is transported to your institution, and on arrival, the nurse performs four-extremity blood pressure measurements. The findings are as follows:

Right leg: 40/25
Left leg: 42/22
Right arm: 48/27
Left arm: 72/35

Which of the following is the most likely diagnosis?

A. Coarctation of the aorta

B. Coarctation of the aorta with VSD

C. Truncus arteriosus with pulmonary artery ostial stenosis

D. Coarctation of the aorta with supravalvar mitral ring

E. Coarctation of the aorta with aberrant right subclavian artery

63. A 30-year-old woman presents for a fetal echocardiogram. You note in her history that she was treated with retinoic acid during early pregnancy. Which of the following categories of congenital heart anomalies is of particular concern for this fetus?

A. Coarctation of the aorta

B. Hypoplastic left heart syndrome

C. Ebstein anomaly

D. Laterality defects

E. Conotruncal defects

64. A 6-year-old boy presents with shortness of breath, which has worsened in the past year. He denies any chest pain or cough. His past medical history is otherwise unremarkable. While performing an echocardiogram, you note the following Doppler flow pattern in the descending aorta (Fig. 3.6). Which of the following is the most likely diagnosis?

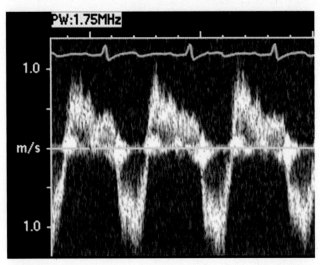

FIGURE 3.6

A. Ascending aorta dilation

B. Mitral regurgitation

C. Aberrant right subclavian artery from the descending aorta

D. Patent ductus arteriosus

E. Anomalous right coronary artery from the left sinus

ANSWERS

1. (B) Fibromas are typically single, firm, intramural tumors involving the ventricular free wall or septum. Clinical manifestations depend largely on the location of the tumor; however, ventricular arrhythmias are frequently seen in these patients and may be the presenting symptom. The presence of ventricular arrhythmias in the vignette should prompt one to think about fibroma as the answer. Successful surgical excision has occurred in some patients, while patients with extensive involvement of critical structures have occasionally been treated with transplantation.

2. (D) Tetralogy of Fallot with absent pulmonary valve is associated with aneurysmal pulmonary artery dilatation. This may cause compression of the bronchi. Up to 40% to 50% of patients may have respiratory distress at birth, some with lobar emphysema. In the acute setting, prone positioning may help by allowing the aneurysmal pulmonary arteries to fall forward and away from the bronchi. Patients with significant respiratory distress requiring surgery at birth have a worse outcome compared to those who do not need respiratory intervention early after birth.

3. (A) The murmur described is that of dynamic outflow tract obstruction. This murmur is typically increased by anything that increases the gradient. Thus, it will be louder with exercise, standing (particularly after squatting), and with the straining portion of the Valsalva maneuver. Systemic vasodilation with nitroglycerine or administration of isoproterenol will also increase the gradient. Administration of phenylephrine, or stimulation of the alpha-adrenergic system, will increase the afterload pressure, decreasing the gradient and thus the intensity of the dynamic outflow murmur.

4. (B) Specific heart defects associated with maternal PKU include left-sided heart defects (coarctation, hypoplastic left heart syndrome), tetralogy of Fallot, and sepal defects. The other defects listed are not commonly seen in maternal PKU. The degree of elevation of the maternal serum phenylalanine level has been shown to be predictive of congenital heart disease in the fetus.

5. (C) This child has Williams syndrome. Of patients with Williams Syndrome, 90% have a deletion identifiable at chromosome 7q11. This may not be readily identifiable on routine karyotype, but can be seen on FISH or microarray testing. Deletions on chromosome 11q23 cause Jacobsen syndrome. Deletions on chromosome 22q11.2 cause the constellation of disorders including DiGeorge syndrome and velocardiofacial syndrome. Both 1p36 and 8p23.1 are lesser recognized deletion syndromes that may result in patients with congenital heart disease.

6. (C) Holt–Oram syndrome is an autosomal dominant disorder caused by mutations of the *TBX5* gene. Patients most often present with abnormalities of the carpal bones of the wrist, which can include a malformed or missing thumb. Around 75% of patients have cardiac manifestations, the most common form being atrial septal defects.

7. (D) The most common viral causes of myocarditis are adenovirus and the enteroviruses, most commonly the Coxsackie viruses. CMV, parvovirus, influenza A, HSV, EBV, HIV, and RSV are other rare viral causes of myocarditis.

8. (C) Patients with DiGeorge syndrome have an increased risk of conotruncal abnormalities compared to the other syndromes listed, particularly interrupted aortic arch and truncus arteriosus. The most common type of interrupted aortic arch in these patients is the type B interruption, between the second carotid and the ipsilateral subclavian artery.

9. (E) The click described is an aortic ejection click, heard commonly in patients with bicuspid aortic valves. If accompanied by a suprasternal notch thrill, the stenosis is more likely to be valvular than subvalvar or supravalvular. A pulmonary valve ejection click may present similarly but with respiratory variation (louder with expiration). A nonejection systolic click may be heard in early systole in mitral valve prolapse with the patient standing, but will occur later in systole with squatting or supine position.

10. (C) The vignette is describing a patient with LEOPARD syndrome, characterized by (L) lentigines, (E) electrocardiographic conduction defects, (O) ocular hypertelorism, (P) pulmonary stenosis, (A) abnormal genitals, (R) retarded growth with subsequent short stature, and (D) deafness. LEOPARD syndrome is an autosomal dominant disorder and overlaps in many features with Noonan syndrome. Similar to Noonan syndrome, mutations in PTPN11 and RAF1 have been implicated in LEOPARD syndrome.

11. (C) The murmur described is a Still's murmur, a common innocent systolic murmur of childhood. Chest x-ray and electrocardiography are normal. The murmur is best heard when the patient is supine.

12. (A) Pericardiocentesis should be performed in patients with clinical tamponade (hypotension, low cardiac output, or pulsus paradoxus >10 mm Hg) and patients with bacterial pericarditis, with immunocompromised hosts, or for diagnosis when the etiology of an effusion is unclear. Asymptomatic effusions in patients with known diagnoses do not require pericardiocentesis unless in hemodynamic compromise. The diagnosis of viral pericarditis is not by itself an indication. In patients with bacterial pericarditis, the fluid may often be too thick to drain or may be loculated within the pericardium. In this case, a surgical intervention (pericardial window, pericardiectomy) should be considered.

Pulsus paradoxus is defined as a decrease in systolic blood pressure of greater than 10 mm Hg during inspiration. Normally during inspiration, systolic blood pressure decreases by 4 to 6 mm Hg due to decreased intrathoracic pressure and increased capacity of the pulmonary venous bed. With tamponade, the left ventricular diastolic volume is restricted by increased pericardial pressure, decreased pulmonary venous return, and shifting of the ventricular septum.

13. (B) Kartagener syndrome is an autosomal recessive disorder including situs inversus, bronchiectasis, and immotility of cilia in the respiratory tract. As a result, these patients have poor mucociliary clearance, increasing their risk of having lower and upper respiratory infections, particularly sinusitis, bronchitis, pneumonia, and otitis. Patients with DiGeorge syndrome may have an increased risk of infection secondary to T-cell dysfunction. Wiskott–Aldrich is an X-linked disorder characterized by thrombocytopenia, eczema, and immune deficiency. Carney complex is an autosomal dominant syndrome of skin hyperpigmentation, endocrine overactivity, and myxomas of the skin and heart.

14. (A) Type A interrupted arch occurs more commonly in patients with aortopulmonary septation defects and accounts for around one-third of patients with interrupted arch. Type B interruptions occur more commonly in patients with DiGeorge syndrome. Type C is much more rare than types A and B, accounting for <1% of patients with interrupted arch. The so-called type D is incompatible with life. See Figure 3.7.

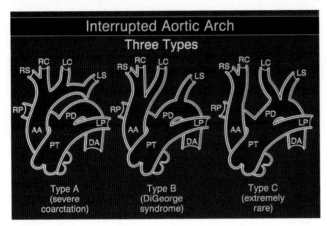

Interrupted Aortic Arch
Three Types

Type A
(severe
coarctation)

Type B
(DiGeorge
syndrome)

Type C
(extremely
rare)

FIGURE 3.7 PT = pulmonary trunk, AA = ascending aorta, PD = patent ductus, LP = left pulmonary artery, RP = right pulmonary artery, RS = right subclavian, RC = right carotid, LC = left carotid, LS = left subclavian, DA = descending aorta. Image courtesy of Dr. William Edwards, Mayo Clinic.

15. (C) Common causes of left axis deviation in infants include the AV canal defects (complete or partial) and tricuspid atresia, with or without transposition of the great vessels. Many patients with AV canal defects may have a more superior axis (−60 degrees to −100 degrees). Right axis deviation may be indicative of right ventricular hypertrophy in certain patients.

16. (D) When presented with a teenage patient with a persistent sinus tachycardia, common things to consider may include hyperthyroidism, substance abuse, pheochromocytoma, autonomic dysfunction, and tachyarrhythmias. Patients with eating disorders more commonly present with bradycardia. Hyperthyroidism is an important cause of resting tachycardia in a teenager and may present with heat intolerance, sweating, palpitations, weight loss, insomnia, and irritability. Pheochromocytoma will present with episodic symptoms of sweating hypertension, and tachycardia. If any dysmorphisms are present, consideration should be given for ordering a karyotype. Diabetes can produce an autonomic neuropathy which may involve an inappropriate tachycardia.

17. (D) The findings listed above are common in rheumatic fever. The nonpruritic lesions on her trunk refer to erythema marginatum, one of the major criteria for rheumatic fever. Other major criteria include carditis, chorea, polyarthritis, and subcutaneous nodules. Minor criteria include fever, arthralgias, prolongation of the PR interval on ECG, and elevated acute phase reactants (CrP, ESR).

18. (A) With coarctation, the blood pressures in the legs are typically lower than those in the upper extremities. The similar blood pressures in the right and left arm imply that the right and left subclavian arteries originate proximal to the coarctation. If there were a low blood pressure in the right arm (but not the left arm), there could be an aberrant right subclavian artery. Patients with AV canal defects and tetralogy of Fallot do not typically present with blood pressure discrepancies between the upper and lower extremities.

19. (E) There is a higher risk of developing necrotizing enterocolitis (NEC) in patients with truncus arteriosus and hypoplastic left heart syndrome. This is thought to be secondary to the relatively tenuous balance between systemic and pulmonary blood flow in these patients prior to surgical palliation or repair. Changes in physiology can markedly reduce the amount of systemic flow (due to preferential pulmonary flow) and cause gut ischemia and NEC.

20. (D) The patient is presenting with Beck's triad, including hypotension, muffled or distant heart sounds, and jugular venous distension, indicative of cardiac tamponade. Patients will be tachycardic and will show evidence of pulsus paradoxus.

21. (B) Pericardial effusions can result as a secondary process of many diseases, including rheumatic fever, lupus, and renal failure, or secondary to a lupus-like reaction to a medication like isoniazid or hydralazine. With this clinical vignette, the patient has a significant effusion with tamponade physiology (pulsus paradoxus is present), but has an unexpected bradycardia. In addition to the recent weight gain and fatigue, this is highly suggestive of hypothyroidism.

22. (A) The gene *NKX2.5* is located on chromosome 5q. Mutations in *NKX2.5* have been identified in familial cohorts of patients with atrial septal defects and conduction anomalies including heart block. Mutations in *TBX5* cause Holt–Oram syndrome, with associated large atrial septal defects and radial anomalies. Mutations in *MLL2* have been implicated in Kabuki syndrome. Mutations in *JAG1* cause Alagille syndrome. *PTNP11* is one of several genes which have been implicated in Noonan syndrome.

23. (A) The physical examination findings are consistent with an atrial septal defect with a large left to right shunt (as indicated by the diastolic flow rumble). In the presence of a diastolic rumble, the $Q_p:Q_s$ is at least 1.5:1 and likely higher. This type of large atrial septal defect will present more commonly with right-sided enlargement and is unlikely to close spontaneously. The expected right atrial enlargement may cause peaked p-waves seen on ECG.

24. (C) The patient is presenting with critical aortic stenosis, with a systolic ejection murmur, a prominent LV impulse, and poor peripheral perfusion. The current standard of care for these patients is a balloon aortic valvuloplasty to be performed in the cath lab. Use of an afterload reducer such as milrinone will result in worsening of the gradient.

25. (E) The most common type of cardiac tumor in children, and especially infants, is rhabdomyomas. Rhabdomyomas are well-circumscribed, noncapsulated, intramural, or intracavitary nodules that can occur in any location in the heart, most typically the ventricles. They may occur singly, but often several are found in the same patient. They have a characteristic "bright" appearance on echo.

26. (D) In patients with mild or moderate aortic stenosis, there is normal physiologic splitting of the S_2 sound. With severe aortic stenosis, there may be a single heart sound due to prolongation of left ventricular ejection time. In extremely severe cases, there may be paradoxical splitting of the S_2 sound.

27. (B) Patients with myxomas often present with a classic triad of symptoms: cardiac obstruction (80% of patients), embolism (~70% of patients), and systemic illness (~60% of patients). The masses are most often pedunculated and friable and occur most commonly in the left atrium. Myxomas can be found attached to the foramen ovale or either ventricle.

28. (D) The patient has Marfan syndrome, based on his enlarged aortic root/sinus of Valsalva and his systemic features. If he had a positive family history of Marfan syndrome, the aortic enlargement would be all that was needed to make a definitive diagnosis in him, even in the absence of systemic features. He should be followed with serial echocardiography for the remainder of his life (at least annually now that his aorta is dilated) and may be referred for surgery. He should have an eye examination to look for ectopia lentis. The normal extra-aortic vessels indicate that we are not likely dealing with Loeys–Dietz syndrome, though there is considerable overlap between all of the thoracic aortopathies.

29. (E) Patients with congenitally corrected transposition of the great arteries (CC-TGA) and those with polysplenia are most at risk for developing high-grade AV block. Patients with CC-TGA should be monitored closely over follow-up with regular ECGs and Holter monitors. Patients with polysplenia, or bilateral left-sidedness, often have other anatomical findings including dextrocardia, ventricular inversion, and an interrupted IVC. Due to underdevelopment of right-sided structures in polysplenia, nodal and conduction tissue is often affected in these patients, placing them at a high risk for complete AV block. This occurs more commonly in patients with polysplenia than patients with asplenia.

30. (C) The patient has been diagnosed with congenital polyvalvular dysplasia, a valvular developmental disorder that results in thickened leaflets with significant regurgitation and prolapse. It typically involves two or more valves, but can involve all four valves of the heart. This disorder most commonly occurs in patients with trisomy 18. In fact, at least 90% of patients with trisomy 18 have some form of valvular dysplasia. Many patients will have an associated ventricular septal defect or other congenital lesion.

31. (D) Patients with Turner syndrome and Noonan syndrome have a higher incidence of partial anomalous venous return. Additionally, patients with visceral heterotaxy, polysplenia, and asplenia have a high incidence of anomalous venous return.

32. (A) Depending on the study, up to 10% of patients with hypertrophic cardiomyopathy may have evidence of preexcitation. The other form of congenital heart disease with an increased incidence of WPW is Ebstein anomaly. Between 20% and 30% of patients with Ebstein anomaly will have Wolff–Parkinson–White syndrome, with left axis deviation and preexcitation, suggesting a right-sided accessory pathway.

33. (E) With worsening of pulmonary stenosis, the systolic murmur peaks later in systole and the split of the S_2 sound widens (the P2 sound is delayed). Once there is severe stenosis, the murmur spills over into diastole and the S_2 sound may become inaudible.

34. (B) The family history is consistent with Noonan syndrome, of whom up to 85% of patients may have congenital heart disease (most commonly pulmonary valvular stenosis, ASD, partial AV canal, coarctation, and hypertrophic cardiomyopathy). The right ventricular lift and short systolic ejection murmur suggest mild pulmonary valve stenosis, likely secondary to a thickened pulmonary valve. Bicuspid aortic valves and coarctation are common in Turner syndrome, and supravalvular pulmonary and aortic stenosis are common in Williams syndrome. Pulmonary branch stenosis is seen commonly in Alagille syndrome.

35. (D) Venous murmurs are more often benign and heard best over the upper chest. They change with head position or compression of the jugular vein and vary with respiration. The murmur is often heard loudest in the standing position.

36. (A) The murmur of aortic stenosis increases after a premature ventricular contraction (PVC). This is secondary to an increased gradient across the aortic valve, produced by enhanced diastolic filling during the compensatory pause of the PVC.

37. (A) Around 30% of patients with Turner syndrome have congenital heart disease, mostly involving the left-sided cardiac structures. Bicuspid aortic valve is the most common (15%), followed by coarctation (10%), and rarely mitral valve anomalies and hypoplastic left heart syndrome (<5%). Aortic root and ascending aorta dilatation are an issue as Turner patients get older, as there is a risk of aortic dissection and sudden death. As such, guidelines for management of patients with Turner syndrome advocate for routine screening with echocardiography, even in the absence of prior congenital heart disease.

38. (B) The chest radiograph displays rib notching bilaterally, as well as the "figure of 3" sign in the upper chest. These are relatively specific for the diagnosis of coarctation of the aorta. Urine metanephrines may be ordered if one is concerned for a pheochromocytoma, which may present with intermittent hypertensive, flushing, tachycardic, sweating episodes. If the arch is unable to be adequately visualized by transthoracic echo, then a stress echocardiogram is unlikely to provide further information.

39. (C) Around 80% of patients with congenitally corrected transposition will have a ventricular septal defect. These defects are typically perimembranous and subpulmonary and are due to atrial and septal malalignment. LVOT (subpulmonary ventricular outflow tract) obstruction occurs in 30% to 50% of patients. Morphologic tricuspid valve dysplasia is common as well in CC-TGA.

40. (D) In the presence of a normal coronary artery origins and a normal ventricular wall thickness, the most likely cause of death in this patient is long QT syndrome. The history of seizures and syncope are important, and the history of a drowning in the family also is more likely to implicate long QT syndrome. Any episode of syncope during maximal exertion requires evaluation for potential pathology.

41. (A) Due to variations in the location of the VSD and great arteries, double outlet right ventricle can present in several different ways. This patient is presenting with cyanosis but mildly increased pulmonary vascular markings. If the VSD were subaortic, there typically will not be cyanosis. If there were pulmonary stenosis, the pulmonary vascular markings should be normal or decreased. This patient therefore most likely has the Taussig–Bing anomaly, double outlet right ventricle with side-by-side great arteries and a subpulmonary VSD.

42. (B) Alagille syndrome is an autosomal dominant disorder that presents with particular facial features including a triangular-shaped face, broad forehead, and deep-set eyes. They tend to have butterfly vertebrae, a paucity of bile ducts, and many will require liver transplantation. The most common cardiac manifestations include peripheral pulmonary stenosis and tetralogy of Fallot.

43. (C) The murmur of obstruction heard in HCM will typically be increased with exercise, standing, and Valsalva maneuver. Increasing the systemic afterload pressure (handgrip, phenylephrine) will decrease the gradient and thus the intensity of the dynamic outflow murmur. Amyl nitrate is a potent vasodilator that can decrease afterload and increase the gradient, increasing the intensity of the murmur.

44. (D) The differentiation between HCM and "athlete's heart" can be difficult. Factors that favor the diagnosis of HCM include the presence of irregular hypertrophy (as opposed to pure concentric hypertrophy), normal sized LV diastolic dimensions, left atrial enlargement, abnormal ECG, abnormal LV diastolic function, family history of HCM, and female gender. A test of deconditioning can be performed, after which the LV thickness will resolve in those with the diagnosis of "athlete's heart."

45. (C) A severe form of myocarditis can be a complication of Chagas disease, caused by *Trypanosoma cruzi*. Chagas is endemic throughout much of Latin and South America, but is rarely seen in the United States except in recent immigrants.

46. (C) In restrictive cardiomyopathy, the atria are markedly enlarged. RVSP is often greater than 50 mm Hg, as opposed to constrictive pericarditis, where it is typically less than 50 mm Hg. The other options, including the presence of a septal bounce, equal RVEDP and LVEDP, and normal pulmonary vascular resistance index are more typical of constriction. Patients with restrictive cardiomyopathy will rarely show changes in Doppler flow velocities with inspiration and expiration.

47. (B) The murmur of rheumatic heart involvement of the mitral valve is typically high-pitched, holosystolic, heard best at the apex and radiating to the left axilla. The murmur will be heard best at the end of expiration while the patient is lying in the left lateral decubitus position.

48. (E) The clinical vignette is describing a patient with cri-du-chat syndrome (Lejeune syndrome), caused by a deletion of the short arm of chromosome 5 (5p–). The most common cardiac manifestations of cri-du-chat are VSDs, ASDs, PDAs, and tetralogy of Fallot.

49. (A) The major criteria for rheumatic fever (RF) may include erythema marginatum, carditis, chorea, polyarthritis, and subcutaneous nodules. Minor criteria include fever, arthralgias, prolongation of the PR interval on ECG, and elevated acute phase reactants (CrP, ESR). Migratory polyarthritis is the most common manifestation, affecting 40% to 70% of cases of RF. Carditis is also relatively common, affecting 30% to 60% of patients. Chorea is present in 10% to 30% of patients, while the two dermatologic findings occur in less than 10% of patients each.

50. (D) Ellis–van Creveld syndrome occurs most commonly among the Pennsylvania Amish community and includes skeletal and ectodermal dysplasias, including short stature, short limbs, hypoplastic or dysplastic fingernails, postaxial polydactyly, and neonatal or small teeth. It is caused by mutations in the *EVC* and *EVC2* genes on chromosome 4. Over half of these patients have congenital heart disease, of whom most have a large atrial septal defect or common atrium.

51. (A) Common training-related ECG findings include sinus bradycardia, first-degree AV block, incomplete right bundle branch block, early repolarization, and isolated QRS voltage criteria for LVH. Studies have reported that up to 10% to 40% of high school or college athletes may meet voltage criteria for LVH, despite having normal echoes. Left bundle branch block is uncommon and mandates further evaluation.

52. (C) The characteristic cardiac tumor in patients with tuberous sclerosis is rhabdomyoma. These patients are often asymptomatic, but may present with symptoms of obstruction if the tumors are large. The vast majority of these tumors will resolve without intervention. Surgical excision can be performed in patients with hemodynamic compromise or arrhythmia secondary to their rhabdomyomas.

53. (E) While most patients with tetralogy of Fallot do not have an identifiable genetic cause, 22q11.2 is the most commonly *identified* genetic cause, occurring in 20% of patients. Most deletions are de novo, but the inheritance pattern is autosomal dominant. Up to 10% are familial, with variable expressivity and incomplete penetrance.

54. (D) The double aortic arch commonly presents in infancy or in the first few months of life. The presentation will be earlier if both arches are widely patent and is later if one of the arches is hypoplastic. Patients with a retroesophageal left subclavian artery with right aortic arch do not have a technical vascular ring and rarely require treatment in the absence of other concerns. A retroesophageal right subclavian artery with a left aortic arch is the most common arch anomaly, occurring in 0.5% of the general population, but does not commonly cause symptoms in infancy. Left pulmonary artery slings will result in anterior indentation of the esophagus on barium swallow, but typically present with respiratory distress and stridor in the first few years of life. Persistent fifth aortic arch is extremely rare and may present incidentally on an imaging study, incidentally in conjunction with other congenital heart disease, or a pattern similar to coarctation.

55. (D) The typical friction rub is loudest when the heart is closest to the chest wall; this occurs when the patient leans forward, kneels, and inspires. The absence of a rub does not exclude pericarditis, especially in the presence of a large effusion.

56. (D) This child has Jacobsen syndrome, characterized by distinctive facial features (wide-spaced eyes, ptosis, small ears, short stature) and thrombocytopenia. Patients have a tendency to have life-threatening hemorrhages and are often followed in hemophilia clinics. Patients with Jacobsen syndrome can have ventricular septal defects, left-sided lesions (primarily involving the mitral and aortic valve), and other forms of congenital heart disease. This syndrome has also been named the "11q23 deletion syndrome."

57. (A) Pulmonary stenosis and patent ductus arteriosus are the two most common cardiac defects diagnosed in patients with congenital rubella syndrome. Patients may also present with ventricular septal defects or tetralogy of Fallot.

58. (C) The question is describing the click and murmur of mitral valve prolapse. In this setting, the murmur is typically preceded by the click. The click is heard in early or midsystole with the patient in the standing position, but moves later in systole with squatting or supine position. The aortic ejection click of a patient with a bicuspid valve is heard most often early in systole after S_1. A pulmonary valve ejection click may present similarly but with respiratory variation (louder with expiration). A rub is typically present in both systole and diastole.

59. (B) Up to 95% of patients with trisomy 18 will have some form of congenital heart disease (CHD), including polyvalvular dysplasia, ventricular septal defects, outlet abnormalities (tetralogy of Fallot, double outlet right ventricle), and AV canal defects. Patients with Down syndrome have a 40% chance of having CHD. Around 25% of Turner syndrome patients will have CHD, as will 80% of patients with 22q11 deletion (DiGeorge syndrome, velocardiofacial syndrome). Patients with 5p−, or cri-du-chat syndrome, have a 20% risk of having CHD.

60. (E) At least 50% of patients with interrupted aortic arch type B have a 22q11.2 deletion, compared to 35% of patients with truncus arteriosus, 24% of patients with isolated arch anomalies, 15% of patients with tetralogy of Fallot, and 10% of patients with perimembranous ventricular septal defects. Of all patients with a 22q11.2 deletion, around 80% are estimated to have some form of congenital heart disease.

61. (C) Hypertrophic cardiomyopathy is the most common cause of sudden death in athletes in the United States, affecting up to 44% of patients. Coronary artery anomalies are implicated in a further 17%, with myocarditis affecting 6% of patients. The ion channelopathies are implicated in 3% of cases.

62. (E) With coarctation, the blood pressures in the legs are typically lower than those in the upper extremities. A low blood pressure in the right arm (but not the left arm) suggests that the right subclavian artery originates distal to the coarctation, as occurs with an aberrant right subclavian artery.

63. (E) Retinoic acid, including other forms such as isotretinoin and etretinate, is commonly used in adolescents and young adults with acne and other skin conditions. Strict guidelines have been enacted due to the high risk of complex congenital heart anomalies (particularly conotruncal defects) in exposed fetuses. Extracardiac defects are also common.

64. (D) The diagram above shows evidence of large flow reversals in the descending aorta. This can be caused by a large ductus arteriosus, severe aortic insufficiency, or an intracranial arteriovenous malformation such as a vein of Galen malformation. Another potential cause of this is a large LV–aorta tunnel, which may arise above the right aortic sinus of Valsalva. Mitral regurgitant flow would be at a much higher velocity than is shown here.

Cardiac Catheterization and Angiography

Jason Anderson and Nathaniel W. Taggart

QUESTIONS

1. An 8-year-old boy was referred for a hemodynamic catheterization due to concern for pulmonary hypertension. The patient is sedated and intubated prior to the case on mechanical ventilation. Based upon the data in Table 4.1, which of the following best represents this patient's cardiac output?

   A. 2.2 L/min/m²
   B. 2.6 L/min/m²
   C. 3.2 L/min/m²
   D. 3.6 L/min/m²
   E. Unable to determine

2. A 6-month-old infant is referred for cardiac catheterization due to an inability to visualize the left pulmonary artery on transthoracic echocardiography. The angiograms in Figure 4.1 were obtained. What is the most likely diagnosis for this patient?

   A. Pulmonary atresia with VSD
   B. Tetralogy of Fallot
   C. Transposition of the great arteries
   D. Isolated ventricular septal defect
   E. Isolated branch pulmonary artery stenosis

TABLE 4.1 Cardiac Catheterization Data

Location	Pressure (mm Hg)	SpO₂ (%)
Superior vena cava		72
Inferior vena cava		70
Right atrium	Mean 5	70
Right ventricle	33/8	70
Left pulmonary artery	Mean 12	70
Left ventricle	80/10	99
Ascending aorta	84/50/68	99
Femoral artery	86/50/70	99
VO₂ (assumed) = 150 mL/min/m²		
ABG (femoral) = pH 7.35; pCO₂ 36; pO₂ 37		
Hemoglobin = 12 g/dL		

Ventricular pressures are shown as systolic/end-diastolic. Arterial pressures are shown as systolic/diastolic/mean.

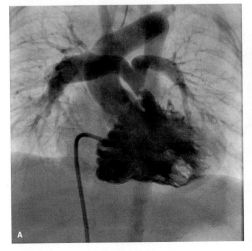
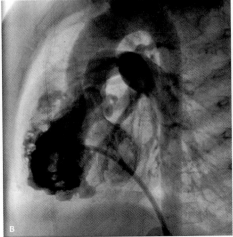

FIGURE 4.1

3. A 6-year-old boy with complex congenital heart disease (atrial situs solitus, visceral situs ambiguous, polysplenia, dextrocardia, single left SVC, partial AV canal defect) has undergone surgical baffling of the left SVC to the right atrium and subsequent stent implantation due to baffle stenosis. He is referred for catheterization. Based on the catheter course demonstrated in Figure 4.2, what additional diagnosis is likely present for in this patient?

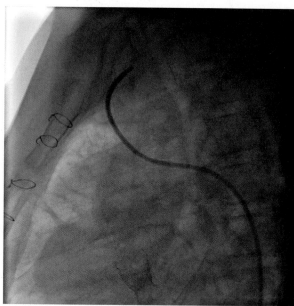

FIGURE 4.2

A. Interrupted aortic arch type A
B. Interrupted aortic arch type B
C. Interrupted aortic arch type C
D. Interrupted inferior vena cava
E. Fontan procedure

4. Which of the following abnormalities would most likely result in a prominent V wave on right atrial pressure tracing?

A. Tricuspid valve stenosis
B. Hypertrophic cardiomyopathy with severe septal hypertrophy
C. Atrial septal defect
D. Pulmonary valve regurgitation
E. Gerbode defect

5. A 17-year-old boy is undergoing an interventional cardiac catheterization when he manifests a change in the arterial pressure waveform (Fig. 4.3) and marked jugular venous distention. Which of the following interventions is most likely indicated at this time?

A. Removal of the guidewire
B. Repositioning of the endotracheal tube
C. Pericardiocentesis
D. External defibrillation
E. Lidocaine administration

6. An 18-year-old woman experiences headaches and urticaria 72 hours after implantation of a Amplatzer septal occluder device for closure of a moderate ASD. The only medication recommended postoperatively was aspirin,

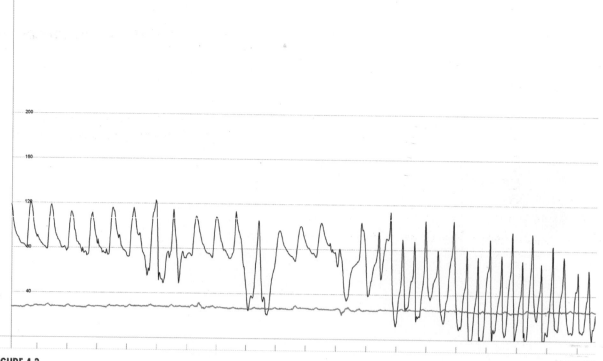

FIGURE 4.3

which she has tolerated without complication in the past. An allergic reaction to which of the following compounds would best explain her symptoms?

A. Titanium
B. Selenium
C. Copper
D. Stainless steel
E. Nickel

7. A 13-year-old boy undergoes ASD device closure utilizing a 22-mm Amplatzer septal occluder device with subsequent atrial tachycardia to 280 beats per minute with 2:1 AV conduction block. Which of the following statements is true regarding conduction abnormalities following ASD device closure?

A. Most resolve within the first 24 hours of device placement
B. Most resolve 2 weeks after device placement
C. Complete heart block occurs in approximately 5% of patients
D. Aspirin therapy should be continued indefinitely for any device-induced conduction abnormality
E. Friction from the device can cause extranodal AV pathways to develop

The following scenario applies to Questions 8 to 12:

Cardiac catheterization is performed on a 4-month-old infant from South America with an unrepaired congenital heart defect; hemodynamic data are shown in Table 4.2.

TABLE 4.2 Cardiac Catheterization Data

Location	Pressure (mm Hg)	SpO$_2$ (%)
Superior vena cava		64
Right atrium	12/14/10	68
Right ventricle	77/12	72
Left pulmonary artery	70/28/42	83
Right pulmonary artery	69/28/42	83
Left ventricle	69/12	95
Left atrium	12/13/11	99
Ascending aorta	76/34/49	83
Femoral artery	82/33/48	83
VO$_2$ (assumed) = 150 mL/min/m^2		
ABG (femoral) = pH 7.35; pCO$_2$ 36; pO$_2$ 51		
Hemoglobin = 17.4 g/dL		

Atrial and pulmonary capillary wedge pressures are shown as a-wave/v-wave/mean. Ventricular pressures are shown as systolic/end-diastolic. Arterial pressures are shown as systolic/diastolic/mean.

8. Based upon the hemodynamic data in Table 4.2, what is this patient's Q_p/Q_s?

A. 0.8
B. 1.2
C. 1.6
D. 2.0
E. Unable to calculate

9. Based upon the hemodynamic data in Table 4.2, which of the following most closely represents the volume of this patient's *left-to-right* shunt?

A. 0.8 L/min/m^2
B. 1.5 L/min/m^2
C. 2.2 L/min/m^2
D. 2.8 L/min/m^2
E. Unable to calculate

10. Based upon the hemodynamic data in Table 4.2, which of the following most closely represents the volume of this patient's *right-to-left* shunt?

A. 0.8 L/min/m^2
B. 1.5 L/min/m^2
C. 2.2 L/min/m^2
D. 2.8 L/min/m^2
E. Unable to calculate

11. Based upon the hemodynamic data in Table 4.2, what is this patient's pulmonary arteriolar resistance?

A. 4.2 Woods units × m^2
B. 7.8 Woods units × m^2
C. 9.1 Woods units × m^2
D. 14.1 Woods units × m^2
E. Unable to calculate

12. Which of the following diagnoses is most consistent with this clinical scenario?

A. Truncus arteriosus
B. Tetralogy of Fallot
C. Patent ductus arteriosus with Eisenmenger syndrome
D. Interrupted aortic arch with patent ductus arteriosus
E. D-transposition of the great arteries with large atrial septal defect

13. An 8-year-old patient with history of congenital heart disease undergoes cardiac catheterization. The angiogram in Figure 4.4 is obtained. Which of the following disorders is most commonly associated with the defect shown?

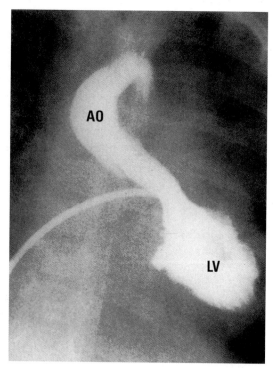

FIGURE 4.4 LV, left ventricle; Ao, aorta.

A. Marfan syndrome
B. Loeys–Dietz syndrome
C. Williams syndrome
D. Down syndrome
E. Ellis–van Creveld

14. A cyanotic newborn was taken for cardiac catheterization emergently. Angiography was performed (Fig. 4.5). Which of the following was the most likely indication for catheterization?

A. Balloon angioplasty of the aortic coarctation

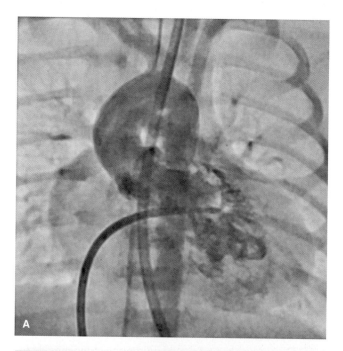

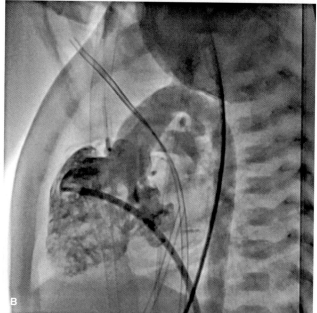

FIGURE 4.5

B. Balloon atrial septostomy
C. Balloon valvuloplasty of the aortic valve
D. Balloon valvuloplasty of the pulmonary valve
E. Delineation of the source of pulmonary blood flow

15. A 19-year-old man with dyspnea on exertion is referred for hemodynamic cardiac catheterization. Because of some abnormal hemodynamic findings, the angiogram in Figure 4.6 was obtained. Which of the following is demonstrated in the angiogram?

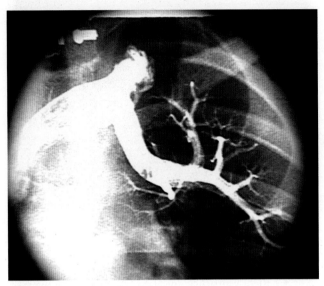

FIGURE 4.6

    A. Left SVC connecting to the coronary sinus
    B. PAPVC of the left upper pulmonary vein to the left SVC
    C. PAPVC of the left upper pulmonary vein to the innominate vein

    D. PAPVC of the left upper pulmonary vein to the coronary sinus
    E. MAPCA from the aortic arch to the left upper pulmonary artery

The following clinical scenario applies to Questions 16 to 19:

A 17-year-old girl presents with syncope during exertion. Physical examination is significant for a right ventricular lift and a single, loud S_2. Echocardiogram demonstrates a small ASD with small right-to-left shunt and a dilated, hypertrophied right ventricle with moderately decreased systolic function. Cardiac catheterization is performed, and the data are shown in Table 4.3.

16. Which of the following defects best explains the clinical and hemodynamic findings?

    A. Primary (idiopathic) pulmonary hypertension
    B. Anomalous pulmonary venous connections
    C. Ventricular septal defect
    D. Patent ductus arteriosus
    E. Anomalous right pulmonary artery from the ascending aorta

17. Based upon the hemodynamic data in Table 4.3, which of the following most closely represents Q_p/Q_s on room air?

    A. 0.3
    B. 0.5
    C. 0.7
    D. 0.9
    E. Unable to calculate

TABLE 4.3 Cardiac Catheterization Data

Location	Room Air Pressure (mm Hg)	Room Air SpO$_2$ (%)	Room Air pO$_2$ (mm Hg)	100% FiO$_2$ Pressure (mm Hg)	100% FiO$_2$ SpO$_2$ (%)	100% FiO$_2$ pO$_2$ (mm Hg)
IVC		68			74	
SVC		76			84	
RA	15/17/13	74		16/17/14	81	
RV	130/14	73		124/15	82	
MPA	126/88/107	72	35	120/82/100	78	44
LPA	125/87/106	72	35	119/80/99	78	44
RPA	127/86/106	72	35	121/77/99	78	44
LA	12/14/10	94		13/14/11	99	
LUPV		99	97		100	394
RUPV		99			100	
LV	114/11	96		106/11	98	
Asc Ao	110/76/88	96	83	102/71/83	98	93
Desc Ao	108/74/87	84		101/72/83	92	
VO$_2$ (assumed)	125 mL/min/m^2			125 mL/min/m^2		
Blood gas (pulm vein)	pH 7.38; pCO$_2$ 38; pO$_2$ 98; hemoglobin 12.5 g/dL			pH 7.40; pCO$_2$ 41; pO$_2$ 394; hemoglobin 12.5 g/dL		

18. Based upon the hemodynamic data in Table 4.3, which of the following most closely represents pulmonary vascular resistance on *room air*?

    A. 28 Woods units $\times$ m^2
    B. 31 Woods units $\times$ m^2
    C. 35 Woods units $\times$ m^2
    D. 42 Woods units $\times$ m^2
    E. Unable to calculate

19. Based upon the hemodynamic data in Table 4.3, which of the following most closely represents pulmonary vascular resistance on *100% FiO$_2$*?

    A. 19 Woods units $\times$ m^2
    B. 26 Woods units $\times$ m^2
    C. 31 Woods units $\times$ m^2
    D. 34 Woods units $\times$ m^2
    E. Unable to calculate

20. A child is referred for preoperative cardiac catheterization. The angiogram in Figure 4.7 is obtained. Which of the following connections is demonstrated in this angiogram?

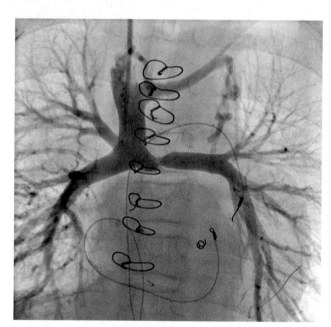

FIGURE 4.7

    A. Classic Blalock–Taussig shunt
    B. Modified Blalock–Taussig shunt
    C. Classic Glenn shunt
    D. Bidirectional Glenn shunt
    E. Damus–Kaye–Stansel anastomosis

21. A 12-month-old boy undergoes cardiac catheterization. The angiogram shown in Figure 4.8 is obtained. Which of the following is shown in the angiogram?

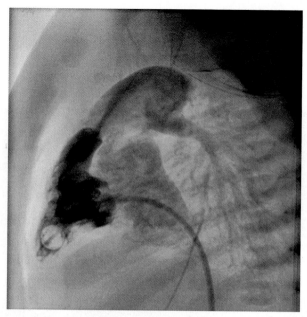

FIGURE 4.8

    A. Severe dynamic infundibular obstruction
    B. Poststenotic pulmonary artery dilation
    C. Right ventricular apical diverticulum
    D. Right ventricular outflow tract pseudoaneurysm
    E. Diverticulum of Kommerell

22. The angiogram shown in Figure 4.9 is obtained in an otherwise healthy, asymptomatic 8-month-old girl with an enlarged cardiac silhouette on chest x-ray. Based on these findings, which of the following is recommended for the patient?

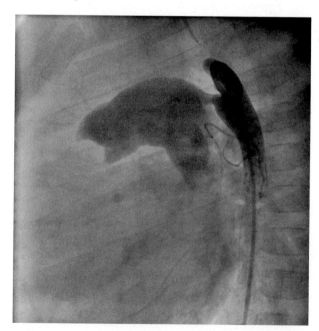

FIGURE 4.9

A. No further cardiology follow-up is necessary
B. Repeat catheterization in 6 to12 months
C. Transcatheter intervention
D. Oral diuretic therapy
E. Surgical referral for operative management

The following clinical scenario applies to Questions 23 and 24:

A 4-year-old boy with a history of surgical repair of anomalous origin of the right pulmonary artery from the ascending aorta developed proximal right pulmonary artery stenosis. Mean Doppler gradient across the stenosis is 13 mm Hg. Lung perfusion scan demonstrates 60% flow to the left lung and 40% to the right lung.

He undergoes cardiac catheterization. Hemodynamic catheterization performed prior to intervention produces the data shown in Table 4.4.

TABLE 4.4 Hemodynamic Cardiac Catheterization Data

Location	Pressure^a (mm Hg)	SpO$_2$ (%)
SVC		75
RA	7/6/5	78
RV	32/6	72
MPA	31/14/20	73
LPA	30/15/20	73
RPA	16/10/12	73
PCWP	10/12/8	
Femoral artery	108/74/87	99
VO$_2$ (assumed)	140 mL/min/m^2	
Blood gas (pulm vein)	pH 7.40; pCO$_2$ 40; pO$_2$ 100; hemoglobin 10.8 g/dL	

^{a}Pressures shown are a/v/mean for atrial/wedge pressures, systolic/end diastolic for ventricular pressures, and systolic/diastolic/mean for arterial pressures.

23. Based upon the hemodynamic data in Table 4.4, which of the following most closely represents this patient's cardiac index?
A. 3.2 L/min/m^2
B. 3.7 L/min/m^2
C. 4.0 L/min/m^2
D. 4.6 L/min/m^2
E. Unable to calculate

24. Based upon the hemodynamic data in Table 4.4, which of the following most closely represents this patient's pulmonary vascular resistance?
A. 1.8 Woods units × m^2
B. 2.2 Woods units × m^2
C. 2.7 Woods units × m^2
D. 3.2 Woods units × m^2
E. Unable to calculate

25. After assisting with an ASD closure utilizing a Gore Cardioform septal occluder in an adult patient, the primary team asks for follow-up recommendations prior to discharge. A chest x-ray was obtained on the morning of discharge (Fig. 4.10). Which of the following would you advise?

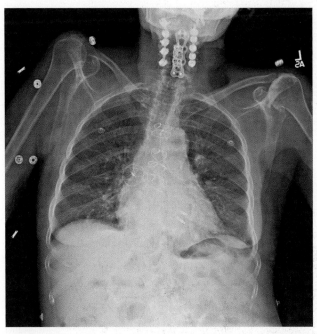

FIGURE 4.10

A. Continue aspirin therapy for 6 months
B. Continue aspirin therapy for 6 months and clopidogrel for 1 month
C. Initiate warfarin therapy
D. Device retrieval
E. Perform emergent pericardiocentesis

26. A newborn with Williams syndrome is referred for catheterization with angiography due to an inability to visualize the LPA on echocardiography. The patient is known to have severe supravalvar aortic stenosis and severe supravalvar pulmonary stenosis. This patient has an elevated risk over the general population for which of the following complications?
A. Access site complications
B. Cardiac perforation
C. Supraventricular tachycardia
D. Sudden death
E. None of the above

27. An adult congenital patient is referred for preoperative right and left heart catheterization. Prior to beginning the case, the patient is noted to be taking NPH insulin for diabetes. Which of the following agents should be avoided in this patient?

A. Fentanyl
B. Heparin
C. Lorazepam
D. Papaverine
E. Protamine

The following scenario applies to Questions 28 and 29:

A 12-year-old boy undergoes hemodynamic cardiac catheterization. Hemodynamic data obtained are shown in Table 4.5.

TABLE 4.5 Hemodynamic Cardiac Catheterization Data

Location	Pressure (mm Hg)	SpO₂ (%)
Inferior vena cava		70
Left innominate vein		92
Superior vena cava		80
Right atrium	8/6/4	74
Right ventricle	24/7	76
Main pulmonary artery	24/13/18	75
Left pulmonary artery	23/12/17	75
Right pulmonary artery	24/14/18	75
Left pulmonary capillary wedge	7/7/6	
Right pulmonary capillary wedge	12/11/10	
Left ventricle	97/11	99
Femoral artery	108/68/76	99

Atrial and pulmonary capillary wedge pressures are shown as a/v/mean. Ventricular pressures are shown as systolic/end diastolic. Arterial pressures are shown as systolic/diastolic/mean.

28. Which of the following defects best explains the discrepancy between right and left pulmonary capillary wedge pressures?

A. Anomalous pulmonary venous connection
B. Right pulmonary vein stenosis
C. Left pulmonary vein stenosis
D. Increased flow through the right pulmonary artery
E. Technical or equipment error

29. Which of the following additional findings is most likely based upon these hemodynamic data?

A. Sinus venosus atrial septal defect
B. Pulmonary sequestration
C. Left vertical vein
D. Unroofed coronary sinus
E. Right ventricular enlargement

30. A 12-year-old boy is referred for device closure of a secundum atrial septal defect. The preliminary plan is to close the lesion utilizing an Amplatzer septal occluder device in the cath lab. As part of the consent process, what is the appropriate incidence to cite for the complication of device erosion as a complication of the procedure?

A. 1 in 1,000,000
B. 1 in 100,000
C. 1 in 10,000
D. 1 in 1000
E. 1 in 100

31. A 10-year-old boy is referred for coarctation of the aorta. In considering the treatment options, which of the following early- to mid-term complications is more likely to occur from balloon angioplasty than aortic stent implantation or surgical repair?

A. Acute aortic wall injury
B. Arrhythmias
C. Access site arterial injury
D. Need for planned re-intervention
E. Need for unplanned re-intervention

32. An 18-year-old woman undergoes cardiac catheterization secondary to severe right ventricular enlargement with findings consistent with pulmonary hypertension on echocardiography. Figure 4.11 was obtained. What is the most commonly associated defect with this finding?

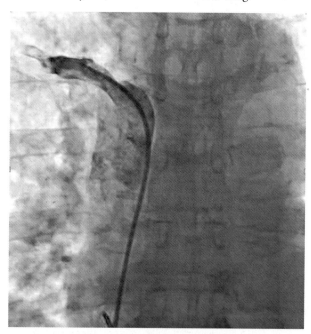

FIGURE 4.11

A. Scimitar syndrome
B. Secundum atrial septal defect
C. Sinus venosus atrial septal defect
D. Membranous ventricular septal defect
E. Partial AV canal defect

33. A 3-day-old male infant with d-TGA is referred for atrial septostomy. Following completion of the procedure, the aortic root angiogram in Figure 4.12 was obtained to define the coronary artery anatomy. Which of the following coronary artery arrangements is present?

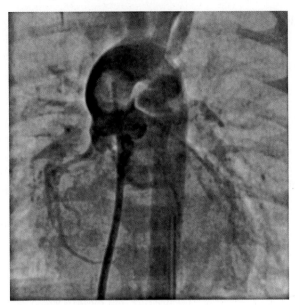

FIGURE 4.12

   A. Anomalous left coronary artery from the pulmonary artery
   B. Circumflex arising from the RCA
   C. LAD arising from the RCA
   D. Single origin of the coronary arteries
   E. Normal branching pattern of d-TGA

TABLE 4.6 Hemodynamic Cardiac Catheterization Data

Location	Pressure (mm Hg)	SpO$_2$ (%)
Superior vena cava		53
Right atrium	11/10/8	57
Left pulmonary vein	10/8/7	100
Left pulmonary vein wedge	Mean 14	
Right pulmonary vein	9/9/7	100
Right pulmonary vein wedge	Mean 14	
Left atrium	10/9/7	94
Left ventricle	84/9	82
Femoral artery	89/58/68	82

VO$_2$ (assumed) = 150 mL/min/m^2
ABG (femoral) = pH 7.37; pCO$_2$ 35; pO$_2$ 50
Hemoglobin = 16.2 g/dL

Atrial and pulmonary capillary wedge pressures are shown as a/v/ mean. Ventricular pressures are shown as systolic/end diastolic. Arterial pressures are shown as systolic/diastolic/mean.

The following scenario applies to Questions 34 and 35:

A 5-month-old girl with tricuspid atresia and normally related great arteries undergoes cardiac catheterization prior to bidirectional cavopulmonary anastomosis. Hemodynamic data are shown in Table 4.6.

34. Based upon the hemodynamics above, what is the Q_p/Q_s?
   A. 0.6
   B. 1.0
   C. 1.6
   D. 2.0
   E. Unable to calculate

35. What is this patient's pulmonary vascular resistance?
   A. 1.1 Woods units × m^2
   B. 1.4 Woods units × m^2
   C. 1.6 Woods units × m^2
   D. 1.8 Woods units × m^2
   E. Unable to calculate

36. A 3-year-old girl with tricuspid atresia and normally related great arteries post bidirectional cavopulmonary anastomosis and ligation of the main pulmonary artery undergoes cardiac catheterization prior to total cavopulmonary anastomosis. Hemodynamic data are shown in Table 4.7. Which of the following most closely represents this patient's Q_p/Q_s?

TABLE 4.7 Hemodynamic Cardiac Catheterization Data

Location	Pressure (mm Hg)	SpO$_2$ (%)
Superior vena cava	Mean 12	53
Left pulmonary artery	Mean 12	53
Right pulmonary artery	Mean 12	53
Right atrium	11/10/8	57
Left pulmonary vein	10/9/8	100
Right pulmonary vein	9/9/8	100
Left atrium	10/9/8	94
Left ventricle	84/9	82
Femoral artery	89/58/68	82

VO$_2$ (assumed) = 150 mL/min/m^2
ABG (femoral) = pH 7.37; pCO$_2$ 35; pO$_2$ 50
Hemoglobin = 16.2 g/dL

Atrial and pulmonary capillary wedge pressures are shown as a/v/ mean. Ventricular pressures are shown as systolic/end diastolic. Arterial pressures are shown as systolic/diastolic/mean.

   A. 0.6
   B. 0.8
   C. 1.2
   D. 1.6
   E. Unable to calculate

37. An infant is referred for preoperative cardiac catheterization and the angiogram in Figure 4.13 is obtained. What finding is demonstrated in this angiogram?

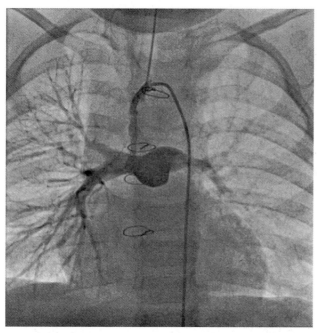

FIGURE 4.13

A. BT shunt
B. Sano shunt
C. Bidirectional Glenn
D. Extracardiac Fontan
E. Damus–Kaye–Stansel anastomosis

38. A 4-month-old male infant is referred for preoperative cardiac catheterization and the angiogram in Figure 4.14 is obtained. This angiogram demonstrates which of the following?

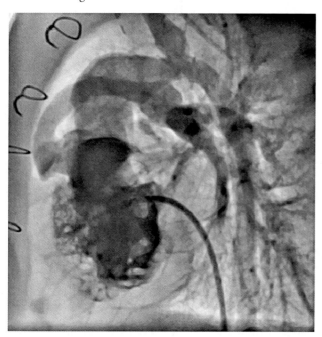

FIGURE 4.14

A. Classic Blalock–Taussig shunt
B. Modified Blalock–Taussig shunt
C. Sano shunt
D. Potts shunt
E. Waterston shunt

39. A 4-year-old boy with a history of repaired complete AV canal has severe left AV valve regurgitation. Accentuation of which of the following would be expected on the pulmonary capillary wedge tracing?

A. A wave
B. C wave
C. V wave
D. X descent
E. Y descent

40. On the RA waveform, the C wave corresponds to which of the following cardiac event?

A. Tricuspid valve closure with bowing of the valve into the atrium
B. Opening of tricuspid valve
C. Atrial filling with closed AV valve
D. Atrial contraction
E. Descent of AV valve ring into the ventricle

41. Which of the following events will decrease the hemoglobin affinity for oxygen?

A. Decrease in temperature
B. Decrease in 2,3-biphosphoglycerate levels
C. Decrease in pH
D. Decrease in pCO_2
E. Decrease in serum glucose concentration

42. During a routine right heart catheterization, the hemodynamic data in Table 4.8 are obtained. What is the most likely cause for the abnormal results obtained?

TABLE 4.8 Routine Right Heart Catheterization: Hemodynamic Data		
Location	**Pressure (mm Hg)**	**SpO$_2$ (%)**
Superior vena cava	Mean 5	74
Inferior vena cava	Mean 5	78
Right atrium	Mean 6	45
Right ventricle	37/13	75
Left pulmonary artery	Mean 12	75
Right pulmonary artery	Mean 12	75
Right pulmonary capillary wedge	Mean 6	99
VO$_2$ (assumed) = 150 mL/min/m^2		

Ventricular pressures are shown as systolic/end diastolic.

A. Improper catheter position
B. Anemia
C. Acidosis
D. Right-to-left shunt at the atrial level
E. Arteriovenous malformation

43. During a routine right heart catheterization, the hemodynamic data in Table 4.9 are obtained. What is the most likely cause for the abnormal results obtained?

TABLE 4.9 Routine Right Heart Catheterization: Hemodynamic Data

Location	Pressure (mm Hg)	SpO$_2$ (%)
Superior vena cava	Mean 5	64
Inferior vena cava	Mean 5	68
Right atrium	Mean 6	85
Right ventricle	37/13	85
Left pulmonary artery	Mean 12	85
Right pulmonary capillary wedge	Mean 6	99
Femoral artery	89/58/68	99
VO$_2$ (assumed) = 150 mL/min/m^2		
Cardiac output by thermodilution = 3 L/min/m^2		
Cardiac output by Fick = 2 L/min/m^2		

Ventricular pressures are shown as systolic/end diastolic. Arterial pressures are shown as systolic/diastolic/mean.

A. Technical error
B. Anemia
C. Acidosis
D. Left-to-right shunt at the atrial level
E. Nonsteady hemodynamic state

44. A 13-year-old boy from South America with pulmonary atresia and VSD with hypoplastic, confluent pulmonary arteries is referred for preoperative cardiac catheterization to evaluate the distribution of MAPCAs. Precath laboratory data demonstrate a hematocrit of 75%. Which of the following is the next best step to pursue?

A. Cancel the procedure; the risk of stroke is too high
B. Give the patient a dose of warfarin the evening prior to procedure
C. Admit the patient for IV fluid hydration the evening before procedure
D. No special precautions need to be taken
E. Perform the entire procedure on 100% FiO$_2$

The following scenario applies to Questions 45 and 46:

A 22-year-old with tetralogy of Fallot (TOF) had a complete repair at 5 years of age. The native pulmonary valve was initially preserved, but subsequently (age 14 years) he developed significant valvular stenosis and regurgitation, and the valve was replaced with a 27-mm porcine bioprosthesis. That valve has now developed severe regurgitation, and he undergoes cardiac catheterization with the plan to insert a transcatheter valve within the pulmonary bioprosthesis. The data in Table 4.10 are obtained during the study. No residual shunts were identified during the study.

TABLE 4.10 Cardiac Catheterization Data

Position	Pressure (mm Hg)
RA	Mean = 5
RV	60/8
MPA	60/8
PCWP	Mean = 20
LV	120/24

RA, right atrium; RV, right ventricle; MPA, main pulmonary artery; PCWP, pulmonary capillary wedge pressure; LV, left ventricle.

45. The data presented in Table 4.11 are most consistent with which of the following?

TABLE 4.11 Cardiac Data

Location	Pressure (mm Hg)	SpO$_2$ (%)
Superior vena cava		72
Right atrium	Mean 13	70
Right ventricle	60/16	70
Left pulmonary artery	60/12/34	70
Left pulmonary capillary wedge	Mean 18	99
Left ventricle	120/22	98
Ascending aorta	122/64/84	98
Femoral artery	124/64/86	98
VO$_2$ (assumed) = 150 mL/min/m^2		
ABG (femoral) = pH 7.35; pCO$_2$ 36; pO$_2$ 51		
Hemoglobin = 13 g/dL		

Atrial and pulmonary capillary wedge pressures are shown as mean. Ventricular pressures are shown as systolic/end diastolic. Arterial pressures are shown as systolic/diastolic/mean.

A. Mild pulmonary regurgitation
B. Moderate pulmonary valve stenosis
C. Restrictive physiology
D. Cardiac tamponade
E. Severe tricuspid regurgitation

46. Which of the following findings on the RA waveform would be consistent with a diagnosis of restrictive cardiomyopathy rather than constrictive pericarditis?

A. Presence of M waves
B. Inspiratory rise in RA pressure
C. Normal respiratory variation in mean RA pressure
D. Equalization of mean RA pressure with RVEDP, PA diastolic, PCWP, and LVEDP
E. Absence of the A wave

47. A 6-year-old boy is referred for a hemodynamic right heart catheterization secondary to progressive right atrial and right ventricular enlargement with no identifiable cause on echocardiography. An arterial blood gas was performed at the start of the case demonstrating hemoglobin of 12.5 gm/dL and pO_2 of 74 mL/dL. The oximetry data in Table 4.12 were obtained during the study. What is the ratio of pulmonary blood flow to systemic blood flow?

TABLE 4.12 Blood Oximetry Data

Site	Sat (%)
High right SVC	63
Low right SVC	88
Right atrium	73
Right ventricle	73
MPA	73
RPA	73
Femoral artery	98

A. 0.4
B. 0.7
C. 1.0
D. 1.4
E. 2.5

48. A 16-year-old patient from Africa has the chest radiograph in Figure 4.15. Which of the following pressure measurements would you expect to find during cardiac catheterization?

A. Mean RA pressure 10 mm Hg
B. RVSP 70 mm Hg
C. Mean PA pressure 20 mm Hg
D. PCWP 18 mm Hg
E. Ascending aorta 152/84 mm Hg

49. The following oxygen saturation data were obtained during a baseline hemodynamic study in an intubated 5-year-old patient: SVC, 72%; RA, 85%; RV, 83%; MPA = 83%; RPA = 84%; LA = 92%; RPV = 99%; LPV = 83%. Which of the following is the best next step?

A. Perform an LV angio to look for a VSD
B. Perform a PA angiogram to evaluate for a pulmonary AV fistula
C. Reevaluate the endotracheal tube position
D. Continue with the ASD device closure
E. Reverse his sedation

50. A 30-year-old woman with a history of tricuspid atresia and nonfenestrated Fontan procedure at age 5 years presents with a 2-year history of dyspnea on exertion and cyanosis that is worse when in the standing position. Which of the following is the most likely cause of her symptoms?

A. Hepatic arteriovenous malformation (AVM)
B. Vein of Galen malformation
C. Lower extremity AVM
D. Upper extremity AVM
E. Pulmonary AVM

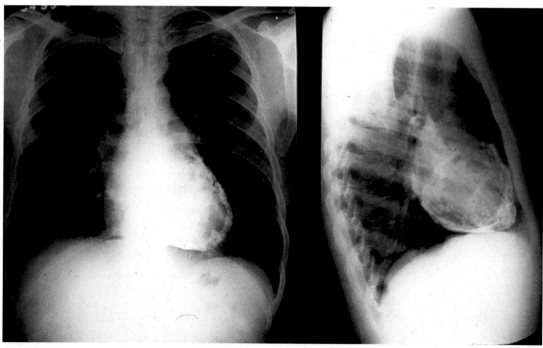

FIGURE 4.15

51. Which of the following patients has the strongest indication for catheter-based intervention?

  A. 20-year-old patient, asymptomatic, pulmonary valve mean Doppler gradient = 24 mm Hg

  B. 30-year-old patient with refractory migraines and a PFO

  C. 40-year-old patient, asymptomatic, pulmonary valve peak-to-peak gradient = 54 mm Hg

  D. 25-year-old patient, asymptomatic, with a continuous murmur and small PDA on echo

  E. 28-year-old patient with a small membranous VSD and recurrent endocarditis

52. A 6-month-old infant with severe aortic valve stenosis is undergoing cardiac catheterization with consideration of aortic valvuloplasty. His aortic valve annulus diameter is 9 mm. Which of the following balloon diameters is most appropriate for initial valvuloplasty?

  A. 6 mm

  B. 8 mm

  C. 10 mm

  D. 12 mm

  E. 14 mm

53. A 6-month-old infant with severe pulmonary valve stenosis is undergoing cardiac catheterization with consideration of pulmonary valvuloplasty. Her pulmonary valve annulus diameter is 9 mm. Which of the following balloon diameters is most appropriate for initial valvuloplasty?

  A. 8 mm

  B. 9 mm

  C. 10 mm

  D. 12 mm

  E. 15 mm

54. A full-term infant with complete TGA and a pH of 7.1 is in the cath lab for balloon atrial septostomy. After vascular access is obtained, which of the following is the best management of this situation?

  A. Balloon atrial septostomy should be performed promptly

  B. Obtain mixed venous saturation in the RA

  C. Perform RV angiography to evaluate coronary anatomy

  D. Perform RA angiography to assess right-to-left shunt

  E. The procedure is not required when patients have a coexistent VSD

55. In an asymptomatic 6-year-old girl the transthoracic echocardiographic images in Figure 4.16 were obtained.

  You are counseling the parents regarding type and timing of intervention. Based upon the images shown, what would you say to the patient?

  A. This is a sinus venosus defect and therefore not amenable to device closure

  B. The defect is well centered and should be easily closed with a device

  C. Closure is not indicated at this time due to the absence of significant right ventricular enlargement

  D. The defect is large and some rims are deficient preventing device closure

  E. Surgery is indicated to repair the anomalous pulmonary vein(s)

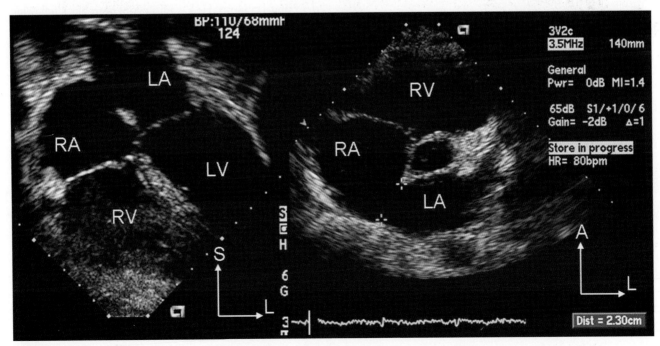

FIGURE 4.16 RA, right atrium; RV, right ventricle; LA, left atrium; LV, left ventricle.

56. You are assessing a 5-year-old girl for possible PDA closure. Echocardiogram shows a large PDA with bidirectional shunting. There is no murmur on examination. Her echo is otherwise normal with no tricuspid regurgitation and no chamber enlargement. Her parents report she is a quiet child but does not seem to be limited in any way. What is the next best step?

  A. Surgical closure of her PDA
  B. Transcatheter closure of her PDA
  C. Return in 3 years for follow-up echo evaluation
  D. Return in 6 to 12 months for follow-up echo
  E. Hemodynamic cardiac catheterization

57. A newborn with an in utero diagnosis of pulmonary atresia with intact ventricular septum is admitted to the NICU. An echocardiogram confirms the diagnosis. The infundibulum appears unobstructed. There is a mild pulmonary valve hypoplasia with no systolic or diastolic flow across the annulus. The RV is small with systolic pressure. The tricuspid valve is hypoplastic with a Z score = −2.5 with moderate regurgitation. The left ventricle has normal size and function. The coronary arteries were not well identified. A large ASD with right-to-left shunting is noted. The patient has a cardiac catheterization to perform radiofrequency perforation and balloon valvuloplasty. The angiogram in Figure 4.17 was obtained. What should be the next step for this patient?

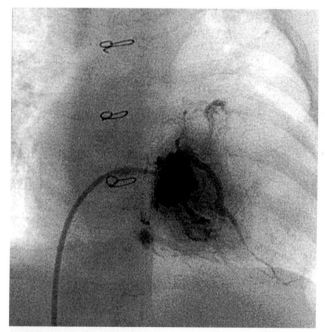

FIGURE 4.17

  A. Dilation of the right coronary artery
  B. Balloon atrial septostomy
  C. Abort perforation and balloon valvuloplasty
  D. Refer for surgical pulmonary valvotomy
  E. Perform pulmonary valvuloplasty with MPA stent placement

58. A 17-year-old patient with no significant past medical history presents with a transient ischemic attack. She had a similar episode 2 years prior but failed to report that event. During the workup, she is found to have a 5-mm secundum ASD with predominant left-to-right shunt, but does have transient right-to-left shunt. Tests for hypercoagulable disorders were negative. The patient is a Jehovah Witness. According to the AHA guidelines, what would you recommend for management of the ASD?

  A. Recommend device closure of the ASD
  B. Recommend observation and treatment with aspirin
  C. Recommend observation alone
  D. Recommend observation and treatment with warfarin
  E. Recommend surgical closure

59. Which of the following lesions with a restrictive atrial communication would be at highest risk of complication with balloon atrial septostomy?

  A. Hypoplastic left heart syndrome
  B. d-TGA with intact ventricular septum
  C. Tricuspid atresia
  D. d-TGA with VSD
  E. Total anomalous pulmonary venous connection

60. A 25-year-old man presents to your clinic with exertional cyanosis. He has a history of heart block following Mustard palliation of d-TGA and required intravenous pacemaker lead placement. He has an echo which reveals a small SVC baffle leak with bidirectional shunting. Which of the following is the most appropriate next step for this patient?

  A. Attempt transcatheter closure of the baffle leak
  B. Surgical closure of the baffle leak
  C. Initiate warfarin therapy indefinitely
  D. Pacemaker externalization
  E. No additional treatment is necessary

61. During cardiac catheterization, a child with coarctation of the aorta is found to have a systolic gradient <20 mm Hg, meeting criteria for a mild coarctation. Which of the following findings may result in underestimation of the severity of coarctation by gradient alone?

   A. CI = 1.5 L/min/m^2 by thermodilution
   B. Right pulmonary capillary wedge pressure of 8 mm Hg
   C. Right pulmonary artery stenosis with inability to pass a wire to the distal RPA
   D. LV end diastolic pressure of 12 mm Hg
   E. ABG demonstrating pCO$_2$ of 68 mm Hg at the start of the case

62. A colleague requests a cardiac catheterization on an infant with diastolic heart failure due to dilated cardiomyopathy in association with 3-methylglutaconic aciduria type II. Prior to proceeding with cardiac catheterization, which of the following laboratory abnormalities should be ruled out?

   A. Thrombocytopenia
   B. Thrombocytosis
   C. Anemia
   D. Neutropenia
   E. Hyperglycemia

ANSWERS

1. (C) In order to solve this problem, the Fick principle must be incorporated. It is absolutely vital to know this equation, and the scenarios to follow throughout the chapter will continue to expand on the utility of this principle. This equation is listed below for systemic flow but can be adapted to pulmonary blood flow in the presence of a shunt by interchanging pulmonary vein (PV) – pulmonary artery (PA) for systemic artery (SA) – mixed venous (MV).

$$\text{Systemic flow (indexed)} = \frac{O_2 \text{ consumption (VO}_2)}{\text{oxygen content}_A - \text{oxygen content}_V}$$

$$\text{Systemic flow (indexed)} = \frac{O_2 \text{ consumption (VO}_2)}{(SA - MV)O_2 \times O_2 \text{ bound to Hgb} + \text{dissolved } O_2}$$

$$\text{Systemic flow (indexed)} = \frac{O_2 \text{ consumption (VO}_2)}{(SA - MV)O_2 \times Hgb \times 1.36 \times 10}$$

$$\text{Systemic flow (indexed)} = \frac{150 \text{ mL/min/m}^2}{(0.99-0.70)O_2 \times 12 \text{ g/dL} \times 1.36 \times 10 \text{ dL/L}}$$

$$\text{Systemic flow (indexed)} = \frac{150 \text{ mL/min/m}^2}{46.6 \text{ mL } O_2/L}$$

$$\text{Systemic flow (indexed)} = 3.2 \text{ L/min/m}^2$$

If the patient is not on supplemental oxygen, the dissolved pO_2 can be ignored as it will be negligible to the final result. The value 1.36 represents the Hüfner factor (oxygen-binding capacity of human hemoglobin). By utilizing the given VO_2 and hemoglobin, along with the systemic arterial sat (LV of 99%; SA = 0.99) and mixed venous sat (RPA of 70%; MV = 0.70), the systemic flow is calculated as 3.2 L/min/m².

2. (B) The catheter course from the IVC to the RA and to the anterior ventricle is consistent with a right ventricular angiogram. There is moderate enlargement of the RV with severe RV outflow tract obstruction at the subpulmonary and pulmonary valve levels with hypoplasia of the main and branch pulmonary arteries. There is right-to-left shunting through the VSD with opacification of the aorta. These findings in constellation are consistent with a diagnosis of tetralogy of Fallot.

3. (D) Figure 4.2 is taken from a straight lateral projection. The catheter in this image is located quite posterior (well over the vertebral bodies) and courses cranially, eventually taking an anterior turn. This position is posterior to the descending aorta, which is located along the anterior aspect of the vertebral bodies, as demonstrated on an LV angiogram from the same case (Fig. 4.18). The catheter is coursing through an azygous vein with the anterior turn located at the anastomosis with the superior vena cava. Azygous continuation into the right or left SVC is seen with interrupted IVC occurring embryologically due to failure to form the right subcardinal-hepatic anastomosis. This venous malformation does not result in clinical manifestations but can complicate interventional cath and EP procedures.

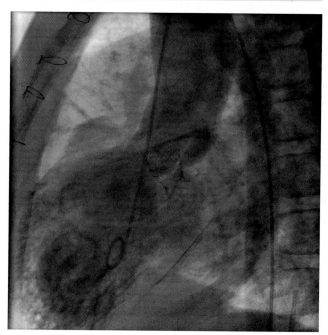

FIGURE 4.18

4. (E) The congenital left ventricle to right atrial shunt (Gerbode defect) would result in enhanced right atrial filling during AV valve closure through ventricular systole. The same finding would be expected in the presence of severe tricuspid valve regurgitation, as seen with Ebstein anomaly. A prominent A wave would be expected for lesions causing RV diastolic dysfunction or obstruction to RV inflow, such as tricuspid valve stenosis.

5. (C) This waveform demonstrates rapid onset hypotension and tachycardia consistent with impaired cardiac output due to cardiac tamponade. The cause is likely hemopericardium due to a complication from catheterization. Sudden circulatory collapse warrants immediate pericardiocentesis and may necessitate drain placement.

6. (E) The metal frame of the Amplatzer® device is made from nitinol, a nickel–titanium alloy. Detectable levels of nickel have been identified in the bloodstream after successful Amplatzer device placement, and allergic reactions have been reported, albeit rarely. The estimated rate for nickel hypersensitivity in the general population is 15%.

7. (A) ECG abnormalities after ASD closure device placement have been reported in 5% to 10% of patients. The incidence appears higher in older patients as compared to children and the vast majority of these abnormalities resolve, especially in children, typically resolving within 24 hours of the procedure. Heart block is a very rare complication from ASD device closure.

8. (B) In room air, Q_p/Q_s can be calculated if you know the mixed venous saturation (MV), systemic arterial saturation (SA), pulmonary venous saturation (PV), and pulmonary arterial saturation (PA) by using the following equation: $Q_p/Q_s = (SA - MV)/(PV - PA)$. For this patient, superior vena cava is the best choice for MV (right atrium is not a mixed chamber), and left atrium can be used at PV because the saturation is near 100%. If left atrial saturation is low (e.g., less than 96%) then one must consider the possibility of a right-to-left shunt at the atrial level. Using these values, $Q_p/Q_s = (0.83 - 0.64)/(0.99 - 0.83) = 1.18$.

9. (C) To calculate shunt volume or shunt percentage, you need to know the *effective pulmonary blood flow* (Q_{ep}), which is the volume of systemic venous blood that goes to the lungs. Left-to-right shunt volume (Q_{L-R}) is then calculated by subtracting Q_{ep} from Q_p. Q_{ep} is calculated by dividing VO_2 by the difference in pulmonary venous (PV) and mixed systemic venous (MV) oxygen content. For this patient, VO_2 is 150 mL/min/m^2. Ignoring dissolved oxygen, the PV − MV oxygen content difference is $1.36 \times 10 \times 17.4 \times (0.99 - 0.64) = 83$ mL/L. Therefore, $Q_{ep} = 150/83 = 1.8$ L/min/m^2. Q_p is $150/[1.36 \times 10 \times 17.4 \times (0.99 - 0.83)] = 4.0$ L/min/m^2. Q_{L-R} is the difference between Q_p and Q_{ep}, or *2.2 L/min/m^2*.

10. (B) Since effective pulmonary blood flow (Q_{ep}) = effective systemic blood flow (Q_{es}) = 1.8 L/min/m^2, right-to-left shunt volume (Q_{R-L}) can be calculated in a similar manner to that described in the previous answer. Using the superior vena cava as mixed venous saturation and ignoring dissolved oxygen, $Q_s = 150/[1.36 \times 10 \times 17.4 \times (0.83 - 0.64)] = 3.3$ L/min/m^2. Q_{R-L} is the difference between Q_s and Q_{es}, or *1.5 L/min/m^2*.

11. (B) Pulmonary arteriolar resistance is calculated by dividing the mean pressure gradient through the pulmonary bed (PA$_{mean}$ − LA$_{mean}$) by Q_p. In this case the transpulmonary gradient is $42 - 10 = 31$ mm Hg and $Q_p = 4.0$ L/min/m^2, so PVR = 7.8 Woods units × m^2.

12. (A) There are four main hemodynamic abnormalities present—pulmonary hypertension, increased pulmonary artery saturation (left-to-right shunting), systemic arterial desaturation (right-to-left shunting), and a widened pulse pressure. The fact that right ventricular and left ventricular saturations are significantly different, but pulmonary artery and aorta saturations are the same, tells us that most of the mixing is occurring at the level of the great arteries, as is seen with truncus arteriosus. Tetralogy of Fallot will have differential systemic and pulmonary artery saturations due to preferential streaming of blood in the ventricles to the ipsilateral great artery. PDA with Eisenmenger syndrome can produce right-to-left shunting, but ascending aorta saturation would be expected to be higher than descending aorta. Interrupted aortic arch with PDA can cause pulmonary hypertension and descending aorta desaturation, but ascending aorta saturation should be relatively normal in the absence of other defects. Transposition of the great arteries with a large ASD can cause mixing of systemic and pulmonary venous blood, but not typically enough that aortic and pulmonary artery saturations are the same.

13. (D) The catheter is advanced from the RA across an ASD to the LA and subsequently the LV. The angiogram demonstrates elongation of the LV outflow tract (the "goose neck" deformity). This finding is present in patients with an AVSD due to the anterior displacement of the aortic valve, creating an elongated LVOT and predisposing the patient to progressive subaortic obstruction. Roughly 40% to 45% of children with Down syndrome will have

congenital heart disease, with approximately 45% having an AVSD. The other answer choices reference primary aortic disease (Marfan and Loeys–Dietz), supravalvar AS and branch PA stenoses (Williams), and large ASD that commonly causes a common atrium (Ellis–van Crevald).

14. (B) The catheter traverses from the IVC to the RA and to the anterior ventricle. The angiogram demonstrates that the anterior ventricle gives rise to the aortic outflow tract, consistent with transposition of the great arteries and the question stem is consistent with TGA with intact ventricular septum and inadequate intercirculatory mixing. Catheterization is not indicated for a newborn with TGA, unless there is severe hypoxia with an inability to provide oxygenation via the native atrial communication or a patent ductus arteriosus with PGE1 administration. In this clinical scenario, balloon atrial septostomy precedes early arterial switch procedure.

15. (C) The left upper pulmonary vein was injected demonstrating a PAPVC with drainage of the LUPV via a vertical vein to the left innominate vein. The innominate vein is the usual site for connection of an anomalous left pulmonary vein. The vertical vein demonstrated in this angiogram is separate embryologically from a left-sided SVC, with a LSVC located directly posterior to the left atrial appendage and draining to the coronary sinus. Much less common sites of PAPVC of the left pulmonary veins would include the coronary sinus, right SVC, left SVC, and azygous vein.

16. (D) This patient has severe pulmonary hypertension both clinically and hemodynamically. While there is a small atrial level shunt (demonstrated echocardiographically and by a small "step-down" in saturation from pulmonary vein to left atrium and left ventricle), the striking hemodynamic abnormalities are suprasystemic pulmonary artery pressure and a significant "step-down" in saturation from ascending aorta to descending aorta." The most likely explanation for this finding is a right-to-left shunt between the ascending and descending aorta, such as a PDA or aortopulmonary window. Primary (idiopathic) pulmonary hypertension would be a consideration in the absence of a significant shunt lesion. The saturation step-down occurs at the level of the great arteries, making anomalous pulmonary veins (an "atrial" level shunt) and ventricular septal defect less likely. Anomalous origin of the right pulmonary artery from the aorta (so called "hemitruncus") can result in pulmonary hypertension/Eisenmenger syndrome, but invasive hemodynamics would demonstrate right pulmonary artery saturation equal to aortic, and a lower left pulmonary artery saturation.

17. (E) While there are sufficient data to calculate Q_p, the available data are inadequate to calculate Q_s. Just like the Fick principle cannot be used to calculate pulmonary blood flow in situations where there are multiple sources of pulmonary blood flow, each with different oxygen content (e.g., tetralogy of Fallot with a surgical aortopulmonary shunt), in this patient, systemic arterial blood flow is derived from both the ascending aorta (higher oxygen content) and the ductus arteriosus (lower oxygen content). Without knowing the proportion of blood flowing to the brachiocephalic arteries relative to the proportion flowing to the descending aorta, we cannot account for this difference in oxygen content by the Fick equation alone.

18. (C) Pulmonary arteriolar resistance is calculated by dividing the pressure difference through the pulmonary bed by pulmonary blood flow (Q_p). The pressure difference through the pulmonary bed is calculated by subtracting the *mean* pulmonary artery pressure (in this case RPA = LPA = 106 mm Hg) from the mean left atrial (10 mm Hg) or pulmonary capillary wedge pressure. Q_p is calculated using the Fick equation, where oxygen consumption (VO_2) is divided by the change in blood oxygen content across the pulmonary capillary bed. The change in oxygen content is calculated by multiplying Hüfner factor for the oxygen-binding capacity of hemoglobin (1.36 mL O_2/g hemoglobin) by the hemoglobin concentration in blood (12.5 g/dL), multiplied by a factor of 10 (to convert dL to L), multiplied again by the difference in hemoglobin saturation before (pulmonary artery = 72% or 0.72) and after (pulmonary vein = 99% or 0.99) the capillary bed. On room air, a small amount of oxygen is dissolved in blood (pO_2); this can be disregarded. In the presence of a higher concentration of inhaled oxygen, pO_2 can be significantly greater and should be included in the calculation. For this patient, the denominator of the Fick equation is $1.36 \times 12.5 \times 10 \times (0.99 - 0.72) = 45.9$. Dividing 125 ($VO_2$) by 45.9 results in an indexed $Q_p = 2.72$ $L/min/m^2$. Pulmonary vascular resistance is then calculated by dividing 96 mm Hg by 2.72 L/min/m² = *35.2 Woods units* $\times$ m².

19. (D) When inhaled oxygen is increased, the relative contribution of dissolved oxygen to total blood oxygen content likewise increases and should be factored into the Fick equation for calculating Q_p. Dissolved oxygen is calculated as $0.003 \times pO_2$. For this patient pulmonary vein oxygen content is $1.36 \times 12.5 \times 10 \times (100\%) + 0.03 \times 394 = 182$ mL O_2/L blood. Pulmonary artery oxygen content is $1.36 \times 12.5 \times 10 \times (78\%) + 0.03 \times 44 = 134$ mL O_2/L blood. Dividing VO_2 by the difference in oxygen content = $125/(182 - 134) = 2.60$ $L/min/m^2$. Pulmonary vascular resistance is then calculated by dividing the pressure difference (99 mm Hg − 11 mm Hg) by Q_p; 88/2.60 = *34 Woods units* $\times$ m².

20. (D) The angiogram demonstrates an injection of the right SVC with a cavopulmonary anastomosis communicating with the right and left pulmonary arteries, consistent with a bidirectional Glenn shunt. There is also stenosis along the left side of the PA insertion of the SVC, a common complication encountered following this procedure. The other options are incorrect and include the classic BT shunt (right subclavian to RPA anastomosis with native vessel), modified BT shunt (right subclavian to RPA anastomosis with artificial material), classic Glenn shunt (RSVC to distal RPA anastomosis supplying a single lung), and DKS anastomosis (transected MPA anastomosed with the ascending aorta).

21. (B) This lateral projection demonstrates an RV injection with pulmonary valve stenosis causing a small, anteriorly directed jet streaming to the MPA with poststenotic dilation of the MPA. The exact mechanism for poststenotic dilation remains controversial, but is likely a result of multiple hemodynamic factors including high velocity and turbulent blood flow accompanied by remodeling of the vascular wall. The other options (A, C, D) address RV pathology, with a normal appearing RV on this angiogram. The diverticulum of Kommerell is a term referencing the bulbous configuration of the origin of an aberrant left subclavian artery in a right-sided aortic arch or aberrant right subclavian artery in the setting of a left-sided aortic arch.

22. (C) The angiogram is a lateral projection demonstrating retrograde access for a left heart catheterization with an angiogram performed in the proximal descending aorta. There is left-to-right shunting through a patent ductus arteriosus to the left pulmonary artery. All symptomatic PDAs with left-to-right shunting and asymptomatic PDAs with LA or LV enlargement should be closed, regardless of age.

23. (B) As described previously, cardiac output (index) is calculated using the Fick equation. Oxygen consumption (VO_2) is divided by the difference in blood oxygen concentration across the capillary bed. In this case cardiac index is $140/1.36 \times 10.8 \times 10 \times (0.99 - 0.73) = 3.7$ $L/min/m^2$.

24. (A) In the presence of unequal branch pulmonary artery pressures, the Fick equation can still be used to calculate Q_p, but consideration of the proportion of flow going to one lung or the other is needed to calculate an accurate pulmonary arteriolar resistance. To accomplish this, we use the data from the lung perfusion scan (40% flow to the right lung; 60% to the left) and calculate the resistance for each lung individually. The flow to the right lung is 40% of 3.7 L/min/m² or 1.5 L/min/m². The arteriolar resistance of the right lung (R_{right}) is 2.7 Woods units $\times$ m². Similarly, the flow to the left lung is 2.2 L/min/m² and the resistance (R_{left}) is 5.5 Woods units $\times$ m². Because the lungs form a parallel circuit, total pulmonary arteriolar resistance is calculated by the following equation: $1/R_{total} = 1/R_{right} + 1/R_{left}$. Thus the total resistance is $(1/2.7 + 1/5.5)^{-1} = 1.8$ Woods units $\times$ m².

25. (D) The ASD closure device has embolized to the right pulmonary artery. This is demonstrated by the device borders extending beyond the borders of the cardiac silhouette. Emergency retrieval is indicated and may be performed percutaneously or via an open surgical approach.

26. (D) A thorough preoperative evaluation is recommended for patients with Williams syndrome to identify those with anatomical abnormalities which may result in coronary artery involvement. Even without evidence of coronary abnormalities on preoperative imaging, these patients remain at risk for sudden cardiac arrest and death, which must be considered when discussing the risk–benefit ratio of cardiac catheterization or any procedure that requires sedation. During sedation or anesthetic induction, patients with supravalvar aortic stenosis can experience coronary artery malperfusion and ischemia, leading to ventricular dysfunction and impaired cardiac output. If not promptly recognized and treated, death can occur.

27. (E) Patients taking NPH insulin are at an increased risk of hypersensitivity reaction to protamine, with an incidence of a reaction in 27% of patients compared to 0.5% in patients with no history of taking insulin. Reactions to protamine can range from back/flank pain, flushing, and peripheral vasodilation to vasomotor collapse, which may be fatal.

28. (A) This patient has an anomalous left pulmonary vein draining to the left innominate vein. This manifests as elevated left innominate vein saturation, representing drainage of the anomalous vein(s) to the innominate vein via a vertical vein. Because the right pulmonary veins drain to the left atrium, the right capillary wedge pressure will

CHAPTER 4 CARDIAC CATHETERIZATION AND ANGIOGRAPHY • 93

reflect left atrial pressure. The left pulmonary vein(s), on the other hand, ultimately drain to the right atrium. Therefore, left capillary wedge pressure will reflect right atrial pressure (in the absence of vertical vein obstruction). Right or left pulmonary vein stenosis would manifest as a gradient between ipsilateral pulmonary capillary wedge pressure and left atrial pressure or left ventricular diastolic pressure. In addition, pulmonary vein stenosis would not explain the elevated innominate vein saturation. There is no evidence to suggest increased right pulmonary artery flow or technical error.

29. (C) As explained in the answer to the previous question, this patient has evidence of anomalous pulmonary vein drainage to the left innominate vein. Therefore, the patient is almost certain to have a draining left vertical vein. Sinus venosus atrial septal defect is much more common with anomalous right pulmonary veins draining directly to the superior vena cava or right atrium. Pulmonary sequestration is often seen in Scimitar syndrome, in which the anomalous pulmonary vein typically drains inferiorly to the inferior vena cava. An unroofed coronary sinus is rare and is more commonly associated with a persistent left superior vena cava. Right ventricular enlargement may occur as a result of significant left-to-right shunt over time, but this patient's overall shunt volume is relatively small, as evidenced by the minimal elevation in pulmonary pressures.

30. (D) Device erosion with the Amplatzer® device occurs in around 0.1% of implants. Speculation regarding oversizing and impingement on the wall of the aorta has been debated. However, erosions have still been reported with smaller devices (20 mm). The newer Gore Helex™ has not been associated with erosion.

31. (A) Forbes et al. (*JACC* 2011) reported a multivariate analysis comparing surgical, stent, and balloon angioplasty treatment of coarctation of the aorta. This study demonstrated that in a select age range of patients (6 to 12 years), balloon angioplasty is more likely to result in an acute aortic wall injury of any type in comparison to stent implantation or surgical repair. Stent patients reported the lowest rate for acute complications, but there are several limitations to the study, including the overrepresentation of surgical patients necessitating a tube graft interposition or patch reconstruction rather than an isolated end-to-end anastomosis.

32. (C) This angiogram demonstrates an injection in an anomalous right upper pulmonary vein with contrast entering the right SVC and returning to the right atrium. Right upper PAPVC is most commonly associated with a superior sinus venosus ASD (deficiency of the common wall between the right SVC and the RUPV resulting in the LA orifice of the RUPV with an unroofed pulmonary vein). Occasionally, a secundum ASD is also present. The other occasional accompanying finding is persistence of the left SVC. Scimitar syndrome was first described by Neill et al. in 1960 and results from anomalous drainage of the RPVs to the IVC, just above or below the diaphragm with several other frequently encountered associated anomalies.

33. (B) A fundamental component to the success of surgical correction of TGA involves the identification of the origin and course of the coronary arteries. This AP projection demonstrates the circumflex arising from the region of the right-facing sinus

and coursing leftward. The LAD arises from the left-facing sinus. The lateral projection would further assist in defining the anterior–posterior course. Based on the information provided, the only answer choice consistent with this angiogram is the circumflex arising from the RCA.

34. (C) The available data are adequate to calculate Q_p/Q_s. With this anatomy, aortic and pulmonary artery saturation will be the same. Using SVC as mixed venous (the right atrium is not a well-mixed chamber), $Q_p/Q_s = (0.82 - 0.53)/(1.00 - 0.82) = 1.6$.

35. (D) For this patient, Q_p can be calculated using femoral artery saturation as pulmonary artery saturation (see answer above). Dividing VO_2 by the pulmonary venous and pulmonary arterial oxygen content difference results in $Q_p = 150/[1.36 \times 16.2 \times 10 \times (1.00 \times 0.82)] = 3.8$ L/min/m^2. The pulmonary vein wedge pressure can be used as a surrogate of mean pulmonary artery pressure; thus, the transpulmonary gradient is $14 - 7 = 7$ mm Hg. PVR = 7 mm Hg/3.8 L/min/m^2 = 1.8 Woods units × m^2.

36. (A) Even though this patient has the same mixed venous, systemic arterial and pulmonary venous saturation and the same hemoglobin as the patient in the previous scenario, her pulmonary arterial saturation is lower, reflecting a lower, but more efficient rate of pulmonary blood flow. For her, $Q_p/Q_s = (0.82 - 0.53)/(1.00 - 0.53) = 0.6$.

37. (A) The catheter is coursing from the aorta to the first brachiocephalic branch allowing for a hand injection in a right-sided BT shunt. Also demonstrated is LPA stenosis with preferential flow through the RPA. The alternative answer choices have been previously described.

38. (C) This RV angiogram was performed in a patient with HLHS following a Norwood procedure and demonstrates a Sano shunt arising from the anterior wall of the single ventricle providing an RV-PA shunt. The other options are incorrect and include the classic BT shunt (right subclavian to RPA anastomosis with native vessel), modified BT shunt (right subclavian to RPA anastomosis with artificial material), Potts shunt (direct descending aorta to LPA anastomosis), and Waterston shunt (direct ascending aorta to RPA anastomosis).

39. (B) Usually the A wave in the RA is slightly higher than the V wave, with the opposite true for the LA (V wave is slightly higher than the A wave). The V wave is due to atrial filling with a closed AV valve during LV contraction. In the setting of left AV valve regurgitation, the V wave will be increased when blood flows back to the LA through the regurgitant orifice. An increased A wave would be expected in mitral valve stenosis or LV diastolic dysfunction.

40. (A) There are five key components to the RA waveform which should be well understood. These include

A wave—atrial contraction
C wave—closure of the AV valve with bowing of the AV valve into the atrium during the start of the ventricular contraction
X descent—descent in pressure as the AV valve ring is pulled into the ventricle
V wave—passive filling of the atrium with a closed AV valve
Y descent—descent due to AV valve opening and passive atrial emptying

41. (C) The oxygen–hemoglobin dissociation curve plots hemoglobin saturation (*y*-axis) against oxygen tension (*x*-axis). A decrease in the hemoglobin affinity for oxygen would be represented by a rightward shift of the oxyhemoglobin curve, resulting in an increased partial pressure of oxygen in the tissue. The events that result in a rightward shift would include an increase in pCO_2, 2,3-BPG, hydrogen ion production (decreased pH = acidosis), and body temperature. Glucose is not a factor in this calculation.

42. (A) The hemodynamic data demonstrate a clear discrepancy between the RA sat and the upstream/downstream sat trend. This sample was most likely obtained from the coronary sinus, consistent with improper catheter position. Coronary artery O_2 extraction is the highest in order to supply the myocardial oxygen demands. Hence, venous saturation from the coronary sinus (coronary venous drainage) is the lowest of any systemic venous structure entering the right atrium. Coronary sinus return makes up ~5% to 7% of systemic venous return. A typical saturation runs between 25% and 45% and if oversampled can misrepresent mixed venous saturation when there is no shunt lesion.

43. (D) Thermodilution, introduced in 1950, utilizes a temperature indicator and fixed volume of fluid to measure a downstream change in temperature. The area under the temperature–time curve is used to determine cardiac output. There are multiple advantages to this method including accurate and reproducible results, short steady-state time requirement, and only the need for venous access. There are several sources of error, however, with discrepancies occurring in the presence of low cardiac output, AV valve regurgitation, and intracardiac shunting. Thermodilution does not accurately reflect systemic cardiac output in shunt physiology ($Q_p \neq Q_s$), as is present in this patient with an ASD and left-to-right shunt.

44. (C) Polycythemia is defined as a hematocrit over 65% and is commonly encountered in patients with cyanotic heart disease. Polycythemia increases the O_2-carrying capacity while decreasing the cardiac output and O_2 delivery to tissues. It also significantly increases the risk of thrombosis and emboli and warrants prehydration 24 hours prior to the procedure with consideration of phlebotomy in the cath lab. Prehydration is further prudent in this patient as renal insufficiency may be further exacerbated by prolonged NPO status and angiography.

45. (C) The data demonstrate a markedly elevated RVEDP and LVEDP, not an unexpected finding in a patient with two prior cardiopulmonary bypass exposures. The pulmonary pulse pressure is wide and consistent with severe pulmonary regurgitation. The RA pressure is similar to the RVEDP, making severe tricuspid regurgitation unlikely. The final issue to address is whether this patient is experiencing restrictive filling or constrictive physiology (typically observed in patients with cardiac tamponade or constrictive pericarditis). The following features are more suggestive of restriction rather than constrictive pericarditis or tamponade: RVSP >50 mm Hg, LVEDP − RVEDP >4 mm Hg, PCWP − mean RAP >4 mm Hg, and RVEDP/RVSP <0.3.

46. (C) There will continue to be respiratory variation in the mean RA pressure in restrictive cardiomyopathy rather than constrictive pericarditis. CP will result in an inspiratory rise or lack of a

decline in RA pressure, which is Kussmaul sign. M waves can be seen in both CP and RCM. Equalization of pressures as listed in option (D) is diagnostic for CP. Absence of A waves should raise concerns for an arrhythmia, specifically atrial fibrillation or flutter.

47. (D) This question expands on the prior information related to calculating Q_p/Q_s and demonstrates the importance of utilizing a proper mixed venous saturation. This patient has PAPVR with a step-up at the low right SVC. Therefore, the appropriate selection for the mixed venous sat is the high right SVC (63%). Q_p/Q_s = (98% − 63%)/(98% − 73%) = 35/25 = 1.4.

48. (D) The chest radiograph demonstrates a heavily calcified pericardium. One would expect this person to have constrictive physiology with elevated LVEDP, mean PCWP, RVEDP, and mean RA pressure. The only answer choice consistent with elevated intracardiac filling pressures is an elevated PCWP. Systemic hypertension is not necessarily a part of constriction; in fact, patients frequently are hypotensive.

49. (C) The left pulmonary venous saturations are unexpectedly low. The right pulmonary veins are fully saturated. If the ET tube is in the right mainstem bronchus, the left lung may be ineffectively ventilated and oxygenated. Pulmonary venous desaturation may be caused by other things, such as pulmonary arteriovenous malformation, but the first step in this situation would be to confirm correct positioning of the endotracheal tube.

50. (E) Pulmonary arteriovenous malformations occur commonly in patients following Fontan procedures. Dyspnea on exertion and orthostatic or exertional cyanosis in Fontan patients can occur due to right-to-left shunting at a widely patent fenestration or can be due to right-to-left shunting from pulmonary arteriovenous malformations. These most commonly occur in the basal region of the lung.

51. (C) Interventional catheterization in adult congenital heart disease. *Circulation.* 2007;115:1622–1633 is an excellent review of indications for catheter-based therapy in adults with congenital heart disease. The 40-year-old patient, asymptomatic, pulmonary valve catheter gradient = 54 mm Hg is the only class I indication listed. Asymptomatic adults with mean Doppler or catheter peak-to-peak gradient >40 mm Hg should undergo pulmonary balloon valvuloplasty. Interventions have been recommended for the other answers but they are class II indications.

52. (B) During balloon aortic valvuloplasty, the balloon size should not exceed the annulus dimension. The risk of significant postprocedure valve regurgitation may occur if the balloon exceeds 100% of the annulus diameter.

53. (D) The general recommendation is that pulmonary balloon valvuloplasty should be performed with a balloon that is 120% of the annulus diameter and should not exceed 140% of the annulus diameter. The risk of significant postprocedure valve regurgitation is increased when the balloon size exceeds 140% of the annulus diameter.

54. (A) The patient is acidotic; hence, balloon septostomy should be performed promptly. RV angiography and other diagnostic procedures may be performed later if the patient's systemic arterial oxygen saturations improve dramatically. Mixing primarily occurs at atrial level in patients with complete TGA, and those with a VSD may still be profoundly cyanotic and acidotic requiring a septostomy.

55. (D) The defect is large (23 mm) particularly for a small child. The anterior-superior and the posterior rim are small or deficient making device closure unlikely, and this patient likely is best treated with surgical closure.

56. (E) AHA Pediatric Catheterization Guidelines—In patients with a large PDA and bidirectional flow due to pulmonary vascular disease, occlusion may be beneficial only if the pulmonary lung bed shows some reactivity to pulmonary vasodilator therapy. These patients should undergo hemodynamic assessment and pulmonary vasoreactivity testing before consideration for ductal occlusion. However, data on this group of patients are scant, and long-term follow-up data are unknown. Should pulmonary vascular disease continue to progress, the ductus will no longer be available to prevent the RV pressures from becoming supersystemic. Class III: Transcatheter PDA occlusion should not be attempted in a patient with a PDA with severe pulmonary hypertension associated with bidirectional or right-to-left shunting that is unresponsive to pulmonary vasodilator therapy (level of evidence: C).

57. (C) Patients with pulmonary atresia and intact ventricular septum (PA-IVS) have increased risk of coronary abnormalities such as right ventricular sinusoids, coronary-cameral fistulae, and coronary stenosis or atresia. RV-to-coronary artery fistulae and RV-dependent coronary circulation (significant portion of LV is supplied by fistulae fed by hypertensive RV) are present in 5% to 35% of PA-IVS patients. Decompression of the RV in the setting of significant RV-dependent myocardial circulation can result in irreversible myocardial ischemia and is usually fatal. See Table 4.13 for recommendations for pulmonary valvuloplasty.

58. (A) Recommendations for device closure of secundum atrial septal defects are listed in Table 4.14. Given that the patient has experienced recurrent TIAs, she meets criteria for closure as a Class IIa indication.

59. (A) BAS is performed to improve atrial mixing (simple d-TGA or d-TGA with VSD) or to treat atrial septal defect restriction in the setting of significant obstruction or stenosis of an atrioventricular valve (HLHS being the most common). It is rarely needed in right heart obstructive lesions, that is, tricuspid atresia (one must be aware that performing a balloon septostomy in a redundant atrial septum, such as in tricuspid atresia, is challenging and one may disrupt the RA/IVC junction with aggressive techniques). It is not performed in patients with TAPVR. This is a lesion that will be surgically corrected at the time of diagnosis and the atrial septum is not typically the location of "obstruction" of the venous return pathway.

The procedure is usually straightforward in patients with d-TGA where the flap of the fossa ovalis is thin and easy to tear with the balloon catheter. BAS can be performed up to a few weeks of age; after this time the atrial septum may be too thick to balloon successfully in any lesion without significant risk of disruption of normal tissue. A blade septostomy will then be needed. The exception to this is the neonate with HLHS and

TABLE 4.13 Recommendations for Pulmonary Valvuloplasty

Class I
1. Pulmonary valvuloplasty is indicated for a patient with critical valvar pulmonary stenosis (defined as pulmonary stenosis present at birth with cyanosis and evidence of patent ductus arteriosus dependency), valvar pulmonic stenosis, and a peak-to-peak catheter gradient or echocardiographic peak instantaneous gradient of ≥40 mm Hg or clinically significant pulmonary valvar obstruction in the presence of RV dysfunction (*level of evidence: A*)

Class IIa
1. It is reasonable to perform pulmonary valvuloplasty on a patient with valvar pulmonic stenosis who meets the above criteria in the setting of a dysplastic pulmonary valve (*level of evidence: C*)
2. It is reasonable to perform pulmonary valvuloplasty in newborns with pulmonary valve atresia and intact ventricular septum who have favorable anatomy that includes the exclusion of RV-dependent coronary circulation (*level of evidence: C*)

Class IIb
1. Pulmonary valvuloplasty may be considered as a palliative procedure in a patient with complex cyanotic CHD, including some rare cases of tetralogy of Fallot (*level of evidence: C*)

Class III
1. Pulmonary valvuloplasty should not be performed in patients with pulmonary atresia and RV-dependent coronary circulation (*level of evidence: B*)

TABLE 4.14 Recommendations for Transcatheter Device Closure of Secundum ASD

Class I
1. Transcatheter secundum ASD closure is indicated in patients with hemodynamically significant ASD with suitable anatomic features (*level of evidence: B*)

Class IIa
1. It is reasonable to perform transcatheter secundum ASD closure in patients with transient right-to-left shunting at the atrial level who have experienced sequelae of paradoxical emboli such as stroke or recurrent transient ischemic attack (*level of evidence: B*)
2. It is reasonable to perform transcatheter secundum ASD closure in patients with transient right-to-left shunting at the atrial level who are symptomatic because of cyanosis and who do not require such a communication to maintain adequate cardiac output (*level of evidence: B*)

Class IIb
1. Transcatheter closure may be considered in patients with a small secundum ASD who are believed to be at risk of thromboembolic events (e.g., patients with a transvenous pacing system or chronically indwelling intravenous catheters, patients with hypercoagulable states) (*level of evidence: C*)

restrictive atrial septum, where the tissue may be very thick, with minimal or no opening at the time of delivery. This procedure is usually performed emergently and immediately after delivery. It may require various techniques, including transseptal or radiofrequency access to the left atrium, the use of dilation balloon (cutting balloon), and stent placement for complete relief of obstruction. A simple balloon septostomy in HLHS with thick, restrictive atrial septum may avulse the pulmonary veins (i.e., the tissue with the least resistance will give way) during the BAS.

60. (B) Patients with a history of Mustard palliation may present with either SVC or IVC baffle obstruction, or with baffle leaks in both the SVC and IVC segments. If large enough, these can cause significant right-to-left shunt with exercise and produce exertional cyanosis. The most appropriate treatment of a symptomatic baffle leak is an attempted closure, either by surgery or catheterization. Recent advances in septal occluding devices have allowed for many of these patients to have their leaks closed in the cath lab with success. Stent placement is indicated in patients with baffle obstruction.

61. (A) Several factors may affect the pressure gradient across the coarctation site. These include LV dysfunction with low cardiac output, a large PDA, or multiple collaterals decompressing the aorta.

62. (D) The patient in this stem has 3-methylglutaconic aciduria type II (Barth syndrome), which is an X-linked disease characterized by DCM, endocardial fibroelastosis, proximal skeletal myopathy, growth failure, neutropenia, and organic aciduria. Prior to catheterization, documentation of the patient's leukocyte count with consideration for G-CSF administration and appropriate antibiotic prophylaxis is indicated.

CHAPTER 5

Noninvasive Cardiac Imaging

Benjamin W. Eidem and M. Yasir Qureshi

QUESTIONS

1. Which statement is correct regarding the Doppler examination?

    A. Pulsed-wave (PW) Doppler requires one crystal to transmit the sound wave and another crystal to receive the reflected sound wave
    B. The maximum frequency shift that can be measured accurately by PW Doppler is termed pulse repetition frequency (PRF)
    C. Nyquist limit = PRF/2
    D. Nyquist limit can be extended by using higher frequency transducer
    E. High PRF is a technique to increase Nyquist limit without range ambiguity

2. In which of the following scenarios is it most appropriate to use the simplified Bernoulli equation to estimate a change in pressure?

    A. Severe pulmonary valve stenosis
    B. Aortic coarctation with bicuspid aortic valve
    C. Patent ductus arteriosus
    D. Subaortic stenosis and aortic stenosis
    E. Blalock–Taussig shunt

3. The Doppler pattern in Figure 5.1 is consistent with which of the following?

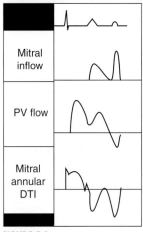

FIGURE 5.1

    A. Normal pattern
    B. Grade 1 diastolic dysfunction (impaired relaxation)
    C. Grade 2 diastolic dysfunction (pseudonormalization)
    D. Grade 3 diastolic dysfunction (restrictive physiology)
    E. Grade 4 diastolic dysfunction (severe irreversible restrictive physiology)

4. A patient has coarctation of the aorta. PW Doppler reveals a peak velocity of 2.0 m/s proximal to the coarctation. A continuous wave (CW) Doppler across the coarctation reveals a peak Doppler velocity of 4.0 m/s. What is the pressure gradient across the coarctation?

    A. 8 mm Hg
    B. 9 mm Hg
    C. 36 mm Hg
    D. 48 mm Hg
    E. 64 mm Hg

5. The Doppler tracing of the descending aorta in Figure 5.2 was obtained in a patient with suspected aortic regurgitation. What is the degree of regurgitation?

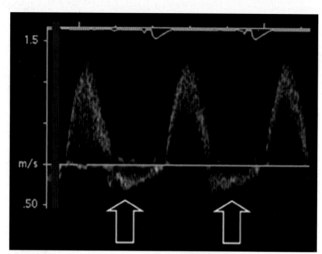

FIGURE 5.2

 A. Unable to determine degree of regurgitation
 B. Trivial
 C. Mild
 D. Moderate
 E. Severe

6. Which of the following statements is correct concerning contrast echocardiography?

 A. Contrast agents utilize microbubbles that are 50 to 100 microns in size
 B. In the normal heart, contrast agents should opacify the right heart but not the left heart
 C. Contrast agents can pass through the pulmonary circulation to opacify the left atrium and left ventricle
 D. Acoustic impedance of contrast agents is higher than that of the blood pool
 E. Contrast effect persists for 10 to 15 seconds in the normal heart

7. Which of the following is correct concerning echocardiographic use of agitated saline injections?

 A. Microbubbles are 1 to 10 microns in size and easily traverse the pulmonary bed to the left heart
 B. In the presence of an intrapulmonary shunt, the majority of these bubbles appear in the left atrium within one to two cardiac cycles.
 C. A negative bubble study (i.e., no bubbles imaged within the left heart) with agitated saline rules out a right-to-left shunt
 D. Indications for agitated saline studies include unexplained cyanosis and stroke
 E. Bubbles cannot be present in the left heart in the normal circulation without the presence of a left-to-right shunt

8. Which of the following is MOST helpful to diagnose the severity of aortic insufficiency?

 A. Degree of left ventricular (LV) dilatation
 B. Length of the color Doppler regurgitant jet into the LV
 C. Amount of diastolic Doppler flow reversal in the ascending aorta
 D. Vena contracta width of the regurgitant jet
 E. Comparison of the forward flow Doppler time velocity integral (TVI) to reverse flow TVI in the abdominal aorta

9. Which of the following formulas is correct for the myocardial performance index (i.e., Tei index):

 A. [ICT + IRT]/ET
 B. PEP/ET
 C. E/E_a
 D. [Pulmonary venous atrial reversal duration] – [mitral inflow atrial duration]
 E. [LVEDD – LVESD]/LVET

10. Which echocardiographic scan plane is *most* optimal to define a *secundum atrial septal defect*?

 A. Suprasternal long-axis view
 B. Parasternal long-axis view
 C. Parasternal short-axis view
 D. Subcostal four-chamber view
 E. Apical four-chamber view

11. Which of the following is the *most* common associated cardiac defect found with a *sinus venosus atrial septal defect*?

 A. Anomalous right pulmonary venous connection
 B. Inlet ventricular septal defect
 C. Bicuspid aortic valve
 D. Persistent left superior vena cava
 E. Coarctation of the aorta

12. Which of the following findings on echocardiography is consistent with constriction?

 A. E/A ratio of mitral Doppler inflow <1.0
 B. Decreased E_a velocity on tissue Doppler of the lateral mitral annulus
 C. Increased respiratory variation in mitral inflow E-wave velocity >30%
 D. Increased hepatic venous atrial systolic Doppler flow reversals during inspiration
 E. Increased E-wave deceleration time on mitral inflow Doppler

13. Which of the following parameters is consistent with restrictive LV physiology?

 A. Mitral inflow E/A Doppler ratio <1
 B. Increased lateral mitral annular E_a velocity
 C. Mitral inflow deceleration time <80 ms
 D. Increased systolic/diastolic ratio of pulmonary venous Doppler
 E. Lateral mitral annular E/E_a ratio <10

14. Which of the following associated congenital heart lesions is *most* common in a patient with Down syndrome and an *atrioventricular septal defect* (AVSD)?

    A. Coarctation of the aorta
    B. Total anomalous pulmonary venous connection
    C. Aortic valve stenosis
    D. Tetralogy of Fallot
    E. Left ventricular hypoplasia

15. Which of the following is the *most* common *anatomic finding* in a *complete AVSD*?

    A. Cleft in posterior leaflet of mitral component of AV valve
    B. Medial rotation of left ventricular papillary muscles
    C. Ratio of left ventricular inlet to outlet distance >1.0
    D. Left ventricular outflow tract (LVOT) is "sprung" anteriorly
    E. Left and right atrioventricular valve attachments are present at different levels

16. Which of the following statements is TRUE regarding *M-mode*?

    A. Has a low PRF
    B. Has excellent temporal resolution
    C. *X*-axis represents distance from transducer
    D. *Y*-axis represents time
    E. Utilizes two imaging crystals to transmit and receive impulses

17. Which of the following statements regarding *spatial resolution* in echocardiography is CORRECT?

    A. Spatial resolution is defined as the smallest distance between two points distinguishable as separate points
    B. Axial resolution is the ability to differentiate points perpendicular to the ultrasound beam path
    C. Lateral resolution is the ability to differentiate between points along the path of the ultrasound beam
    D. Lateral resolution is better than axial resolution
    E. Image resolution is best where the ultrasound beam is widest

18. Which of the following is the most likely *source of error* in calculation of Doppler flow velocity?

    A. Angle of incidence of the ultrasound beam
    B. Depth of the vascular structure
    C. Frequency of the transducer
    D. Presence and degree of imaging artifact
    E. Variation in heart rate

19. Which of the following is true regarding *CW Doppler*?

    A. Utilizes a single ultrasound crystal that continuously transmits and receives
    B. No limit to maximal velocity measured
    C. Excellent range resolution
    D. Less dependent on angle of incidence compared to PW Doppler
    E. Lower Nyquist limit compared to PW Doppler

20. Which of the following statements regarding *PW Doppler* is CORRECT?

    A. Utilizes two ultrasound crystals that continuously transmit and receive
    B. No limit to maximal velocity measured
    C. Excellent range resolution
    D. Lower PRF than color Doppler
    E. PRF is fixed

21. Which of the following is a CORRECT statement regarding the *Nyquist limit*?

    A. Represents the highest frequency shift that can be unambiguously detected and displayed
    B. Is equal to the PRF
    C. Is higher with PW Doppler versus CW Doppler
    D. Remains the same with all transducer frequencies
    E. Is lower at more shallow depths of interrogation

22. Which of the following is a TRUE statement regarding *color Doppler*?

    A. Color Doppler represents the mean velocity of blood flow
    B. Intensity of color represents peak Doppler flow velocity
    C. 2D image content is unchanged with color Doppler imaging
    D. Nyquist limit is increased with color Doppler imaging
    E. Utilizes a single ultrasound beam with multiple sampling sites along that beam

23. Which of the following is the *optimal* echocardiographic view to delineate a *subpulmonary ventricular septal defect*?

    A. Parasternal long-axis view
    B. Apical four-chamber view
    C. Suprasternal long-axis view
    D. Parasternal short-axis view
    E. Apical five-chamber view

24. Which of the following is the *most* characteristic *acquired cardiac lesion* resulting from a subpulmonary ventricular septal defect?

    A. Aortic regurgitation
    B. LVOT obstruction
    C. Right ventricular outflow tract obstruction
    D. Pulmonary valve stenosis
    E. Aortic valve stenosis

25. Which of the following is the *most* characteristic *physiologic effect* of a large ventricular septal defect?

    A. Right ventricular volume overload
    B. Low pulmonary arterial pressure
    C. Equal right ventricular and left ventricular systolic pressure
    D. Increased systemic blood flow
    E. Decreased pulmonary blood flow

26. Which of the following is the BEST morphologic marker of the *right atrium*?

    A. Broad-based triangular appendage
    B. Receives superior vena cava (SVC)
    C. Chamber is connected to morphologic RV
    D. Presence of the valve of the fossa ovalis
    E. Connected to tricuspid valve

27. The *atrial septum* is BEST imaged in which scan plane?

    A. Suprasternal
    B. Subcostal
    C. Parasternal long axis
    D. Parasternal short axis
    E. Apical four chamber

28. Which of the following is a typical echocardiographic feature of the *morphologic right ventricle*?

    A. Ellipsoid shape
    B. More apical insertion point of atrioventricular valve
    C. Smooth superior septal surface
    D. Finely trabeculated apical portion
    E. Lack of atrioventricular valve septal attachments

29. Which of the following is a typical echocardiographic feature of the *morphologic left ventricle*?

    A. Heavily trabeculated inflow portion
    B. Triangular shape
    C. Trabeculated septal surface
    D. Lack of atrioventricular valve septal chordal attachments
    E. More apical insertion of atrioventricular valve

30. A neonate with *pulmonary valve stenosis* has a peak Doppler velocity by CW Doppler of 4.0 m/s. Which of the following is the estimated maximum instantaneous Doppler gradient?

    A. 64 mm Hg
    B. 77 mm Hg
    C. 72 mm Hg
    D. 50 mm Hg
    E. Cannot be calculated

31. Which of the following is the *most* common anatomic type of *subaortic stenosis*?

    A. Tunnel type
    B. Discrete membrane
    C. Asymmetric septal hypertrophy
    D. Systolic anterior motion of mitral valve
    E. Anomalous mitral chordal insertion within the LVOT

32. The *most* common associated cardiac abnormality in the patient with *coarctation of the aorta* is:

    A. Bicuspid aortic valve
    B. Ventricular septal defect
    C. Atrial septal defect

    D. Pulmonary valve stenosis
    E. Coronary artery anomaly

33. In patients with *coarctation of the aorta*, systemic arterial pressure begins to be significantly affected when the overall aortic lumen is narrowed by:

    A. 20% of aortic diameter
    B. 30% of aortic diameter
    C. 50% of aortic diameter
    D. 75% of aortic diameter
    E. 90% of aortic diameter

34. Which of the following is the most diagnostic echo finding in *pericardial effusion with cardiac tamponade*?

    A. Diastolic right atrial wall collapse
    B. 10% variation in mitral inflow Doppler velocities with respiration
    C. Diastolic right ventricular wall collapse
    D. Effusion >25 mm circumferentially
    E. 15% variation in tricuspid inflow Doppler velocities with respiration

35. Which of the following methods of assessing LV systolic function is *most independent of loading conditions*?

    A. Ejection fraction
    B. Shortening fraction
    C. Myocardial performance index
    D. Rate-corrected velocity of circumferential fiber shortening
    E. Stress–velocity index

36. Normal left ventricular shortening fraction is *maximal* at which age?

    A. 2 weeks old
    B. 18 years old
    C. 2 years old
    D. 10 years old
    E. No significant change in shortening fraction occurs with age

37. Holodiastolic *Doppler flow reversal* in the abdominal aorta can be attributed to which of the following?

    A. Bidirectional cavopulmonary anastomosis
    B. Large patent ductus arteriosus
    C. Moderate aortic insufficiency
    D. Sano shunt
    E. High output state

38. Which of the following is the *most* common type of *ventricular septal defect* that is associated with *coarctation of the aorta*?

    A. Apical muscular
    B. Anterior malalignment
    C. Perimembranous
    D. Inlet
    E. Subpulmonary

39. The Doppler finding often seen in patients with supravalvar aortic stenosis has been demonstrated to be a high-velocity poststenotic jet that hugs the aortic wall and preferentially transfers kinetic energy into the right innominate artery. Which of the following best describes this Doppler finding?

   A. Coanda effect
   B. Ohm law
   C. Continuity equation
   D. Poiseuille law
   E. Bernoulli equation

40. In the simplified Bernoulli equation, which *component* of the complete equation is *not* ignored?

   A. Flow acceleration
   B. Convective acceleration
   C. Viscous friction
   D. Proximal Doppler velocity
   E. Vessel length

41. Which of the following is true about an *overriding* atrio-ventricular valve?

   A. Has chordal attachments into both ventricles
   B. Must have chordal attachments to the ventricular septal crest
   C. Empties into two ventricles
   D. Cannot coexist with straddling
   E. Is never associated with malalignment type of VSD

42. Which of the following is true about a *straddling* cardiac valve?

   A. Cannot coexist with overriding
   B. Is always associated with malalignment type of VSD
   C. Frequently involves the aortic valve
   D. Is a common component of tetralogy of Fallot
   E. Involves anomalous insertion of chordae tendineae

43. Which statement is correct regarding *polysplenia syndrome*?

   A. The situs of abdominal viscera is always ambiguous
   B. The spleen are multiple and located on both left and right sides
   C. Inferior vena cava (IVC) fails to join the heart directly with azygos continuation
   D. Multiple gallbladders common
   E. Biliary atresia never occurs

44. Which statement is correct regarding the orientation of the *great arteries* in patients with levocardia?

   A. A right anterior aorta is most frequently associated with congenitally corrected transposition of the great arteries (L-TGA)
   B. A left anterior aorta is most frequently associated with complete transposition (D-TGA)
   C. A right posterior aorta is frequently found in double inlet left ventricle

   D. A left posterior aorta is commonly found in either type (L- or D-) of TGA
   E. Normal hearts are characterized by a right posterior aorta

45. *Tricuspid atresia* is an example of which of the following?

   A. Common inlet
   B. Double inlet
   C. Single inlet
   D. Absent inlet
   E. Ambiguous AV connection

46. Where does a *type A* interruption of the aortic arch occur?

   A. Between the right innominate and left common carotid arteries
   B. Proximal to the right innominate artery
   C. Between the left common carotid and left subclavian arteries
   D. Distal to the left subclavian artery
   E. Just distal to the sinotubular junction in the ascending aorta

47. Which of the following statements is correct concerning *venous return* to the normal heart?

   A. When the IVC is interrupted, venous return to the SVC is from the thebesian veins
   B. When a persistent left SVC drains to a severely dilated coronary sinus, the brachiocephalic vein is typically small or absent
   C. The connection of the right SVC to the right atrium confidently identifies the morphologic right atrium
   D. It is more common for the right pulmonary veins than the left pulmonary veins to merge into a single vein that enters the left atrium
   E. Interruption of the IVC is more common in asplenia versus polysplenia syndrome

48. Which of the following is the most reliable feature that distinguishes the mitral valve from the tricuspid valve?

   A. Shape of the orifice
   B. Atrioventricular valve—semilunar valve continuity
   C. Presence of septal chordal attachments
   D. Level of attachment of atrioventricular valve at cardiac crux
   E. Number of leaflets

49. How many organ systems are characterized by situs or sidedness (i.e., these organ systems do NOT exhibit bilateral mirror image symmetry)?

   A. 2
   B. 3
   C. 4
   D. 5
   E. All organ systems are characterized by sidedness

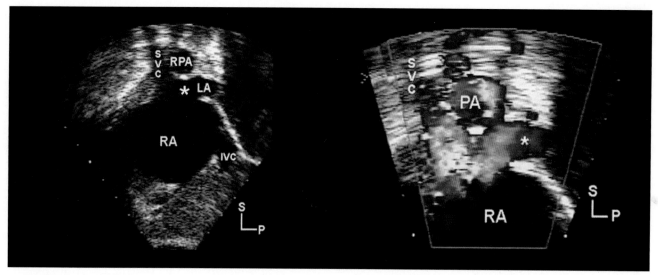

FIGURE 5.3 RA, right atrium; IVC, inferior vena cava; SVC, superior vena cava; RPA, right pulmonary artery.

50. A 9-year-old patient presents with decreased exercise tolerance and cardiomegaly on chest x-ray. An echocardiogram was subsequently performed. What is the defect designated by the asterisk in Figure 5.3?

A. Secundum atrial septal defect
B. Coronary sinus atrial septal defect
C. Sinus venosus atrial septal defect
D. Persistent left superior vena cava to unroofed coronary sinus
E. Primum atrial septal defect

51. Which of the following congenital heart defects is demonstrated in Figure 5.4?

A. Partial AVSD
B. Unroofed coronary sinus
C. Complete AVSD
D. Total anomalous pulmonary venous connection
E. Large inlet ventricular septal defect

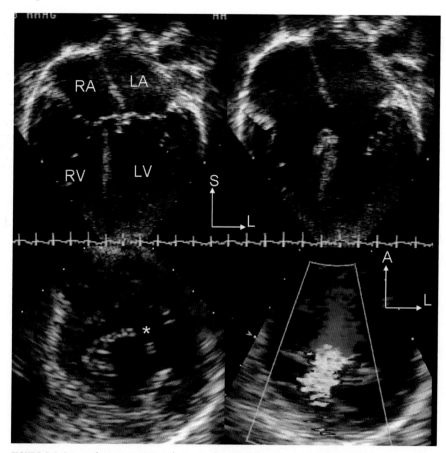

FIGURE 5.4 RA, right atrium; RV, right ventricle; LA, left atrium; LV, left ventricle.

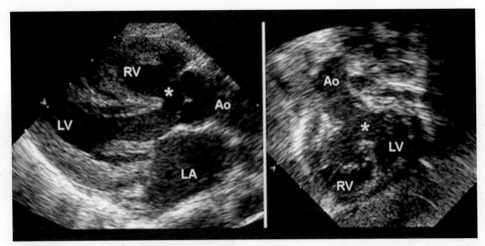

FIGURE 5.5 RV, right ventricle; LV, left ventricle; LA, left atrium; Ao, Aorta.

52. Which of the following congenital heart lesions is NOT consistent with the images in Figure 5.5?

A. Tetralogy of Fallot
B. Pulmonary atresia with ventricular septal defect
C. Truncus arteriosus
D. Large malalignment ventricular septal defect
E. D-TGA

53. A 6-month-old child presents with failure to thrive and the echocardiographic image (Fig. 5.6) is obtained. What is the congenital heart defect demonstrated?

A. Muscular VSD
B. Membranous VSD
C. Infundibular VSD
D. Inlet VSD
E. Doubly committed VSD

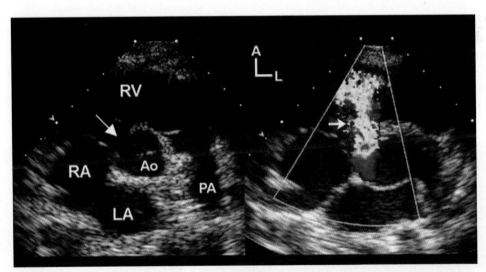

FIGURE 5.6 RA, right atrium; RV, right ventricle; LA, left atrium; PA, Pulmonary artery; Ao, Aorta.

54. Which of the following diagnoses is most consistent with the echocardiographic image in Figure 5.7?

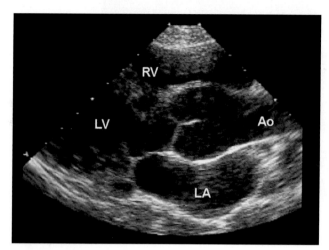

FIGURE 5.7 RV, right ventricle; LV, left ventricle; LA, left atrium; Ao, Aorta.

    A. Down syndrome
    B. DiGeorge syndrome
    C. Marfan syndrome
    D. Noonan syndrome
    E. Williams syndrome

55. What is the most likely etiology of the echocardiographic image in Figure 5.8?

    A. Thrombus
    B. Myxoma
    C. Fibroma
    D. Rhabdomyoma
    E. Secondary metastasis

56. An 8-year-old patient has a resuscitated sudden cardiac death event while playing soccer. An echocardiogram performed in the emergency room displays the image in Figure 5.9. What is the most likely diagnosis?

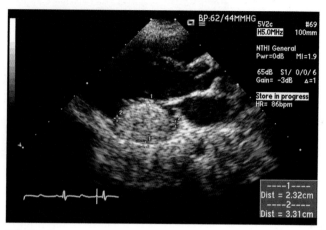

FIGURE 5.9

    A. Rhabdomyoma
    B. Myxoma
    C. Fibroma
    D. Fibroelastoma
    E. Sarcoma

57. Doppler flow studies in the human fetus have shown that the ratio of right-to-left ventricular combined output is about which of the following?

    A. 10%/90%
    B. 25%/75%
    C. 55%/45%
    D. 25%/75%
    E. 90%/10%

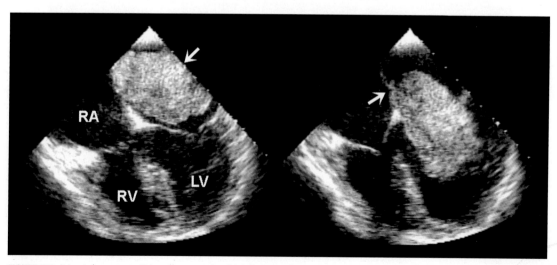

FIGURE 5.8 RA, right atrium; RV, right ventricle; LV, left ventricle.

58. Fetal echocardiography demonstrates tachycardia. You and your colleagues agree that the fetus has sustained ventricular tachycardia (VT) and evidence of hydrops fetalis. The mother desires that "everything be done" for the fetus. The fetus is at 22 weeks gestation. What is your recommendation?

A. Give betamethasone immediately

B. Order anti-SSA/Ro and anti-SSA/La antibody panels and treat with prednisolone if positive

C. Start sotalol 80 mg PO BID

D. Load with digoxin 10 mcg IV

E. Observe only

59. The fetal four-chamber view is inadequate to exclude which of the following congenital heart lesions?

A. AVSD

B. Hypoplastic left heart syndrome

C. Tricuspid atresia

D. D-TGA

E. Ebstein anomaly

60. What is the normal range for fetal cardio-thoracic area ratio?

A. <20%

B. 25% to 35%

C. 40% to 50%

D. 55% to 70%

E. >70%

61. What is the most common fetal arrhythmia?

A. Premature atrial contractions (PAC)

B. Premature ventricular contractions (PVC)

C. Supraventricular tachycardia (SVT)

D. Atrial flutter

E. Complete heart block

62. From the fetal Doppler interrogation in Figure 5.10, what interval is being measured between the parallel lines?

A. PP interval

B. RR interval

C. QT interval

D. PR interval

E. VA interval

63. While performing a fetal echocardiogram, you notice flow reversal across the ductus arteriosus. Which of the following defects is most likely to explain this finding?

A. D-TGA

B. AVSD

C. Critical aortic stenosis

D. Total anomalous pulmonary venous connection

E. Pulmonary atresia with intact ventricular septum

64. While performing a fetal echocardiogram, you notice retrograde flow into the aortic arch. Which of the following defects is most likely to explain this finding?

A. D-TGA

B. AVSD

C. Critical aortic valve stenosis

D. Total anomalous pulmonary venous connections

E. Pulmonary atresia with intact ventricular septum

65. The *normal fetal heart* rate ranges from which of the following?

A. 80 to 120 bpm

B. 60 to 100 bpm

C. 120 to 180 bpm

D. 140 to 220 bpm

E. 100 to 140 bpm

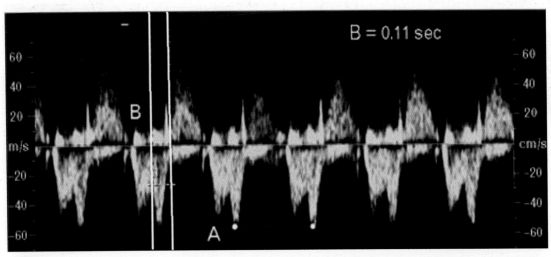

FIGURE 5.10

66. The *normal fetal cardiac axis* is between which of the following?

    A. 30 degrees and 60 degrees
    B. 60 degrees and 90 degrees
    C. 90 degrees and 150 degrees
    D. 60 degrees and 180 degrees
    E. 0 degrees and 90 degrees

67. What percentage of fetal cardiac output at term perfuses the *lungs*?

    A. 10%
    B. 30%
    C. 50%
    D. 75%
    E. 100%

68. Match the fetal *teratogen* and its most commonly associated fetal congenital heart lesion:

    A. Ductal constriction   **1.** Lithium
    B. VSD   **2.** Fetal alcohol syndrome
    C. Coarctation of the   **3.** Indomethacin
        aorta   **4.** Fetal hydantoin
    D. Ebstein anomaly   syndrome
    E. D-TGA   **5.** Isotretinoin

69. Match the *chromosomal anomaly* with its most common congenital heart lesion:

    A. Truncus arteriosus   **1.** Turner syndrome (XO)
    B. VSD   **2.** DiGeorge syndrome
    C. Coarctation of aorta   (22q11–)
    D. AVSD   **3.** Trisomy 21
    E. Supravalvar aortic   **4.** Trisomy 13
        stenosis   **5.** Williams syndrome

70. Which of the following is least commonly associated with *fetal bradycardia*?

    A. Maternal systemic lupus
    B. Umbilical cord compression
    C. Fetal heterotaxy syndrome
    D. Fetal congenitally corrected TGA
    E. Fetal tetralogy of Fallot

71. Which congenital heart lesion should be excluded in the fetus with *SVT*?

    A. Ebstein anomaly
    B. Ventricular septal defect
    C. Coarctation of aorta
    D. D-TGA
    E. AVSD

72. Which of the following is the calculation for the *pulsatility index* (s = peak systolic Doppler velocity, d = minimum diastolic Doppler velocity) in the umbilical artery?

    A. $(s - d)/s$
    B. s/d
    C. $(s - d)/$mean velocity
    D. $(s + d)/s$
    E. $(s + d)/$mean velocity

73. Which of the following is NOT a common echocardiographic sign of congestive heart failure in the fetus?

    A. Abnormal umbilical venous Doppler
    B. Mitral valve regurgitation
    C. Increased pulsatility index in umbilical artery
    D. Increased pulsatility index in middle cerebral artery
    E. Tricuspid valve regurgitation

74. Which of the following fetal lesions would *not* be expected to have significant *ventricular hypertrophy* demonstrated in utero?

    A. Recipient twin in twin–twin transfusion
    B. Fetus of diabetic mother
    C. Fetal hypertrophic cardiomyopathy (HCM)
    D. Fetal tetralogy of Fallot
    E. Fetal Noonan syndrome

75. Insulin-dependent maternal diabetes is a maternal risk factor for congenital heart disease. Which of the following statements regarding this referral for fetal echocardiography is *false*?

    A. The incidence of congenital heart disease is lower than referrals with a family history of congenital heart disease
    B. The most common cardiac lesions include D-TGA
    C. A hemoglobin A1C above 8% predicts a high risk of congenital heart disease
    D. The incidence of congenital heart disease is 3% to 7%
    E. The cardiomyopathy is usually reversible

76. The presence of which of the following devices is a relative contraindication to performing a cardiac magnetic resonance imaging study?

    A. Stainless steel vascular occluding coil
    B. Hemostatic vascular clip
    C. Temporary pacemaker lead without a generator
    D. Atrial septal occluder device
    E. AICD

77. Which of the following devices would generate the most prominent imaging artifact with cardiac magnetic resonance imaging?

    A. Atrial septal occluder device
    B. Permanent pacemaker lead
    C. Stainless steel PDA coil
    D. Nonferromagnetic stent
    E. PDA clip

78. Blood appears *black* on which cardiac magnetic resonance imaging technique?

A. Spin echo
B. Gradient echo cine images
C. Isotropic 3D steady-state free precession (SSFP) images
D. Cardiac-triggered, navigator-gated free-breathing 3D SSFP
E. Contrast-enhanced MRA

79. Which of the following would be the optimal technique to calculate $Q_p:Q_s$ by cardiac magnetic resonance imaging in a patient with a large secundum atrial septal defect?

A. Spatial modulation of magnetization (SPAMM)
B. Contrast-enhanced MR angiogram
C. Velocity-encoded cine (VEC) images
D. Myocardial perfusion study
E. Spin echo images

80. Which of the following is correct regarding the *spin echo* cardiac magnetic resonance imaging technique?

A. Produces bright blood images
B. Low tissue contrast
C. Images acquired during a single cardiac cycle
D. Facilitates tissue characterization of myocardial walls and cardiac tumors
E. Increased imaging artifact with metallic implants compared to other CMR techniques

81. Which of the following is characteristic of the "gradient echo" cardiac magnetic resonance imaging technique?

A. Produces bright blood images
B. Images take longer to acquire than "spin echo" technique
C. High tissue contrast
D. Relatively slow imaging speed compared to spin echo technique
E. Less imaging artifact with metallic implants compared to other CMR techniques

82. Which of the following is the best cardiac magnetic resonance technique to assess *myocardial viability*?

A. Myocardial delayed enhancement (MDE)
B. First-pass myocardial perfusion
C. Dobutamine stress CMR
D. ECG-gated VEC MRI sequence
E. SPAMM

83. Which of the following sequences of cardiac MRI can be done without intravenous administration of contrast agent?

A. Conventional MR angiogram
B. Phase-contrast (velocity-encoded) cine imaging
C. Delayed myocardial enhancement
D. Myocardial perfusion imaging
E. Time-resolved imaging of contrast kinetics (TRICKS)

84. Which of the following sequences allows best assessment of myocardial edema?

A. MR angiogram
B. T1-weighted black-blood imaging
C. T2-weighted black-blood imaging
D. Myocardial perfusion imaging
E. Steady-state free precession imaging

85. Which of the following tests is best to establish a diagnosis of anomalous origin of left coronary artery from right sinus of Valsalva with intramural course?

A. Contrast-enhanced MR angiogram
B. Computed tomography angiography (CTA) without ECG gating
C. CTA with ECG gating
D. Invasive coronary angiography
E. Thallium scan

86. Which advanced imaging modality is best to assess coarctation of aorta?

A. Retrospective ECG-gated CTA
B. Conventional MRA
C. Transesophageal echocardiogram
D. Stress echocardiogram
E. Thallium scan

87. Which of the following statements is TRUE regarding MRI scanners?

A. The magnet is always on
B. The magnet is only on during bright blood imaging
C. The magnet is only on during black-blood imaging
D. The magnet is only on when any imaging is being performed
E. It makes a noise when the magnet is on

88. Which of the following is true for cardiac MRI performed on a patient with acute myocarditis?

A. Myocardial edema is best seen on SSFP cine images
B. T2-weighted sequences can show fatty infiltrate of myocardial wall
C. Early myocardial enhancement is due to impaired perfusion
D. Distribution of delayed myocardial enhancement can help in distinguishing infarction from myocarditis
E. MR angiogram can show filling defect in myocardium

89. Which of the following allows best assessment of pericardial calcification in a patient with pericardial constriction?

A. Noncontrast CT
B. Non–ECG-gated CTA
C. MRA
D. Delayed enhancement on MRI
E. Transthoracic echocardiography

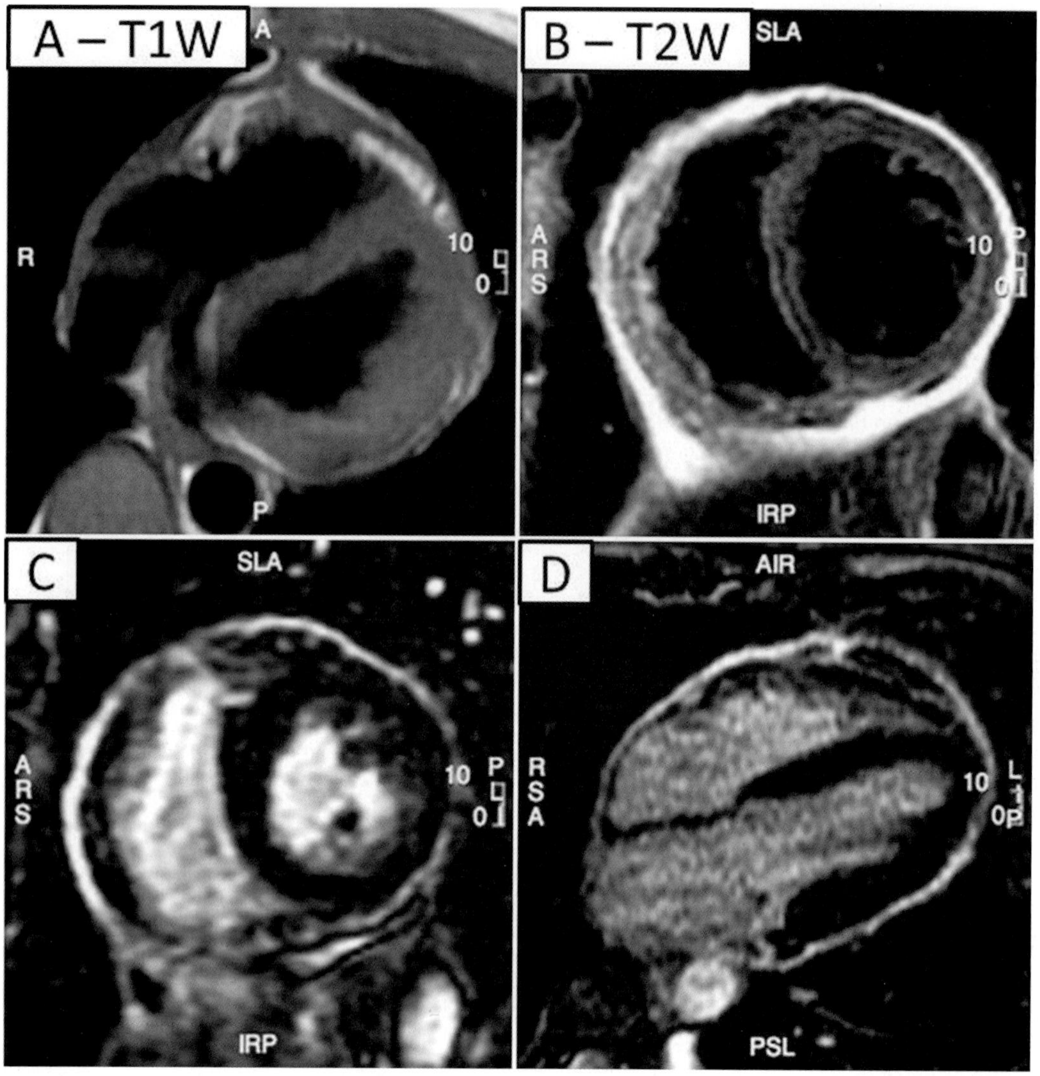

FIGURE 5.11

90. Which of the following MRI sequence allows assessment of myocardial iron overload in patients with thalassemia?

  A. Myocardial T2* quantification
  B. T1-weighted sequences of myocardium
  C. T2-weighted sequences of myocardium
  D. Delayed myocardial enhancement
  E. T1 mapping

91. What is the likely diagnosis on the MRI (Fig. 5.11) of this 17-year-old who presented to emergency room with a 2 day history of chest pain?

  A. Cocaine abuse
  B. Myocardial infarction
  C. Myocarditis
  D. Pericarditis
  E. Musculoskeletal chest pain

92. What is the likely diagnosis on this coronal reformat of CT angiogram (Fig. 5.12) in a 27-year-old acyanotic man presenting with easy fatigability?

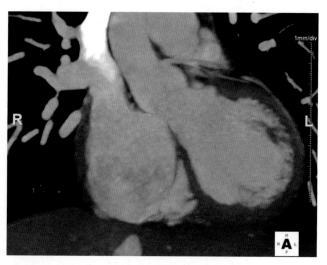

FIGURE 5.12

A. Total anomalous pulmonary venous connection
B. Partial anomalous pulmonary venous connection
C. Anomalous origin of right coronary artery
D. Anomalous origin of left coronary artery
E. Tricuspid atresia

93. Which was the most likely surgery performed on this patient (Fig. 5.13)?

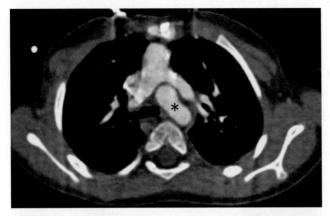

FIGURE 5.13

A. Norwood procedure
B. Glenn procedure
C. Fontan procedure
D. Atrial switch operation
E. Arterial switch operation

94. What is an additional imaging finding in this patient with tetralogy of Fallot (Fig. 5.14)?

A. Anomalous origin of left coronary artery from pulmonary artery
B. Single left coronary artery
C. Single right coronary artery
D. Coronary atherosclerosis
E. Prominent conal branch of right coronary artery anterior to the pulmonary valve

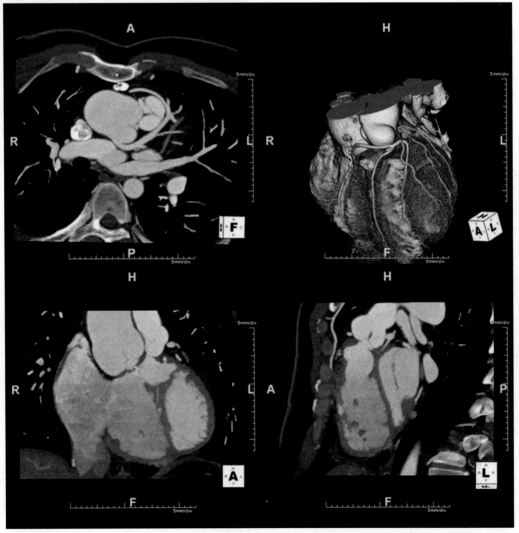

FIGURE 5.14

95. What is the name of the surgical shunt shown on this MR angiogram (Fig. 5.15)?

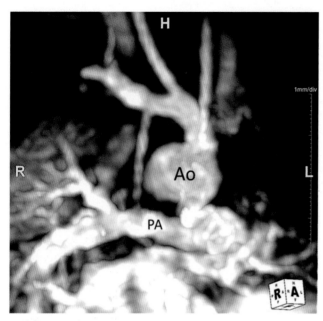

FIGURE 5.15 Ao, aorta; PA, pulmonary artery

    A. Waterston shunt
    B. Potts shunt
    C. Classic Blalock–Taussig shunt
    D. Modified Blalock–Taussig shunt
    E. Central shunt

96. What is the likely diagnosis in this 32-year-old patient (Fig. 5.16)?

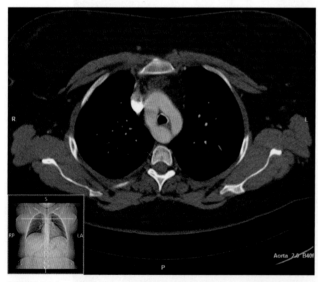

FIGURE 5.16

    A. Left aortic arch with normal branching pattern
    B. Left aortic arch with aberrant left subclavian artery origin
    C. Right aortic arch with mirror image branching pattern
    D. Right aortic arch with aberrant left subclavian artery origin
    E. Double aortic arch

97. What is the likely diagnosis in this 47-year-old patient (Fig. 5.17) with reduced exercise tolerance?

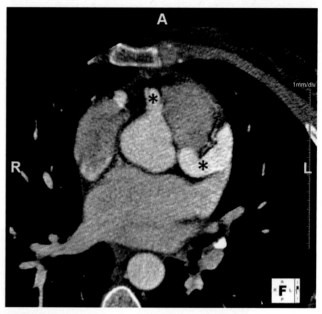

FIGURE 5.17

    A. Anomalous origin of right coronary artery from left aortic sinus
    B. Anomalous origin of left coronary artery from right aortic sinus
    C. Anomalous origin of left coronary artery from pulmonary artery
    D. Coronary artery fistula
    E. Long-term complication of Kawasaki disease

98. What is the likely diagnosis in this 12-year-old (Fig. 5.18) who had Fontan procedure?

99. What is the most common additional coexisting diagnosis in the patient with this CTA finding (Fig. 5.19)?

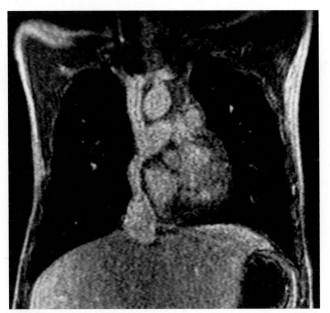

FIGURE 5.18

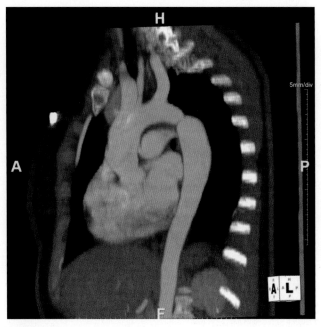

FIGURE 5.19

A. Stenosis of superior cavopulmonary anastomosis
B. Stenosis of inferior cavopulmonary anastomosis
C. Stenosis of IVC-Fontan conduit anastomosis
D. Stenosis of Fontan conduit
E. Thrombosis in Fontan circuit

A. Atrial septal defect
B. Ventricular septal defect
C. Common AV valve
D. Tetralogy of Fallot
E. Anomalous pulmonary vein connection

ANSWERS

1. (C) PW Doppler utilizes one crystal that both emits and receives the sound pulses. The maximal frequency shift that can be determined by PW Doppler is equal to one-half the PRF and is termed the Nyquist limit. This Nyquist limit can be extended by using lower frequency transducers. High PRF lacks range gating resulting in range ambiguity.

2. (A) The simplified Bernoulli equation ignores the components of flow acceleration and viscous friction. Doppler velocities across a patent ductus arteriosus or Blalock–Taussig shunt will likely be underestimated due to viscous friction in these tortuous connections and difficulties with proper ultrasound beam alignment. Multiple obstructions in series, such as multiple sites of LVOT obstruction (subvalvar, valvar, coarctation), will need to account for flow acceleration proximal to the distal site(s) of obstruction. Isolated valvar stenoses would be an appropriate use of the simplified Bernoulli equation.

3. (B) These Doppler patterns are consistent with impaired relaxation. Mitral inflow Doppler demonstrates an $E:A$ ratio <1 while mitral annular tissue Doppler imaging also demonstrates a decreased early annular velocity and abnormal E'/A' ratio <1. Pulmonary venous Doppler shows a systolic dominance and a prominent atrial reversal wave, consistent with grade 1 diastolic dysfunction (Fig. 5.20).

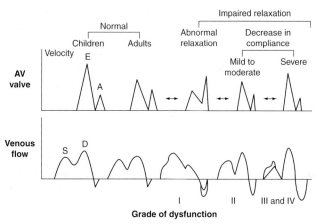

FIGURE 5.20

4. (D) The pressure gradient can be predicted by using the "expanded" Bernoulli equation, $P_1 - P_2 = 4(V_2^2 - V_1^2)$, utilizing the Doppler velocities proximal and distal to the coarctation: $4([4.0]^2 - [2.0]^2) = 48$ mm Hg.

5. (E) The presence of holodiastolic flow reversal in the abdominal aorta is consistent with severe aortic regurgitation.

6. (C) Contrast agents are designed to pass through the pulmonary capillary bed to opacify the left heart structures. The typical size of these microspheres is 1 to 10 microns. The acoustic impedance of contrast agents is much lower than that of the blood pool. The contrast effect persists for 3 to 5 minutes with most contrast agents.

7. (D) Microbubbles created with agitated saline range in size from 10 to 100 microns and do not pass through the pulmonary capillary bed. These microbubbles opacify the right atrium and right ventricle but not left heart structures in the absence of an intracardiac or intrapulmonary shunt. They can be helpful to identify an intracardiac right-to-left shunt that may be an etiology in stroke or unexplained cyanosis. In the presence of an intrapulmonary shunt the microbubbles typically appear in the left heart in three to five cardiac cycles compared to one to two cardiac cycles for an intracardiac shunt. A negative bubble study does not definitively exclude the presence of an intermittent right-to-left shunt.

8. (D) The width of the regurgitant jet (vena contracta) and the ratio of the vena contracta dimension to the aortic annulus dimension are quantitative measures to grade aortic regurgitation. The degree of left ventricular dilatation is a semiquantitative measure and is most consistent with the duration of aortic regurgitation in addition to its severity. The length of the regurgitant jet into the left ventricle is influenced by many factors in addition to regurgitant severity including LV end diastolic pressure and eccentricity of the jet. The degree of Doppler flow reversal in the abdominal aorta is an excellent predictor of regurgitation degree as is the forward to reverse flow TVI ratio in the distal transverse aortic arch.

9. (A) The myocardial performance index (MPI) is a ratio of the total time spent in isovolumic activity (isovolumic contraction and isovolumic relaxation times) divided by the time spent in ventricular ejection (Fig. 5.21).

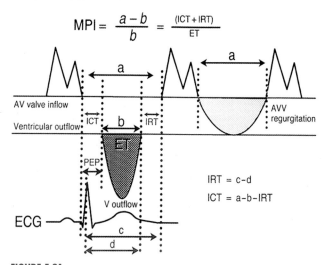

$$MPI = \frac{a - b}{b} = \frac{(ICT + IRT)}{ET}$$

$$IRT = c - d$$
$$ICT = a - b - IRT$$

FIGURE 5.21

10. (D) The subcostal imaging window is optimal to demonstrate the atrial septum and any associated atrial septal defects that may be present. To visualize the atrial septum without potential drop-out, the imaging plane of sound should be perpendicular to the cardiac structure of interest. With respect to the atrial septum, the imaging plane that is optimally perpendicular is the subcostal four-chamber and sagittal views. Atrial septal defects can be demonstrated in other imaging windows including

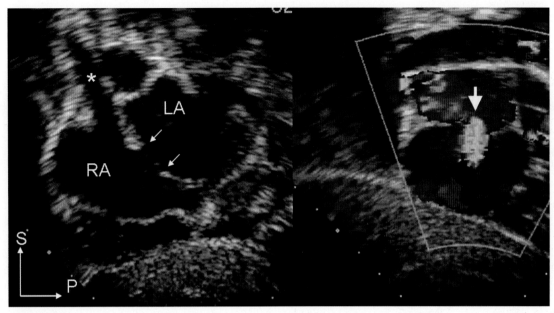

FIGURE 5.22 RA, right atrium; LA, left atrium.

the parasternal short-axis, apical four-chamber, and high right parasternal views but care must be taken not to diagnose an atrial septal defect when the plane of sound is more parallel to the atrial septum creating the potential for false drop-out in the 2D image. The addition of color Doppler and spectral Doppler interrogation in these views will also facilitate the diagnosis of an atrial septal defect (Fig. 5.22).

11. (A) Sinus venosus atrial septal defects are most commonly associated with anomalous connection of the right pulmonary veins. Either a single right upper pulmonary vein or the right upper and middle pulmonary veins insert anomalously to the superior vena cava or the SVC–right atrial junction. Sinus venosus defects are found most commonly in the superior portion of the atrial septum creating a "biatrial" insertion of the superior vena cava. These defects can also be located inferiorly near the entrance of the inferior vena cava into the right atrium.

12. (C) Constrictive pericarditis is characterized by increased respiratory variation in mitral inflow Doppler velocities by >25%. Transmitral Doppler often demonstrates an increased *E:A* ratio and a shortened E-wave deceleration time. Lateral mitral tissue Doppler velocities are usually normal. Hepatic venous Doppler will demonstrate increased atrial systolic flow reversals during expiration.

13. (C) Echocardiographic hallmarks of restrictive LV physiology in adults include an increased mitral inflow Doppler *E:A* ratio >2.0, shortened mitral E-wave deceleration time <160 msec, decreased lateral mitral E_a velocity, and an increased E/E' ratio >15. Pulmonary venous Doppler demonstrates decreased systolic to diastolic pulmonary venous filling wave ratio with significantly increased atrial reversal wave velocity and duration.

14. (D) Patients with Down syndrome (trisomy 21) have an almost 50% incidence of congenital heart disease, with AVSD being the most common cardiac anomaly in this cohort. AVSD in association with tetralogy of Fallot is a common constellation of

cardiac anomalies in patients with Down syndrome. Obstruction of the LVOT and coarctation of the aorta are also common cardiac abnormalities in patients with AVSD but are not as common in Down syndrome patients. Left ventricular hypoplasia can also occur in the setting of AVSD ("unbalanced AVSD with right ventricular dominance") but is less commonly seen in this cohort. Aortic valve stenosis and anomalous pulmonary venous connections are uncommon.

15. (D) Anatomic hallmarks of AVSD include a cleft in the anterior leaflet of the left atrioventricular valve, lateral rotation of the left ventricular papillary muscles, and attachments of the left and right atrioventricular valves at the same level at the cardiac crux. In addition, due to the absence of the atrioventricular septum in these defects, the left ventricular inflow is shortened and the left ventricular outflow is elongated ("goose-neck deformity") creating a ratio of LV inlet to LV outlet ratio <1. Owing to the presence of a common atrioventricular valve, the aortic valve is no longer "wedged" between the tricuspid and the mitral valves and is pushed anteriorly ("sprung").

16. (B) M-mode has excellent temporal resolution and a high fixed PRF. The *x*-axis represents time while the *y*-axis represents distance from the transducer. M-mode utilizes a single imaging crystal.

17. (A) Spatial resolution is defined as the smallest distance between two points that are distinguishable from one another. Axial resolution is the ability to differentiate points along the ultrasound beam and is equal to its wavelength. Lateral resolution is the ability to resolve points perpendicular to the ultrasound beam and is dependent on beam width, with the best resolution found where the beam is the narrowest. Axial resolution is better than lateral resolution.

18. (A) Doppler velocity is calculated as follows: $V = [c(f_d)]/[2f_o \cos \theta]$. The speed of sound (c) and the transmitted ultrasound frequency (f_o) are constant while the frequency shift (f_d) can be

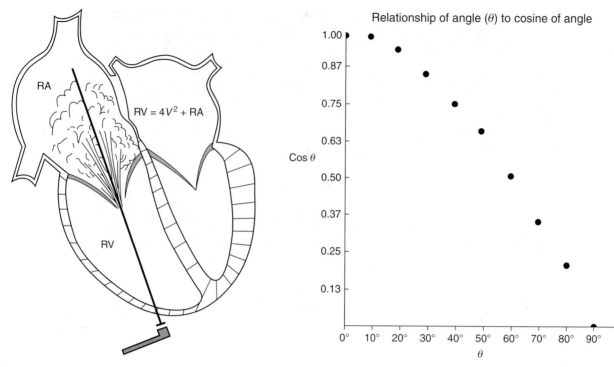

FIGURE 5.23 RA, right atrium; RV, right ventricle.

measured very accurately. Therefore, the main source of error in velocity calculation is the angle of incidence (θ) between the ultrasound beam and the moving structure or blood. When the angle of incidence is <20 degrees, the Doppler velocity is not significantly underestimated (Fig. 5.23).

19. (B) CW Doppler utilizes two crystals, one that is continuously transmitting and one that is continuously receiving, making the sampling rate infinite so that there is no limit to the detection of the maximal frequency shift. A disadvantage is that there is no range gating resulting in lack of range resolution (the maximal Doppler velocity can be anywhere along the ultrasound beam path). Both CW and PW Doppler are equally dependent on the angle of incidence for accurate velocity determination (Fig. 5.24).

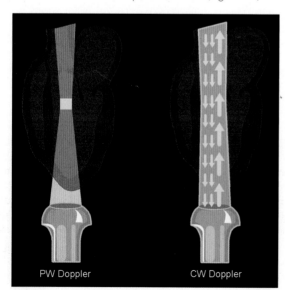

FIGURE 5.24

20. (C) PW Doppler utilizes one crystal that intermittently transmits and receives. The time between transmission and reception allows the determination of the depth of the signal providing excellent range resolution. However, the maximal detectable frequency shift is limited resulting in a lower Nyquist limit than CW Doppler. Spectral Doppler has a higher PRF than color Doppler. PRF varies with the depth of the sample volume with PW Doppler, with a higher PRF with more shallow sample volumes.

21. (A) The Nyquist limit is the maximal frequency shift detectable by PW Doppler and is equal to one-half of the PRF. The Nyquist limit is lower with PW Doppler and is increased with lower frequency transducers and at shallower depths of interrogation.

22. (A) Color Doppler utilizes multiple sampling sites along multiple ultrasound beams to generate frequency shifts that are converted into a digital format and autocorrelated into a color scheme. Color Doppler is a mean velocity of blood flow with the intensity of color representing mean Doppler flow velocities. The Nyquist limit is lower with color Doppler compared to spectral Doppler. Color Doppler is superimposed on 2D images resulting in less resolution.

23. (D) Subpulmonary ventricular septal defects are located adjacent to the pulmonary valve and aortic valve. These VSDs have been termed subpulmonary, supracristal, or doubly committed defects. These defects can be best demonstrated in the parasternal short-axis scan plane but can also be demonstrated from the subcostal and apical windows with appropriate angulation into the right ventricular outflow tract.

24. (A) Aortic regurgitation is the most common associated abnormality because of prolapse of the aortic cusp into a subpulmonary ventricular septal defect. While this associated prolapse

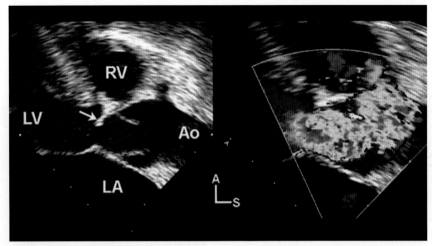

FIGURE 5.25 RV, right ventricle; LV, left ventricle; LA, left atrium; Ao, aorta.

of aortic tissue limits the size of the VSD and can lessen the left-to-right shunt, the progression of aortic insufficiency due to distortion of the aortic valve is well recognized. If this regurgitation is significant and progresses, then surgical closure of the ventricular septal defect is indicated (and is not dependent on the size of the left-to-right shunt).

25. (C) Large ventricular septal defects result in equalization of right and left ventricular pressures as well as elevated pulmonary arterial pressure. Left-to-right shunting at ventricular level results in a substantial increase in pulmonary blood flow with left atrial and left ventricular volume overload. Overall systemic blood flow is not significantly increased in this setting.

26. (A) The best morphologic hallmarks of the right atrium are the broad-based right atrial appendage and the connections of the inferior vena cava and coronary sinus. Superior vena caval connection(s) have significant anatomic variability. Atrioventricular relationships can also vary and are not hallmarks of right atrial morphology. The valve of the fossa ovalis is septum primum and a left atrial structure. The atrioventricular valve is a hallmark of ventricular morphology, with the morphologic tricuspid valve being the anatomic hallmark of the right ventricle.

27. (B) The best imaging plane to define the entire atrial septum is the subcostal imaging plane because it is perpendicular to this anatomic structure. False drop-out can occur in imaging planes that are more parallel to the atrial septum.

28. (B) The best anatomic hallmark of the morphologic right ventricle is the connection of the tricuspid valve with a more apical insertion at the cardiac crux compared to the morphologic mitral valve. The tricuspid valve is "septophilic" with attachments to the ventricular septum. The right ventricle is more crescent in shape with prominent trabeculations.

29. (D) A higher insertion of the morphologic mitral valve at the cardiac crux and lack of atrioventricular valve chordal attachments to the ventricular septum ("septophobic") are excellent anatomic hallmarks of the morphologic left ventricle. The LV is elliptical in shape with fine trabeculations, mainly toward the cardiac apex.

30. (A) Utilizing the modified Bernoulli equation to obtain the peak instantaneous gradient across the pulmonary valve, $4 \times$ (velocity)^2, then $4 \times (4.0)^2 = 64$ mm Hg.

31. (B) The most common type of subaortic stenosis is related to a discrete membrane proximal to the aortic valve within the LVOT (Fig. 5.25). This membrane is most often circumferential and can be adherent to both the aortic valve and the anterior leaflet of the mitral valve. LVOT obstruction in the setting of hypertrophic cardiomyopathy (HCM) is often related to asymmetric septal hypertrophy in combination with systolic anterior motion of the mitral valve chordal and leaflet tissue. Anomalous mitral chordal insertions within the LVOT can be isolated or found in association with congenital heart disease and may result in obstruction but are not as common as discrete membranes (Fig. 5.25).

32. (A) Bicuspid aortic valve is the most commonly associated cardiac finding in patients with simple coarctation with some studies showing as high as an 80% occurrence in patients with coarctation. Atrial and ventricular septal defects are also common in patients with coarctation. Pulmonary valve stenosis and coronary arterial anomalies are much less frequent in this cohort.

33. (C) The aortic lumen must be narrowed by at least 50% to significantly affect systemic arterial pressure; 50% narrowing = 10 mm Hg gradient.

34. (C) Cardiac tamponade occurs when increasing fluid in the pericardial space causes a rise in intrapericardial pressure (typically greater than intracardiac pressure) compromising systemic venous return to the right atrium. Diastolic right atrial and right ventricular wall collapse occurs when intrapericardial pressure exceeds intracardiac pressure, with collapse of the right ventricle more sensitive to identify tamponade physiology. Pulsed-wave Doppler is more sensitive to identify cardiac tamponade with respiratory changes in Doppler flow across the tricuspid valve (>30%) and mitral valve (>25%) being most characteristic due to ventricular interdependence. While the overall size of the pericardial effusion is important, how quickly the fluid accumulates has more of an effect on intrapericardial pressure due to the relative compliance of the pericardium in the acute and chronic settings.

35. (E) The relationship between velocity of circumferential fiber shortening and end systolic wall stress is independent of heart rate and preload and incorporates afterload making it a quantitative measure of ventricular contractility. Ejection fraction, shortening fraction, and the myocardial performance index are all significantly impacted by both preload and afterload.

36. (A) SF = (LV EDD − LV ESD)/LV EDD. Left ventricular shortening fraction is maximal during the first month of life (range 35% to 45%). Mean LV shortening fraction in children is 36% and ranges from 28% to 40%.

37. (B) The presence of holodiastolic Doppler flow reversal is consistent with a significant run-off from the descending aorta including a large patent ductus arteriosus, severe aortic valve regurgitation, systemic-to-pulmonary artery shunts, and large arteriovenous fistula.

38. (C) The most common ventricular septal defect associated with coarctation is a perimembranous defect. While less common, a posterior malalignment VSD often results in severe coarctation or interruption of the aortic arch. Muscular VSD as well as inlet VSD can also occur in the setting of coarctation, in particular with an unbalanced RV-dominant AVSD.

39. (A) The systolic jet in patients with supravalvar aortic stenosis propagates further than the jet originating with aortic valvar stenosis and has a tendency to be entrained along the aortic wall thereby transferring its kinetic energy into the right innominate artery. This physical principle, termed the Coanda effect, often is expressed clinically in these patients by marked discrepancy in upper arm blood pressures, with the right arm pressure higher than the left arm blood pressure.

40. (B) In the simplified Bernoulli equation, convective acceleration is calculated while flow acceleration and viscous friction are ignored. To accurately utilize the simplified equation, the proximal Doppler velocity must be negligible (Fig. 5.26).

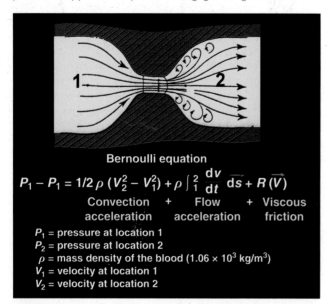

Bernoulli equation

$$P_1 - P_1 = 1/2\, \rho\, (V_2^2 - V_1^2) + \rho \int_1^2 \frac{dv}{dt}\, \vec{ds} + R\,(\vec{V})$$

Convection + Flow + Viscous
acceleration   acceleration   friction

P_1 = pressure at location 1
P_2 = pressure at location 2
ρ = mass density of the blood (1.06×10^3 kg/m^3)
V_1 = velocity at location 1
V_2 = velocity at location 2

FIGURE 5.26

41. (C) An overriding atrioventricular valve empties into two ventricles. It is committed to the ventricle to which >50% of its orifice is directed (Fig. 5.27). This connection is always associated with a malalignment VSD. Valves that override can also straddle by having chordal attachments to the contralateral ventricle (Fig. 5.27).

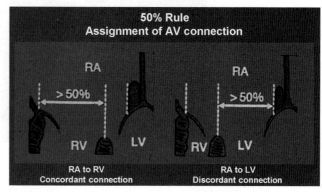

50% Rule
Assignment of AV connection

RA   RA

>50%   >50%

RV   LV   RV   LV

RA to RV   RA to LV
Concordant connection   Discordant connection

FIGURE 5.27 AV, atrioventricular; RA, right atrium; RV, right ventricle; LV, left ventricle.

42. (E) A straddling atrioventricular valve has anomalous chordal insertions or papillary muscles in the contralateral ventricle. Straddling and override often coexist. Straddling is associated with the presence of a ventricular septal defect but does not require a malalignment type of defect. Semilunar valves do not have chordae or papillary muscles so they do not straddle. Straddling is not a common feature of tetralogy of Fallot.

43. (C) Interruption of the intrahepatic portion of the inferior vena cava with azygous vein continuation to the superior vena cava is a common feature of polysplenia syndrome (left atrial isomerism). The abdominal situs is variable and can be ambiguous, inversus, or solitus. The spleens are usually multiple and are characteristically located on the same side. A single gall bladder is most typical but biliary atresia can and does occur.

44. (E) In the normal heart the aorta is located in a rightward and posterior location relative to the pulmonary artery. In D-transposition, the aorta is typically anterior and rightward. In L-transposition (congenitally corrected TGA), the aorta is most commonly anterior and leftward. The aorta is also most commonly leftward and anterior in double inlet left ventricle.

45. (C) Tricuspid atresia is an example of a single inlet atrioventricular valve connection (Fig. 5.28).

46. (D) Type A interruption of the aortic arch occurs distal to the origin of the left subclavian artery. Type B interruption occurs between the left common carotid and left subclavian arteries. Type C interruption occurs between the right innominate and the left common carotid arteries.

47. (B) When a persistent left superior vena cava drains to the coronary sinus, the size of the coronary sinus is inversely proportional to the size of the bridging innominate vein. When the coronary sinus is severely dilated, the innominate vein is most commonly very small or absent. When the inferior vena cava is interrupted, venous return is directed from the azygous vein to the superior vena

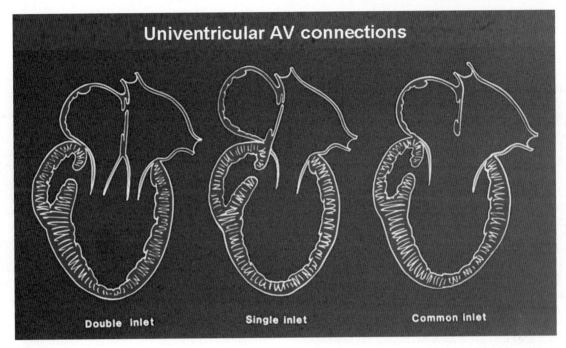

Univentricular AV connections

Double inlet   Single inlet   Common inlet

FIGURE 5.28

cava. Interruption of the IVC is more common in polysplenia syndrome versus asplenia syndrome. Superior vena caval connections are variable and are not an anatomic hallmark of the morphologic right atrium. The left pulmonary veins more commonly merge than the right veins as they connect to the left atrium.

48. (D) While all these are features that distinguish the morphologic tricuspid valve from the mitral valve, the most reliable anatomic hallmark is the level of attachment of the atrioventricular valve at the cardiac crux. The atrioventricular valves are invariably associated with their appropriate morphologic ventricle (tricuspid valve with the right ventricle and mitral valve with the left ventricle) and are the best marker for atrioventricular connection and ventricular morphology.

49. (B) Organ systems with sidedness include the cardiac, pulmonary, and gastrointestinal systems. Cardiac sidedness is determined by the position of the right atrium. Pulmonary situs is defined by the positions of the morphologic right and left lungs. Abdominal situs is characterized by the location of the liver and stomach.

50. (C) Subcostal images demonstrate a sinus venosus atrial septal defect with partial anomalous pulmonary venous connection to the superior vena cava. The defect is located in the superior/posterior portion of the atrial septum adjacent to the superior vena cava. The right upper and middle pulmonary veins are often anomalous and most commonly connect to the superior vena cava.

51. (A) These images demonstrate the classic features of a partial AVSD (Fig. 5.29). There is a large primum atrial septal defect with a large left-to-right atrial level shunt. Owing to lack of the atrioventricular septum, both atrioventricular valves are inserted at the same level at the cardiac crux. The inlet ventricular septum is

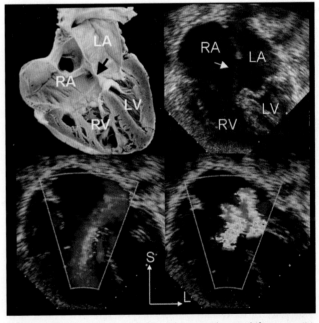

FIGURE 5.29 RA, right atrium; RV, right ventricle; LA, left atrium; LV, left ventricle.

intact. Color Doppler also demonstrates significant mitral regurgitation, most likely related to a cleft in the anterior leaflet.

52. (E) Both the parasternal and the subcostal images demonstrate a large anterior malalignment ventricular septal defect with approximately 50% aortic override of the VSD. This anatomy can be consistent with tetralogy of Fallot, pulmonary atresia with VSD, or truncus arteriosus with additional imaging of the right ventricular outflow tract, the pulmonary arteries, and aortic arch helping to differentiate these diagnoses.

53. (B) This parasternal short-axis scan demonstrates a large membranous VSD with a large left-to-right shunt.

54. (C) This parasternal long-axis scan demonstrates significant aortic root dilatation consistent with Marfan syndrome. Classic echocardiographic features of Marfan syndrome include aortic root dilatation and mitral valve prolapse. Hallmark cardiac findings in Down syndrome include AVSD and VSDs. Most common cardiac lesions in DiGeorge syndrome include aortic arch anomalies and conotruncal defects. Noonan syndrome typically has right ventricular outflow and pulmonary artery anomalies as well as atrial septal defects and HCM. Williams syndrome classically presents with supravalvar aortic stenosis and supravalvar/branch pulmonary arterial stenoses.

55. (B) Cardiac myxomas are the most common adult cardiac tumor and the second most common childhood cardiac tumor. The majority (75%) are located in the left atrium and are typically attached to the fossa ovalis. When large, they can obstruct atrioventricular valve inflow leading to symptoms including positional dyspnea, syncope, and even death. Constitutional symptoms include weight loss, malaise, arthralgias, and myalgias. Carney syndrome is a familial form of myxoma and is associated with lentigines and endocrine abnormalities.

56. (C) This parasternal long-axis scan shows a large homogeneous echogenic mass in the posterior wall of the left ventricle consistent with a cardiac fibroma. Fibromas are firm, white, nonencapsulated tumors. They are typically located in the left ventricle within the posterior wall or septum and commonly at the cardiac apex. They are often large and can result in cavitary obstruction or impair atrioventricular valve function. These tumors also have a significant risk of sudden death due to ventricular arrhythmias.

57. (C) The right ventricle ejects 55% to 60% of combined fetal cardiac output while the left ventricle ejects 40% to 45%. Cardiac output increases significantly during gestation, but the relative amounts of output from these two parallel circulations remain relatively the same.

58. (C) This fetus has significant hemodynamic compromise by the underlying fetal tachycardia. Starting sotalol is the most effective therapy to treat this hydropic fetus. Digoxin has poor maternal fetal transfer in the hydropic fetus and is not the first-line drug therapy in this clinical scenario. Maternal lupus is associated with fetal heart block and bradycardia; hence, evaluation of ant-SSA/Ro and anti-SSA/La antibodies is not indicated. At 22 weeks, delivery of a live fetus is not an optimal strategy either, so pretreatment of the mother with betamethasone is not indicated.

59. (D) Evaluation of the outflow tracts is necessary to exclude D-TGA because the four-chamber view is often normal in these fetuses. The remainder of the listed congenital heart lesions is readily diagnosed in the fetal four-chamber view.

60. (B) The normal fetal heart comprises about one-third of the fetal thorax, ranging from 25% to 35%.

61. (A) Fetal arrhythmias occur in 1% to 3% of all pregnancies. PAC comprise the largest percentage of these rhythm abnormalities followed by PVC. Fetal SVT, atrial flutter, and complete heart block account for <10% of all reported fetal arrhythmias.

62. (D) This is the mechanical PR interval, measured from the beginning of atrial inflow (mitral A-wave) to the beginning of ventricular ejection.

63. (E) With lack of antegrade flow across the atretic pulmonary valve, fetuses with pulmonary atresia with intact ventricular septum often have reversal of flow across the ductus arteriosus into the hypoplastic main pulmonary artery and branch pulmonary arteries. The other listed congenital heart lesions all typically have a normally functioning pulmonary valve with antegrade flow into the main pulmonary artery and ductus arteriosus.

64. (C) Because of limited antegrade blood flow across the critically stenotic aortic valve, flow within the aortic arch is supplied retrograde from the ductus arteriosus. The other listed congenital heart lesions all typically have a normally functioning aortic valve with antegrade flow into the ascending aorta and transverse aortic arch and antegrade flow from the ductus arteriosus to the descending aorta.

65. (C) The normal fetal heart rate ranges from 100 to 180 bpm throughout gestation. Fetal bradycardia is defined as a sustained heart rate less than 100 bpm while fetal tachycardia as a sustained rate greater than 180 bpm.

66. (A) The normal leftward axis of the fetal heart (relative to the midline) ranges from 30 degrees to 60 degrees.

67. (A) At term, 10% of fetal cardiac output perfuses the lungs. The remainder of this deoxygenated blood is directed through the ductus arteriosus to the descending aorta and placenta for oxygenation.

68. (1-D, 2-B, 3-A, 4-C, 5-E) Lithium has been shown in studies to be associated with fetal Ebstein anomaly as well as atrial septal defects and atrioventricular valve atresia. Fetal alcohol syndrome has been commonly associated with septal defects including atrial and ventricular septal defects and is less commonly associated with coarctation and conotruncal defects. Indomethacin is a potent ductal constrictor. Coarctation of the aorta and LVOT obstruction have been described in fetal hydantoin syndrome. Exposure to isotretinoin during gestation has been associated with fetal D-TGA as well as septal defects and conotruncal anomalies.

69. (1-C, 2-A, 3-D, 4-B, 5-E) Turner syndrome is most commonly associated with coarctation of the aorta and aortic stenosis with bicuspid aortic valve. Other less common defects in Turner syndrome include atrial and ventricular septal defects. DiGeorge syndrome is characterized by interrupted aortic arch and conotruncal defects, including truncus arteriosus. The hallmark lesion associated with trisomy 21 is an AVSD; other lesions include secundum atrial septal defect, ventricular septal defect, tetralogy of Fallot, and aortic arch obstruction. Trisomy 13 has a very high incidence of congenital heart disease, namely ventricular septal defects. Also associated is hypoplastic left heart syndrome, tetralogy of Fallot, and AVSD. Williams syndrome is most commonly associated with supravalvar aortic stenosis and branch pulmonary artery stenosis and also with septal defects and aortic arch anomalies.

70. (E) Maternal systemic lupus is associated with complete heart block in the fetus. Umbilical cord compression can result in transient fetal bradycardia or even brief asystole. Both heterotaxy syndrome and congenitally corrected transposition (L-TGA) are also associated with complete heart block and fetal bradycardia. Tetralogy of Fallot is not a frequent association with fetal conduction abnormalities.

71. (A) Ebstein anomaly is associated with a 15% to 20% incidence of rhythm abnormalities, most notably Wolff–Parkinson–White syndrome and SVT.

72. (C) Doppler velocities within the umbilical artery reflect downstream resistance within the placenta. The pulsatility index is defined as the peak systolic velocity minus the end diastolic velocity divided by the mean velocity.

73. (D) In fetuses with congestive heart failure, the cerebral resistance typically falls ("brain-sparing effect") resulting in a decreased pulsatility index in the middle cerebral artery. A concomitant increase in the umbilical artery pulsatility index is a common finding. Pulsations within the umbilical vein or flow reversal in the ductus venosus are ominous signs in the fetus with heart failure and compromised cardiac output. Atrioventricular valve regurgitation is common in fetal heart failure.

74. (D) While right ventricular hypertrophy is one of the salient features of tetralogy of Fallot, it is usually secondary to RV outflow obstruction and develops postnatally. Prominent hypertrophy during fetal life is present in the recipient twin in twin–twin transfusion syndrome as well as in poorly controlled maternal diabetes in late gestation fetuses. Both fetal HCM and Noonan syndrome have variable expression of ventricular hypertrophy (from absent to massive hypertrophy).

75. (A) The incidence of congenital heart disease in maternal diabetes (4% to 10%) is higher than those with a previous family history of congenital heart disease (2% to 4%). The most common cardiac lesions in fetuses of diabetic mothers include D-TGA, truncus arteriosus, and tetralogy of Fallot. Risk of congenital heart disease in the fetus has been directly associated with the maternal hemoglobin A1C level during early gestation. HCM associated with poor maternal glucose control is most often reversible within weeks or months post delivery.

76. (E) Most implanted metallic objects, including coils, clips, pacemaker leads, and occluder devices, are weakly ferromagnetic and are relatively immobile after implantation. Pacemakers and AICDs are a relative contraindication to a cardiac MR examination, but recent reports suggest that even these devices may be safe for the MR examination.

77. (C) Stainless steel objects, such as PDA coils, cause the most imaging artifact with MR imaging. Occluder devices including the Amplatzer ASD device also cause significant imaging artifact. Pacemaker leads, PDA vascular clips, and nonferromagnetic stents cause less artifact with MR imaging.

78. (A) With spin echo, there is a relatively long time period between spin excitation and data sampling resulting in blood flow leaving the imaging plane when the signal is sampled. This produces an image where blood appears black and surrounding cardiac tissue is encoded in shades of gray or white. Spin echo sequences provide still images for anatomy and tissue characterization. Blood appears bright in gradient echo, steady-state free precession, and contrast-enhanced images.

79. (C) VEC MRI is a gradient echo sequence that can measure blood flow velocity and quantify blood flow. The other sequences do not provide any quantifiable flow or velocity information.

80. (D) Spin echo cardiac magnetic resonance imaging is a black-blood technique where the blood pool is black and the surrounding cardiac tissue is encoded in shades of gray or white. Signal acquisition is performed over several cardiac cycles. This technique produces high tissue contrast and has less imaging artifact with metallic implants compared to other cardiac MR techniques. Spin echo applications include imaging myocardial and blood vessel walls, cardiac masses and tumors, and the pericardium. T1- and T2-weighted sequences in spin echo imaging can help in tissue characterization.

81. (A) Gradient echo sequences have less time between spin excitation and signal detection resulting in a faster acquisition than spin echo sequences. Therefore, the gradient echo technique results in high imaging speed with multiple images acquired during each cardiac cycle. The signal from slower moving tissue is gray and has less contrast compared to spin echo images and is more susceptible to imaging artifacts. Faster moving blood has a stronger signal resulting in bright blood images.

82. (A) MDE has become the primary cardiac MR technique to assess myocardial viability. Washout of gadolinium contrast agents is delayed in necrotic myocardium as well as areas of fibrotic tissue. Nonviable myocardium therefore appears bright when compared to viable myocardium. MDE has been shown to be very effective in determining the presence, size, and transmurality of myocardial infarctions as well as in the identification of the presence and extent of myocardial fibrosis in patients with HCM.

83. (B) Phase-contrast (or velocity-encoded) cine imaging is used for flow quantification and does not require any contrast administration. Conventional MRA is performed with contrast; however, newer noncontrast MRA sequences do not require contrast agents. Intravenous contrast administration is needed for myocardial perfusion, delayed enhancement, and TRICKS.

84. (C) T2-weighted sequences are fluid-sensitive and can best detect myocardial edema such as in a patient with acute myocarditis. First-pass perfusion imaging may or may not show a hypo-attenuated filling defect in the area of myocardial edema. Other sequences do not help in assessment of myocardial edema.

85. (C) ECG-gated CTA is the best test to assess intramural course of anomalous coronary artery origin. MRA does not have the spatial resolution to confirm this diagnosis. CTA without ECG gating does not allow assessment of coronary arteries. Invasive coronary angiography cannot assess the intramural course of anomalous coronary artery. Thallium scan can only show myocardial areas of hypoperfusion.

86. (B) Conventional MRA can assess the coarctation of aorta. CTA can also do the assessment; however, ECG gating is not needed for this purpose. Retrospective ECG-gated CTA has highest dose of radiation. TEE, stress echo, and thallium scan are not optimal tests for coarctation assessment.

87. (A) *The magnet is always on!* This is an important fact for MRI safety. Ferromagnetic objects brought into the room can act as projectiles and may cause injury to patient or personnel. The magnet is always on, even when not in use.

88. (D) Delayed myocardial enhancement is typically subepicardial or midmyocardial and patchy in myocarditis. In infarction, the delayed enhancement is typically subendocardial or transmural. Myocardial edema is best seen on T2-weighted black-blood images. Fatty infiltrates can be seen on T1-weighted images and are not a hallmark of myocarditis. Early myocardial enhancement is due to hyperemia of the inflamed areas. MR angiogram does not help in myocardial assessment.

89. (A) Noncontrast CT is the best test to assess pericardial calcification. Contrast enhancement and ECG gating are not needed for this purpose. The other imaging modalities do not help in this assessment.

90. (A) T2* quantification is required for measurement of iron in myocardial tissue in patients with thalassemia or other chronic blood transfusion recipients. Other sequences cannot be used to quantify tissue iron load.

91. (D) MR images show typical features of pericarditis. Panel A shows thickened pericardium on T1-weighted double-inversion recovery sequence. Panel B shows pericardial edema and a small effusion on T2-weighted sequence. Panels C and D show diffuse postcontrast delayed enhancement of the pericardium. Myocardium has normal appearance in all these images.

92. (B) CTA shows anomalous drainage of right upper and right middle pulmonary veins draining to superior vena cava.

The left coronary artery seems to be originating normally in this view, whereas the right coronary is not seen. This single coronal plane does not show the tricuspid valve, right ventricle, and the left pulmonary veins but the clinical history of acyanosis precludes the diagnoses of TAPVC and tricuspid atresia.

93. (E) Asterisk marks the aortic arch. The image shows the main pulmonary artery anterior to the aorta with the branch pulmonary arteries "draped-over" the aorta. This is consistent with the LeCompte maneuver performed with an arterial switch operation in patients with D-TGA. In atrial switch procedures the great arterial relationship remains transposed.

94. (B) The images show single left coronary artery with the right coronary branch traveling anterior to the pulmonary valve. This is important if transannular patch augmentation of pulmonary valve is intended. To avoid trauma to RCA, a RV-PA conduit may be needed to relieve the RV-PA gradient.

95. (D) The image shows a shunt placed between the right subclavian artery and the pulmonary artery, which is consistent with a modified BT shunt. Classic BT shunt is direct end-to-side anastomosis of subclavian artery to the PA. Waterston shunt is direct side-to-side anastomosis of ascending aorta to the right pulmonary artery. Potts shunt is direct side-to-side anastomosis of descending aorta to the left pulmonary artery. Central shunt is a small conduit from aorta to pulmonary artery.

96. (E) The single axial image of this CT angiogram shows aortic arches on both sides of trachea, consistent with double aortic arch. The branching pattern is not seen on this image. Typical branching pattern for double aortic arch is separate origin of four aortic arch branches. The right common carotid and right subclavian arteries arise from the right aortic arch, whereas the left common carotid and the left subclavian arteries arise from the left aortic arch.

97. (C) The CT angiogram shows anomalous origin of left coronary artery from the pulmonary artery. Asterisks mark the right and left coronary arteries. With chronic run-off of blood from the LCA into the pulmonary artery, the main coronary arteries become dilated over time due to increased flow from RCA to LCA via collaterals.

98. (D) The MR angiogram shows a coronal plane with Fontan conduit stenosis. This is a common finding in patients who received a conduit made of biologic material such as aortic homograft. The anastomotic sites appear patent without any thrombi in the Fontan circuit.

99. (B) The CTA shows coarctation of aorta. VSD and bicuspid aortic valve are common coexisting diagnoses in patients with coarctation of aorta.

ACKNOWLEDGMENT

Figures 5.3, 5.4, 5.5, 5.8, 5.9, 5.20, 5.21, 5.23, 5.24, 5.26, 5.27, 5.28, and 5.29 are from Eidem BW, Cetta F, O'Leary PW. Echocardiography in Pediatric and Adult Congenital Heart Disease. Philadelphia, PA: Lippincott Williams & Wilkins, 2010. © Mayo Foundation for Medical Education and Research. All rights Reserved.

SUGGESTED READINGS

Allen HD, Driscoll DJ, Shaddy RE, et al. *Moss and Adams' Heart Disease in Infants, Children, and Adolescents.* 7th ed. Philadelphia, PA: Lippincott Williams & Wilkins; 2008.

Didier D, Ratib O, Beghetti M, et al. Morphologic and functional evaluation of congenital heart disease by magnetic resonance imaging. *J Magn Reson Imaging.* 1999;10:639–655.

Drose JA. *Fetal Echocardiography.* 2nd ed. St Louis, MO: Saunders Elsevier; 2010.

Eidem BW, Cetta F, O'Leary PW. *Echocardiography in Pediatric and Adult Congenital Heart Disease.* Philadelphia, PA: Lippincott Williams & Wilkins; 2010.

Hance-Miller W, Fyfe DA, Stevenson JG, et al. Indications and guidelines for performance of transesophageal echocardiography in the patient with pediatric acquired or congenital heart disease. A report from the Task Force of the Pediatric Council of the American Society of Echocardiography. *J Am Soc Echocardiogr.* 2005;18:91–98.

Kilner PJ, Geva T, Kaemmerer H, et al. Recommendations for cardiovascular magnetic resonance in adults with congenital heart disease from the respective working groups of the European Society of Cardiology. *Eur Heart J.* 2010;31:794–805.

Lai WW, Geva T, Shirali GS, et al.; Task Force of the Pediatric Council of the American Society of Echocardiography. Pediatric Council of the American Society of Echocardiography. Guidelines and standards for performance of a pediatric echocardiogram: a report from the Task Force of the Pediatric Council of the American Society of Echocardiography. *J Am Soc Echocardiogr.* 2006;19:1413–1430.

Lang RM, Bierig M, Devereux RB, et al. Recommendations for chamber quantification: a report from the American Society of Echocardiography's Guidelines and Standards Committee and the Chamber Quantification Writing Group, developed in conjunction with the European Association of Echocardiography, a branch of the European Society of Cardiology. *J Am Soc Echocardiogr.* 2005;18:1440–1463.

Lopez L, Colan SD, Frommelt PC, et al. Recommendations for quantification methods during the performance of a pediatric echocardiogram: a report from the Pediatric Measurements Writing Group of the American Society of Echocardiography Pediatric and Congenital Heart Disease Council. *J Am Soc Echocardiogr.* 2010;23:465–495.

Oh JK, Seward JB, Tajik AJ. *The Echo Manual.* 3rd ed. Philadelphia, PA: Lippincott Williams & Wilkins; 2006.

Prakash A, Powell AJ, Krishnamurthy R, et al. Magnetic resonance imaging evaluation of myocardial perfusion and viability in congenital and acquired pediatric heart disease. *Am J Cardiol.* 2004;93:657–661.

Prakash A, Powell AJ, Geva T. Multimodality noninvasive imaging for assessment of congenital heart disease. *Circ Cardiovasc Imaging.* 2010;3:112–125.

Rychik J, Ayres N, Cunco B, et al. American Society of Echocardiography guidelines and standards for performance of the fetal echocardiogram. *J Am Soc Echocardiogr.* 2004;17:803–810.

CHAPTER 6

Cardiac Electrophysiology

Bryan C. Cannon, Philip Wackel, and Andrew Schneider

QUESTIONS

1. A fetal ultrasound performed at 32-week gestation reveals fetal SVT at a rate of 250 beats per minute (bpm) with 1:1 AV relationship. There is no evidence of hydrops fetalis and the ventricular function is good. Over the next 24 hours, the fetus is observed and tachycardia persists. You would advise which of the following:

   A. Adenosine administration via cordocentesis through umbilical vein
   B. Continued observation
   C. Atenolol
   D. Digoxin
   E. Immediate delivery

2. A patient presents after an irregular heart beat was noted on a preparticipation sports physical. The electrocardiogram (ECG) is shown in Figure 6.1. There is no murmur and he has an otherwise normal examination. He is asymptomatic. What would you advise?

   A. He can participate in all sports
   B. No competitive sports
   C. He may participate in all sports if the rhythm can be normalized by an antiarrhythmic medication
   D. He may participate in all sports if he undergoes a successful ablation procedure
   E. He may participate in low-impact sports such as golf

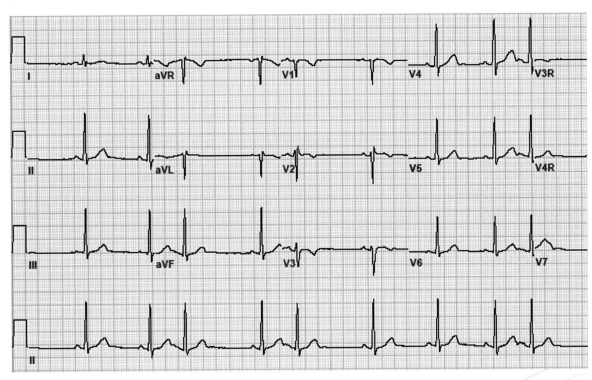

FIGURE 6.1

3. A 3-year-old asymptomatic boy is referred to you after an ECG is obtained on preoperative screening prior to a tonsillectomy. There is no family history of sudden death. The ECG is shown in Figure 6.2. What would be the most appropriate therapy?

A. Implant an ICD
B. Begin β-blocker therapy
C. Perform an electrophysiology study
D. Start amiodarone
E. Direct current cardioversion

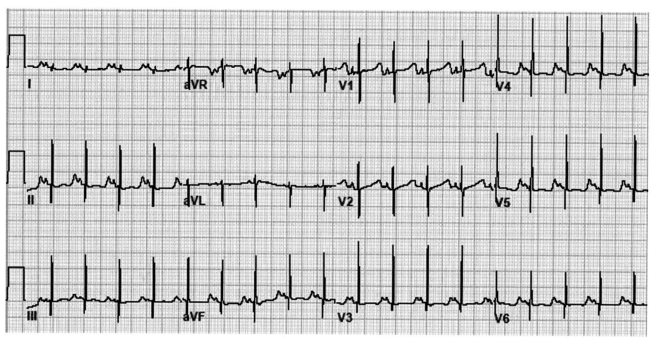

FIGURE 6.2

4. A newborn presents with a heart rate of 210 bpm shortly after birth. The prenatal course was unremarkable. An ECG is obtained and is shown in Figure 6.3. What would be the next most appropriate step?

A. Oral amiodarone
B. Vagal maneuvers
C. Intravenous amiodarone
D. Oral propranolol
E. Direct current cardioversion

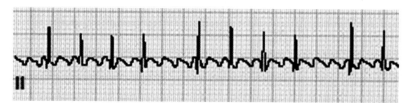

FIGURE 6.3

5. An 8-year-old patient with a repaired VSD presents with a new onset seizure. The rhythm strip shown in Figure 6.4 was obtained during the seizure episode and sent to you for review. Which of the following therapies is most appropriate?

A. Direct current cardioversion
B. IV lidocaine drip
C. Oral β-blocker
D. No therapy
E. IV amiodarone

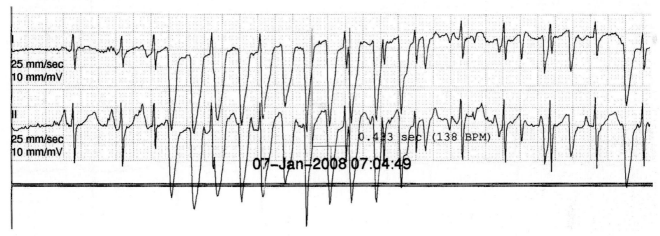

FIGURE 6.4

6. A 14-year-old boy presents for evaluation of a murmur and is noted to have left ventricular septal hypertrophy on his echocardiogram consistent with hypertrophic cardiomyopathy. Which of the following additional factors most increases the risk of sudden death?

A. Marked left ventricular hypertrophy on the ECG (R wave 50 mm in V6)
B. Left ventricular septal wall thickness of 1.7 cm in systole
C. Left ventricular outflow gradient of 20 mm Hg
D. Family history of multiple sudden deaths
E. Chest pain with exercise

7. A 14-year-old patient with dilated cardiomyopathy is on digoxin, furosemide, and enalapril for his heart failure. He is now starting to have frequent episodes of supraventricular tachycardia (SVT) and you would like to start him on amiodarone. Which medication adjustment will most likely be required?

A. Decrease the dose of digoxin
B. Increase the dose of digoxin
C. Increase the dose of furosemide
D. Decrease the dose of enalapril
E. Make no changes in any of the medications

8. An 8-year-old boy has been complaining of episodes of fast heart rates lasting 15 to 20 minutes. These typically occur with exercise. He has an episode every 3 months. A 24-hour Holter monitor shows variability in the QRS morphology as shown in Figure 6.5. The etiology of his symptoms is most likely to be which of the following?

A. Ventricular tachycardia
B. Junctional tachycardia
C. Reentrant supraventricular tachycardia
D. Atrial flutter
E. Automatic focus atrial tachycardia

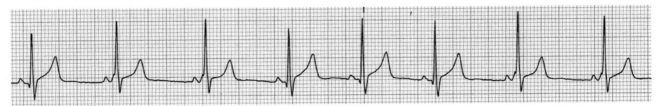

FIGURE 6.5

9. A 14-year-old girl presents with a rash with central clearing, nonspecific joint pain, and the ECG shown in Figure 6.6. The treatment of choice would be:

A. Gentamicin
B. Doxycycline
C. Vancomycin
D. Intravenous immune globulin (IVIG)
E. β-Blocker

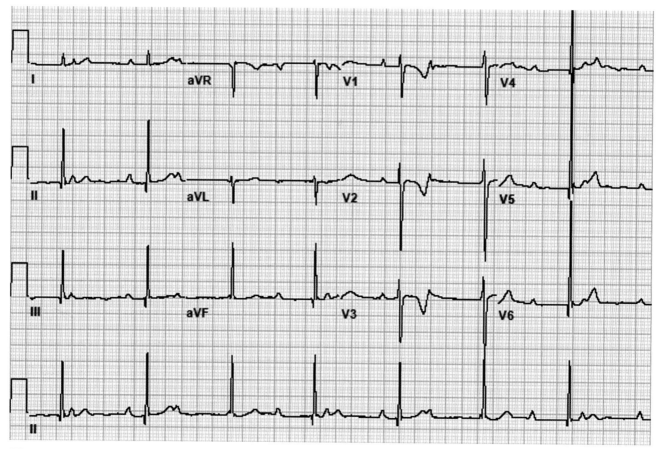

FIGURE 6.6

10. A 15-year-old girl presents following a syncopal episode. Upon further investigation you find out that she had been standing on a hot day in church and felt lightheaded before passing out. The event was witnessed and her parents describe a brief episode of jerking of her arms following her syncope. She awoke within 10 seconds and was oriented to time and place, but did have a headache. Her ECG and physical examination were normal. What is the next most appropriate step?

A. Implantable loop recorder placement
B. 24-Hour ambulatory monitoring
C. Recommend increased fluid intake
D. EP study
E. Neurology referral

11. A 16-year-old football player comes to you for evaluation of palpitations and dizziness. The ECG shown in Figure 6.7 is obtained. What would you do?

A. Perform a 24-hour Holter monitor. If there are no arrhythmias, let him play

B. Permanently disqualify him from all competitive sports based on the ECG
C. Let him play as the ECG findings are a normal variant
D. Not let him play until evaluation including an echocardiogram is performed
E. Let him play and repeat the ECG in 6 months

12. A 14-year-old girl is referred to your office after she was noted to have a first-degree AV block, a right bundle branch block, and a left anterior fascicular block on a 12-lead ECG. On your examination, you also note drooping eyelids and ataxia. What would be the most logical next step?

A. Implant a pacemaker
B. IV steroid administration
C. Perform an electrophysiologic study
D. Initiate medical therapy with theophylline
E. Implant an implantable cardioverter defibrillation (ICD)

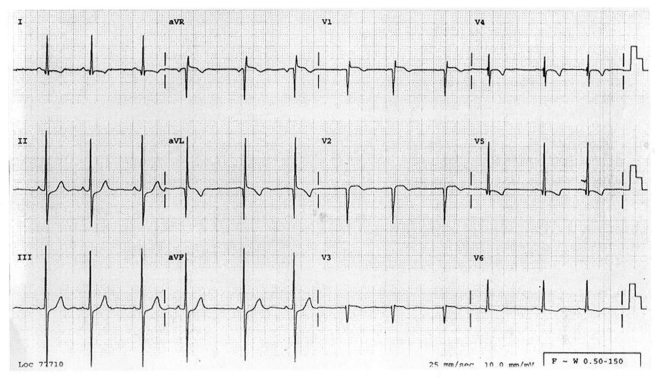

FIGURE 6.7

13. A 1-week-old child gets a 12-lead ECG for bradycardia. The ECG recordings are shown in Figure 6.8. The patient is asymptomatic with a good blood pressure and an average heart rate of 65 bpm. How would you treat the child?

A. Initiation of a β-blocker only
B. Pacemaker placement
C. Follow-up in 2 months with a repeat ECG and 24-hour Holter monitor
D. Isoproterenol drip
E. Initiation of amiodarone

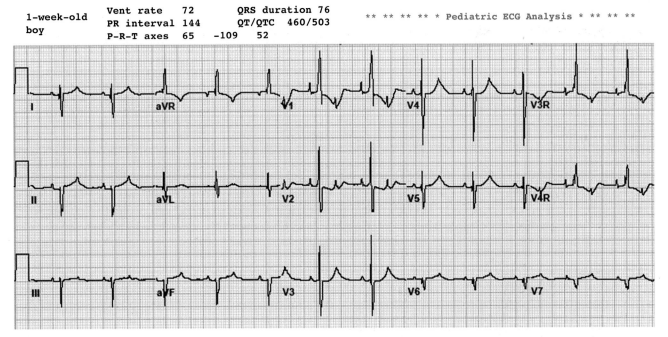

FIGURE 6.8

14. What is the relationship of the conduction system to the ventricular septal defect in a patient with an AV canal?

   A. Posterior and superior to the ventricular septal defect
   B. Posterior and inferior to the ventricular septal defect
   C. Anterior and superior to the ventricular septal defect
   D. Anterior and inferior to the ventricular septal defect
   E. On the left side of the heart

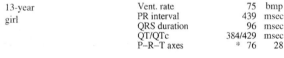

15. Which of the following findings at 37-week gestation is cause for greatest immediate concern?

   A. Fetal heart rate of 110 bpm with no variability on internal fetal monitoring
   B. Fetal heart rate of 160 bpm during obstetrical visit
   C. Fetal heart rate of 90 bpm heard during an office visit with pulsatile umbilical artery flow
   D. Fetal heart rate that decelerates early and synchronously with uterine contractions
   E. Fetal heart rate that varies randomly between 120 and 150 bpm during labor

16. Risk of sudden death in patients who have had repair of tetralogy of Fallot is highest in those with which of the following?

   A. QRS duration of 190 msec with residual right ventricular hypertension
   B. Frequent premature ventricular contractions
   C. Sinus bradycardia on 24-hour Holter monitoring
   D. Neonatal primary repair with right ventricular outflow tract patch
   E. Sinus node dysfunction with right bundle branch block and left anterior hemiblock

17. A 10-year-old child with polyarthritis has the ECG shown in Figure 6.9. The patient will also likely have:

   A. Choreiform movements of the hands
   B. Coronary artery aneurysms
   C. A dilated ascending aorta
   D. Glomerulonephritis
   E. Bifid uvula

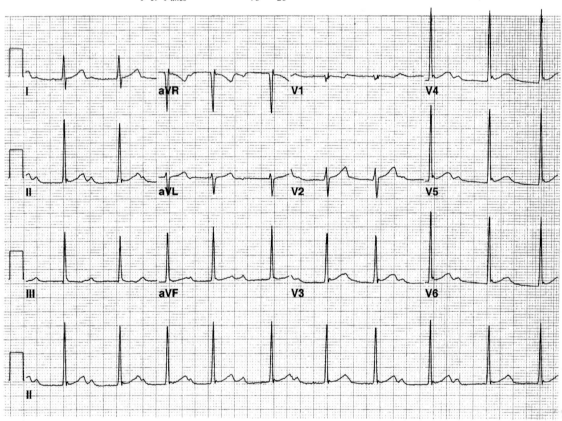

13-year girl	Vent. rate	75	bmp
	PR interval	439	msec
	QRS duration	96	msec
	QT/QTc	384/429	msec
	P–R–T axes	* 76	28

FIGURE 6.9

18. Irregular fetal heart sounds are heard during a routine prenatal visit at 32-week gestation. Results of fetal ultrasonography suggest appropriate fetal size and development, normal ventricular function, and no evidence of hydrops. A fetal echocardiographic M-mode tracing shows frequent premature atrial beats, some of which are not conducted to the ventricle with the heart rate intermittently dropping into the 60s. The most appropriate management is:

A. Maternal digoxin therapy
B. Maternal sotalol therapy
C. Maternal flecainide therapy
D. Immediate delivery
E. Observation only

19. A 7-year-old boy has had three episodes of SVT in the past month. Apart from some palpitations and mild dizziness, he does not have any symptoms. He has a documented heart rate of 240 bpm. The tachycardia is able to be terminated by one dose of adenosine, intravenously. An ECG is obtained following conversion to sinus rhythm and is shown in Figure 6.10. Which of the following drugs should be recommended to decrease the chance of a recurrence?

A. Verapamil
B. Oral amiodarone to be taken only after tachycardia starts
C. Digoxin
D. Mexiletine
E. Propranolol

20. Which of the following statements most accurately describes the normal change in the ECG during the first week after birth?

A. An increase in the size of the R wave in lead V1
B. A shift in the QRS frontal plane axis from greater than +135 degrees to less than +30 degrees
C. A change in T-wave polarity from positive to negative in lead V1
D. Development of a Q wave in lead V1
E. Shortening of the PR interval

21. In an 8-year-old girl who has permanent junctional reciprocating tachycardia, electrocardiography during an episode of tachycardia would most likely show:

A. Deeply negative P waves in leads II, III, and aVF
B. No visible P waves
C. Two P waves for every QRS complex
D. P waves that are positive in lead aVF and negative in lead I
E. A P-wave axis identical to sinus rhythm

22. A 5-year-old child with diabetic ketoacidosis has a heart rate of 140 bpm. Serum potassium concentration is 8.5 mEq/L. The ECG rhythm strip would be expected to demonstrate which of the following?

A. Low-amplitude T wave
B. Prominent Q wave
C. Prolonged QRS duration
D. Short PR interval
E. High-amplitude P wave

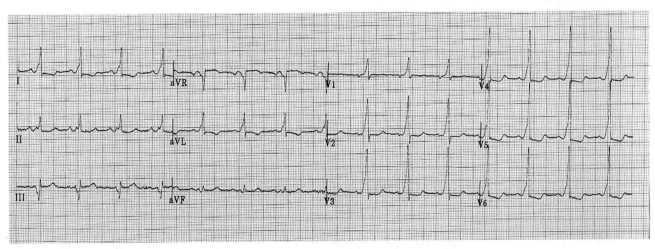

FIGURE 6.10

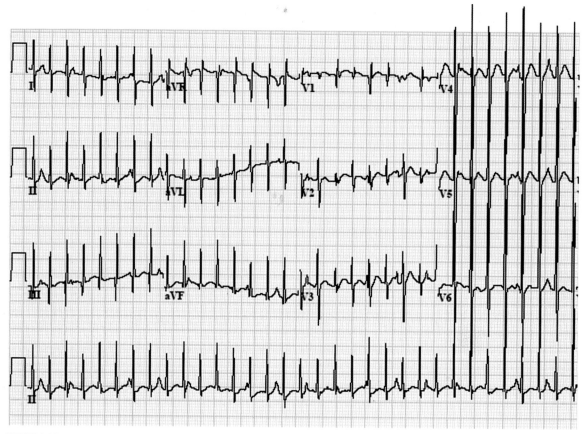

FIGURE 6.11

23. A 6-month-old presents with tachycardia immediately following complete repair for tetralogy of Fallot. The ECG is shown in Figure 6.11. The most likely diagnosis is:

- **A.** Atrial flutter with variable AV conduction
- **B.** Ventricular tachycardia
- **C.** Reentry supraventricular tachycardia using an accessory pathway
- **D.** Ectopic atrial tachycardia
- **E.** Junctional ectopic tachycardia

24. Which of the following coronary artery abnormalities is most likely to be present in an asymptomatic 16-year-old high-school athlete who dies suddenly on the court during a basketball game?

- **A.** Left circumflex coronary artery arising from the right coronary artery
- **B.** Right coronary artery arising from the pulmonary artery
- **C.** Left main coronary artery originating from the right sinus of Valsalva and passing between the aorta and the pulmonary artery
- **D.** Right coronary artery-dominant circulation
- **E.** Single left coronary artery

25. Which of the following is most likely a result of maternal treatment with amiodarone during pregnancy?

- **A.** Neonatal hypothyroidism
- **B.** Neonatal jaundice
- **C.** Neonatal pulmonary fibrosis
- **D.** Neonatal cataracts
- **E.** Neonatal renal dysfunction

26. A 4-year-old is noted to have a murmur and an ECG is obtained and shown in Figure 6.12. Which of the following diagnoses is most likely?

- **A.** Primum atrial septal defect
- **B.** Secundum atrial septal defect
- **C.** Sinus venosus atrial septal defect
- **D.** Unroofed coronary sinus
- **E.** Patent foramen ovale

27. Which of the following drugs is relatively contraindicated in a patient with congenital long QT syndrome?

- **A.** Lidocaine
- **B.** Amoxicillin with clavulanate
- **C.** Verapamil
- **D.** Erythromycin
- **E.** Metoprolol

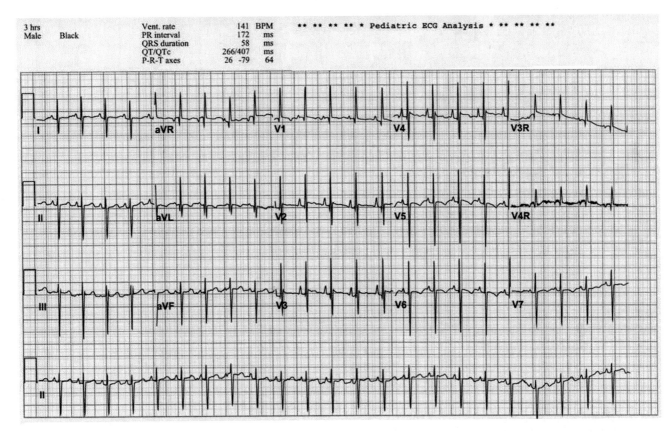

FIGURE 6.12

28. On a routine physical examination, a 1-month-old infant has a heart rate of 240 bpm. There is no murmur and heart size is normal. There is no tachypnea, and blood pressure and perfusion are normal. ECG documents tachycardia with a normal QRS duration and an unvarying RR interval. Ice is applied to the infant's face without change in the cardiac rhythm. The next most appropriate step in management would be:

   A. IV amiodarone
   B. IV verapamil
   C. IV adenosine
   D. IV propranolol
   E. IV digoxin

29. A 3-hour-old infant weighing 4 kg is noted to be in atrial flutter. The blood pressure is 75/40 mm Hg and perfusion to the extremities is good. A synchronized direct current cardioversion is attempted with 4 J. The patient remains in atrial flutter following delivery of energy. Which of the following is the next most appropriate treatment for this patient?

   A. Attempt unsynchronized cardioversion with 4 J
   B. Attempt synchronized cardioversion with 8 J
   C. Wait 1 hour, then repeat cardioversion with 4 J
   D. IV adenosine
   E. IV amiodarone

30. Which of the following ECG findings constitutes a class I indication for cardiac pacemaker implantation in a 1-day-old male infant with complete AV block, no structural heart disease, and normal cardiac function?

   A. Ventricular rate of 60 bpm and QRS duration of 60 msec
   B. Atrial rate of 70 bpm and ventricular rate of 70 bpm
   C. Atrial rate of 140 bpm and ventricular rate of 80 bpm
   D. Ventricular rate of 70 bpm and rare uniform premature ventricular contractions
   E. Ventricular rate of 75 bpm and a QRS duration of 130 msec

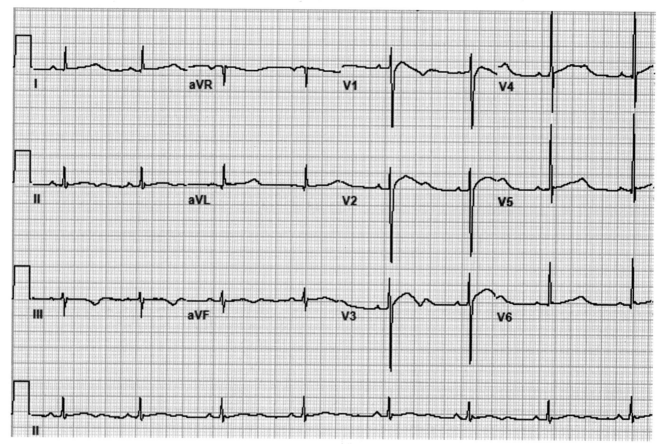

FIGURE 6.13

31. A 14-year-old previously healthy girl collapses while playing soccer. Following successful cardiopulmonary resuscitation, the ECG in Figure 6.13 was obtained. Which of the following is the most likely test to define her diagnosis?

   A. Cardiac MRI
   B. Measurement of AH and HV intervals on intracardiac electrophysiology study
   C. Echocardiogram
   D. Genetic testing for KCNQ1 mutation
   E. Procainamide challenge

32. In order for reentry to occur in cardiac muscle and to result in dysrhythmia, which of the following must also be present?

   A. An area of conduction delay
   B. Delayed repolarization
   C. Entrainment
   D. Triggered activity
   E. Increased automaticity

33. A 16-year-old girl underwent closure of a VSD at 8 months of age. She did well until the present examination when a slow irregular heart rate was noted. The patient has had no symptoms. An ECG shows Mobitz type II block and a heart rate of 70 bpm. Which of the following is most appropriate management for this patient's condition?

   A. Theophylline therapy
   B. Amiodarone therapy
   C. Digoxin therapy
   D. Permanent pacemaker placement
   E. Observation

34. A 13-year-old boy presents with the rhythm in Figure 6.14. He underwent an atrial septal defect repair 1 day ago. Blood pressure is 90/56 mm Hg. Which of the following will most likely terminate this arrhythmia?

   A. IV adenosine
   B. IV labetalol
   C. Rapid atrial pacing through atrial pacing wires
   D. Oral propranolol
   E. Correction of hypokalemia

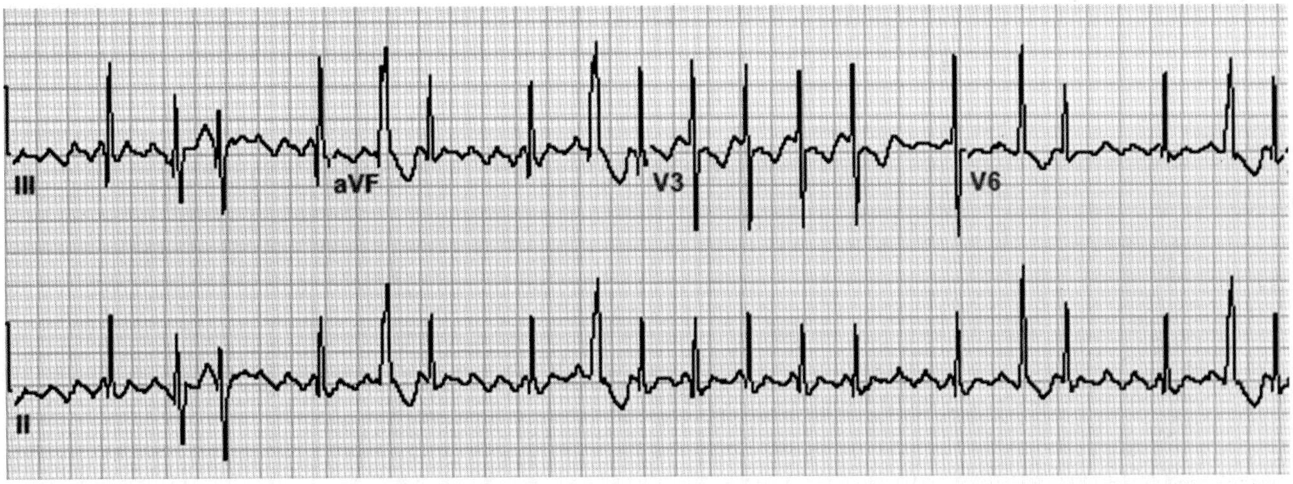

FIGURE 6.14

35. A 9-year-old boy who is pacemaker dependent is being evaluated by you for the first time. He developed complete AV block postoperatively after VSD repair. His ECG demonstrates 100% pacing in the ventricle at a rate of 65 bpm and there is no atrial sensing. His parents tell you that his pacemaker has been DDD at a rate of 75 bpm for the past 5 years. Which of the following is the most probable cause for this rate change?

   A. Intrinsic variation in the operation of a normal pacemaker
   B. Rate-responsive pacing
   C. Intermittent failure of the pacemaker to capture
   D. Elective replacement indicator (ERI) of the pacemaker
   E. Unintentional reprogramming of the pacemaker

36. Cardiovascular manifestations of hyperthyroidism include which of the following?

   A. Heart block
   B. Atrial fibrillation
   C. Narrow pulse pressures
   D. Decreased ejection fraction
   E. Low voltage on ECG

37. In pediatric patients, sick sinus syndrome is most likely to be associated with which of the following?

   A. Surgery for congenital heart disease
   B. Lyme disease
   C. Maternal systemic lupus erythematosus (SLE)
   D. Cardiomyopathy
   E. Myocarditis

38. A 12-year-old patient presents for follow-up several years after a sinus venosus atrial septal defect (SVASD) that was repaired surgically. The patient has signs and symptoms of intermittent dizziness. An ECG during symptoms will most likely show:

   A. Complete AV block
   B. Sinus bradycardia
   C. Ventricular tachycardia
   D. Junctional tachycardia
   E. Mobitz type II second-degree AV block

39. A 7-year-old has a pacemaker implanted for complete heart block following his surgery. A dual chamber pacemaker is implanted with the lower rate set at 60. On examination, you note the patient's heart rate to be 85 bpm and regular. What is the most likely mode of this pacemaker at this time?

   A. AAI
   B. VVI
   C. DDI
   D. DDD
   E. DOO

40. Which of the following is the most likely side effect of β-blocker therapy in children?

   A. Hypothyroidism
   B. Behavioral changes
   C. Rash
   D. Headache
   E. Weight loss

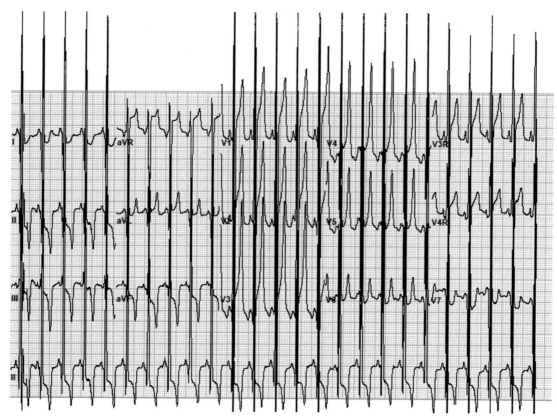

FIGURE 6.15

41. An 8-month-old patient has the ECG shown in Figure 6.15. Which of the following is the most likely metabolic disorder?

A. Hunter
B. Hurler
C. Pompe disease
D. Phenylketonuria
E. Maple syrup urine disease

42. A 12-year-old patient has congenitally corrected transposition (L-transposition) of the great arteries but has not undergone any surgical intervention. This patient is at most risk for which of the following?

A. Sinus node dysfunction
B. Complete AV block
C. Junctional ectopic tachycardia
D. Atrial flutter
E. Torsades de pointes (TdP)

43. It is standard practice to measure the baseline conduction intervals at the beginning and the end of every electrophysiology study. A normal HV interval is usually between which of the following?

A. 120 and 160 msec
B. 40 and 100 msec
C. 70 and 110 msec

D. 35 and 55 msec
E. 0 and 100 msec

44. During an electrophysiology study, an atrial extrastimulus protocol is performed where a train of 8 paced beats in the atrium at 600 msec (S_1) is followed by a premature beat (S_2) at sequentially decreasing intervals. The AH interval is measured after each prematurely paced (S_2) beat. This sequence in Figure 6.16 demonstrates:

A. AV node effective refractory period (ERP)
B. A jump in the AH interval indicating dual AV nodal physiology
C. Atrial muscle effective refractory period
D. Wenckebach
E. AV node conduction disease

45. In Figure 6.17, a single ventricular extrastimulus protocol is being performed as described in Question 44. The drive train (S_1) and premature ventricular beat (S_2) are labeled. This tracing shows:

A. VA Wenckebach
B. Failure of ventricular output
C. Retrograde effective refractory period (ERP) of an accessory pathway
D. Ventricular muscle ERP
E. Retrograde ERP of AV node

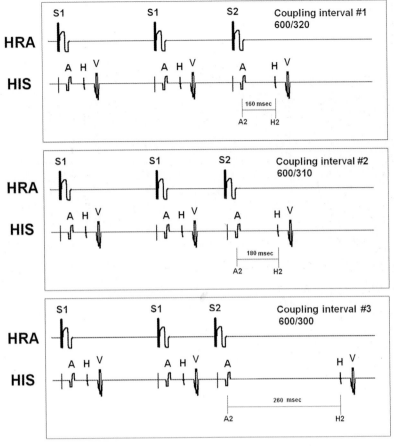

FIGURE 6.16

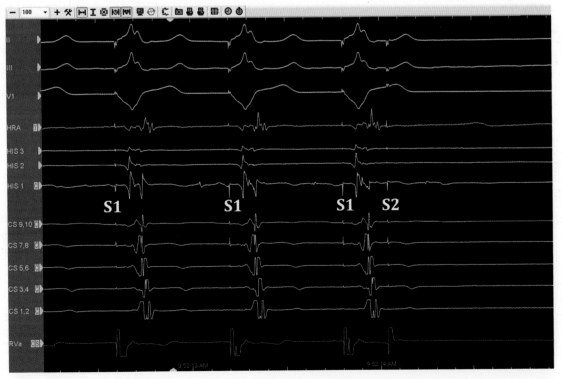

FIGURE 6.17

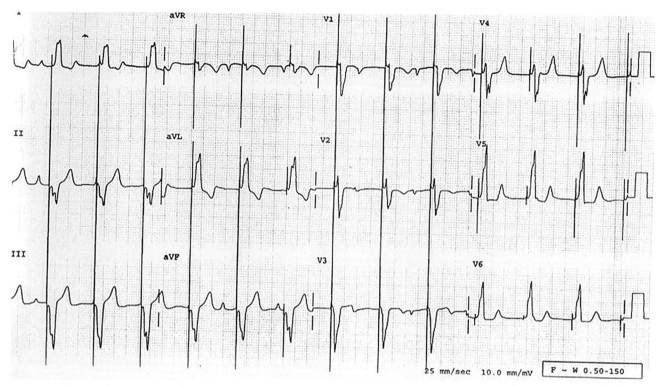

FIGURE 6.18

46. The ECG in Figure 6.18 was obtained from a patient with a permanent pacemaker. According to the ECG, the pacemaker is working in what mode?

   A. AAI
   B. DDD
   C. VVI
   D. DOO
   E. VDD

47. A 12-year-old boy has had documented heart rate of 250 bpm. He is brought to the EP lab where a tachycardia is induced with cardiac stimulation. The catheters are in the following positions: RV, right ventricular apex; CS, proximal coronary sinus (CS) with CS 9–10 in the right atrium outside the mouth of the CS; His, bundle of His. The intracardiac tracings in Figure 6.19 are recorded. These are most consistent with which of the following?

   A. Ventricular tachycardia
   B. AV reentry tachycardia using an accessory pathway
   C. AV nodal reentry tachycardia
   D. Ectopic atrial tachycardia
   E. Complete AV block

48. A 3-day-old baby presents with saturations of 76% on 100% oxygen. An ECG is obtained and shown in Figure 6.20. The ECG is most suggestive of:

   A. Tetralogy of Fallot
   B. Pulmonary atresia with intact ventricular septum
   C. Truncus arteriosus
   D. Total anomalous pulmonary venous return
   E. Large patent ductus arteriosus

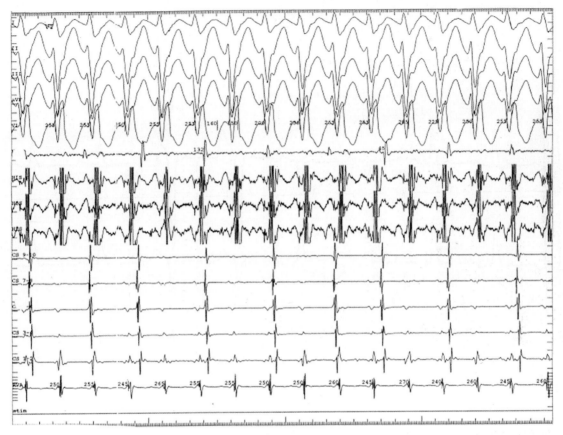

FIGURE 6.19

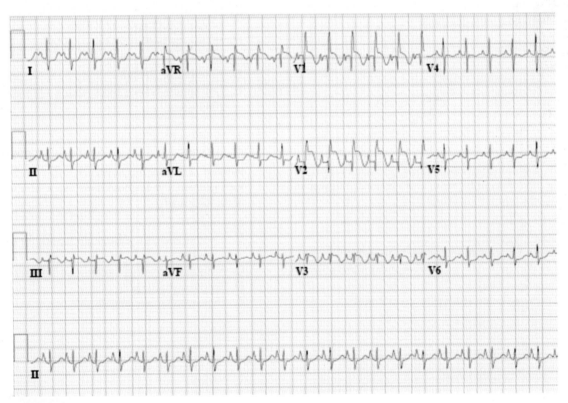

FIGURE 6.20

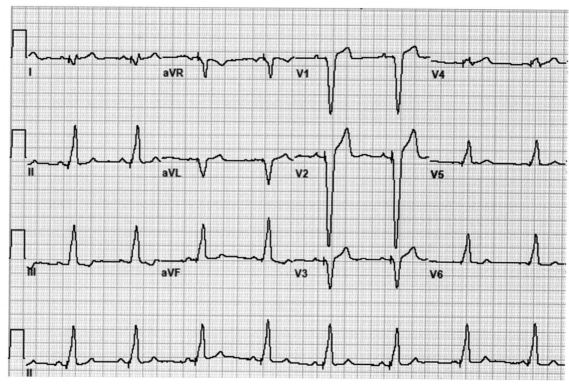

FIGURE 6.21

49. A 12-lead ECG is obtained on a patient with a permanent pacemaker (Fig. 6.21). The lower rate limit is set at 60, but no information is available on the pacemaker. You conclude that the pacemaker is most likely programmed in which of the following mode?

   A. DDD
   B. VVI
   C. AAI
   D. VOO
   E. DOO

50. A 3-year-old boy is noted to be bradycardic in the immediate postoperative period after a VSD repair. He is otherwise stable and his blood pressure is within the normal range. The ECG in Figure 6.22 is obtained. You would advise which of the following?

   A. Start epinephrine
   B. Start isoproterenol
   C. Implant a permanent epicardial pacemaker
   D. Use the temporary epicardial pacemaker and observe for at least 7 days
   E. Discharge home with follow-up in 2 weeks

51. Which of the following is an indication for placement of a permanent pacemaker in a patient with no symptoms?

   A. PR interval of 300 msec
   B. Progressive prolongation of the PR interval followed by a dropped beat
   C. No change in the PR interval followed by a dropped beat
   D. Sinus rate of 30 bpm
   E. Left bundle branch block with a QRS duration of 200 msec

52. A 12-year-old boy has a cardiac arrest while riding his bicycle. He is appropriately resuscitated and brought to the intensive care unit. You notice the rhythm in Figure 6.23 with agitation. His diagnosis is most consistent with which of the following?

   A. Long QT syndrome
   B. Catecholaminergic polymorphic ventricular tachycardia (CPVT)
   C. Arrhythmogenic right ventricular dysplasia
   D. Brugada syndrome
   E. Hypertrophic cardiomyopathy

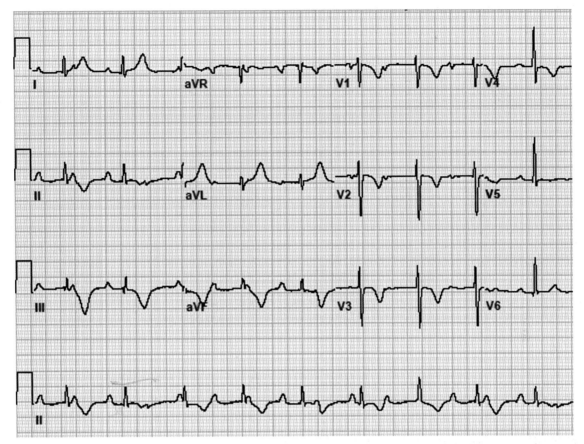

FIGURE 6.22

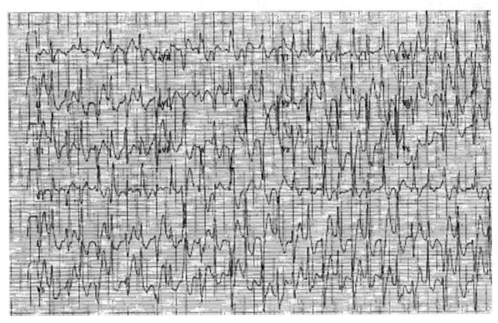

FIGURE 6.23

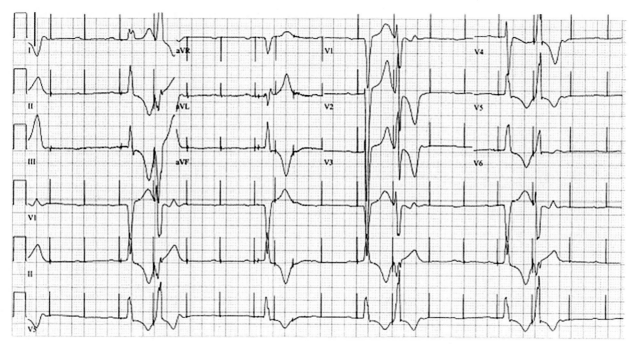

FIGURE 6.24

53. A 4-year-old child with Down syndrome had repair of a VSD at 6 months of age and subsequently developed complete heart block. A permanent epicardial pacemaker was implanted. He now presents with irritability and decreased oral intake for 1 day. You obtain the ECG in Figure 6.24. This ECG is most consistent with which of the following?

A. Oversensing

B. Magnet placement over the pacemaker

C. Pacemaker at elective replacement indicator (ERI)

D. Pacemaker self-test

E. Intermittent capture of ventricular lead

54. A 16-year-old patient is being started on amiodarone. The family asks you about potential side effects with this medicine. You would advise them that potential adverse effects of amiodarone include all of the following *EXCEPT*:

A. Photosensitivity

B. Thyroid dysfunction

C. Peripheral neuropathy

D. Corneal microdeposits

E. Renal dysfunction

55. A 6-month-old child has SVT at a rate of 240 bpm and a grade 3/6 pansystolic murmur best heard at the right lower sternal border. She has had no previous cardiac operations The resting ECG is shown in Figure 6.25. What is the most likely underlying heart disease?

A. Ventricular septal defect

B. Ebstein anomaly

C. Pulmonary stenosis

D. Corrected transposition of the great arteries

E. Dilated cardiomyopathy

56. A 16-year-old girl presents with dizziness with postural changes, but no syncope. On Holter monitoring, you document a 3.5-second pause during a documented episode of dizziness. The rest of her evaluation including echocardiography and baseline ECG is normal. What do you do next?

A. Electrophysiology study

B. Tilt table testing

C. Liberalize fluid intake in addition to regular exercise

D. Recommend pacemaker implantation

E. Recommend ICD implantation

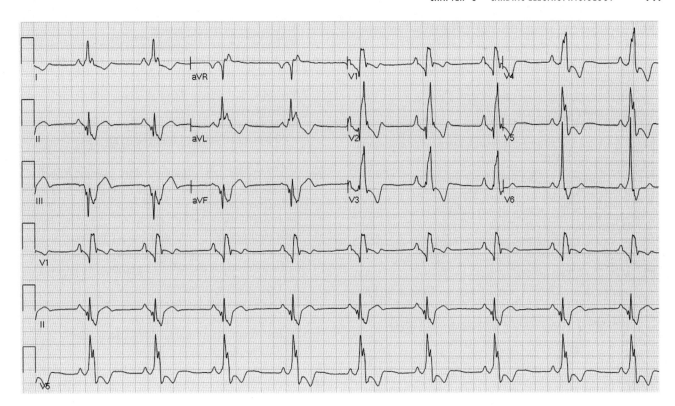

FIGURE 6.25

57. A 4-year-old child presents with digoxin toxicity, 2:1 heart block, and periods of complete heart block. You would consider all the following in the management options in this patient except:

A. Administration of oxygen
B. Place a temporary transvenous pacemaker
C. Digoxin immune Fab
D. Lidocaine for ventricular arrhythmias
E. Induce hypokalemia

58. A 14-year-old boy en route to the hospital by ambulance following his collapse in the street has the rhythm in Figure 6.26. In addition to defibrillation, what would you consider?

A. Digoxin IV
B. Atropine IV
C. Magnesium sulfate IV
D. Potassium IV
E. Adenosine IV

59. You are called down to the emergency department to help manage a hemodynamically stable 10-year-old with a known history of AV node reentry tachycardia who presented with palpitations and a narrow complex tachycardia at a rate of 240 bpm. His palpitations began 4 hours prior to presenting to the emergency department. The patient's weight is 30 kg. The ED physician has already attempted, unsuccessfully, to terminate the tachycardia via vagal maneuvers. He gave two separate doses of adenosine (3 and 6 mg, respectively), administered through a 24-gauge IV in the left hand followed by a 5-cc saline flush. The IV appears to be functioning well. There is no change in the tachycardia with administration of adenosine. The most likely reason that the adenosine was not effective is due to:

A. The mechanism of tachycardia
B. The size and position of the IV
C. The dose of adenosine
D. The duration of his tachycardia
E. The saline flush following the adenosine

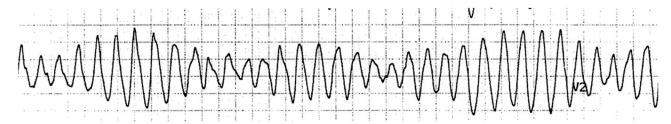

FIGURE 6.26

60. What does the "R" in DDDR, VVIR, or AAIR represent?

  A. Automatic reprogram
  B. Biventricular pacing
  C. Reverse polarity
  D. Rate response
  E. Rapid pacing

61. What would be an appropriate indication for programming a pacemaker AAIR?

  A. Third-degree (complete) heart block
  B. Type I second-degree heart block
  C. Type II second-degree heart block
  D. Sinus node dysfunction
  E. Intermittent third-degree heart block

62. A patient's implantable cardioverter defibrillator (ICD) is programmed at VVI with a lower rate limit of 80 bpm with a ventricular fibrillation zone of 180 bpm. Under what circumstance will the patient receive a shock?

  A. The heart rate drops below 80 bpm
  B. A wide complex rhythm is detected at a rate >80 bpm
  C. Sinus tachycardia occurs at 190 bpm
  D. Ventricular tachycardia occurs at a rate of 160 bpm
  E. Atrial flutter occurs with an atrial rate of 220 bpm with 2:1 AV conduction

63. A 13-year-old patient with a pacemaker for complete heart block and no underlying escape rhythm is undergoing surgery for resection of a mass in the abdomen. The surgeon anticipates use of electrocautery during the procedure. A recommendation is made to place a magnet over the pacemaker during the procedure. Which of the following is the reason for making this recommendation?

  A. Improves sensing during the procedure
  B. Avoids inappropriate pacemaker inhibition due to oversensing from electrocautery during surgery
  C. Makes the pacemaker more rate responsive during surgery
  D. Deflects the electrical energy from entering the pacemaker generator
  E. Prevents overheating of the pacemaker generator

64. A 16-year-old patient has an ICD for hypertrophic cardiomyopathy and cardiac arrest. When asked about the effects of placement of a magnet over an ICD, you would advise that all following are correct except:

  A. Disables all shock therapy
  B. Enables asynchronous pacing in programmed mode
  C. Avoids inappropriate shocks due to oversensing from electrocautery during surgery
  D. Stops appropriate shock delivery due to ventricular tachycardias
  E. The effects are temporary and present only as long as the magnet is placed over the ICD

65. A 15-year-old boy collapses while playing basketball. An AED is placed and he is in ventricular fibrillation and receives an appropriate shock which converts him into normal sinus rhythm. His ECG, EST, echo, cardiac MRI, and neurologic examination are normal. His drug screen is negative as is the rest of his evaluation. Which of the following is the MOST appropriate next step?

  A. Discharge on amiodarone
  B. Discharge on β-blocker therapy
  C. Hemodynamic catheterization
  D. Placement of an implantable loop recorder
  E. ICD implantation

66. A newborn is suspected of having congenital heart disease and an ECG is performed and shown in Figure 6.27. The ECG shown is most closely associated with:

  A. Hypoplastic left heart syndrome
  B. Tricuspid atresia
  C. Truncus arteriosus
  D. Transposition of the great arteries
  E. Tetralogy of Fallot

67. A newborn baby presents with complete AV block with a narrow complex junctional escape rhythm. Which of the following is the most likely finding in the mother?

  A. Serum potassium of 8
  B. Ventricular septal defect
  C. Low platelet count
  D. 22q11 deletion
  E. Anti-Ro (SSA) and anti-La (SSB) antibodies

68. The most likely electrolyte abnormality with the ECG in Figure 6.28 is:

  A. Sodium
  B. Potassium
  C. Calcium
  D. Magnesium
  E. Lead

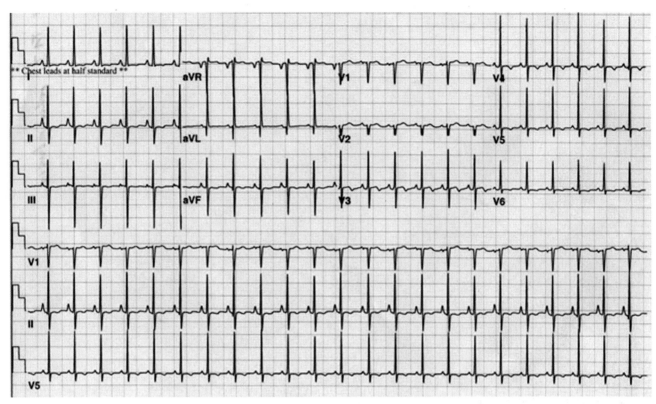

FIGURE 6.27

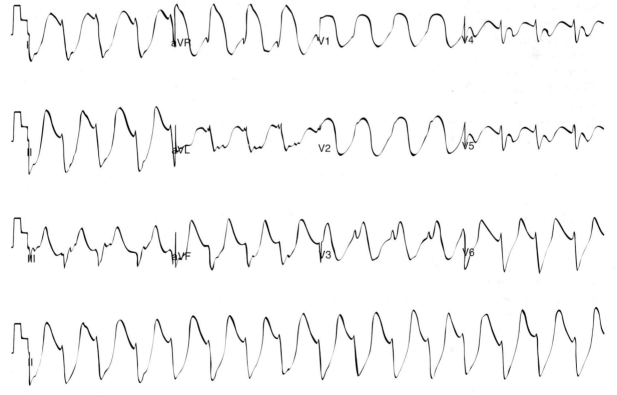

FIGURE 6.28

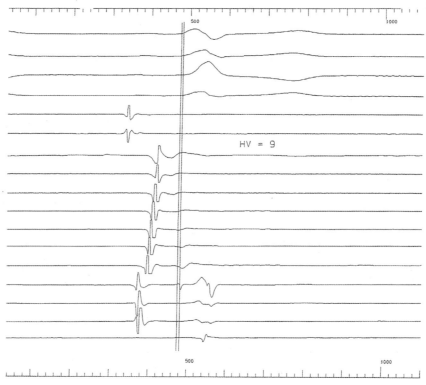

FIGURE 6.29

69. The intracardiac electrogram in Figure 6.29 shows an HV of 9 msec. What does this indicate?

A. First-degree AV block
B. Dual AV node physiology
C. Infra-Hisian conduction delay
D. Preexcitation
E. Bundle branch block

70. A 6-year-old boy presents with the ECG shown in Figure 6.30. He is defibrillated back into sinus rhythm.

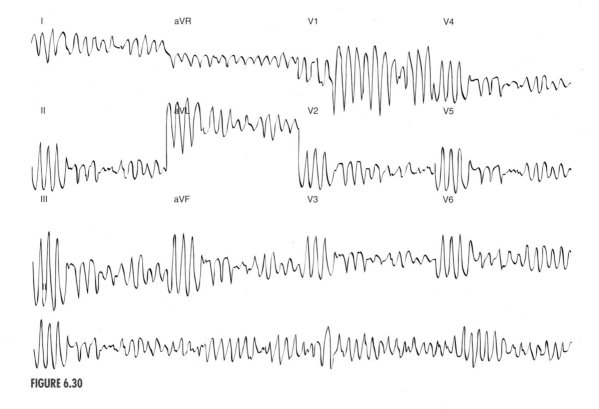

FIGURE 6.30

Heart Rate: 202 BPM

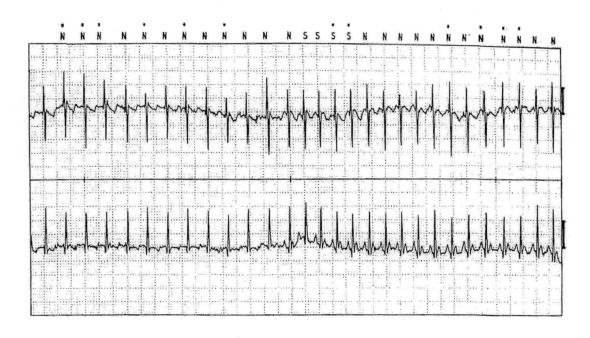

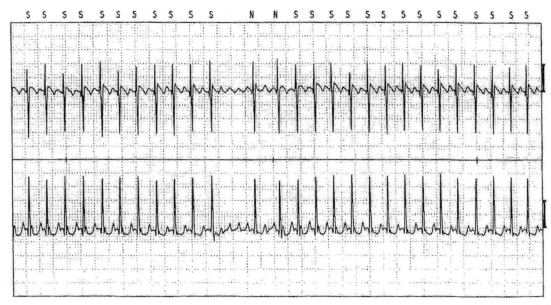

FIGURE 6.31

Which drug should be avoided in the future in the patient who presented with this ECG?

A. Propranolol
B. Enalapril
C. Coumadin
D. Lidocaine
E. Erythromycin

71. The next most appropriate step for the newborn patient with the ECG in Figure 6.31 is which of the following?

A. Cardioversion
B. Adenosine
C. Ventricular pacing
D. Lidocaine
E. Verapamil

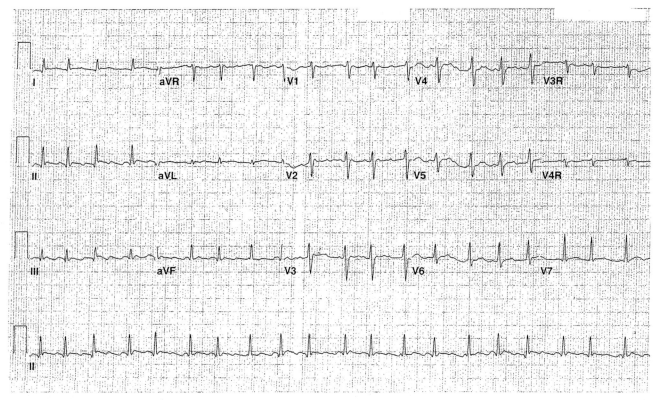

FIGURE 6.32

72. The neonate with the ECG in Figure 6.31 most likely has:

  A. Complete AV canal
  B. Ventricular septal defect
  C. Electrolyte abnormality
  D. No structural heart disease
  E. Absence of the radius on radiograph

73. The patient with the ECG in Figure 6.32 is most at risk for which of the following?

  A. Stroke
  B. Torsade de pointes
  C. Liver failure
  D. Complete AV block
  E. Pulmonary fibrosis

74. An asymptomatic 14-year-old patient with a normal examination and resting ECG has a 24-hour Holter showing the finding in Figure 6.33 while sleeping. The rest of the Holter is normal. Which of the following is the next most appropriate step?

  A. EP study
  B. Exercise treadmill test
  C. Reassurance
  D. Cardiac MRI
  E. Pacemaker implantation

75. An asymptomatic 10-year-old patient has the ECG shown in Figure 6.34 during an exercise treadmill test. His resting ECG shows preexcitation. What does this tracing indicate?

  A. The patient is at low risk for sudden death
  B. The patient is at high risk for sudden death
  C. The patient is at low risk for supraventricular tachycardia
  D. The patient is at high risk for supraventricular tachycardia
  E. The patient has ventricular tachycardia rather than preexcitation

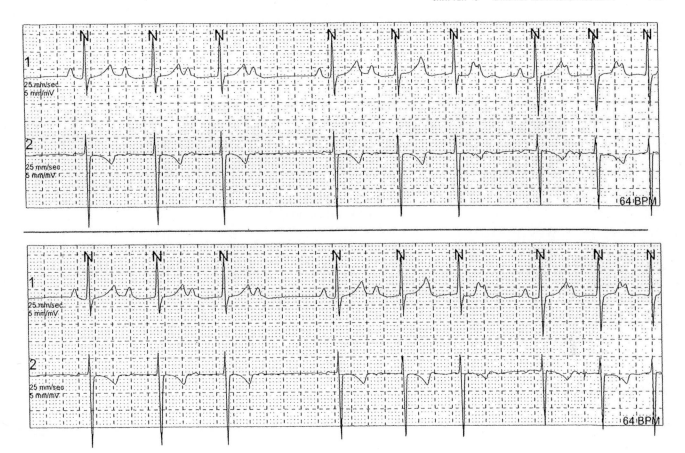

FIGURE 6.33

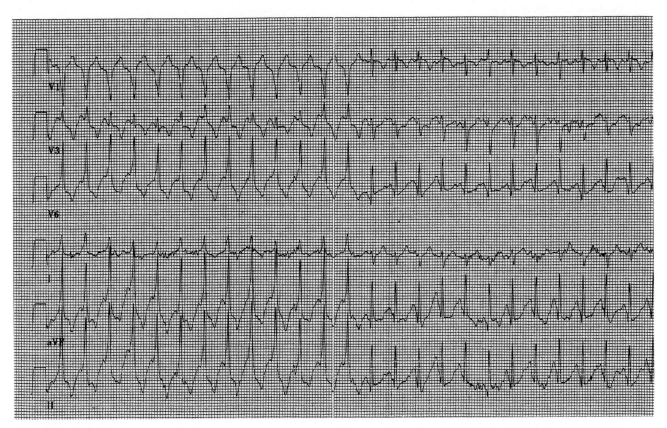

FIGURE 6.34

MAX RR

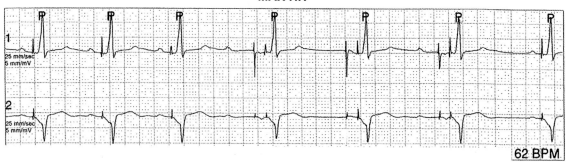

FELT SKIPPED BEATS

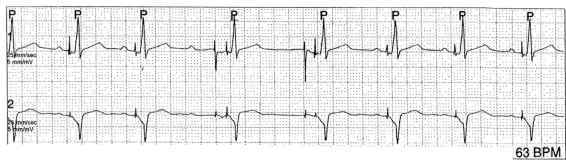

FIGURE 6.35

76. The patient with the tracing in Figure 6.35 likely has which of the following?

   A. Normally functioning DDD pacemaker
   B. Atrial lead dysfunction
   C. Ventricular lead dysfunction
   D. Atrial and ventricular lead dysfunction
   E. Biventricular pacemaker

77. The underlying diagnosis in the patient in Figure 6.36 is most likely to be which of the following?

   A. Wolff–Parkinson–White
   B. Renal failure
   C. Atrial septal defect
   D. Thyroid storm
   E. Anorexia nervosa

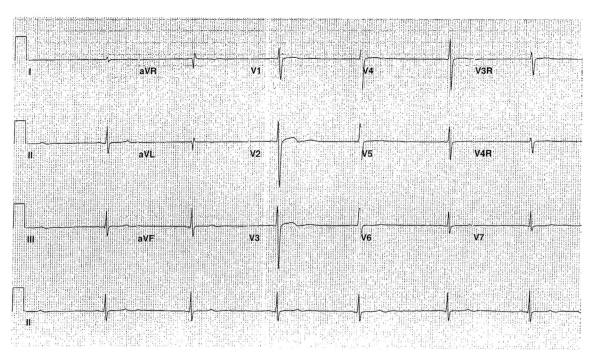

FIGURE 6.36

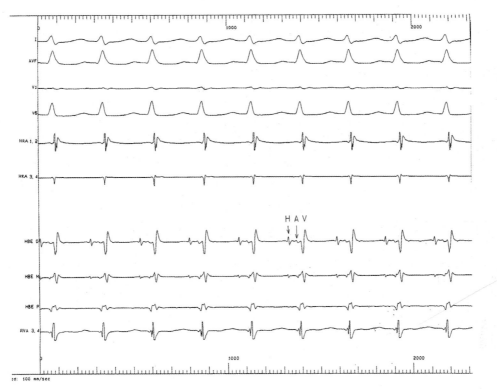

FIGURE 6.37

78. The intracardiac tracing in Figure 6.37 shows which of the following?

   A. Atrial flutter with 2:1 conduction
   B. SVT using an accessory pathway
   C. Atypical AV node reentry tachycardia
   D. Typical AV node reentry tachycardia
   E. Normal sinus rhythm

79. A newborn infant presents with abnormal facies and the ECG in Figure 6.38. Which of the following is the most likely cardiac diagnosis?

   A. Truncus arteriosus
   B. Total anomalous pulmonary venous return
   C. Tetralogy of Fallot
   D. Coarctation of the aorta
   E. Complete AV canal

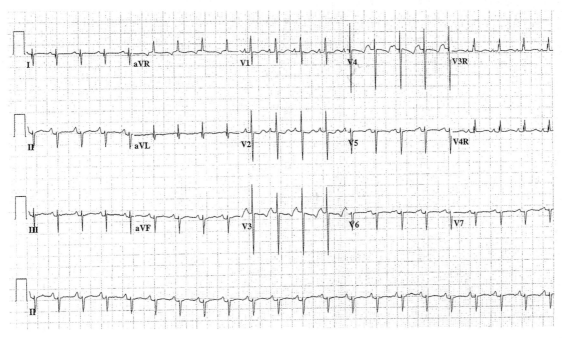

FIGURE 6.38

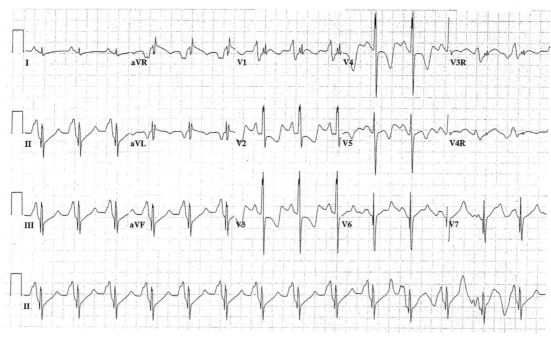

FIGURE 6.39

80. The patient with the ECG in Figure 6.39 is most at risk for which of the following?

   A. Pulmonary hypertension
   B. AV node reentry tachycardia
   C. Intracranial tumor
   D. Polysplenia
   E. Aortic regurgitation

81. The patient with the ECG in Figure 6.40 most likely will have which of the following?

   A. Hypertonia
   B. Hepatomegaly
   C. Widely spaced nipples
   D. Aniridia
   E. Hematuria

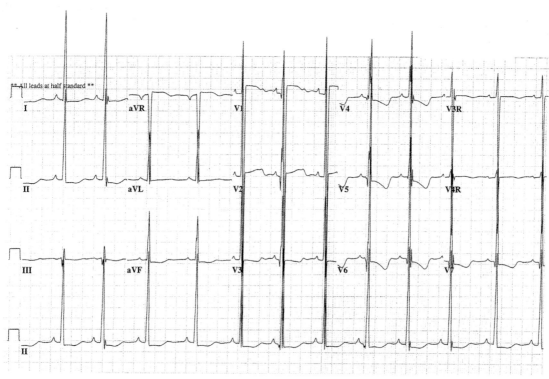

FIGURE 6.40

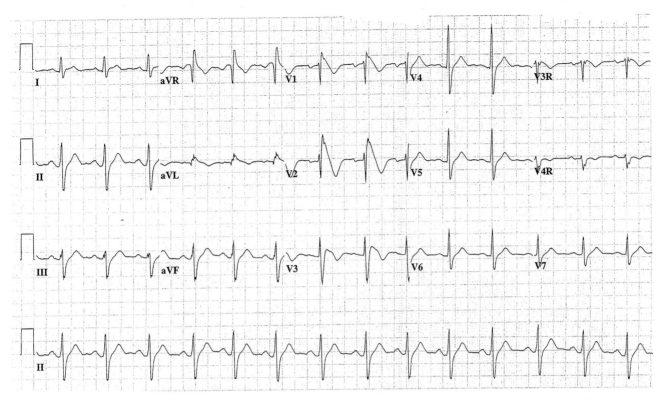

FIGURE 6.41

82. A 17-year-old patient presents with two episodes syncope with no warning signs and no underlying discernible cause. He has the ECG shown in the Figure 6.41. What is the next most appropriate step?

  A. Cardiac catheterization with coronary angiography
  B. Initiation of atenolol
  C. ICD
  D. Initiation of amiodarone
  E. Reassurance and discharge from clinic

83. The most likely genetic defect with the ECG in Figure 6.41 is which of the following?

  A. HERG mutation
  B. KCNQ1 mutation

  C. 22q11.2 deletion
  D. Trisomy 21
  E. SCN-5A mutation

84. Which of the following is the drug most likely to bring out this finding on ECG (Fig. 6.41)?

  A. Epinephrine
  B. Lidocaine
  C. Esmolol
  D. Adenosine
  E. Procainamide

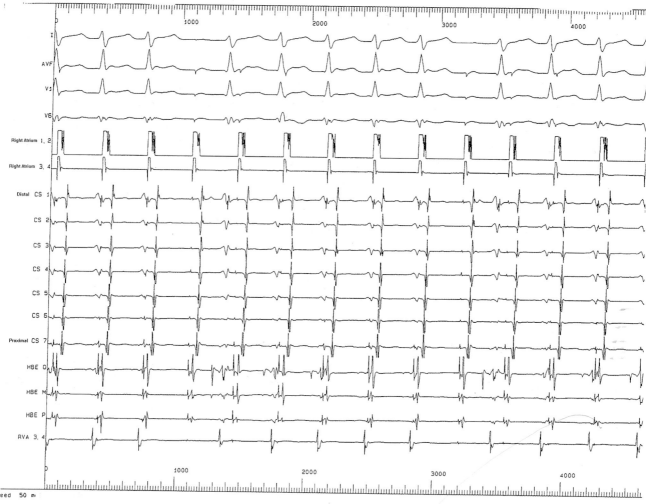

FIGURE 6.42

85. The intracardiac tracing in Figure 6.42, performed during atrial pacing in the high right atrium (HRA), shows which of the following?

   A. Wenckebach (Mobitz type I second-degree AV block)
   B. Initiation of supraventricular tachycardia
   C. AH jump (ERP of the fast pathway of the AV node)
   D. Loss of preexcitation
   E. Initiation of atrial fibrillation

86. A 17-year-old boy presents with chest pain and the ECG tracing in Figure 6.43. The most likely etiology of the ECG findings is:

   A. Cocaine
   B. Myosin heavy chain mutation
   C. Increased intracranial pressure
   D. Coxsackie virus
   E. Erythromycin

87. A previously asymptomatic patient presents with the ECG shown in Figure 6.44. The patient most likely has an underlying diagnosis of which of the following?

   A. Ebstein anomaly
   B. Atrial septal defect
   C. LQTS
   D. Arrhythmogenic right ventricular dysplasia
   E. Truncus arteriosus

88. Which drug is relatively contraindicated with this ECG (Fig. 6.44)?

   A. Amiodarone
   B. Adenosine
   C. Flecainide
   D. Fentanyl
   E. Diphenhydramine

17-yr
Male   Black

Vent. rate   141   BPM
PR interval   132   ms
QRS duration   76   ms
QT/QTc   276/423 ms
P-R-T axes   73 90 35

Test ind:CHEST PAIN

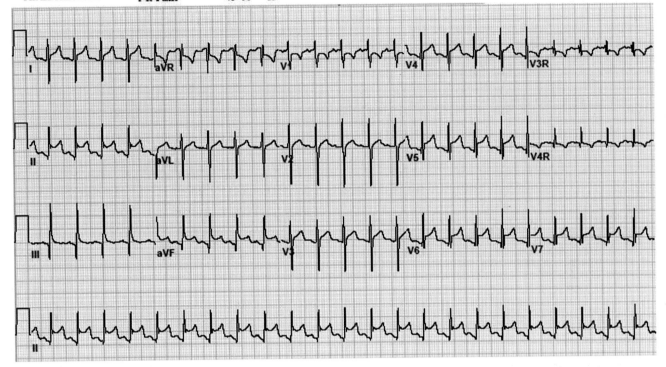

FIGURE 6.43

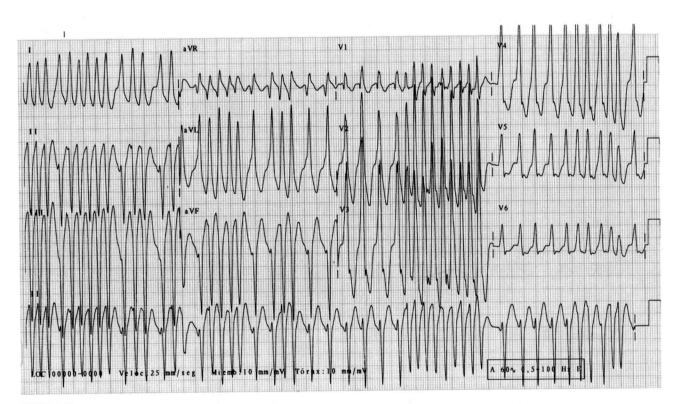

FIGURE 6.44

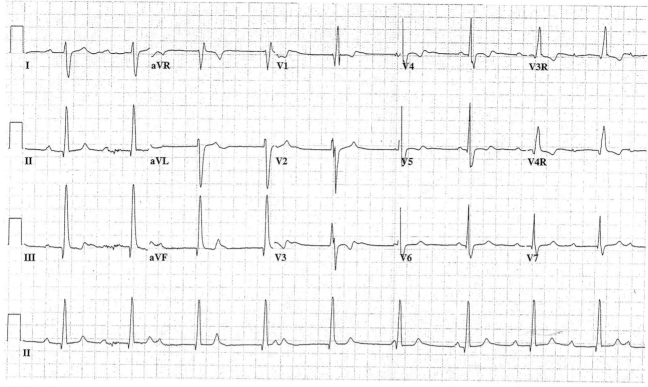

FIGURE 6.45

89. A 13-year-old patient presents with fatigue and exercise intolerance with a normal echocardiogram. The presenting ECG is shown in Figure 6.45. This patient will most likely require which of the following?

   A. Pacemaker
   B. ICD
   C. β-Blocker therapy
   D. Left stellate ganglionectomy
   E. Cardiac transplantation

90. Which of the following is NOT associated with the ECG in Figure 6.45?

   A. Chagas disease
   B. Congenitally corrected transposition of the great arteries
   C. Maternal Ro and La antibodies
   D. Hypertrophic cardiomyopathy
   E. Endocarditis with abscess formation

91. With adenosine, the tachycardia in the ECG (Fig. 6.46) will likely:

   A. Continue with only P waves in a saw tooth configuration
   B. Terminate followed by several sinus beats, then restart

   C. Slow transiently, then speed up
   D. Have no changes
   E. Widen transiently, then narrow

92. Which of the following is NOT in the differential diagnosis for a long RP tachycardia?

   A. Atypical AV node reentry tachycardia
   B. Atrial tachycardia
   C. Mahaim fiber tachycardia
   D. Permanent form of junctional reciprocating tachycardia (PJRT)
   E. Atrial flutter

93. The intracardiac tracing in Figure 6.47 was obtained in a patient after placement of catheters. The proximal coronary sinus (CS) catheter is placed 2 mm inside the mouth of the CS. The tracing shows which of the following?

   A. Supraventricular tachycardia due to a right-sided accessory pathway
   B. Supraventricular tachycardia due to a left-sided accessory pathway
   C. Atypical AV node reentry tachycardia
   D. Normal sinus rhythm
   E. Wenckebach

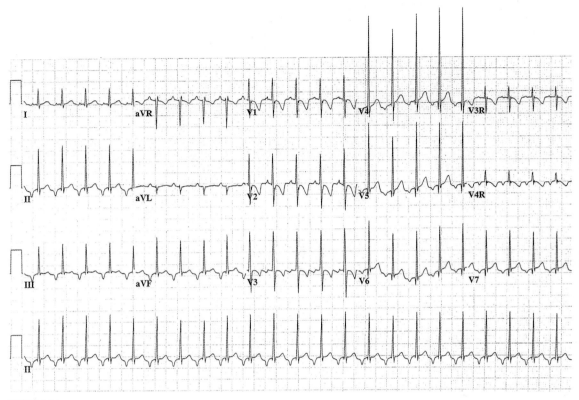

FIGURE 6.46

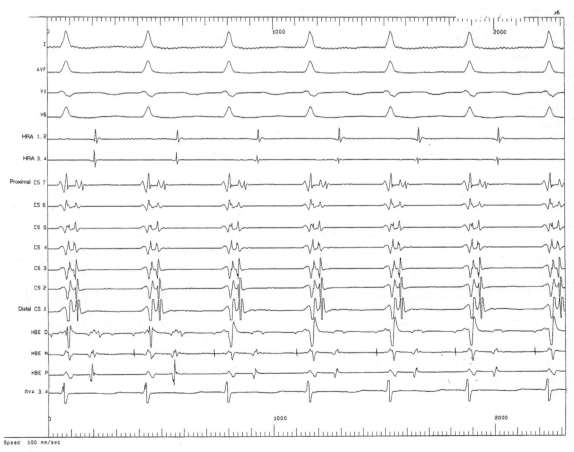

Speed: 100 mm/sec

FIGURE 6.47

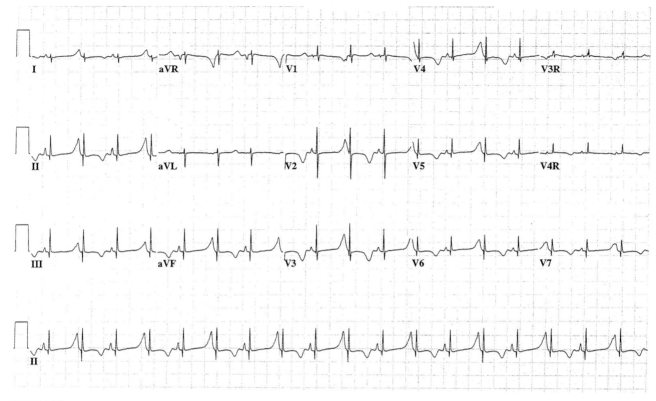

FIGURE 6.48

94. Which of the following is NOT true in the patient with the ECG in Figure 6.48?

    A. Patient is at risk for sudden death
    B. Patient should NOT be given methadone
    C. Family members should be screened for the same condition
    D. The underlying problem is likely due to a mutation in a calcium channel
    E. The patient is at risk for 2:1 AV block

95. An 18-year-old man underwent repair of a sinus venosus atrial septal defect at the age of 12. He developed sinus node dysfunction and underwent implantation of a single chamber atrial pacemaker set AAIR at a rate of 60. He also has a history of atrial ectopic tachycardia and atrial fibrillation requiring cardioversion. He notices that every day when driving on the bumpy road to his job on a farm, his heart rate steadily increases and he feels uncomfortable. He has an old truck and carries multiple electronic devices in the back seat. The most likely source of his increased heart rate is:

    A. The rate-responsive feature of the pacemaker
    B. An atrial arrhythmia
    C. Electromagnetic interference to the pacemaker
    D. Pacemaker oversensing
    E. Magnet response of the pacemaker

96. A 5-year-old boy is diagnosed with Brugada syndrome by genetic testing after his father was diagnosed with Brugada syndrome. His initial ECG is normal but you tell the family that the classic ECG findings in Brugada syndrome will most likely become evident during:

    A. Emotional stress
    B. Fever
    C. Hypertension
    D. Dehydration
    E. Sleep

97. Which of the following is a class I indication for chronic resynchronization therapy (CRT or biventricular pacing)?

    A. Left bundle branch block pattern, ejection fraction 25%, QRS duration 140 msec
    B. Left bundle branch block pattern, ejection fraction 40%, QRS duration 200 msec
    C. Left bundle branch block pattern, ejection fraction 30%, QRS duration 170 msec
    D. Right bundle branch block pattern, ejection fraction 25%, QRS duration 190 msec
    E. Right bundle branch block pattern, ejection fraction 30%, QRS duration 180 msec

ANSWERS

1. (D) Fetal arrhythmias occur in 1% to 2% of pregnancies and account for 10% to 20% of referrals to pediatric cardiologists. Of these arrhythmias 80% to 90% are premature atrial contractions with only around 10% of the arrhythmias being sustained. SVT may limit diastolic filling time and result in hydrops or decreased ventricular function. Treatment is recommended for sustained arrhythmia (typically >50% SVT burden) or evidence of hydrops. Digoxin is usually first-line agent if no hydrops is present, with case series reports of 60% to 80% positive responders. It takes a relatively high digoxin level (typically around 2) to achieve adequate fetal transfer (0.6 fetal transfer rate). The fetal transfer rate decreases by around 50% in the presence of hydrops. Other agents used in the treatment of atrial flutter include flecainide, sotalol, and amiodarone. Both flecainide and sotalol have an excellent fetal transfer (0.8 to 1). These medications are used when SVT is refractory to digoxin or in the presence of hydrops. Amiodarone can also be used and may have a role in very hydropic infants, but the maternal transfer is poor (0.1 to 0.3). In the patient described, continued observation is not the best option as the fetus will likely develop hydrops (usually within 48 hours) if the tachycardia is sustained. At 32-week gestation on no therapy, immediate delivery is not indicated. Atenolol is very poorly transported across the placenta and is not typically used in the treatment of fetal SVT. Adenosine has a half-life of 3 to 5 seconds and would be metabolized prior to reaching the fetus. Administration of adenosine to the fetus via direct injection in the umbilical vein has been reported, but carries some risk to the fetus performing the injection and would only be used in extreme cases if medical management fails.[1]

2. (A) Premature atrial contractions (PACs) are a benign finding and are present in many, otherwise healthy adolescents. Although a very small percentage may have an atrial tachycardia, the finding of isolated premature atrial contractions does not require any restriction for athletic participation in a patient who is asymptomatic. In general, minimal workup is required for asymptomatic PACs and an echo is not typically required if the examination is normal. No treatment is required and the patient may participate in competitive sports without restrictions.

3. (B) The ECG shows a prolonged corrected QT interval (around 520 msec) consistent with a diagnosis of long QT syndrome (LQTS). β-Blockers are the first-line therapy for LQTS. β-Blockers have been shown to decrease the incidence of sudden cardiac death and syncope in LQTS, particularly in long QT syndrome type 1. Risk factors for sudden cardiac death in LQTS are length of the QT interval (with QT intervals over 500 being the highest risk) and previous episodes of syncope. A prophylactic ICD is not indicated in most cases of LQTS. In this 3-year-old, placement of an ICD would be technically challenging and would have a high incidence of long-term complications. Given the lack of symptoms, a β-blocker would be a better first line of therapy. There is no indication for a routine electrophysiology study in LQTS as the diagnosis can be made based on the ECG. Amiodarone would be relatively contraindicated in LQTS as it prolongs the QT interval. A cardioversion is not indicated as the patient is in sinus rhythm.

4. (E) The rhythm strip demonstrates 2:1 atrial flutter converting to 4:1 atrial flutter. Although digoxin can be used to slow the ventricular response with atrial flutter, it typically will not terminate the arrhythmia. Direct current cardioversion is the most effective method for terminating this arrhythmia. Vagal maneuvers are unlikely to terminate the tachycardia but may slow the ventricular rate and make the flutter more visible. Sotalol, β-blockers, or amiodarone can be used but may take a period of time to be effective and may not convert the rhythm. Cardioversion has an extremely high likelihood of quick conversion to sinus rhythm and is therefore the most reasonable option. In infants, atrial flutter has a low incidence of recurrence and typically will not require any short- or long-term antiarrhythmic medication.

5. (D) The rhythm strip (Fig. 6.49) shows artifact mimicking a wide complex tachycardia. Any motion of the ECG leads during recording may create an artifact that may initially appear to be supraventricular or ventricular tachycardia. However, in this tracing, the QRS complexes can be marched through the tracing (shown by the *red arrows*) and show an underlying sinus rhythm. The *red circle* shows two very closely spaced deflections. It would not be physiologically possible to have two QRS complexes that

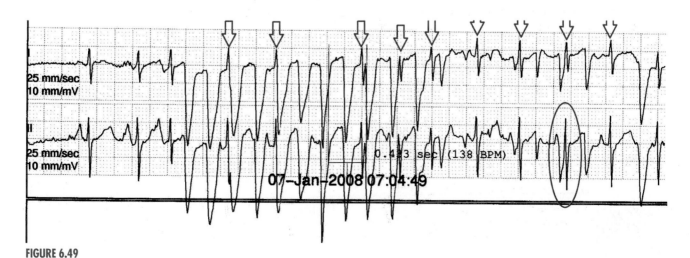

FIGURE 6.49

are so closely coupled as the ventricular myocardium needs time to repolarize prior to contracting again. With all of the evidence showing artifact, no therapy is necessary.

6. (D) A number of risk markers are used to assess the risk for sudden death in patients with hypertrophic cardiomyopathy, the strongest of which are a family history of premature sudden death and a septal thickness >30 mm. Other risk factors include non-sustained ventricular tachycardia, unexplained (not neurally mediated) syncope, and a blood pressure decrease or inadequate increase during exercise testing. Late gadolinium enhancement on an MRI scan of the heart may also carry an increased risk of sudden death. The magnitude of left ventricular hypertrophy on ECG does not help in risk stratification. It is controversial whether or not the outflow tract gradient predisposes a patient to sudden death, but a gradient of 20 mm Hg is relatively mild and not helpful in risk stratification.[2]

7. (A) Amiodarone increases warfarin effect, digoxin and phenytoin levels, and class I antiarrhythmic toxicity. Digoxin is excreted primarily by the kidneys. Digoxin dose should be reduced when given in conjunction with amiodarone. There is no significant interaction between ACE inhibitors or furosemide with amiodarone.

8. (C) This patient is at risk for having episodes of supraventricular tachycardia. The ECG tracing shows intermittent preexcitation (short PR interval and delta wave). In patients with Wolff–Parkinson–White syndrome (WPW) the preexcitation can often be intermittent and picked up when monitoring for longer periods such as on a Holter monitor. Patients with WPW are at risk for having episodes of supraventricular tachycardia. Although it is possible that these are premature ventricular contractions, the PR interval is exactly the same on all of the beats with the wider QRS complex, making preexcitation much more likely. There is no evidence of an atrial arrhythmia.

9. (B) The ECG shows complete AV block. In combination with the classic rash with central clearing (erythema migrans with a bull's eye rash), this patient likely has Lyme disease caused by the spirochete *Borrelia burgdorferi*. The infection is transmitted to humans by tick bites. In patients with Lyme disease, the incidence of cardiac involvement has been estimated to be 8% and usually occurs within a few weeks of the onset of the illness. The most common feature of Lyme carditis is atrioventricular block. The AV block usually resolves gradually with normalization of the PR interval in 1 to 2 weeks. Persistence of AV block requiring a pacemaker is unusual. Prompt treatment with antibiotics is the treatment of choice, but temporary pacing may be necessary if the heart rate is very slow. Treatment is usually with doxycycline, but cephalosporins and amoxicillin can also be used. Gentamicin and vancomycin are not typically used. IVIG is used for Kawasaki disease which typically does not present with AV block. Myocarditis can also present with AV block, but the clinical picture is more consistent with Lyme disease.[3]

10. (C) Neurocardiogenic syncope is very common in the teenage years. These patients may have a myoclonic jerk resembling a seizure or may actually have a seizure when syncopal. In the presence of a single episode and clear history suggesting neurocardiogenic syncope, no further workup may be necessary.

Recommending liberalization of fluid intake may be adequate. A neurology referral is not necessary if history is strongly suggestive of neurocardiogenic syncope. Myoclonic jerks are occasionally seen with syncope and may be mistaken for seizures. The lack of a postictal phase goes against (but does not exclude) seizures. A 24-hour ambulatory monitor is unlikely to capture sporadic episodes. An implantable loop recorder is effective at ruling out arrhythmias in patients with syncope, but is typically used in patients with multiple episodes of syncope with no discernable cause and is not indicated for a single episode of syncope classic for neurocardiogenic syncope.

11. (D) The ECG shows left ventricular hypertrophy and T-wave inversion. T-wave inversion on an ECG may be a marker for abnormal ventricular myocardium. The ECG is most consistent with hypertrophic cardiomyopathy. T-wave inversion in the left precordial leads (V5 and V6) is almost always an abnormal finding. In addition, the T waves are inverted in leads I and aVL, which is also an abnormal finding. The forces are suggestive of increased left ventricular hypertrophy (notice that the ECG is half standard in the precordial leads). A complete workup including an echocardiogram to evaluate the coronary arteries is necessary before clearing the patient for sports.

12. (A) The Kearns–Sayre syndrome (characterized by its onset before the age of 20 years, chronic ophthalmoplegia, pigmentary retinal degeneration, and at least one of the following symptoms: ataxia, heart block, and high protein content in the cerebrospinal fluid) is a severe variant of chronic progressive external ophthalmoplegia with frequent rearrangements of the mitochondrial DNA (mtDNA). Patients typically present with a bundle branch block and prolonged QT interval that progress to complete heart block. Prophylactic pacemaker therapy is advisable in patients suffering from the Kearns–Sayre syndrome, who have bifascicular block on the precordial ECG as they may rapidly progress to complete AV block.[4] Although they are at risk for AV block, there is no indication for a prophylactic implantable cardioverter defibrillator. Steroids or an electrophysiology study is of no benefit.

13. (B) The ECG demonstrates long QT syndrome (LQTS) with 2:1 AV block (more appropriately termed pseudo 2:1 AV block as the AV node has normal function). Note the prominent P waves in leads V1 and V2 that fall in the middle of the T wave and are not conducted. Because of the bradycardia and severity of the phenotype, long QT syndrome with 2:1 AVB has a poor prognosis with up to 50% mortality rate in infancy. Mutations of cardiac ion channel genes cause LQTS, manifesting as increased risk of ventricular tachycardia and sudden death. The prognosis is generally poor. β-Blocker therapy alone can have side effects including enhancing the AV block. Hence, β-blocker therapy along with pacemaker implantation is recommended, although a β-blocker may be added to decrease the chance of ventricular arrhythmias. There is no indication for isoproterenol in a stable patient with a reasonable underlying rate. Amiodarone may lengthen the QT interval and is relatively contraindicated in LQTS.[5]

14. (B) The course of the AV node and His–Purkinje system in endocardial cushion defects passes through the central fibrous body beneath the crest of the VSD. It is therefore displaced posteriorly and inferiorly. In the frontal plane, the initial QRS vector forces are usually directed inferiorly to the right, and the QRS loop moves counterclockwise, superiorly and to the left resulting in left axis deviation. The mean QRS axis in the frontal plane ranges between −30 degrees and −180 degrees, with most axes directed between −30 degrees and −120 degrees.[6]

15. (A) The normal baseline heart rate of the human fetus falls between 120 and 160 bpm. Normal short-term variability consists of beat-to-beat variability of 2 to 3 bpm around the baseline. Long-term variability consists of fluctuations in baseline heart rate occurring 3 to 5 times per minute, with an amplitude of 5 to 20 bpm. Normally, an increase in fetal blood pressure (such as during labor) leads to bradycardia by initiating a vagal nerve reflex. Fetal hypoxemia can have a direct depressing effect on the function of the central nervous system and fetal myocardium, which can result in decrease or loss of fetal heart rate variability.

16. (A) Predictors of long-term survival after tetralogy of Fallot repair include older age at operation, significant residual hemodynamic abnormalities after surgery, use of an outflow tract patch, a QRS duration >180 msec, elevated left ventricular end diastolic pressure, and poor left ventricular function.[7,8] The presence of premature ventricular contractions does not increase the risk of sudden death. Atrial tachycardia is found in 20% to 30% of patients in long-term follow-up and may predispose to sudden death. However, there is no correlation between sinus bradycardia and sudden death. Right bundle branch block and left anterior hemiblock were initially thought to be risk factors for long-term development of complete AV block, but this has not been proven to be true.

17. (A) The ECG shows a prolonged PR interval of around 400 msec. ECG evidence of PR interval prolongation is a minor Jones criteria for acute rheumatic fever. To make a diagnosis of acute rheumatic fever, you need two major or one major and two minor criteria. The clinical manifestations of acute rheumatic fever follow the inciting group A streptococcal infection after a period of latency of about 3 weeks. Rheumatic fever is a multisystem disease affecting primarily the heart, the joints, the brain, and the cutaneous and subcutaneous tissues. Carditis associated with acute rheumatic fever is seen in about 50% of the patients. Tachycardia is one of the early signs of myocarditis. Complete heart block is not usually seen in rheumatic carditis.[9] Choreiform movements are rapid jerking movements of the hands, face, and feet and are characteristics of rheumatic fever. Kawasaki disease resulting in coronary artery aneurysms, Marfan syndrome resulting in a dilated ascending aorta, and juvenile rheumatoid arthritis do not typically give a prolonged PR interval. Systemic lupus erythematosus and scleroderma may also be associated with a prolonged PR interval. Glomerulonephritis is not associated with acute rheumatic fever and does not affect the PR interval. A bifid uvula is associated with Loeys–Dietz syndrome which does not result in PR prolongation.

18. (E) Premature atrial beats are common in the fetus and the neonate and do not warrant any therapy. Blocked premature atrial contractions may result in temporary decreases in the heart rate, but these are not concerning in the fetus with good ventricular function and no hydrops. Early delivery is not indicated. The incidence of premature beats detected in utero is approximately 2%, with less than 10% of these arrhythmias persisting in the newborn.

In the fetus, PACs account for 80% to 90% of premature beats. In the newborn, premature ventricular contractions are recognized in approximately 30% of infants with extrasystoles.[10,11]

19. (E) The ECG demonstrates findings consistent with Wolff–Parkinson–White syndrome (WPW). Propranolol is frequently the first-line therapy for SVT in patients with WPW. Digoxin and verapamil are relatively contraindicated in the presence of WPW as it may increase the risk for ventricular fibrillation.[12] Flecainide is a second-line agent if the patient is not responsive to β-blockers. Mexilitine is a class IB antiarrhythmic not indicated for SVT. Amiodarone has a very long half-life and takes several days to build up a therapeutic level orally. Therefore a "pill in pocket" strategy of taking medications only after SVT starts will likely not be effective.

20. (C) A change in T-wave polarity from positive to negative in the right precordial leads describes the normal maturation of change in the ECG during the first week of life. The positive T wave in lead V1 in the first days of life most likely results from the early appearance of repolarization in the left ventricle and the late termination of depolarization in the right ventricle. An overall left ventricle to right ventricle sequence results, and this accounts for the upright T wave in lead V1 in the normal term infant.[13] The axis will shift to the left, but not to less than 55 degrees. There are decreased right ventricular forces so the R wave will typically get smaller in lead V1. The PR interval remains the same, although it will lengthen with age.

21. (A) Permanent junctional reciprocating tachycardia (PJRT) is an accessory pathway-mediated tachycardia due to a slowly conducting accessory pathway typically located in the right posterior septum. The position of the pathway creates P waves with a purely negative polarity in leads II, III, and aVF with a P-wave axis of −90 degrees.[14] Because the accessory pathway conducts slowly, P waves are usually easily visible on the ECG. Because it is an accessory pathway-mediated tachycardia, there is a 1:1 relationship of the ventricles to the atria. PJRT tends to be an incessant form of tachycardia and may cause a cardiomyopathy. PJRT tachycardia rates tend to be slower (150 to 200 bpm) than other accessory pathway-mediated tachycardias, which makes them more difficult to detect clinically.

22. (C) At K of 5.5 to 6.5 mEq/L, the T waves become tall and peaked. At serum K level above 6.6 mEq/L, QRS widening along with ST segment elevation is noted. Above 8.5 mEq/L the P waves disappear. At ~9 mEq/L, arrhythmias begin: AV block, ventricular tachycardia, and ventricular fibrillation.[15] Q waves are indicative of infarction and are not typically seen with elevated potassium.

23. (E) Junctional ectopic tachycardia is the most common arrhythmia in the acute postoperative period following congenital heart surgery. It is a focal tachycardia with gradual warm-up and cool-down and rate variability. The P waves may be visible in the terminal portion of or shortly after the QRS complex or be completely dissociated. The rate may be constant or fluctuate with increases and decreases in the catecholamine state.[16] The ECG shown demonstrates VA dissociation with the ventricular rate being faster than the atrial rate. As the ventricular rate is faster than the atrial rate, this excludes atrial flutter and ectopic atrial tachycardia as the cause. In a reentrant SVT using an accessory pathway, there should be a 1:1 relationship between the atria and ventricles. Although VA dissociation can be seen in ventricular tachycardia, the QRS complex is narrow, essentially excluding ventricular tachycardia as a cause.

24. (C) The most common coronary anomaly, accounting for one-third of all coronary anomalies, is the origin of the left circumflex coronary artery from the right main coronary artery. This finding is usually incidental and has no clinical significance. Much less common (accounting for 1% to 3% of coronary anomalies) but of greater clinical significance is the origin of the left main coronary artery from the right sinus of Valsalva. The left coronary can take four potential pathways: (1) posterior to the aorta, (2) anterior to the RVOT, (3) within the ventricular septum beneath the RV infundibulum, and (4) between the aorta and the pulmonary artery. When the LMCA passes between the aorta and the pulmonary artery, it may cause sudden cardiac death.[17] A right dominant coronary artery system is a normal variant. Pulmonary origin of the right coronary artery and a single left coronary artery are very rare variants and much less likely than an anomalous origin of the left coronary artery.

25. (A) Neonatal thyroid abnormalities (hyperthyroidism or hypothyroidism) are the most common sequelae of maternal treatment with amiodarone. There is no significant impact to the neonatal liver, lungs, eyes, or kidneys.[18]

26. (A) The ECG shown demonstrates left axis deviation (axis of −80 degrees). This is seen in patients with a primum ASD. The ECG also demonstrates right ventricular hypertrophy (Q wave in lead V1) and right atrial enlargement (P wave taller than three boxes). Other types of atrial septal defects (secundum, sinus venosus, and unroofed coronary sinus) typically show a normal to rightward axis, and older patients will frequently have an rSR' pattern in lead V1. A prolonged PR interval may be seen in all types of ASDs. A PFO is seen in 20% to 30% of the normal population and does not result in any changes on the ECG.

27. (D) Erythromycin is associated with prolongation of the QT interval. In patients with baseline-prolonged QT intervals, care should be taken to avoid administration of any medications that have been implicated in drug-induced torsades de pointes, including QT-prolonging antiarrhythmic drugs, tricyclic antidepressants, erythromycin, ondansetron, and chloral hydrate.[19] The other drugs shown do not have a significant effect on the QT interval.

28. (C) Adenosine has a half-life of 2 to 10 seconds and is an excellent drug for acute termination of reentry SVT or diagnosis of atrial arrhythmias such as atrial flutter. DC cardioversion would be indicated in a hemodynamically unstable patient. Verapamil is relatively contraindicated in infants less than 1 year of age. Propranolol is used for long-term prevention of SVT and would not be a first-line IV treatment before adenosine is attempted. Amiodarone may be used when other first-line agents have failed or if the patient is unstable and there is around a 30% chance of significant hypotension with rapid IV administration. IV digoxin may be proarrhythmic and is not generally given as a first-line agent.

29. (B) DC cardioversion would be used as a first-line therapy for neonatal atrial flutter. The recommended energy is 0.5 to 1 J/kg.

However, frequently in neonates, a higher dose is required as the energy is not delivered as efficiently through small neonatal pads or patches. If energy delivery of 1 J/kg is unsuccessful, the energy should be increased and cardioversion reattempted. In a stable rhythm with a pulse, synchronized cardioversion is indicated, as unsynchronized cardioversion may result in a shock on a T wave inducing ventricular fibrillation. There is no indication to wait and repeat cardioversion as another 4 J shock is not likely to be successful. IV adenosine will only create temporary AV block and is not helpful in converting atrial flutter. It is important to differentiate failure to convert an arrhythmia and successful cardioversion with immediate reinitiation of the arrhythmia. If cardioversion is successful in restoring sinus rhythm but the tachycardia reinitiates shortly after cardioversion, it may be necessary to begin an antiarrhythmic agent like amiodarone. However, in this instance, where the cardioversion was not successful, the next most appropriate step would be increasing the energy dose.

30. (E) A wide QRS escape rhythm in a patient with complete heart block is a class I indication for a pacemaker. The class I recommendations for permanent pacing in children, adolescents, and patients with congenital heart disease are as follows[20]:

1. Advanced second- or third-degree AV block associated with symptomatic bradycardia, ventricular dysfunction, or low cardiac output.
2. Sinus node dysfunction with correlation of symptoms during age-inappropriate bradycardia. The definition of bradycardia varies with the patient's age and expected heart rate.
3. Postoperative advanced second- or third-degree AV block that is not expected to resolve or persists at least 7 days after cardiac surgery.
4. Congenital third-degree AV block with a wide QRS escape rhythm, complex ventricular ectopy, or ventricular dysfunction.
5. Congenital third-degree AV block in the infant with a ventricular rate less than 50 to 55 bpm or with congenital heart disease and a ventricular rate less than 70 bpm.
6. Sustained pause-dependent VT, with or without prolonged QT, in which the efficacy of pacing is thoroughly documented.

In this patient, a QRS duration of 130 msec constitutes a wide complex escape, which may be unstable, and therefore requires pacemaker placement. The atrial rate is not important in determining the need for a pacemaker. Although complex ventricular ectopy is an indication for pacemaker placement, rare PVCs would not meet this criterion. In a stable patient and in the absence of congenital heart disease, a heart rate of 60 would not warrant immediate pacemaker placement.

31. (D) Long QT syndrome type 1, the most common form of long QT, presents as syncope or arrhythmias with exercise. The ECG in this patient clearly shows a prolonged QT interval. Genetic testing may reveal a cause in about 75% of patients with a high index of suspicion for long QT syndrome. An echocardiogram may be helpful in identifying hypertrophic cardiomyopathy but the ECG does not suggest hypertrophy. Magnetic resonance imaging may be helpful in identifying arrhythmogenic ventricular cardiomyopathy or myocarditis, but the ECG is consistent with long QT syndrome rather than either of these diagnoses. There are typically no abnormalities of the AH or HV intervals in patients with long QT syndrome and there is no suggestion of conduction disease of the AV node based on the ECG. Procainamide challenge may be helpful in bringing out Brugada syndrome, but there is no indication of Brugada syndrome on the ECG, and procainamide will further prolong the QT which may precipitate ventricular arrhythmias.

32. (A) For SVT to occur, there need to be two pathways with differences in conduction properties and refractory periods separated by an area of nonconduction. Entrainment is a form of mapping reentry tachycardias, and triggered activity and increased automaticity are properties of focal tachycardias.

33. (D) One of the long-term complications that can manifest in patients who have had surgery for congenital heart disease is the development of heart block. This is more common in patients who had temporary AV block in the immediate postoperative period. Late development of AV block may play a role in sudden cardiac death. The presence of Mobitz type II second-degree heart block implies conduction system disease placing a patient at risk, and pacemaker placement is warranted even with a good underlying heart rate and no symptoms. However, in the presence of Mobitz type I second-degree heart block (Wenckebach), pacemaker placement is not warranted unless the patient has a slow underlying rate and/or symptoms. Digoxin and amiodarone may worsen AV conduction. There is no indication for theophylline therapy for the treatment of AV block in the current era.

34. (C) Atrial flutter has traditionally been characterized as a macro reentrant arrhythmia with atrial rates between 240 and 400 bpm. The ECG usually demonstrates a regular rhythm, with P waves that can appear saw-toothed, also called flutter waves. Since the atrioventricular (AV) node cannot conduct at the same rate as the atrial activity, one commonly sees some form of conduction block, typically 2:1 or 4:1. This block may also be variable and cause atrial flutter to appear as an irregular rhythm. Atrial flutter is a common manifestation in patients who have undergone atrial surgery. DC cardioversion is the most effective way to terminate atrial flutter and would be indicated in a patient with hemodynamic instability. An alternative is atrial overdrive pacing which may be performed through atrial pacing wires in the postoperative setting. Temporary overdrive pacing can be an effective means of terminating reentry tachycardias such as atrial flutter and paroxysmal supraventricular tachycardia. Typically the pacing rate is set at 10 to 20 bpm faster than the tachycardia rate. Progressively faster rates can be tried with multiple attempts although there is a risk of inducing atrial fibrillation. Adenosine and digoxin will block the ventricular response, but not typically terminate the arrhythmia. Correction of hypokalemia is unlikely to terminate the arrhythmia.

35. (D) The elective replacement indicator (ERI) is set when the battery voltage drops below a certain limit. From this point on, it paces at a rate lower than the set rate. The rate is different for each pacemaker. The pacemaker may change from dual chamber to a single chamber pacing mode as well to conserve battery life. From the point that the ERI is set, the pacemaker will operate at ERI conditions for at least 3 months. As the battery is further depleted, erratic pacing will ensue and the pacemaker is at end-of-life (EOL) mode, and the pacemaker will further conserve battery life by disabling all pacemaker features except pacing. The patient should be scheduled for pacemaker replacement when

the ERI is first reached. Rate-responsive pacing increases the rate in response to increased patient activity. Pacemakers may be set to decrease the pacing rate at night while the patient is sleeping (sleep mode), but otherwise the pacemaker should pace at the set rate. Intermittent failure of capture would result in pacing at the lower rate limit, but there would be pacing spikes that would not be captured on the ECG.

36. (B) Atrial fibrillation occurs in 10% to 15% of patients with hyperthyroidism. Thyroid hormone contributes to arrhythmogenic activity by altering the electrophysiologic characteristics of atrial myocytes by shortening the action potential duration and enhancing automaticity and triggered activity in the pulmonary vein cardiac tissue.[21] Decreased voltages on an ECG can result from hypothyroidism, but not usually in hyperthyroidism. Hyperthyroidism may also be associated with a hyperdynamic state with an increased pulse pressure and hypercontractile function, although ejection fraction may decrease in the face of long-standing hyperthyroidism. Hyperthyroidism typically does not affect conduction and does not cause heart block.

37. (A) Surgery within the atrium can result in damage to the sinus node. The risk for sinus node dysfunction is directly related to the extent of surgery within the atrium. Patients after an atrial switch or Fontan procedure are at greatest risk for sinus node dysfunction. Lyme disease, maternal SLE, and myocarditis are more commonly associated with AV block. Patients with cardiomyopathy may present with atrial and ventricular arrhythmias.

38. (B) Sinus node dysfunction is the most common arrhythmia after sinus venosus ASD repair. Sinus venosus atrial septal defect (SVASD) differs from secundum atrial septal defect by its atrial septal location and its association with anomalous pulmonary venous connection. The SVASDs tend to have a higher incidence of sinus node dysfunction likely due to their proximity to the sinus node with the potential for direct damage or injury to the sinus node artery during repair. In one study, at follow-up after SVASD repair, 6% of patients had sinus node dysfunction, a permanent pacemaker, or both, and 14% of patients had atrial fibrillation.[22]

39. (D) The Heart Rhythm Society and the British Pacing and Electrophysiology Group have developed a code to describe various pacing modes (NBG code). This is a series of letters used to describe how the pacemaker is programmed. The first position denotes the chamber(s) paced, and the second position denotes the chamber(s) sensed (A for atria, V for ventricles, and D for both atria and ventricles). The third position indicates the response of the pacemaker to a sensed event (I for inhibit, T for track, and D for both inhibit and track). In the inhibit mode, when the pacemaker senses an intrinsic cardiac event, it inhibits pacing. In this manner, it allows intrinsic cardiac events to happen without pacing. In the triggered or tracking mode, the pacemaker actively paces in response to a sensed event (e.g., senses an intrinsic atrial contraction then paces the ventricle in response). A DDD pacemaker paces both atrium and ventricle, senses both atrium and ventricle, and both inhibits and tracks in response to a sensed event. As the heart rate of the patient is higher than the set rate limit of the pacemaker, the device is sensing the native atrial rate at a rate of 85 bpm and triggering the ventricle to pace at the same rate. If the patient were set AAI or VVI, it would pace only the atria or ventricles at the lower set rate. If a DDI setting was selected, the patient would sense and pace in both the atria and ventricles, but would not have the capability of tracking an atrial rate above the lower rate limit of the pacemaker as it is only set in the inhibit mode. The DDI mode is helpful in patients with atrial arrhythmias to avoid the pacemaker tracking rapid atrial rates with subsequent rapid pacing in the ventricles. In the DOO mode, the pacemaker would pace the atria and ventricle at the lower rate limit with no sensing (i.e., would pace both the atria and ventricles without regard to the intrinsic cardiac activity).

40. (B) Behavioral changes, depression, and mood swings are the most common side effects of β-blockers in children. Other less common side effects include lightheadedness, tiredness, headaches, nightmares, difficulty sleeping, heartburn, diarrhea, and constipation. Rarely, β-blockers can cause a rash. Hypoglycemia has been reported, but is also rare. β-Blockers can exacerbate asthma. They should also be used in caution in patients with diabetes as they can block hypoglycemic symptoms in these patients. Amiodarone, rather than β-blockers, causes hypothyroidism.

41. (C) The ECG shows marked ventricular hypertrophy with QRS complexes going off the page as well as a short PR interval. There is also evidence of strain with ST segment changes and T-wave inversion in the limb leads. Pompe disease is a glycogen storage disease (type II). The disease is linked to an inherited deficiency of the lysosomal enzyme acid α-glucosidase, which is responsible for the breakdown of glycogen to glucose. The result is intralysosomal accumulation of glycogen, primarily in muscle cells, that leads to a progressive loss of muscle function. It is one of the most severe and lethal form of hypertrophic cardiomyopathy, typically causing death within the first 2 years of life. Babies appear clinically well at birth, but within 6 months start developing hypotonia, severe cardiomegaly, hepatomegaly, poor weight gain, difficulty sucking, and an enlarged protruding tongue. The ECG classically shows a short PR interval and extremely large QRS voltages suggestive of left ventricular hypertrophy.

42. (B) Patients with congenitally corrected transposition (ccTGA) of the great arteries are at risk for development of complete AV block. Because of the displacement of the AV node and the abnormal course of conduction tissue which runs very superficially, there is an increased risk for development of complete AV block. Approximately 10% of the patients may present with heart block. Spontaneous complete heart block occurs at a rate of up to 2% per year in this population. These patients also have an increased risk for Wolff–Parkinson–White. The atria are not generally dilated in the absence of AV valve regurgitation and patients are not at a high risk of atrial flutter or sinus node dysfunction. Junctional tachycardia and torsades are also rare in ccTGA.

43. (D) The normal HV interval is between 35 and 55 seconds. A shorter HV interval is seen with ventricular preexcitation (WPW) and a longer HV interval is suggestive of AV node or His–Purkinje disease and can be seen in patients who have a bundle branch block.

44. (B) By delivering premature atrial stimuli (S_2 @ 320, 310, and 300 msec) after a pacing train (S_1 @ 600 msec), there should be a small decremental change in the AH interval.

However, if there is a large change (>50 msec) in the AH interval with a 10 msec change in the premature atrial stimulus (S_2), this increase in the AH interval is called an "AH jump" and suggests dual AV node pathways (i.e., both a fast pathway and a slow pathway) that may be a substrate for AV nodal reentry tachycardia. If the S_2 captures the atrium but does not conduct to the ventricles, then the AV node effective refractory period has been reached. If the S_2 fails to capture the atrium, the atrial muscle effective refractory period has been reached. Wenckebach is seen during atrial pacing and not during an extrastimulus protocol. The lengthening of the AV conduction time represented by the AH interval is a normal finding (decremental property of the AV node) and does not indicate AV node conduction system disease.

45. (B) The intracardiac ECG shows a drive train of pacing (S_1) followed by a prematurely paced ventricular stimulus (S_2). The paced beat is delivered creating a pacing spike (excluding failure of output). However, this beat does not capture the ventricle (there is a pacing spike but no resulting QRS on the surface ECG) and therefore represents the ventricular muscle ERP. If the premature stimulus captured the ventricle beat but then blocked going to the atrium (ventricular signal on the ventricular catheter and a QRS on the surface ECG) but did not conduct to the atrium, this would represent the AV node retrograde ERP. There is normal atrial activation and no evidence of an accessory pathway. VA Wenckebach occurs during ventricular pacing and not during a ventricular extrastimulus protocol.

46. (C) The ECG demonstrates pacing in the VVI mode. The rate is 75 bpm. The P waves have no relationship to the QRS complex (are dissociated), indicating that there is no sensing of the atrium, eliminating the possibility of DDD or VDD pacing. There are no atrial pacing spikes eliminating the possibility of DOO (asynchronous dual chamber) pacing. There is pacing in the ventricle so AAI is not a possibility. The pacemaker could be pacing VOO or VVI (since no intrinsic beats are seen on the tracing), but VOO was not a choice and therefore VVI is the correct answer.

47. (A) The surface tracings show a wide complex tachycardia. The atrial electrical signals (shown in the coronary sinus tracings) have no relationship to (are dissociated from) the ventricular electrical signals (shown on the bottom two ventricular electrogram tracings). As the atrial rate is slower than the ventricular rate, the tachycardia is originating distal to the AV node and is therefore a ventricular tachycardia. As the atrial rate is slower than the ventricular rate this cannot be an atrial tachycardia. In an accessory pathway-mediated tachycardia, there is a 1:1 relationship between the atria and ventricles as the atria, AV node, ventricles, and accessory pathway are all obligatory parts of the circuit. In AV node reentry tachycardia, the AV relationship is also typically 1:1. As the patient is in a wide complex rhythm with a rapid ventricular rate, although there is VA dissociation, there is no evidence of antegrade complete AV block (to make this diagnosis, the atrial rate must be typically faster than the ventricular rate).

48. (B) This patient has evidence of right ventricular hypertrophy (large Q wave in lead V1) and ST segment elevation consistent with ischemia in V1 and V2. This is consistent with right ventricular ischemia. This can be seen in patients with pulmonary atresia with intact ventricular septum and right ventricle-dependent coronary circulation. The high pressure in the right ventricle creates sinusoidal connections between the right ventricle and coronary artery circulation that may predispose the patient to ischemia. Tetralogy of Fallot and truncus arteriosus can result in RVH, but not typically ischemia. Total anomalous pulmonary venous return may result in RVH and right atrial enlargement, but also does not give signs of ischemia.

49. (A) The ECG demonstrates atrial sensing followed by ventricular tracking and resultant ventricular pacing. This is a dual chamber pacemaker and the pacing mode is either DDD or VDD. The VDD mode is capable of atrial sensing but not pacing in the atrium. Most patients have both an atrial and a ventricular lead placed with a dual chamber pacemaker. However, there are leads that have the capability in a single lead to sense both the atrium and the ventricle as well as pace the ventricle achieving AV synchrony using a single lead set VDD. If the pacemaker was set VVI or VOO, it would pace at the lower rate limit of 60, not the rate of 80 seen in the tracing. If the pacemaker were set DOO (pacing in the atria and ventricles without sensing), both atrial and ventricular pacing spikes would be present in the tracing and would pace through the tracing without any regard to exiting P waves or QRS complexes.

50. (D) The ECG shows complete AV block. AV conduction block is a complication of 1% to 3% of surgical operations for congenital heart disease. Unless treated with an implanted pacemaker, postoperative complete heart block is associated with 28% to 50% mortality, and permanent pacemaker implantation is a class I indication for surgically induced complete AV block regardless of the ventricular escape rate and condition of the patient. Postoperative heart block often proves to be transient, typically resolving within 7 to 10 days of onset, and it is prudent to wait at least 7 days to determine whether AV nodal conduction will return. Once their AV node recovers, however, these patients should be monitored for long-term development of conduction abnormalities.[23,24] In a stable patient with a reasonable escape rate, there is no indication for epinephrine or isoproterenol.

51. (C) Mobitz type I second-degree AV block, also referred to as Wenckebach periodicity, is characterized by progressive PR prolongation, usually owing to changes in the AH interval (reflecting AV node delay), with eventual failure of conduction to the ventricle. In contrast, type II AV block refers to abrupt failure of AV conduction of one or more atrial impulses without prior PR prolongation. Type II block usually occurs below the AV node. In addition to the absence of progressive PR prolongation before block, type II block may abruptly progress to third-degree block with an inadequate escape rhythm and is therefore an indication for a pacemaker, even in the absence of symptoms.[20,25] Sinus bradycardia, Wenckebach, and a prolonged PR interval are not indications for a pacemaker in an asymptomatic patient, but would be an indication if symptoms correlate with the rhythm. Left bundle branch block by itself is not an indication for pacemaker placement, regardless of QRS duration.

52. (B) The ECG shows bidirectional ventricular tachycardia with the QRS changing in every other beat during the VT. This tachycardia is most consistent with CPVT.

Features of CPVT are a catecholamine-driven (typically exercise or emotion) ventricular tachyarrhythmias, a typical pattern of bidirectional ventricular tachycardia during exercise or emotion

with a normal resting ECG and a structurally normal heart. CPVT is a genetic disease related most commonly to mutations in the cardiac ryanodine receptor gene (*RYR2*) or calsequestrin 2 gene (*CASQ2*).[26] Long QT syndrome and Brugada syndrome arrhythmias are typically triggered by an early afterdepolarization with a PVC appearing at the end of the T wave and the classic arrhythmia is torsades. Arrhythmogenic right ventricular cardiomyopathy typically produces VT from the right ventricle and hypertrophic cardiomyopathy patients are at an increased risk of VT, but bidirectional VT is the hallmark feature of CPVT.

53. (E) The findings on this ECG are consistent with intermittent capture of ventricular lead. There are pacing spikes with no capture, ventricular escape beats at a slow rate, and intermittent capture of the ventricle by the pacemaker. This is most consistent with a partial fracture of the ventricular lead. The lead impedance will often be out of the normal range when interrogated. This patient will need to be admitted and have the output of the pacemaker adjusted. If this is not successful or there are other indicators of lead malfunction, the pacing lead will need to be replaced. Undersensing is the inability of the pacemaker to sense spontaneous myocardial depolarization that results in paced complexes in the presence of the heart's intrinsic rhythm. This leads to inappropriate pacing complexes after native QRS beats. There is likely undersensing occurring as the native ventricular escape beats (first QRS on the tracing) do not reset the pacemaker timing cycle (delaying the next paced beat) and the pacemaker continues to pace at the lower rate limit. This is another marker that there is likely a major problem with the lead. Oversensing refers to the pacemaker sensing artifacts and hence not pacing when indicated. The pacemaker is continually pacing in the tracing without inhibiting (withholding pacing), so oversensing is not present. ERI is the point in the pacemaker battery life where replacement is needed but the pacemaker will continue to operate and will still result in ventricular capture. At the end of life when the battery voltage is extremely low, the pacemaker may not be able to generate enough energy to capture the heart which will result in a similar picture to the ECG shown. Placing a magnet over a pacemaker typically causes it to pace asynchronously, but not lose capture. Typically when a pacemaker performs a testing feature, it will not allow loss of capture for even a single beat.

54. (E) Adverse effects of amiodarone include photosensitivity, thyroid dysfunction, weakness, peripheral neuropathy, corneal microdeposits, and elevation of hepatic enzymes. Periodic evaluation of thyroid function and liver function should be performed in patients taking amiodarone chronically. Nausea is common at the initiation of therapy, but generally resolves over time. Photosensitivity is quite common, and patients should be instructed to cover their skin and use skin-blocking agents. Less common but serious side effects include proarrhythmia and pulmonary fibrosis.[27] Corneal microdeposits can also be seen, and a yearly ophthalmology visit is warranted for patients on chronic amiodarone. Renal dysfunction is not a side effect of amiodarone.

55. (B) The ECG shows marked right atrial enlargement with a right bundle branch block as well as suggestion of preexcitation in leads V2 and V3. These findings are most consistent with Ebstein anomaly of the tricuspid valve. WPW is associated with Ebstein anomaly, hypertrophic cardiomyopathy, and congenitally corrected transposition of the great arteries. Around 30%

of patients with Ebstein have preexcitation and 50% of those with an accessory pathway will have more than one accessory pathway. Patients with Ebstein are at risk for reentrant SVT using an accessory pathway, atrial tachycardia and atrial flutter due to the dilated atrium, and atrial fibrillation. A complete AV canal, total anomalous pulmonary venous return, and dilated cardiomyopathy may result in a dilated right atrium, but do not typically have the enormous P waves seen in this ECG and do not usually have a right bundle branch block and preexcitation. Pulmonary stenosis as an isolated finding does not typically result in right atrial enlargement.

56. (C) The patient's presentation is consistent with neurocardiogenic (or vasovagal) syncope. All the therapeutic options can be used for treatment of neurocardiogenic syncope. However, fluid liberalization and behavior modification should be the first steps in the treatment of symptoms. A majority of the patients will improve with this alone and need no further intervention.[28] A tilt table test is useful only when the diagnosis cannot be made by history alone. Although there is a pause of 3.5 seconds, without true episodes of syncope, a pacemaker is not indicated until other therapeutic options have been attempted. In addition, in many patients with neurocardiogenic syncope, there is a combined problem of hypotension and bradycardia, and placing a pacemaker may not alleviate symptoms. An ICD is not indicated in neurocardiogenic syncope. There is no value to an invasive electrophysiology study as this phenomenon is mediated by bradycardia induced by the vagus nerve rather than an arrhythmia.

57. (E) Digoxin toxicity is a relatively rare occurrence and typically occurs in the presence of acute or chronic renal failure. Hypokalemia increases digoxin cardiac sensitivity and should be corrected. Patients with hypomagnesemia, hypokalemia, or both may become cardiotoxic even with therapeutic digitalis levels. Patients with digoxin toxicity should receive IV hydration and oxygen and be admitted to an intensive care unit for monitoring. Arrhythmias play a prominent role in digoxin toxicity. β-Blockers may be helpful for treatment of supraventricular tachyarrhythmias with rapid ventricular rates. In the presence of sinus node suppression or AV node block, however, they may cause further bradycardia and should be used with caution, and a short-acting β-blocker such as esmolol should be the first line of therapy. Lidocaine can suppress ventricular arrhythmias. Phenytoin (which is a class IB antiarrhythmic in addition to being an antiepileptic medication) is also very effective in treating ventricular arrhythmias. The ventricular arrhythmias from digoxin result from early afterdepolarizations (depolarization of the ventricular myocardium during early repolarization). These early afterdepolarizations are also the mechanism of induction of arrhythmias in Long QT syndrome. Temporary pacing is an alternative for patients with severe bradycardia. Digoxin immune fab is made from immunoglobulin fragments from sheep which have been exposed to a digoxin derivative. It irreversibly binds to digoxin, making it unable to act on its target cells, including those in the heart. Just as with any other antibody product, patients must be monitored for anaphylactic shock, but the product is extremely effective. The onset of action ranges from 20 to 90 minutes with a complete response generally occurring within 4 hours.

58. (C) This rhythm strip shows torsades de pointes (TdP), which is a ventricular tachycardia with a varying QRS morphology.

Magnesium sulfate ($MgSO_4$) can be a helpful adjunct in the treatment for TdP. Its use is therefore recommended for therapy of TdP. Magnesium can be given at 5 to 10 mg/kg IV or 1 to 2 g IV in adults initially in a rapid bolus over 30 to 60 seconds. The dose can be repeated in 5 to 15 minutes and a drip can be started at 0.3 to 1 mg/kg/h. Magnesium can be effective even in patients with normal magnesium levels.[29] Defibrillation should be performed in patients with sustained torsades especially if magnesium is not readily available, but magnesium may prevent further recurrences. There is no significant effect of digoxin, atropine, potassium, or adenosine in torsades.

59. (B) Adenosine is used in the diagnosis and treatment of supraventricular arrhythmias. Adenosine works via a specific adenosine receptor linked to the potassium channel. This results in shortening of the action potential duration and sinus bradycardia as well as AV block. It has a very short half-life of 1 to 5 seconds and is metabolized by erythrocytes and endothelial tissue. It must be given by a rapid push in a large vein as close to the heart as possible. The most likely reason that adenosine is not effective is that it was not given by a rapid push in a large vein. In this case, the 24-gauge IV was likely too small to administer the dose rapidly. Adenosine should be effective in converting AV node reentry tachycardia. The dose is usually 0.1 to 0.4 mg/kg so an effect should have been seen at the dose given. Adenosine should be effective regardless of the duration of the tachycardia episode. A saline flush is almost always given with the dose to ensure that the entire dose of adenosine is quickly administered into the bloodstream.

60. (D) The fourth letter of the NBG pacing code represents rate response pacing. The pacemaker uses some type of sensor to detect activity and increases the lower rate limit of pacing in conjunction with the level of activity. When the activity ceases, the pacing returns to the set basal rate. Rate response enables a patient's pacemaker to vary heart rate when the sinus node cannot provide the appropriate rate to meet the body's demands. Rate-responsive pacing is indicated for patients who have chronotropic incompetence (heart rate cannot reach appropriate levels during exercise or to meet other metabolic demands). The fifth letter in the NBG code is occasionally used to signify biventricular pacing (pacing both the left and right ventricles).

61. (C) When the pacemaker is programmed AAIR, it is capable of pacing and sensing only in the atrium. This mode of pacing is indicated only when there is a problem with the sinus node. To correct any degree of heart block, a lead in the ventricle is necessary.

62. (C) The patient will receive a defibrillation shock if the ventricular rate goes at or above the programmed shock rate of 180 bpm. In the ventricular fibrillation zone, the patient will receive a shock if the ventricular rate is above the set rate, even if the rhythm is sinus. A separate ventricular tachycardia zone can be set with discriminators to try to determine if the arrhythmia is a sinus tachycardia or atrial tachycardia and can be programmed to withhold shock therapy if the device determines that the patient is not in ventricular tachycardia. In the ventricular fibrillation zone, these discriminators are not available and the device will deliver therapy purely based on the ventricular rate. In addition, the patient will not receive a shock if a ventricular tachycardia occurs at a rate slower than the set shocking rate (in this case, 180 bpm). Sinus tachycardia falling in the VT zone can lead to inappropriate shocks and is one of the most common reasons for inappropriate shocks in patients with an ICD.

63. (B) Electrocautery can create inappropriate noise and sensing within the pacemaker thus causing it to oversense and prevent necessary pacing. Placement of a magnet over a pacemaker causes an asynchronous pacing (no sensing, just pacing at the pacemaker's magnet rate). This avoids inappropriate pacemaker inhibition due to oversensing from electrocautery during surgery.

64. (B) When a magnet is placed over most ICDs, it disables shock therapy but pacing is not affected. This is different from when a magnet is placed over a pacemaker which enables an asynchronous pacing. By disabling shock therapy, it avoids inappropriate shocks due to oversensing from electrocautery during surgery. However, it also avoids appropriate shocks due to ventricular tachycardias. The effects are temporary and remain there only as long as the magnet is placed over the ICD.

65. (E) The etiology of a cardiac arrest is not always clear despite extensive testing. In the absence of a known reversible or treatable cause of sudden cardiac arrest, ICD is the treatment of choice and a class I indication for ICD placement according to the 2008 Pacemaker/ICD guidelines as this patient is at risk of having another cardiac arrest. β-Blockers and amiodarone are not as effective as an ICD in preventing sudden cardiac death and are not a substitute for ICD placement. An implantable loop recorder is only capable of recording rhythms and not delivering therapy. There is no indication for hemodynamic catheterization in the face of a normal echo and cardiac MRI.

66. (B) The ECG shown demonstrates left axis deviation (axis of 0 degrees), left ventricular hypertrophy, and right atrial enlargement (P wave taller than three boxes) with a marked decrease in right-sided forces. This is most consistent with a diagnosis of tricuspid atresia. Patients with tricuspid atresia may also have a short PR interval without evidence of preexcitation. The major causes of left axis deviation in the pediatric population are complete AV canal, primum ASD, tricuspid atresia, and Wolff–Parkinson–White. Left ventricular hypertrophy only rarely causes left axis deviation in pediatric patients. Hypoplastic left heart syndrome, truncus arteriosus, and tetralogy of Fallot frequently show right axis deviation and right ventricular hypertrophy, but may also be normal in the immediate newborn period. In truncus arteriosus, the axis is typically normal but combined ventricular hypertrophy is commonly seen.

67. (E) Complete heart block (CHB) detected in utero is strongly associated with maternal antibodies to SSA (Ro) and SSB (La). Their pathogenic role in the development of CHB has been established in several studies. The mothers of affected infants frequently have autoimmune disease (systemic lupus erythematosus, Sjögren syndrome) but are frequently asymptomatic. Although the association of anti-SSA/SSB with CHB is widely accepted, the precise mechanism by which these antibodies cause cardiac conduction abnormalities remains to be defined. Fetal and neonatal diseases are presumed to be due to the transplacental passage of these immunoglobulin G (IgG) autoantibodies from the mother into the fetal circulation.[30] Since these antibodies may have a pathogenic role in CHB, screening of infants with isolated CHB or neonatal lupus and their mothers for the presence of anti-SSA and anti-SSB is strongly recommended. Elevated serum potassium does not cause complete AV block without causing QRS widening. Maternal congenital heart disease does not cause isolated complete heart block. 22q11 deletions have been reported in patients with complete heart block, but are a rare cause, and Ro and La antibodies are a much more common finding.

68. (B) The ECG shows a wide complex rhythm at a rate of ~150 bpm. There is a characteristic "sine wave" pattern. In addition, there is no differentiation between the QRS and the T wave. This is seen in patients with hypoxia, acidosis, or hyperkalemia. Initial findings of hyperkalemia are tall-peaked T waves. As the potassium level increases, the T waves become more peaked and an intraventricular conduction delay results in a widened QRS along with PR prolongation. The resultant ECG may resemble a sine wave or wide ventricular tachycardia. At concentrations >9 mEq/L atrial standstill, AV block, and ventricular fibrillation can occur.[31] Increased calcium causes a shortened QT interval. The other electrolytes have minimal effect on the ECG.

69. (D) In Wolff–Parkinson–White, there is an accessory connection between the atria and the ventricles bypassing the AV node. These accessory pathways conduct quickly to the ventricles. It normally takes 35 to 70 msec to get through the AV node and bundle of His. This time is represented by the HV (His to ventricle) interval that can be measured in the EP lab. The HV interval is calculated by measuring the distance from the His deflection to the earliest QRS deflection on any lead on the surface ECG. A short HV interval (<25 to 35 msec) indicates an alternative method of conduction other than the AV node, which is only possible in the presence of an accessory pathway.[32] In some cases, the HV interval may actually be negative, with the ventricular myocardium in close proximity to the site of the accessory pathway being activated prior to the bundle of His. Bundle branch block and infra-Hisian conduction delay result in a prolonged HV interval. First-degree AV block typically has a prolonged AH (atrium to His) interval. Dual AV node physiology is seen during an atrial extrastimulus protocol and results in prolongation of the AH interval.

70. (E) This ECG shows torsades de pointes (TdP). In this type of ventricular tachycardia, the QRS complexes change morphology as if they were rotating around a point. This is the classic arrhythmia seen in patients with long QT syndrome (LQTS). Of the medications on the list, erythromycin is a medicine that prolongs the QT interval and should therefore be avoided in this patient.[33] Propranolol and lidocaine are used in the treatment of long QT syndrome. Enalapril and coumadin have no significant effect on the QT interval.

71. (A) The ECG shows atrial flutter. The treatment of choice for converting this rhythm is cardioversion. Adenosine will only block the AV node, but the atrial flutter will continue. Ventricular pacing will have no effect on this atrial arrhythmia. Lidocaine has minimal effect on atrial arrhythmias. As the newborn heart is very sensitive to calcium, calcium channel blockers such as verapamil should be avoided as they may result in long pauses and have been associated with sudden death with longer term use.[34]

72. (D) The newborn myocardium has unique properties that allow it to conduct impulses very rapidly. Atrial flutter at very fast rates (up to over 400 bpm) can be maintained in the presence of no structural heart disease. Although it is important to perform an echocardiogram on all patients who present atrial flutter, the majority of these patients have no underlying structural heart disease and a low incidence of recurrence of atrial flutter.[34]

73. (A) This ECG shows atrial fibrillation with an irregularly irregular rhythm. This rhythm results in no organized atrial contractions and stasis in the atria. This stasis predisposes patients to thrombi and potential strokes. This risk may persist for some period of time, even after sinus rhythm is restored.[35]

74. (C) This tracing shows Mobitz type I second-degree AV block (Wenckebach) with progressive prolongation of the PR interval followed by a dropped beat. This finding is not uncommon in teenagers and older adults while sleeping, but is rare while awake. If it occurs in an otherwise asymptomatic person while sleeping, it likely has no clinical significance and, as an isolated finding, does not require any therapy or further evaluation.

75. (A) This tracing shows loss of preexcitation *in a single beat* (shown in the middle of the tracing with a change from a wide, preexcited QRS to a narrow QRS). The loss in a single beat on an exercise treadmill test indicates an accessory pathway that will not rapidly conduct to the ventricle in atrial fibrillation and is therefore at a low risk for sudden death. The antegrade conduction seen on a resting ECG has no definitive relationship with the retrograde conduction that causes supraventricular tachycardia, and therefore, the risk of SVT cannot be estimated. There is no evidence of ventricular tachycardia.[36]

76. (B) The tracing shows intermittent atrial undersensing as well as atrial pacing with no evidence of capture. This is indicative of atrial lead dysfunction. The ventricular lead shows capture of all beats and there is no evidence of dysfunction. The variability of the rate is due to atrial lead dysfunction and there is no evidence of oversensing or undersensing of the ventricular lead.[37]

77. (E) This ECG shows severe bradycardia, relatively low-voltage QRS complexes, and low-amplitude T waves with no other significant abnormalities. The body's response to nutritional deprivation is to decrease the heart rate. There is no evidence of Wolff–Parkinson–White. Renal failure typically causes electrolyte disturbances that change the QRS or QT intervals. An atrial septal defect usually does not result in severe bradycardia. Thyroid storm involves hyperthyroidism and an elevated heart rate. This ECG could be consistent with hypothyroidism.[38]

78. (D) The intracardiac tracing shows a pattern of activation through the bundle of His, to the atrium followed by the ventricle. This pattern of activation is the classic pattern seen with typical AV node reentry tachycardia.[32] There is 1:1 AV conduction (one atrial impulse for every ventricular impulse), so this is not atrial flutter with 2:1 conduction. The atrial activation is earlier on the His catheter rather than the high right atrial catheter making sinus rhythm unlikely. An accessory pathway-mediated tachycardia has to go down the AV node through the ventricle up the accessory pathway to the atrium and then back down the AV node. This creates a pattern of His deflection, ventricle followed by an atrial

activation at least 20 to 40 msec following the QRS. Atypical AV node reentry tachycardia is a long RP tachycardia, and this is a short RP tachycardia.

79. (E) This ECG shows left axis deviation with the S wave being larger than the R wave in leads I and aVF giving an axis between −90 degrees and −180 degrees (northwest axis). There are small Q waves in leads I and aVL indicating that the axis went through a counterclockwise vectorcardiogram loop to get to the final axis. This is indicative of extreme left axis deviation. If the axis went through a clockwise vectorcardiogram (through right axis deviation), there would be small Q waves in leads II, III, and aVF. Left axis deviation is the classic finding in patients with complete AV canal, primum atrial septal defect, or tricuspid atresia. The other lesions listed may give right axis deviation, but do not give left axis deviation classically.

80. (A) This ECG shows massive right and left atrial enlargement consistent with restrictive cardiomyopathy. It is very unusual to see this degree of bi-atrial enlargement in any condition other than restrictive cardiomyopathy. Patients with restrictive cardiomyopathy are at risk for pulmonary hypertension. None of the other conditions listed as answers are associated with restrictive cardiomyopathy.[39]

81. (B) This ECG, which is performed at half-standard (any measured voltage should be doubled to determine the true height), shows massive ventricular hypertrophy. There is also a shortened PR interval. These findings are consistent with a glycogen storage disorder, particularly glycogen storage disease type 2 (Pompe disease). These patients present with hepatomegaly.[40,41]

82. (C) This ECG shows the classic pattern for Brugada syndrome with a right bundle branch block pattern and ST segment elevation in leads V1 and V2. This is a channelopathy affecting ion transport (typically sodium) during cardiac conduction. The clinical manifestations of Brugada syndrome are highly variable. Symptomatic patients experience ventricular tachyarrhythmias that may lead to recurrent syncope and/or sudden cardiac death. In symptomatic patients with Brugada syndrome who have either syncope or ventricular arrhythmias, an ICD is the best option.[42,43] β-Blockers are not effective at preventing sudden cardiac death, and amiodarone may exacerbate ventricular arrhythmias. Patients with a spontaneous ECG for Brugada syndrome are thought to be at higher risk for arrhythmias. Although ST segment elevation is present, patients have normal coronary arteries.

83. (E) The genetic defect associated with Brugada syndrome results from a mutation in the SCN-5A channel that is a sodium channel. HERG and KCNQ1 mutations cause LQTS. 22q11.2 deletion is associated with DiGeorge syndrome. Trisomy 21 has no relationship to Brugada syndrome.[44]

84. (E) In patients with Brugada syndrome, Vaughan Williams class I drugs such as procainamide that block the sodium channel may bring out a Brugada-type pattern on ECG. Epinephrine may be useful in identifying patients with LQTS, but not Brugada syndrome.[45]

85. (A) This tracing shows progressive prolongation of the atrium to His (AH interval) and consequentially PR intervals followed by a nonconducted beat. This finding can be created by pacing the atria faster and faster during an atrial pacing protocol. There is no evidence on this tracing of supraventricular tachycardia, atrial fibrillation, an increase in the AH interval, or preexcitation.[32]

86. (D) This tracing shows diffuse ST segment elevation and PR segment depression consistent with pericarditis. Coxsackie virus is the most common cause of viral pericarditis. Cocaine can result in coronary vasospasm and ischemia, but the ECG changes are usually localized to one segment (not diffuse ST segment elevation) and the ECG in cocaine use may appear abnormal without evidence of true acute infarction. A myosin heavy chain mutation may result in hypertrophic cardiomyopathy with subsequent left ventricular hypertrophy with strain, but not the diffuse ST segment elevation and PR depression seen on this ECG. Patients with hypertrophic cardiomyopathy often have a short PR interval due to true preexcitation or pseudo-preexcitation (rapid AV nodal conduction seen in HCM). Increased intracranial pressure can cause T-wave changes and QT prolongation, but not diffuse ST segment elevation. Erythromycin prolongs the QT interval, but does not affect ST or PR segments.

87. (A) This tracing shows an irregular wide complex tachycardia. This is atrial fibrillation in the presence of either a preexisting bundle branch block or preexcitation (Wolff–Parkinson–White). The most likely scenario in a previously asymptomatic patient is atrial fibrillation with WPW. The patient has rapid conduction through the accessory pathway and is at risk for ventricular fibrillation. With the rapid ventricular conduction, the patient should be cardioverted as quickly as possible. As the accessory pathway conducts very rapidly, the patient should undergo an ablation to eliminate conduction in the accessory pathway and, if this is not possible, should be treated with an antiarrhythmic medication such as flecainide or amiodarone that can potentially slow conduction in the accessory pathway. Patients with Ebstein anomaly have an increased incidence of WPW and are at risk for atrial fibrillation because of their dilated atria. WPW is classically associated with Ebstein, congenitally corrected transposition of the great arteries, and hypertrophic cardiomyopathy, not the other conditions listed.[46]

88. (B) In the presence of atrial fibrillation and WPW, any drug that can block the AV node, such as adenosine, digoxin, or a calcium channel blocker, is relatively contraindicated. This may cause preferential conduction down the accessory pathway resulting in rapid conduction to the ventricle and subsequently ventricular fibrillation.[47]

89. (A) This ECG shows complete AV block. There is no relationship between the P waves and the QRS complexes, the atrial rate is faster than the ventricular rate, and there are P waves that should conduct, but do not. There is no significant enough increase in ventricular arrhythmias to warrant implantation of an ICD in the absence of other risk factors. β-Blockers will have little effect and may slow the underlying junctional rate. Left stellate ganglionectomy may have some utility in LQTS, but not complete AV block. Cardiac transplantation is not indicated. A pacemaker is indicated in the presence of symptoms, a wide complex escape rhythm, complex ventricular ectopy, or a heart rate <50 in the absence of congenital heart disease and 70 in the presence of congenital heart disease.[20]

90. (D) Hypertrophic cardiomyopathy is not classically associated with AV block. All the other conditions may result in alterations of AV nodal conduction.

91. (B) This ECG shows a long RP tachycardia (the P wave occurs greater than half the distance between two successive QRS complexes). The P waves are deeply negative in leads II, III, and aVF. This is consistent with either the permanent form of junctional reciprocating tachycardia (PJRT) or atypical AV node reentry tachycardia. PJRT is an accessory pathway-mediated tachycardia due to a slowly conducting accessory pathway typically located in the right posterior septum. Because the accessory pathway conducts slowly, the atrial activation is seen a significant time following the QRS. Both PJRT and atypical AV node reentry tachycardia are dependent on the AV node and will break with adenosine. However, both also tend to be incessant and may reinitiate quickly after termination with adenosine. Atrial flutter will continue with only P waves in a saw-tooth pattern after adenosine. Sinus tachycardia will slow transiently, then speed back up. A sinus tachycardia or atrial tachycardia in the presence of preexcitation may widen transiently as the AV node blocks and there is preferential conduction down the AV node.

92. (C) The differential diagnosis for a long RP tachycardia shown includes an atrial tachycardia, PJRT, or atypical AV node reentry tachycardia. A Mahaim fiber is an accessory pathway fiber that conducts antegrade only. Mahaim fiber tachycardias present with a wide complex tachycardia. Atrial flutter can also present as a long RP tachycardia.[48]

93. (B) This tracing shows a supraventricular tachycardia. The atrial activation is earliest in the mid-CS, which runs along the AV groove between the left atrium and left ventricle. There are no normal structures that connect the atria and the ventricles present in this location. Therefore, this tracing shows supraventricular tachycardia due to a left-sided accessory pathway.[32]

94. (D) This ECG shows prolonged QT syndrome with QRS alternans. This is an alternating pattern of appearance of the T waves. This is a poor prognostic sign, and these patients are at risk for both 2:1 AV block (which this patient has on other tracings) and sudden death. Methadone prolongs the QT interval and should be avoided. Most cases of LQTS are familial; hence, other family members should be screened. The underlying mutation is typically due to a sodium or potassium channel mutation and only very rarely due to a calcium channel mutation. Calcium channel mutations are a common cause of catecholaminergic polymorphic ventricular tachycardia (CPVT).[49]

95. (A) Pacemakers have a feature that allows the pacemaker to increase the pacing rate in response to patient activity. This is called rate responsiveness and is denoted by the R in the fourth letter of the NBG pacing code (AAIR).[37] The most common mechanism for this to occur is through an accelerometer. An accelerometer senses motion and then increases the patient's pacing rate in response. In this particular instance, the bumpy road creates motion that the pacemaker senses and subsequently increases the pacing rate as a response. The pacemaker cannot determine if the motion is due to exercise, physical activity, or other sources of motion. An atrial arrhythmia would be unlikely to happen at the same time each day. Electromagnetic interference may inhibit the function of the pacemaker or make it pace asynchronously, but would not give a gradual increase in heart rate. Oversensing would result in a decrease in the rate from inhibition of pacing. When a magnet is placed over the pacemaker, it asynchronously paces at a set rate determined by the pacemaker manufacturer (the magnet rate). While this may cause an increase in the rate, it would pace at a constant rate and not steadily increase.

96. (B) The classic ECG findings of Brugada are ST segment elevation and a right bundle branch block pattern in leads V1 and V2. A spontaneous Brugada ECG pattern carries the highest risk for arrhythmias. However, some patients may have a normal ECG at rest. Fever can be a trigger for the ECG findings in Brugada syndrome and patients may exhibit an increased incidence of arrhythmias during febrile illnesses. In addition to fever, the ECG findings in Brugada syndrome may be brought out by repeating an ECG with "high-lead" placement of leads V1 and V2 as indicated. This involves moving the two leads up one and/or two intercostal space, in an attempt to bring out characteristic changes in the J-point and ST segments of leads V1 and V2. Procainamide may also be infused to bring out the typical ECG findings in Brugada syndrome. Emotional stress is a typical trigger for long QT syndrome type 2. Dehydration may bring out symptoms in patients with hypertrophic cardiomyopathy.

Hypertension may result in left ventricular hypertrophy with strain on an ECG, but typically does not affect the right-sided leads (V1 and V2). The majority of events in long QT syndrome type 3 happen during sleep, but sleep does not classically bring out the ECG pattern seen in Brugada syndrome.

97. (C) Chronic resynchronization therapy (CRT) also known as biventricular pacing is used to try to promote ventricular synchrony in patients with heart failure and a wide QRS. The 2012 guidelines state that CRT is indicated for patients who have LVEF less than or equal to 35%, sinus rhythm, LBBB with a QRS duration greater than or equal to 150 msec, and NYHA class II, III, or ambulatory IV symptoms on guideline-directed medical therapy (the only class I indication). It is generally only beneficial when the ejection fraction is less than 35% and is only indicated after medical therapy is optimized. There is some evidence that CRT may be beneficial with more narrow QRS durations and in patients with a right bundle branch block pattern, but it tends to have a lower success rate in these patients and is therefore not a class I indication. CRT is NOT recommended for patients with NYHA class I or II symptoms and non-LBBB pattern with QRS duration less than 150 msec. CRT only improves symptoms and does not decrease the incidence of arrhythmias or increase survival.[50]

ACKNOWLEDGMENT

The authors would like to acknowledge Anjan Batra, MD, for his contributions to the first edition of the textbook. Some of the questions included in this edition are modifications of his original questions.

REFERENCES

1. Donofrio MT, Moon-Grady AJ, Hornberger LK, et al. Diagnosis and treatment of fetal cardiac disease: a scientific statement from the American Heart Association. *Circulation.* 2014;129(21):2183–2242.

2. Autore C, Quarta G, Spirito P. Risk stratification and prevention of sudden death in hypertrophic cardiomyopathy. *Curr Treat Options Cardiovasc Med.* 2007;9:431–435.

3. Costello JM, Alexander ME, Greco KM, et al. Lyme carditis in children: presentation, predictive factors, and clinical course. *Pediatrics.* 2009;123:e835–e841.

4. Polak PE, Zulstra F, Roelandt JR. Indications for pacemaker implantation in the Kearns–Sayre syndrome. *Eur Heart J.* 1989; 10:281–282.

5. Goldenberg I, Moss AJ, Peterson DR, et al. Risk factors for aborted cardiac arrest and sudden cardiac death in children with the congenital long-QT syndrome. *Circulation.* 2008;117(17): 2184–2191.

6. Boineau JP, Moore EN, Patterson DF. Relationship between the ECG, ventricular activation, and the ventricular conduction system in ostium primum ASD. *Circulation.* 1973;48:556–564.

7. Murphy JG, Gersh BJ, Mair DD, et al. Long-term outcome in patients undergoing surgical repair of tetralogy of Fallot. *N Engl J Med.* 1993;329(9):593–599.

8. Khairy P, Harris L, Landzberg MJ, et al. Implantable cardioverter-defibrillators in tetralogy of Fallot. *Circulation.* 2008;117:363–370.

9. Balli S, Oflaz MB, Kibar AE, et al. Rhythm and conduction analysis of patients with acute rheumatic fever. *Pediatr Cardiol.* 2013;34(2):383–389.

10. Kleinman CS, Copel JA, Weinstein EM, et al. In utero diagnosis and treatment of fetal supraventricular tachycardia. *Semin Perinatol.* 1985;9:113–129.

11. Kleinman CS. Prenatal diagnosis and management of intrauterine arrhythmias. *Fetal Ther.* 1986;1:92–95.

12. Kugler JD, Danford DA, Gumbiner CH. Ventricular fibrillation during transesophageal atrial pacing in an infant with Wolff–Parkinson–White syndrome. *Pediatr Cardiol.* 1991;12(1): 36–38.

13. Benson DW. The normal electrocardiogram. In: Allen H, Shaddy R, Feltes T, et al., eds. *Moss and Adams' Heart Disease in Infants, Children, and Adolescents: Including the Fetus and Young Adults.* 7th ed. Philadelphia, PA: Lippincott Williams & Wilkins; 2007:152–165.

14. Cannon B, Snyder C. Disorders of cardiac rhythm and conduction. In: Allen HD, Driscoll DJ, Shaddy RE, et al., eds. *Moss and Adams' Heart Disease in Infants, Children, and Adolescents: Including the Fetus and Young Adults.* 8th ed. Philadelphia, PA: Lippincott Williams & Wilkins; 2012:1573.

15. Petrov D, Petrov M. Widening of the QRS complex due to severe hyperkalemia as an acute complication of diabetic ketoacidosis. *J Emerg Med.* 2008;34:459–461.

16. Collins KK, Van Hare GF, Kertesz NJ, et al. Pediatric nonpostoperative junctional ectopic tachycardia medical management

and interventional therapies. *J Am Coll Cardiol.* 2009;53(8): 690–697.

17. Lorenz EC, Mookadam F, Mookadam M, et al. A systematic overview of anomalous coronary anatomy and an examination of the association with sudden cardiac death. *Rev Cardiovasc Med.* 2006;7(4):205–213.

18. Bartalena L, Bogazzi F, Braverman LE, et al. Effects of amiodarone administration during pregnancy on neonatal thyroid function and subsequent neurodevelopment. *J Endocrinol Invest.* 2001; 24(2):116–130.

19. www.crediblemeds.org

20. Epstein AE, DiMarco JP, Ellenbogen KA, et al. ACC/AHA/ HRS 2008 guidelines for device-based therapy of cardiac rhythm abnormalities: a report of the American College of Cardiology/ American Heart Association Task Force on Practice Guidelines (Writing Committee to Revise the ACC/AHA/NASPE 2002 Guideline Update for Implantation of Cardiac Pacemakers and Antiarrhythmia Devices): developed in collaboration with the American Association for Thoracic Surgery and Society of Thoracic Surgeons. *Circulation* 2008;117:e350–e408.

21. Jayaprasad N, Francis J. Atrial fibrillation and hyperthyroidism. *Indian Pacing Electrophysiol J.* 2005;5:305–311.

22. Attenhofer Jost CH, Connolly HM, Danielson GK, et al. Sinus venosus atrial septal defect long-term postoperative outcome for 115 patients. *Circulation.* 2005;112:1953–1958.

23. Batra AS, Wells WJ, Hinoki KW, et al. Late recovery of atrioventricular conduction after pacemaker implantation for complete heart block associated with surgery for congenital heart disease. *J Thorac Cardiovasc Surg.* 2003;125(6):1291–1293.

24. Gross GJ, Chiu CC, Hamilton RM, et al. Natural history of postoperative heart block in congenital heart disease: implications for pacing intervention. *Heart Rhythm.* 2006;3:601–604.

25. Shaw DB, Kekwick CA, Veale D, Gowers J, Whistance T. Survival in second degree atrioventricular block. *Br Heart J.* 1985;53(6):587–593.

26. Laitinen PJ, Brown KM, Piippo K, et al. Mutations of the cardiac ryanodine receptor (RyR2) gene in familial polymorphic ventricular tachycardia. *Circulation.* 2001;103:485–490.

27. Vrobel TR, Miller PE, Mostow ND, Rakita L. A general overview of amiodarone toxicity: its prevention, detection, and management. *Prog Cardiovasc Dis.* 1989;31(6):393–426.

28. Sheldon RS, Grubb BP 2nd, Olshansky B, et al. 2015 Heart Rhythm Society expert consensus statement on the diagnosis and treatment of postural tachycardia syndrome, inappropriate sinus tachycardia, and vasovagal syncope. *Heart Rhythm.* 2015;12(6): e41–e63.

29. Tzivoni D, Banai S, Schuger C, et al. Treatment of torsade de pointes with magnesium sulfate. *Circulation.* 1988;77:392–397.

30. Brito-Zerón P, Izmirly PM, Ramos-Casals M, et al. The clinical spectrum of autoimmune congenital heart block. *Nat Rev Rheumatol.* 2015;11(5):301–312.

31. Viera AJ, Wouk N. Potassium disorders: hypokalemia and hyperkalemia. *Am Fam Physician.* 2015;92(6):487–495.

32. Fogoros R. *Electrophysiologic Testing.* 4th ed. Malden, MA: Wiley Blackwell Publishers; 2012.

33. Cubeddu LX. Iatrogenic QT abnormalities and fatal arrhythmias: mechanisms and clinical significance. *Curr Cardiol Rev.* 2009;5(3): 166–176.

34. Wren C. Cardiac arrhythmias in the fetus and newborn. *Semin Fetal Neonatal Med.* 2006;11(3):182–190. Epub 10 March 2006.

35. Olsson SB, Halperin JL. Prevention of stroke in patients with atrial fibrillation. *Semin Vasc Med.* 2005;5(3):285–292.

36. Bricker JT, Porter CJ, Garson A Jr, et al. Exercise testing in children with Wolff–Parkinson–White syndrome. *Am J Cardiol.* 1985;55:1001–1004.

37. Ellenbogen KA, Wood MA. *Cardiac Pacing and ICDs.* 5th ed. Hoboken, NJ: Wiley-Blackwell; 2008.

38. Casiero D, Frishman WH. Cardiovascular complications of eating disorders. *Cardiol Rev.* 2006;14(5):227–231.

39. Denfield SW, Rosenthal G, Gajarski RJ, et al. Restrictive cardiomyopathies in childhood. Etiologies and natural history. *Tex Heart Inst J.* 1997;24(1):38–44.

40. Kishnani PS, Hwu W-L, Mandel H, et al. A retrospective, multinational, multicenter study on the natural history of infantile-onset Pompe disease. *J Pediatr.* 2006;148:671–676.

41. Hirschhorn R, Arnold JJR. Glycogen storage disease type II: acid alpha-glucosidase (acid maltase) deficiency. In: Scriver C, Beaudet A, Sly W, et al., eds. *The Metabolic and Molecular Bases of Inherited Disease.* 8th ed. New York: McGraw-Hill; 2001: 3389–3420.

42. Haverkamp W, Rolf S, Eckardt L, et al. Long QT syndrome and Brugada syndrome: drugs, ablation or ICD? *Herz.* 2005;30(2): 111–118.

43. Postema PG, Wolpert C, Amin AS, et al. Drugs and Brugada syndrome patients: review of the literature, recommendations, and an up-to-date website (www.brugadadrugs.org). *Heart Rhythm.* 2009;6(9):1335–1341.

44. Ackerman MJ, Priori SG, Willems S, et al. HRS/EHRA expert consensus statement on the state of genetic testing for the channelopathies and cardiomyopathies: this document was developed as a partnership between the Heart Rhythm Society (HRS) and the European Heart Rhythm Association (EHRA). *Heart Rhythm.* 2011;8(8):1308–1339.

45. Antzelevitch C, Brugada P, Borggrefe M, et al. Brugada syndrome: report of the second consensus conference: endorsed by the Heart Rhythm Society and the European Heart Rhythm Association. *Circulation.* 2005;111(5):659–670.

46. Pietersen AH, Andersen ED, Sandoe E. Atrial fibrillation in the Wolff–Parkinson–White syndrome. *Am J Cardiol.* 1992;70: 38A–43A.

47. Paul T, Guccione P, Garson A Jr. Relation of syncope in young patients with Wolff–Parkinson–White syndrome to rapid ventricular response during atrial fibrillation. *Am J Cardiol.* 1990;65: 318–321.

48. Walsh EP, Saul JP, Triedman J, eds. *Cardiac Arrhythmias in Children and Young Adults with Congenital Heart Disease.* Baltimore, MD: Williams & Wilkins; 2001.

49. Lehnart SE, Ackerman MJ, Benson DW Jr, et al. Inherited arrhythmias: a National Heart, Lung, and Blood Institute and Office of Rare Diseases workshop consensus report about the diagnosis, phenotyping, molecular mechanisms, and therapeutic approaches for primary cardiomyopathies of gene mutations affecting ion channel function. *Circulation.* 2007;116(20):2325–2345.

50. Epstein AE, DiMarco JP, Ellenbogen K, et al. 2012 ACCF/AHA/ HRS focused update incorporated into the ACCF/AHA/HRS 2008 guidelines for device-based therapy of cardiac rhythm abnormalities: a report of the American College of Cardiology Foundation/ American Heart Association Task Force on Practice Guidelines and the Heart Rhythm Society. *Circulation.* 2013;127(3): e283–e352.

CHAPTER 7

Exercise Physiology and Testing

Justin M. Horner and David Driscoll

QUESTIONS

1. What is the most commonly accepted method of indexing maximum oxygen uptake ($\dot{V}O_2$) in clinical exercise testing?

   A. Age
   B. Sex
   C. Lean body mass
   D. Body weight (kilograms)
   E. Exponent of body length

2. Which method of exercise would achieve a higher maximum oxygen uptake ($\dot{V}O_2$max)?

   A. Stationary electronically braked cycle ergometer
   B. Arm crank ergometer
   C. Hand grip ergometer
   D. Treadmill ergometer
   E. Stationary mechanically braked cycle ergometer

3. Which cardiac index has the smallest increase with exercise when measured in the supine position?

   A. Heart rate (HR)
   B. Minute ventilation
   C. Stroke volume
   D. Respiratory rate
   E. Blood pressure

4. What cardiovascular changes would be expected during exercise?

	Cardiac output	HR	EF	Total peripheral resistance	CVP
A.	↑	↑	↑	↑	↑
B.	↑	↑	↑	↓	↑
C.	↑	↑	↑	↑	↓
D.	↑	↑	↑	↓	NC
E.	↑	↑	↑	↑	NC

5. Which blood pressure change would be expected in a normal 15-year-old male patient (resting blood pressure = 110/61 mm Hg) with isometric hand grip exercise?

   A. 150/60 mm Hg
   B. 155/55 mm Hg
   C. 120/40 mm Hg
   D. 170/65 mm Hg
   E. 140/110 mm Hg

6. Which blood pressure change would be expected in a normal 15-year-old male patient (resting blood pressure = 110/72 mm Hg) with isotonic exercise?

   A. 200/100 mm Hg
   B. 130/60 mm Hg
   C. 120/68 mm Hg
   D. 124/76 mm Hg
   E. 200/70 mm Hg

7. What maximum HR and maximum oxygen consumption would best represent a normal 15-year-old male patient during isotonic exercise?

	HR (bpm)	Oxygen consumption ($\dot{V}O_2$max mL/kg/min)
A.	200	40
B.	145	25
C.	190	60
D.	200	20
E.	190	30

8. A healthy 21-year-old woman on no medications just finished a treadmill exercise test. She exercised for a total of 6 minutes. The exercise physiologist technician questioned her effort. However, the patient claimed she "gave it her all." What is her expected maximal HR if she gave an intense effort?

A. 123 bpm
B. 158 bpm
C. 185 bpm
D. 189 bpm
E. 196 bpm

9. As a normal child ages, what ventilatory changes at peak exercise would be expected?

	Maximum RR	Tidal volume	Minute ventilation ($\dot{V}E$)
A.	↑	↑	↑
B.	↓	↑	↑
C.	↑	↓	↑
D.	↓	↑	↓
E.	↓	↓	↑

10. What cardiovascular changes would be expected with improved fitness?

	Stroke volume	HR (resting)	HR (max)	Cardiac output
A.	↑	↓	↑	↑
B.	↓	↑	↑	↑
C.	↑	↑	NC	↓
D.	↓	↓	↑	↓
E.	↑	↓	NC	↑

11. Choose the correct statement:
A. Joule is the standard unit of power
B. Peak $\dot{V}O_2$ and $\dot{V}O_2$max are synonymous

C. Exercise testing utilizes isometric forms of exercise in most centers
D. In the same subject, a higher $\dot{V}O_2$max can be achieved with treadmill testing when compared to cycle testing
E. A "watt" is a unit of work

12. Which condition would be a contraindication for exercise testing?
A. Atrial septal defect (ASD) with left-to-right shunt
B. Ventricular septal defect (VSD) with left-to-right shunt
C. Severe primary pulmonary hypertension
D. Remote history of myocardial infarction
E. Remote history of rheumatic heart disease

13. Which diagram is correct (Fig. 7.1)? Four conditions are depicted.

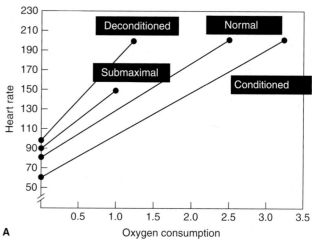

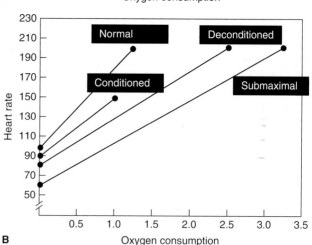

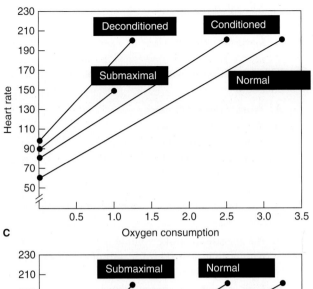

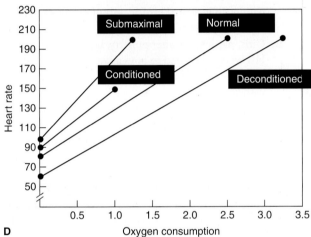

FIGURE 7.1 Oxygen consumption versus heart rate. Modified from Allen HD, Driscoll DJ, Shaddy RE, et al. *Moss & Adams' Heart Disease in Infants, Children, and Adolescents: Including the Fetus and Young Adult.* 8th ed. Philadelphia, PA: Lippincott Williams & Wilkins/Wolters Kluwer; 2013.

14. Identify the correct statement regarding ventilatory anaerobic threshold (VAT):

   A. The VAT is the $\dot{V}O_2$ at which there is a disproportionate decrease in minute ventilation relative to oxygen uptake
   B. VAT is synonymous with the threshold for decompensated metabolic acidosis
   C. There is commonly a relative drop in lactate production when VAT is reached
   D. When VAT is reached, there is a decrease in mixed expired O_2 concentration
   E. During incremental exercise VAT reflects the onset of anaerobic metabolism

15. As compared to an acyanotic patient, an unrepaired, cyanotic patient at peak exercise will exhibit a higher:

   A. HR
   B. Ventilatory equivalent for oxygen
   C. Blood oxygen saturation
   D. Maximum oxygen uptake
   E. Diastolic blood pressure

16. Which statement is correct regarding an exercise protocol?

   A. Duration of exercise test between 12 and 15 minutes
   B. Modified Bruce protocol is appropriate for children with limited exercise capacity
   C. James protocol has relatively small work increments
   D. Ramp protocol has large increases in workload
   E. Ramp protocol is appropriate for assessing steady-state exercise

17. Which statement is correct regarding the ventilatory response to exercise?

   A. Total ventilation increases because of increased rate, while tidal volume remains constant
   B. Tidal volume increases predominately by tapping into the expiratory reserve volume
   C. $\dot{V}E/\dot{V}O_2$ declines early in exercise as a result of better ventilation and blood flow matching in the lungs
   D. Normal subjects terminate exercise because ventilation can increase no further while cardiac output can continue to increase
   E. Diffusion limitation is a common problem during routine clinical exercise testing

18. Which of the following exercise-testing technique statements would be correct?

   A. Circling 60% of the patient's arm with the sphygmomanometer cuff is appropriate
   B. Sphygmomanometer cuff width equals 30% of the upper arm length
   C. The assumption that acetylene–helium technique approximates cardiac output in a patient with a large atrial septal defect and left-to-right shunt
   D. That acetylene–helium technique is dependent on even distribution of inspired gas in the lungs
   E. CO_2 rebreathing technique to measure cardiac output is better tolerated in children than the acetylene–helium technique

19. A 22-year-old male, well-trained college football athlete underwent a treadmill exercise study midseason. Shortly thereafter, he sustained a lower limb injury and was unable to train for 3 months during recovery. He completed a second treadmill exercise test at the start of retraining. Both exercise studies were maximum effort. Which data would best describe his situation?

		Test 1	Test 2
A.	HR (bpm) maximum	200	150
B.	Maximum $\dot{V}O_2$ (L/min)	50	35
C.	Maximum $\dot{V}E$ (L/min)	35	55
D.	Maximum exercise systolic BP (mm Hg)	200	180
E.	Maximum exercise O_2 saturation	92%	98%

20. In a healthy 15-year-old woman without lung disease who gave maximum effort on spirometry before exercise testing, which statement about maximum voluntary ventilation (MVV) is correct?

A. MVV is reliably measured as it is independent of subject effort

B. Maximal $\dot{V}_E$ <70% of resting MVV suggests pulmonary limitation to exercise

C. MVV is ~35 to 40 times FEV_1

D. MVV is typically measured during early exercise

E. MVV can also detect vocal cord dysfunction as a cause for exertional dyspnea

21. In healthy patients, which of the following is a normal physiologic response during exercise?

A. Increased end-systolic volume

B. Increased diastolic pressure during isotonic exercise

C. Among similar-sized children, girls have a higher peak systolic blood pressure than boys

D. African-American children have a higher blood pressure response to exercise when compared to Caucasian children

E. Blood pressure increases during exercise are due to increased systemic resistance

22. Which patient would be a good candidate for the use of acetylene–helium rebreathing technique during exercise testing for the measurement of cardiac output?

A. A 15-year-old boy with Ebstein anomaly and a large secundum ASD with right-to-left shunt

B. A 12-year-old girl s/p Fontan operation with arteriovenous pulmonary fistulas

C. A 14-year-old boy with a patent foramen ovale with trivial left-to-right shunt

D. An 8-year-old boy with a moderate membranous ventricular septal defect with left-to-right shunt

E. A 10-year-old girl with a persistent left superior vena cava and unroofed coronary sinus

23. During exercise stress testing, what direct measurement can be determined by using acetylene–helium rebreathing technique?

A. Systemic blood flow

B. Pulmonary oxygen exchange

C. Cardiac output

D. Shunt volume

E. Effective pulmonary blood flow

24. In a healthy, normal child, what organ system is most commonly responsible for limiting maximal achievable workload?

A. Pulmonary

B. Cardiovascular

C. Musculoskeletal

D. Neurologic

E. Gastrointestinal

25. The calculation of work can be completed with which equation?

A. Work = force × distance

B. Work = force/distance

C. Work = distance/force

D. Work = mass × acceleration

E. Work = mass/acceleration

26. Which statement about exercise-testing physiology is correct?

A. An increase in stroke volume is the major determinant of an increased cardiac output during exercise in a normal patient

B. Girls, particularly after puberty, have a slightly lower HR when compared to boys at any given workload

C. For patients >20 years of age, maximal HR changes with age

D. For patients >20 years of age, maximum HR increases with conditioning

E. Total systemic vascular resistance increases with increased workload

27. Using a cycle exercise protocol which of the following patients, if a maximal effort was achieved, would result in a higher maximal $\dot{V}_{O_2}$ during work?

A. A 17-year-old African-American girl

B. A 17-year-old Caucasian boy

C. An 18-year-old Caucasian anemic boy

D. A 12-year-old Caucasian boy

E. A 12-year-old African-American girl

28. Which of the following echocardiographic findings would be most consistent with the heart of a well-trained, normal athlete?

A. Decreased left ventricular end-diastolic dimension

B. Decreased left ventricular wall thickness

C. Decreased stroke volume

D. Increased left ventricular end-diastolic volume

E. Increased left ventricular end-systolic dimension

29. Which of the following conditions is an absolute contraindication to exercise testing?

A. Second-degree AV block

B. Severe aortic stenosis

C. Catecholaminergic polymorphic ventricular tachycardia

D. Long QT syndrome

E. Anomalous origin of a coronary artery

30. Which of the following statements comparing treadmill exercise testing to cycle ergometry is correct?

   A. Cycle ergometry-derived maximum oxygen uptake ($\dot{V}O_2$) is higher than treadmill testing

   B. Noise and artifact are less during treadmill exercise testing

   C. Cycle ergometry allows for a more accurate work measurement

   D. Cycle ergometry is potentially more dangerous than treadmill ergometry

   E. Younger children (4 to 6 years of age) may have more difficulty using a treadmill ergometry than a cycle ergometry

31. Which statement is most accurate regarding aortic stenosis and exercise stress testing?

   A. Total work performed has a linear relationship with transaortic pressure gradient

   B. Greater increase in systolic blood pressure with exercise when compared to normal patients

   C. The higher the transaortic gradient, the lower the expected ST segment change during exercise

   D. The higher the transaortic gradient, the higher the maximum oxygen uptake ($\dot{V}O_2max$) achievable

   E. Total work performed has an inverse relationship with transaortic pressure gradient

32. Which exercise-testing statement would be most correct in an 8-year-old boy with pulmonary atresia, ventricular septal defect, and a systemic arterial-to-pulmonary arterial anastomosis?

   A. Achievement of normally expected maximum aerobic power

   B. Normal ventilation relative to maximal oxygen uptake ($\dot{V}O_2max$)

   C. Blood oxygen saturation improves with exercise

   D. Complete repair would improve the blood oxygen saturation with exercise

   E. Complete repair would improve exercise time to be superior to normal patients

33. Which statement is consistent with an appropriate exercise technique?

   A. Only two surface electrocardiogram (ECG) leads need to be recorded during the exercise study

   B. A complete 12-lead ECG should be obtained once at rest, at each workload, and several times after completion

   C. The use of skin cleanser, electrode paste, and lead bandaging is necessary for treadmill ergometry but unnecessary for cycle ergometry

   D. Diastolic blood pressure measurement is typically made with ease during treadmill ergometry

   E. Direct blood pressure measurement in the radial artery underestimates the central aortic blood pressure

34. As compared to an acyanotic patient, a cyanotic patient at peak exercise will exhibit a higher:

   A. HR

   B. Ventilatory equivalent for oxygen

   C. Arterial blood oxygen saturation

   D. Arterial pCO_2

   E. Diastolic blood pressure

35. Using the CO_2 rebreathing technique during an exercise study, which statement is most correct?

   A. The CO_2 rebreathing technique is well tolerated by all patients and is noninvasive

   B. The CO_2 concentration in the rebreathing technique does not need to be adjusted for the patient's size and exercise intensity

   C. The CO_2 rebreathing technique does not obtain enough information to use the Fick principle for determining the cardiac output

   D. The instrument dead space in the tubing does not need to be accounted for

   E. The CO_2 rebreathing technique can be completed noninvasively by using the Bohr equation

ANSWERS

1. (D) Maximum oxygen uptake is closely related to cardiac output. The more work/exercise a patient does the more oxygen uptake will be needed. Many methods for indexing $\dot{V}O_2$max have been suggested. Males tend to have a higher lean body mass than females, which causes differences in $\dot{V}O_2$max between the sexes. $\dot{V}O_2$max also changes with increasing age. Previous studies have revealed an exponent of body length (1.5 to 3.21) has also been unreliable. The most commonly accepted method of indexing $\dot{V}O_2$ is body weight.

2. (D) The higher maximum $\dot{V}O_2$ that can be achieved depends on the type of work performed $\dot{V}O_2$, which will be related to the mass of muscle used to exercise and the amount of exercise done. One uses more muscle groups when exercising on a treadmill than when using the ergometers listed in the question.

3. (C) Stroke volume is dependent on the left ventricular end-diastolic volume and ejection fraction. In the supine position, stroke volume will increase normally due to increased volume return (increased end-diastolic volume) to the heart. Thus, the stroke volume is already increased from baseline, and the volume needed to reach maximum stroke volume will be small and limited. Finally, stroke volume primarily increases early in exercise and will increase little thereafter.

4. (D) In the normal patient, exercise is associated with an increase in cardiac output, HR, and ejection fraction. A decrease in the total peripheral resistance will occur, and no change occurs in central venous pressure. These changes primarily are due to the large increase in sympathetic activity during exercise. The decreased total peripheral resistance primarily is due to a decreased skeletal muscle vascular resistance allowing more blood flow to the muscles. Finally, the central venous pressure remains relatively unchanged due to the compensatory mechanisms of the skeletal muscle pump and the respiratory pump that both promote increased venous return and thus no need to increase the central venous pressure.

5. (E) Isometric exercise consists of constant muscle length (no change) against a force/tension. Examples include holding a weight in a fixed position, pushing against a door frame, or hand grip exercise. During isometric exercise, systolic and diastolic blood pressure increase significantly.

6. (E) During isotonic exercise, systolic blood pressure increases. However, diastolic blood pressure remains relatively unchanged (within 10 mm Hg of resting diastolic pressure). Blood pressure changes depend on the patient's size as well as gender. Larger patients and/or males will have a higher blood pressure at rest and during exercise compared to smaller patients and/or females. The systolic blood pressure increase during exercise is attributed to increased cardiac output despite a reduction in total systemic resistance.

7. (A) There is a linear relationship between HR and $\dot{V}O_2$max until maximum workload is reached. Each individual has a maximum HR that is achievable, usually ranging between 195 and 215 bpm in adolescents. Normal oxygen consumption ($\dot{V}O_2$max) is considered to be roughly 35 to 45 mL/kg/min. Therefore, a

HR of 200 bpm and oxygen consumption of 40 mL/kg/min would be normal for a 15-year-old. HR of 145 bpm and oxygen consumption of 1.0 L/min would represent a submaximal exercise test/effort or chronotropic insufficiency.

8. (E) The accepted maximum HR for patients 5 to 20 years of age is roughly 195 to 215 bpm. However, for patients >20 years of age, the equation ($HR_{max} = 210 - 0.65 \times$ age) is the accepted method of determining the maximum HR for each individual. Therefore, this patient's maximum HR is 196 bpm ($HR_{max} = 210 - 0.65 \times 21$).

9. (B) During exercise, minute ventilation increases. This occurs by an increase in both ventilation frequency and tidal volume. These parameters will continue to increase with increasing age. However, the maximum respiratory rate that can be achieved at peak exercise will decrease with increasing age.

10. (E) Repetitive exercise will usually result in improved fitness. Physiologic changes that occur with improved fitness include a decreased resting HR and increased stroke volume and cardiac output with exercise. With conditioning, the decrease in resting HR is likely due to increased stroke volume as well as increased vagal influence at rest. There is no change to maximum HR with improved fitness.

11. (D) A joule is standard unit of work, not of power. Peak $\dot{V}O_2$ is that which a subject can achieve. $\dot{V}O_2$max is the $\dot{V}O_2$ reached when $\dot{V}O_2$ plateaus. Most centers utilize isotonic exercise-testing protocols. A higher $\dot{V}O_2$max can be achieved with treadmill than with cycle exercise because more muscle groups are used when exercising on a treadmill than on a cycle.

12. (C) Of the answers listed, the only contraindication to exercise testing would be severe primary pulmonary hypertension. An atrial septal defect would not be a contraindication to exercise testing. They are relatively common (5% to 10% of the population) and a left-to-right shunt would not cause increased hypoxia with exercise. The same would hold true for a ventricular septal defect. An *acute* myocardial infarction or *acute* rheumatic heart disease would both be contraindications to exercise testing due to fragile myocardial tissue. However, a history of either of these may be an indication for exercise testing to assess symptoms of fatigue and/or exercise intolerance rather than a contraindication.

13. (A) As one becomes better conditioned, rest HR declines and $\dot{V}O_2$max increases but HR_{max} does not change. As one becomes deconditioned, rest HR increases and $\dot{V}O_2$max decreases but HR_{max} remains the same. If one fails to reach predicted HR_{max} either the effort was submaximal or the patient has chronotropic insufficiency.

14. (E) The VAT occurs at the point of exercise when there is a disproportionate increase in minute ventilation ($\dot{V}E$) relative to oxygen uptake. This results in an increased expiration of mixed oxygen concentration. In adults, a disproportionate increase in lactate is also frequently observed. Decompensated acidosis is not synonymous with VAT. Decompensated acidosis occurs later in exercise, after the VAT has occurred.

15. (B) The ventilatory equivalent for oxygen is minute ventilation divided by oxygen uptake ($\dot{V}E/\dot{V}O_2$). Patients with cyanotic heart disease typically have more hypoxemia at rest and during exercise. The presence of a large right-to-left shunt is a major determinant of this abnormal exercise response. At peak exercise, cyanotic patients increase their minute ventilation ($\dot{V}E$) disproportionately to their oxygen uptake ($\dot{V}O_2$), resulting in a higher ventilatory equivalent for oxygen than acyanotic patients. The blood oxygen saturation and maximum oxygen uptake ($\dot{V}O_2$) will be lower than for an acyanotic patient.

16. (B) There is no one "best" exercise protocol. However, in general, a "good" exercise protocol should have nonexcessive increments of workload with a duration lasting no longer than 8 to 12 minutes. The Bruce treadmill protocol and/or the "modified" Bruce protocol are popular with children and those individuals incapable of long exercise due to smaller, frequent increases of workload. The James protocol involves cycle ergometry with relatively large increments of workload. The ramp treadmill protocol is becoming more and more popular due to a constantly increasing workload. This test's workload can be adjusted in order to have the test last 8 to 10 minutes. However, this protocol does not allow assessment of steady-state exercise due to the constant changing workload.

17. (C) As exercise is begun and pulmonary blood flow increases, resting V/Q mismatch is reduced because of more uniform perfusion of the lungs and ventilation. Hence ventilation becomes more efficient and $\dot{V}E/\dot{V}O_2$ decreases. When the ventilator anaerobic threshold is reached, $\dot{V}E/\dot{V}O_2$ will increase. With increased work, the ventilatory response includes increased minute ventilation ($\dot{V}E$), respiratory rate, and tidal volume. As a child grows, the maximum respiratory rate that can be achieved decreases, but the tidal volume and $\dot{V}E$ increases. Normal patients terminate exercise because cardiac output can no longer increase, even though there typically is still ventilatory reserve available. Diffusion limitation is rarely a problem during routine clinical exercise testing.

18. (D) Acetylene–helium rebreathing technique is used to measure cardiac output indirectly by measuring effective pulmonary blood flow in the absence of significant intracardiac shunts. This technique is also dependent upon even distribution of the inspired gas throughout the lungs. It will not be a reliable method for cardiac output measurement in patients with lung disease that involves mismatching of ventilation and perfusion. The sphygmomanometer cuff should have a bladder length that covers at least 80% of the circumference of the upper arm and at least 40% width of the upper arm.

19. (B) With improved fitness, a patient can complete more work; thus, a higher maximum $\dot{V}O_2$ is achieved. Maximum minute ventilation ($\dot{V}E$) also increases with improved fitness. During a maximal effort exercise study, the patient's ability to reach maximum HR and maximum blood pressure will not be limited due to the time of deconditioning. The oxygen saturation should not be low during an exercise test in a highly trained athlete.

20. (C) MVV is obtained at rest, and it is dependent on the patient's effort. MVV has been shown to be ~35 to 40 times the forced expiratory volume (FEV_1). Owing to the dependence on the patient's effort, MVV must cautiously be used for suggesting pulmonary limitation. At the point of exercise termination in a normal patient, minute ventilation ($\dot{V}E$) is 60% to 70% of MVV. Patients with lung disease and pulmonary limitation will achieve a $\dot{V}E >70\%$ by tapping into the ventilatory reserve. Tidal flow-volume loops are a more accurate method of assessing pulmonary limitation to exercise than MVV. Tidal flow-volume loops also have the advantage of assessing vocal cord dysfunction, which is an increasingly common cause for exertional dyspnea.

21. (D) African-American children have a higher blood pressure response to exercise than Caucasian children. The same holds true for larger-sized children when compared to smaller-sized children. Of similar-sized patients, boys have a greater blood pressure response than girls. During exercise, the cardiac output will increase by increasing stroke volume as well as HR. Therefore, the end-systolic volume will decrease. During isotonic exercise, the diastolic pressure remains relatively stable (change <10 mm Hg); however, during isometric exercise the diastolic blood pressure increases. Blood pressure increases during exercise predominately occur by increased cardiac output. The total systemic resistance decreases during exercise.

22. (C) Acetylene–helium rebreathing technique, which is dependent on even distribution of the inspired gas throughout the lungs, is used to measure cardiac output indirectly by measuring effective pulmonary blood flow in the absence of significant intracardiac shunts. It will not be a reliable method of cardiac output measurement in patients with lung disease that involves mismatching of ventilation and perfusion or those patients with significant intracardiac or intrapulmonary shunts. Therefore, the only patient with an insignificant intracardiac shunt of those listed would be the 14-year-old boy with a patent foramen ovale with trivial left-to-right shunt.

23. (E) Acetylene–helium rebreathing technique is noninvasive, and it is usually well tolerated by children. This method directly measures the effective pulmonary blood flow in the absence of significant intrapulmonary or intracardiac shunts. This allows for an effective method to estimate cardiac output. Acetylene diffuses from the alveolus into the pulmonary capillary blood, and thus the acetylene concentration declines relative to the volume of effective pulmonary blood flow. This technique depends on an even distribution throughout the lungs.

24. (B) In the normal, healthy child, the cardiovascular system will be the limiting factor to exercise. Maximum cardiac output will be achieved when the maximum HR limits ventricular filling during diastole and in turn stroke volume. Well-fit patients can continue to exercise at their maximum HR for 1 to 2 minutes. The pulmonary system, in a normal, healthy child, will not limit exercise capacity. Minute ventilation ($\dot{V}E$) and work have a linear relationship until the ventilatory anaerobic threshold (VAT) is achieved. At this point, there is a disproportionate increase in $\dot{V}E$ relative to $\dot{V}O_2$. At the point of exhaustion, $\dot{V}E$ is 60% to 70% of maximum ventilation volume.

25. (A) A few equations for exercise are needed to calculate the total work accomplished as well as the total power achieved. Work is defined by force multiplied by distance or, in other words, the force needed to move a mass a given distance. The unit for work is the Newton-meter or joule (J). Force is mass × acceleration. Power is the work performed per unit of time. The other equations listed are not correct.

26. (C) For patients between the ages of 5 and 20, the estimated HR_{max} is ~195 to 215 bpm. For patients >20 years of age, the maximum HR will decrease with increasing age. A commonly accepted equation to determine a patient's maximum HR is: $HR_{max} = 210 - (0.65 \times age)$. The reason for this decline in HR_{max} is unclear but may be due to fibrosis and scarring of the sinoatrial node. Stroke volume increases early in exercise with little change thereafter. The HR increases, then accounts for increasing cardiac output. With exercise the total systemic vascular resistance declines. Systolic blood pressure will increase with isotonic exercise while the diastolic blood pressure remains relatively unchanged. With isometric exercise, both systolic and diastolic blood pressures rise.

27. (B) Maximal $V\dot{}_{O_2}$ achieved is dependent on age, sex, ethnicity, hemoglobin level, and type of work completed. As age increases in childhood, the maximal $\dot{V}O_2$ achievable also increases. Between the sexes, the maximal $\dot{V}O_2$ achievable is relatively the same before puberty, but thereafter, males have a higher $\dot{V}O_2$max. Anemic patients have a lower achievable $\dot{V}O_2$max than patients with normal hemoglobin. Finally, achievable $\dot{V}O_2$max depends on the type of work completed; the more muscle groups involved, the higher the $\dot{V}O_2$max achievable. Therefore, a higher $\dot{V}O_2$max is achieved with treadmill ergometry > cycle ergometry > arm crank ergometry > hand grip ergometry. Therefore, the older, nonanemic male would achieve the highest $\dot{V}O_2$max during cycle exercise testing.

28. (D) In a well-trained athlete resting HR will decrease while the stroke volume at rest and at maximum HR will increase. On echocardiography, an increased left ventricular end-diastolic dimension/volume will be noted. A decreased left ventricular end-systolic dimension/volume will occur.

29. (B) Of the answers listed, the only contraindication to exercise testing would be severe aortic stenosis. Known exercise-induced arrhythmias can be relative contraindications; however, exercise testing is a useful provocative test as in catecholaminergic polymorphic ventricular tachycardia and long QT syndrome. Therefore, exercise testing can be carried out in these patients. First- and second-degree AV block would not be absolute contraindications to exercise testing. Finally, anomalous origin of a coronary artery would not be an absolute contraindication to exercise testing to help determine the necessity for operative repair.

30. (C) Neither treadmill nor cycle ergometry is superior to the other. However, there are advantages and disadvantages to each type. Treadmill ergometry will allow a patient to derive a higher $\dot{V}O_2$max due to the use of more muscle groups during exercise. Also, most people, even very young children, can walk efficiently but not all can cycle efficiently. However, the treadmill

ergometers are potentially more dangerous due to the potential of the patient falling and there is more noise and artifact while running when compared to stationary cycling. A more accurate and controlled measurement of work can be obtained with cycle ergometry. This is because work/power changes are more easily accomplished and recorded with a mechanically or electronically braked cycle ergometer when compared to a treadmill ergometer. However, this will also depend on the exercise protocol used.

31. (E) Exercise testing in aortic stenosis patients can be helpful in the assessment of mild to moderate stenosis for significant ST segment changes with exercise as well as distinguishing between chest wall pain and more significant causes of chest pain. However, severe aortic stenosis is a contraindication to exercise testing. In aortic stenosis, there is an inverse relationship between the total work performed and transaortic pressure gradient. Also, patients with more severe aortic stenosis (i.e., higher transaortic gradient) have a lower increase in their blood pressure response during exercise than less severe aortic stenosis patients. The higher the transaortic gradient, the more likely the expected ST segment changes to occur. Finally, it has been shown that patients with more severe aortic stenosis achieved a lower $\dot{V}O_2$max.

32. (D) Unrepaired single ventricle patients will have reduced maximum aerobic power and excessive ventilation relative to $\dot{V}O_2$. Specifically, unrepaired patients with pulmonary atresia with VSD have decreased total work, maximal power achieved, exercise time, and maximal oxygen uptake when compared to first-stage repaired or complete repair patients as well as normal patients. Blood oxygen saturation levels in unrepaired and first-stage repaired patients are lower at rest than normal patients and decrease significantly with exercise. After complete repair, patients will have a relatively normal resting blood oxygen saturation level and may have a small decrease with exercise. This is similar to normal, healthy patients who may have little to no decrease with exercise.

33. (B) A complete 12-lead ECG should be obtained once at rest, at each workload, and several times after completion. A typical recording includes at rest sitting, supine, and standing; then at each workload and peak exercise, as well as each minute (1 to 5) of recovery. At least three standard surface ECG leads should be continuously displayed and recorded during the exercise study as well as for 5 to 10 minutes after the study is completed. The operator should have the option of switching between various combinations of those leads (i.e., inferior leads, anterior right, anterior left). Appropriate ECG electrode and lead placement should be used in all types of ergometry to limit artifact. This includes skin cleansing and abrading, electrode paste use, and ECG lead cable securing with an elastic band/knit shirt. Owing to the typical artifact with treadmill exercise testing, the Korotkoff sounds, especially diastolic, can be very difficult to measure accurately. Direct blood pressure measurement, through arterial access, in the peripheral arteries will overestimate the central aortic pressure due to peripheral amplification.

34. (B) Because of the right-to-left shunt and resultant increase in dead space, cyanotic patients overventilate in order to remove additional CO_2. Hence ventilation is disproportionately high relative to $\dot{V}O_2$.

35. (E) The CO_2 rebreathing technique is one of the two most frequently used techniques (other being acetylene–helium rebreathing technique) for measuring cardiac output noninvasively. The CO_2 rebreathing technique is based on the Fick principle for CO_2 {Cardiac output = $\dot{V}_{CO_2}$/[C_vCO_2(mixed venous CO_2) − $CaCO_2$(systemic arterial CO_2)]}. However, arterial CO_2 content needs to be directly measured from systemic arterial blood pCO_2 or, noninvasively, by estimating this by using the Bohr equation.

This is accomplished by solving for $PaCO_2$ (systemic arterial pCO_2): VD/VT = ($PaCO_2$ − $PeCO_2$)/$PaCO_2$. This technique is not well tolerated by all, especially children, because rebreathing CO_2 can cause dyspnea, an unpleasant taste, and a transient headache. This technique involves a few areas of potential error. These include the need to adjust CO_2 concentration used for the patient's size and exercise intensity as well as taking into account the dead space (mouthpiece, etc.).

CHAPTER 8

Outpatient Cardiology

Angela Kelle, Brandon Morrical,
and Adam Putschoegl

QUESTIONS

1. Which of the following is a supplemental lab finding used in the diagnosis of Kawasaki disease?

   A. Hyperalbuminemia
   B. Thrombocytopenia
   C. Thrombocytosis in the first 3 days
   D. Leukopenia
   E. Sterile pyuria

2. You are seeing a 3-year-old patient who is 6 weeks status post diagnosis of Kawasaki disease. At her last echo, 2 weeks after diagnosis, she was found to have a 4 mm aneurysm in the left anterior descending (LAD) coronary artery. The other branches were normal. Her repeat echo today shows complete resolution of the LAD aneurysm. Which of the following should be included as part of her follow-up?

   A. Patient needs to continue high-dose aspirin therapy until 1-year follow-up appointment
   B. Patient can be switched to low-dose aspirin therapy now that there is resolution of the aneurysm
   C. Patient should have no restrictions on her physical activity at this time
   D. Annual follow-up with echo, ECG, and stress test is needed
   E. An echo needs to be repeated at 6 months to look for aneurysm recurrence

3. A 6-year-old boy is referred to pediatric cardiology secondary to an LDL concentration of 170 mg/dL. Pertinent family history includes a grandfather with coronary vascular disease and first myocardial infarction at age 50. The patient has a BMI that puts him in the 90th percentile. Which of the following is the best management step?

   A. Weight management including nutritional counseling and increased physical activity should be started while

initiating a bile acid-binding resin, such as cholestyramine

   B. Single pharmacotherapy with a statin should be initiated
   C. Niacin should be initiated in addition to weight management
   D. Repeat cholesterol screening should be performed at the age of 8
   E. Weight management should be the primary method of control

4. A 17-year-old girl is referred to pediatric cardiology clinic after ascending aortic dilatation was found on an echocardiogram performed secondary to chest pain complaints. The remainder of the echocardiogram was normal. On review of the echocardiogram, the sinus of Valsalva is dilated with a Z-score of +3.4. A physical examination reveals the patient has scoliosis, pectus carinatum, and a hindfoot deformity. Family history is positive for a maternal grandfather with ascending aortic dissection. Which of the following genes should be tested for maximum yield?

   A. Transforming growth factor, β receptor 1 (TGFBR1)
   B. Fibrillin 1 (FBN1)
   C. Collagen, type III, α 1 (COL3A1)
   D. ADAM metallopeptidase with thrombospondin type 1 motif, 10 (ADAMTS10)
   E. Actin, α 2, smooth muscle, aorta (ACTA2)

5. Which of the following medications is *least* likely to be prescribed to a 22-year-old patient with a known FBN1 mutation and sinus of Valsalva dilatation to 42 mm?

   A. Losartan
   B. Enalapril
   C. Digoxin
   D. Atenolol
   E. Amlodipine

6. A 13-year-old boy is referred to pediatric cardiology clinic secondary to hypertension. His blood pressure was recorded as 128/78 at his last health maintenance visit. On the basis of age and height, he is greater than the 95% for systolic and the 90% for diastolic blood pressure. In pediatric cardiology clinic, his blood pressure is 130/80, using auscultation and an appropriate cuff size. Which is the next best step in evaluation and treatment?

   A. Ambulatory blood pressure monitoring
   B. Recommend dietary modifications as a primary therapy
   C. Echocardiogram to evaluate end-organ damage
   D. Renal ultrasound
   E. Initiation of atenolol

7. You are consulting on an 8-year-old boy who is found to have blood pressures in the 92 to 94 percentile range on multiple readings over the past several visits at his pediatrician's office. Which category does this child fall into and what is the next best step?

   A. Stage 2 hypertension; initiate pharmacotherapy
   B. Stage 1 hypertension; echocardiogram
   C. Prehypertension; echocardiogram
   D. Prehypertension; lifestyle changes and repeat BP in 6 months
   E. Normal; yearly blood pressure monitoring

8. A 16-year-old girl is referred to pediatric cardiology clinic secondary to a murmur heard at a sports physical. On auscultation, there is a I–II/VI systolic ejection murmur best heard over the right upper sternal border and a blowing decrescendo diastolic murmur over the right chest radiating toward the apex. What other finding on physical examination might be expected?

   A. Narrowed pulse pressure
   B. Systolic ejection click at the apex
   C. Displaced right ventricular impulse
   D. Elevated diastolic blood pressure
   E. Decreased femoral pulses

9. A 12-year-old girl presents with a high-pitched, blowing, holosystolic murmur heard best over the apex of the chest. An echocardiogram confirms moderate mitral valve regurgitation with thickening of the mitral valve. Suspecting rheumatic heart disease (RHD), you send streptococcal antibody titers, which are elevated. Which of the following additional findings would most strongly support the diagnosis of acute RHD?

   A. Arthralgia
   B. Fever
   C. Elevated ESR or CRP
   D. Prolonged PR interval
   E. Erythema marginatum

10. What is the most appropriate antimicrobial regimen to treat a 5-year-old patient with rheumatic fever if the patient has a penicillin allergy (rash)?

    A. Amoxicillin for 10 days
    B. Cephalexin for 10 days
    C. Azithromycin for 10 days
    D. Vancomycin for 5 days
    E. Clindamycin for 5 days

11. In a patient with a reported syncopal episode, which of the following features would prompt hospitalization or intense outpatient workup?

    A. Syncope with exertion
    B. Syncope after rising from lying to standing position
    C. Family history of bicuspid aortic valve
    D. Previous near-syncopal episode
    E. Loss of bladder control during syncopal episode

12. A 14-year-old girl is referred to your office following two episodes of loss of consciousness, both occurring during soccer practice. Each episode lasted 1 minute, and the patient returned quickly to baseline. She denies any nausea, vomiting, sweating, or blurred vision prior to the episodes but reports that her heart was beating "funny" prior to the episodes. Family history is negative for sudden cardiac death. Physical examination is unremarkable. Which of the following is the next best step in evaluation?

    A. Exercise stress test
    B. Electrocardiogram
    C. Echocardiogram
    D. Holter monitor
    E. In-hospital monitoring

13. Which of the following is considered the gold standard for diagnosis of myocarditis?

    A. Viral cultures and titers
    B. Electrocardiogram
    C. Endomyocardial biopsy
    D. Magnetic resonance imaging (MRI)
    E. Echocardiography

14. Which of the following accounts for the cardiac findings of cardiomegaly, left ventricular hypertrophy (LVH), and a flow murmur observed in patients with sickle cell anemia?

    A. Chronic anemia
    B. Thrombotic crisis
    C. Arrhythmia
    D. Iron overload
    E. Hypertension

15. A 6-year-old boy has been referred by his primary care physician for evaluation of a murmur. His examination reveals a normal precordial impulse with a normal S_1 and S_2 that splits appropriately. The child is >99th percentile for BMI. There is a 2/6 systolic murmur best heard at the LUSB that is accentuated with lying down. The murmur resolves when he sits upright. His blood pressure measures 135/75 in his right upper extremity taken with a child-sized blood pressure cuff. Regarding this patient, which of the following is most likely true?

   A. The blood pressure measurement is likely falsely elevated. His blood pressure should be repeated using a cuff with a bladder size that is at least 80% of the upper arm circumference

   B. The blood pressure measurement is likely falsely elevated. His blood pressure should be repeated using a cuff that is two-thirds the length of the upper arm

   C. The blood pressure measurement is likely falsely elevated. His blood pressure should be repeated with the same cuff and with repositioning his arm to a more inferior level from where the initial measurement was performed

   D. The blood pressure measurement is likely accurate, and the family should be counseled on appropriate nutritional strategies

   E. The blood pressure measurement is likely accurate, and this child should undergo echocardiography to rule out possible coarctation of the aorta

16. A 3-year-old girl is referred to the pediatric cardiology clinic for a murmur. The child is at the 3rd percentile for weight and 45th percentile for height. She has no cyanosis or apparent dyspnea. She has had no syncope. On examination, there is a 3/6 systolic murmur best heard in the left upper sternal border that has a crescendo–decrescendo quality. There is no diastolic murmur. She has a normal S_1 and a fixed split S_2. Pulses are normal. Which of the following is the most likely source of murmur?

   A. Increased flow across the tricuspid valve

   B. Increased flow across the pulmonary valve

   C. Left-to-right shunting at the atrial level

   D. Left-to-right shunting at the ventricular level

   E. Increased flow across the aortic valve

17. A 13-year-old boy was referred for evaluation of an ASD that was diagnosed as an infant. He has been lost to follow up. His last echocardiogram was 10 years ago. Notes reveal that at the time of diagnosis his examination was described as having a fixed split S_2 with a 3/6 crescendo–decrescendo murmur best heard at the LUSB and a soft middiastolic murmur heard at the LLSB. During your examination, he has a normal S_1, his S_2 splits with expiration, and it is prominent. He has a short systolic murmur heard along the LUSB. There is no diastolic murmur. His liver is palpable 1 cm below the costal margin. Which of the following is the best explanation for his physical examination findings?

   A. The absence of the diastolic murmur indicates a decrease in left-to-right shunting as a result of the decreasing size of the ASD

   B. The prominent S_2 indicates he has increased his left-to-right shunt

   C. The absence of a fixed split S_2 and increased S_2 prominence indicates a decrease in left-to-right shunting as a result of increased pulmonary artery pressures

   D. The systolic murmur is from tricuspid regurgitation as a result of RV enlargement

   E. The splitting of his S_2 indicates a decrease in his left-to-right shunting as a result of the decreasing size of the ASD

18. You are evaluating a 2-month-old infant who weighs 3.9 kg. He was full-term and birth weight was 3.6 kg. The infant has a large VSD that was demonstrated on echocardiography obtained soon after birth. Currently his respiratory rate is 60 breaths per minute. The parents report that he is not cyanotic but he does take 40 minutes to complete a 2 oz. bottle of formula. What is the next most appropriate step for this infant?

   A. Dietician referral to increase caloric intake

   B. Cardiology follow-up in 2 months

   C. Begin treatment with furosemide 0.3 mg orally once daily

   D. Begin treatment with furosemide 4 mg orally twice daily

   E. Pulmonary consult to evaluate for noncardiac etiologies of tachypnea

19. A 9-year-old girl is referred to the pediatric cardiology clinic for evaluation of a murmur. She is an otherwise healthy child. There is no parasternal lift. She has a 2/6 early systolic murmur best heard between the apex and left lower sternal border. It is of low pitch and has a musical quality. It is best heard with the bell of the stethoscope. It decreases with Valsalva. Her pulses are normal. What is the most appropriate next step in evaluating this murmur?

   A. Obtain an electrocardiogram

   B. Obtain an echocardiogram

   C. Reassurance only

   D. Obtain a chest x-ray

   E. Obtain a chest x-ray and electrocardiogram

20. A 3-week-old full-term infant is referred for evaluation of a murmur. The pregnancy was complicated by gestational diabetes. There is a 2/6 midsystolic murmur best heard in the axilla and back. The first and second heart sounds are normal. The child has oxygen saturations of 97% in the upper and lower extremities and is at the 30th percentile for weight. What is the most likely cause of the murmur in this child?

   A. Increased blood flow velocity across the pulmonary valve due to subvalvar obstruction
   B. Normal transitioning of the pulmonary vasculature as pulmonary pressures fall
   C. Right to left blood flow across the ventricular septum
   D. Right-to-left shunting across a PDA
   E. Flow through a pulmonary AV fistula

21. In which patient is administration of bacterial endocarditis prophylaxis most appropriate based on the 2007 American Heart Association guidelines?

   A. A 12-year-old patient status post orthotopic heart transplant 3 years ago, now with moderate tricuspid valve regurgitation undergoing teeth cleaning
   B. An 8-year-old patient status post VSD patch closure 5 months ago undergoing a bronchoscopy without biopsy for evaluation of chronic cough
   C. A 15-year-old patient with Ebstein anomaly status post tricuspid valve repair 1 year ago, with residual mild TR undergoing extraction of two wisdom teeth
   D. A 22-year-old patient status post extracardiac Fontan undergoing diagnostic colonoscopy due to intermittent blood in the stool
   E. A 20-year-old female with history of congenital aortic stenosis, status post Ross procedure with an RV-to-PA conduit 10 years ago, undergoing cesarean section for failure to progress

22. An 8-year-old patient with a history of tetralogy of Fallot and placement of a bioprosthetic pulmonary valve will have a tonsillectomy next week. He is penicillin allergic. In this patient, what is the best strategy for IE prophylaxis?

   A. Ceftriaxone IM
   B. Azithromycin PO
   C. Cefepime IV
   D. Vancomycin IV
   E. IE prophylaxis is not indicated in this patient

23. Which of the following is most correct regarding risk of cardiotoxicity related to chemotherapy in children?

   A. Acute cardiotoxicity occurs in 15% of children receiving anthracycline-based chemotherapy regimens
   B. The greatest risk factor for development of cardiotoxicity is total accumulated anthracycline dose
   C. 10% of patients will experience clinical heart failure symptoms within 15 years post receiving anthracycline-based chemotherapy

   D. Children are at an overall lower risk of developing cardiotoxicity related to anthracycline chemotherapy when compared to adults receiving a comparable dose
   E. Early onset cardiomyopathy related to chemotherapy toxicity is usually a transient phenomenon with recovery of cardiac function in the majority of cases

24. A 13-year-old boy with severe pulmonary arterial hypertension (PAH) is seen for follow-up care. He takes sildenafil and bosentan. Which of the following is most correct regarding the natural history of patients with PAH?

   A. 5-Year survival for an untreated child with idiopathic PAH is 50%
   B. Introduction of targeted PAH therapies have improved symptomatology, but have not significantly altered the long-term survival
   C. Children with PAH are more likely to initially present with syncope or near-syncopal episodes than with right heart failure
   D. The least common presentation of PAH in children is dyspnea and fatigue
   E. Patients with acquired PAH (Eisenmenger syndrome) typically have a greater mortality when compared to patients with idiopathic PAH

25. An 11-year-old boy with type 1 diabetes has a persistent serum low-density lipoprotein (LDL) cholesterol concentration of 180 mg/dL. His LDL was 175 mg/dL last year, and at that time better diet and exercise were recommended. On the basis of the current guidelines for management of hyperlipidemia in childhood, which of the following would be the most appropriate next step?

   A. Obtain an echocardiogram
   B. Measure the carotid artery intimal thickness
   C. Enroll the patient in a disciplined exercise training program
   D. Begin statin therapy
   E. Tighten diabetic control

26. A 13-year-old girl who recently immigrated to the United States with her parents is evaluated in a pediatric cardiology clinic. She has a reported history of a VSD. Her examination reveals a parasternal lift over the xiphoid area. She has a 3/6 harsh holosystolic murmur coincident with S_1 best heard at the RLSB. There is a single, loud, palpable S_2 and no diastolic murmur. Her systemic oxygen saturation is 85%. Regarding this patient's examination, which of the following is correct?

   A. The murmur is likely from left-to-right shunting through a large perimembranous VSD
   B. The murmur is likely from right-to-left shunting through a large perimembranous VSD
   C. The murmur is likely from tricuspid regurgitation

D. The lift is from LVH that has developed from the left-to-right shunt

E. The systolic murmur is likely from flow across the pulmonary valve

27. Two sisters present for a second opinion regarding sports participation. They are both competitive swimmers. During routine sports physicals, one sister was found to have a QTc of 490 msec. The other sister's QTc is normal. Neither girl has ever had a cardiac arrest event or syncopal episode. Both girls were subsequently tested and found to be positive for type 1 LQTS mutation. Which of the following is your recommendation regarding sports participation?

A. Neither girl should participate in competitive swimming

B. Both girls may take part in any sport without restrictions, including swimming

C. The sister with a prolonged QTc should be restricted to class IA (low static and dynamic component) sports; her sister (with a normal QTc) may take part in any sport without restrictions

D. The sister with a prolonged QTc should not take part in any competitive sport; her sister (with a normal QTc) may take part in only class IA (low static and dynamic component) sports

E. Both girls should have an ICD placed. Only after ICD placement may they continue competitive swimming

28. Double-chamber RV (DCRV) is associated with a VSD in which of the following?

A. 60% to 90% of patients

B. 40% to 50% of patients

C. 20% to 30% of patients

D. 5% to 10% of patients

E. Less than 5% of patients

29. A 16-year-old young lady presents after two episodes of vasovagal syncope. These symptoms never occur during exercise. The symptoms usually occur in the midmorning, especially after not eating breakfast. There is no family history of sudden death. She has had no prior evaluation for syncope. What is the next appropriate test to order?

A. Echocardiogram

B. 24-Hour Holter monitor

C. 30-Day event monitor

D. ECG

E. Tilt-table test

30. What is the most common cause of chest pain in children?

A. Musculoskeletal chest wall pain

B. Asthma

C. Pneumonitis

D. Coronary insufficiency

E. Gastroesophageal reflux/esophagitis

31. Which of the following is true regarding pulsus paradoxus?

A. Pulsus paradoxus is defined as an exaggeration of the normal BP variation during the expiratory phase of respiration, in which the pulse pressure declines as one exhales and increases as one inhales

B. Pulsus paradoxus is defined as an exaggeration of the normal BP variation during the inspiratory phase of respiration, in which the systolic pressure declines as one inhales and increases as one exhales

C. Pulsus paradoxus is one of the hallmarks of hypovolemia

D. Pulsus paradoxus is indicative of several conditions including aortic stenosis, mitral stenosis, and coarctation of the aorta

E. Pulsus paradoxus results from an accentuated increase of the blood pressure, which leads to the widened pulse pressure

32. A 16-year-old boy has a high-pitched early diastolic murmur heard best with the diaphragm of your stethoscope at the left midsternal border with radiation toward the apex. When the patient leans forward and exhales, the murmur is accentuated. Which of the following is the most likely defect causing this murmur?

A. Pulmonary valve regurgitation

B. Aortic valve regurgitation

C. Mitral valve regurgitation

D. Tricuspid valve stenosis

E. Mitral valve stenosis

33. You are evaluating a teenage athlete who has complained of chest pain with exercise. On further questioning, she recalls that she had a syncopal episode during a basketball game earlier this year. Which of the following is the most common cause of sudden cardiac death in young athletes?

A. Prolonged QT syndrome

B. Arrhythmogenic RV dysplasia

C. Anomalous origin of the right coronary artery from the left sinus of Valsalva

D. Anomalous origin of the left main coronary artery from the right sinus of Valsalva

E. Hypertrophic cardiomyopathy

34. In a patient with anomalous left coronary artery arising from the pulmonary artery (ALCAPA), what associated defect may protect the patient from LV dysfunction?

A. Pulmonary valve stenosis

B. Large PDA with large left-to-right shunt

C. Tricuspid regurgitation

D. Mitral regurgitation

E. LVH

35. You are evaluating a 7-year-old boy with restrictive cardiomyopathy (RCM). Which is the most likely etiology of his RCM?

   A. Glycogen-storage disease
   B. Thiamin deficiency
   C. Amyloidosis
   D. Muscular dystrophy
   E. Collagen vascular disease

36. Which patient with rheumatic carditis is most likely to develop persistent rheumatic heart disease (RHD)?

   A. A 13-year-old girl with acute aortic and mitral regurgitation
   B. A 3-year-old girl with acute aortic and mitral regurgitation
   C. A 3-year-old girl with acute isolated mitral regurgitation
   D. A 13-year-old boy with acute aortic and mitral regurgitation
   E. A 3-year-old boy with acute aortic and mitral regurgitation

37. What is the most common clinical finding in a 7-year-old patient with an anomalous right coronary artery from the left sinus?

   A. Palpitations
   B. Chest pain with exertion
   C. No symptoms
   D. Congestive heart failure
   E. Syncope

38. A 10-year-old boy with a bicuspid aortic valve is scheduled for repair of a dental cavity. On the basis of the 2007 ACC/AHA endocarditis guideline statement, administration of which of the following antibiotics for this boy would be in closest accordance with current recommendations for endocarditis prophylaxis?

   A. None
   B. Procaine penicillin, 1 million units intramuscularly (IM), immediately prior to the procedure
   C. Amoxicillin, 50 mg/kg orally, 1 hour prior to the procedure
   D. Amoxicillin, 50 mg/kg orally, immediately after the procedure
   E. Clindamycin, 20 mg/kg IM, immediately prior to the procedure

39. On the basis of the 2007 ACC/AHA endocarditis guidelines, which of the following conditions (all 5 years after intervention or infection) would warrant antibiotic prophylaxis against infectious endocarditis (IE) before a dental procedure?

   A. Small residual ventricular septal defect after primary surgical closure
   B. Heart transplantation

   C. Bicuspid aortic valve with mild aortic regurgitation and a history of IE
   D. Device closure of a secundum atrial septal defect
   E. Extended end-to-end coarctation repair with a 10 mm Hg residual gradient

40. A 13-year-old boy presents with a newly discovered large ASD with left-to-right shunt. He asks about clearance for sports participation. In which of the following sports can he participate competitively?

   A. He cannot participate in sports
   B. Baseball
   C. Football
   D. Golf
   E. Table tennis

41. A local family medicine doctor asks you about a recent ECG performed on one of his teenage male patients, a state championship high-school football player. Which of the following ECG findings would be most concerning in this patient?

   A. First-degree AV block
   B. T-wave inversion in limb leads
   C. Incomplete RBBB
   D. Early repolarization
   E. QRS voltage criteria for LVH

42. A 13-year-old patient with multiple chronic symptoms, newly diagnosed with SLE, is referred to your clinic. A screening echocardiogram was performed prior to the visit. What is the most likely abnormal finding on this patient's echocardiogram?

   A. Myocarditis
   B. Pericardial effusion
   C. Tricuspid regurgitation
   D. Valvular vegetation
   E. Coronary arteritis

43. A 15-year-old boy is being seen in your clinic for a sports preparticipation evaluation for football. He has had one episode of syncope, which happened after standing up quickly after a nap. He has a history of mild asthma, and he has occasional shortness of breath after intense training which resolves with albuterol. His paternal grandfather died of a heart attack at the age of 61, and his older brother drowned while swimming competitively last year. On cardiac examination, he has a 2/6 systolic vibratory murmur that is more prominent when supine. Which of the following features of his exam and history are most concerning and likely requires further workup?

   A. Episode of syncope
   B. Shortness of breath with exercise
   C. Grandfather's heart attack
   D. Brother's death
   E. Heart murmur

44. You are seeing a 4-week-old female infant for a murmur, and based on your examination you refer the patient for echocardiography, which identifies a 5mm secundum ASD. The mother wants to know if this means her baby will need surgery. What are you most likely to tell her?

   A. The ASD probably gets larger as she grows
   B. The ASD is likely to close on its own
   C. The ASD should be closed via device in the cath lab soon to prevent symptoms
   D. The ASD stays the same size
   E. She will probably need surgical closure by 1 year of age

45. A 20-year-old man you have followed for several years is about to move and transition to an adult practice. His history is remarkable for coarctation of the aorta, discovered when he was 13 years of age and repaired soon after. He has done well on follow-up aside from occasional difficulty with blood pressure control. He is otherwise healthy. He asks if he is at risk for any other complications. Which of the following is he at higher risk for developing?

   A. Renal injury
   B. Intracranial aneurysms
   C. DVTs
   D. Liver damage
   E. Retinal hemorrhages

46. A 9-year-old boy with a history of HLHS, currently with Fontan physiology and doing well from a symptomatic standpoint, has been struggling in school. His parents are concerned about his difficulties and feel like he is falling more behind his peers. Which of the following is true regarding neurodevelopmental outcomes in children with congenital heart defects?

   A. Children with cyanotic lesions and acyanotic lesions have the same degree of learning difficulties
   B. If a child has complete repair of a cyanotic lesion, developmental outcomes will normalize
   C. Longer duration of cyanosis is associated with greater decline in cognitive ability
   D. Visual–spatial skills are often intact, even if there are other learning difficulties
   E. Children with d-TGA have the highest risk of adverse developmental outcomes

47. You are seeing a 7-year-old male patient with 6 days of fever >101 degrees F, an injected pharynx, edema of both his hands and feet, polymorphous rash, a CRP of 88 (normal <10) and a cervical lymph node measuring 2 cm. Echocardiogram is unremarkable. When will the patient be able to completely stop his aspirin therapy, assuming he responds well to initial treatment?

   A. When his CRP level reaches 44
   B. 7 days after completion of his IVIG
   C. When his echo 10 days after diagnosis is negative for coronary artery aneurysm
   D. When his CRP is less than 3
   E. When his echo 6 weeks after diagnosis is negative for coronary artery aneurysm

48. You are seeing a 3-year-old patient who has evidence of left axis deviation on a screening EKG. Which of the following should remain at the top of your differential diagnosis?

   A. Bicuspid aortic valve
   B. Secundum ASD
   C. Wolff–Parkinson–White syndrome
   D. Hypertrophic cardiomyopathy
   E. Muscular VSD

49. You are seeing a 12-month-old, previously formula-fed baby who is being treated with a sodium channel blocker for AVNRT diagnosed shortly after birth. Mom states that the baby is doing well and she has no concerns. You order an EKG. What findings on EKG would be of concern to you?

   A. Inverted T waves in leads V1–V3
   B. Prolonged PR interval
   C. RSR′ pattern in V1
   D. Heart rate of 140 bpm
   E. Dominant R waves in V1–V3

50. You are called by a local pediatrician regarding a 2-week-old male infant with a history of poor prenatal care, now presenting with somnolence, poor feeding, and failure to gain weight. The infant is tachycardic with a prominent RV impulse, liver edge 2 cm below the costal margin, and a bruit at the anterior fontanelle. Cranial ultrasound is suspicious for vein of Galen malformation. Which of the following is true regarding these defects?

   A. Intracardiac defects are not commonly associated with this lesion
   B. Fetuses are typically unaffected and presentation is typically as pulmonary vascular resistance drops
   C. Intracranial hemorrhage is common
   D. Retrograde diastolic flow can be seen in the descending thoracic aorta on echocardiography
   E. Surgical ligation of anomalous vessels is the preferred therapy

51. You are seeing an 8-year-old girl in your clinic. When reviewing family history, the patient's mother tells you that the patient's uncle had a myocardial infarction last year at the age of 56 and that the patient's grandmother also had a heart attack many years ago at the age of 67. The patient's mother recently had a cholesterol panel checked and remembers her total cholesterol level being elevated at 230 mg/dL. There is no other pertinent family history. On examination, the patient appears well with a BMI at the 62nd percentile. The remainder of her exam is unremarkable. Based on the above data, what do you recommend regarding cholesterol screening for your patient?

A. No need to check a cholesterol level until the patient is 25 years old
B. No need to check a cholesterol level until the patient is 17 years old
C. Check a fasting lipid profile now
D. Check a nonfasting lipid profile at the age of 9 and calculate a non-HDL cholesterol
E. Check a fasting lipid profile now and again in 4 weeks

52. You are asked to see a patient in your clinic who was initially adopted from China at the age of 6 months and is seeing you today just after his 12th birthday. His previous records show that a murmur has been heard intermittently by his pediatrician but recently it seemed more prominent so the pediatrician ordered an echo. This showed a ventricular septal defect in the outlet septum. LV is of normal size and function with mild aortic valve regurgitation. The right ventricle appears normal with a right ventricular systolic pressure of 28 mm Hg. As you consider further follow-up for this patient, at what point would you consider surgical referral for repair of his underlying heart defect?

A. Refer now, given the location of the defect
B. Refer if cardiac catheterization shows a $Q_p:Q_s$ of 1.75:1
C. Refer if follow-up echocardiogram shows moderate aortic valve regurgitation
D. Refer if patient develops pneumonia within the next year
E. No referral due to high likelihood of spontaneous closure.

53. You are counseling a family regarding their infant's new diagnosis of a complete atrioventricular septal defect. The child is scheduled to undergo complete repair, and the family asks if additional surgeries will be needed in the future. What is the most common indication for reoperation?

A. Right AV valve regurgitation
B. Left AV valve regurgitation
C. Left AV valve stenosis
D. Residual ventricular septal defect
E. Left ventricular outflow tract obstruction

54. A 2-month-old male neonate with HLHS status post Norwood procedure presents to clinic for a follow-up visit. The patient's father asks about expected neurodevelopment. You discuss that:

A. Overall IQ is typically below the normal range
B. Frequency of ADHD is similar to age-matched controls
C. Less than 15% of patients receive special education services
D. More than 15% of patients demonstrate behavior problems
E. No specific developmental follow-up will be necessary

55. A patient comes to your clinic for a second opinion following a diagnosis of Brugada syndrome. Which of the following is true?

A. Estrogen is thought to be contributory, and arrhythmic events are more common in females
B. Inheritance is typically autosomal recessive
C. ICD implantation is indicated in asymptomatic patients with a drug-induced type I ECG if there is a family history of sudden cardiac death
D. Symptoms commonly occur during exercise
E. SCN5A mutations are found in <30% of clinically diagnosed Brugada syndrome patients

56. An 18-year-old woman is referred to your clinic due to a family history of Marfan syndrome (MFS) in her brother. An echocardiogram performed just prior to the visit shows aortic root dilation with a Z-score of 3.0. She is otherwise healthy. Which of the following is true regarding this patient?

A. She has "potential MFS" based on the Revised Ghent Criteria
B. She should undergo yearly echocardiograms
C. β-Blocker therapy should be initiated at this time
D. Baseline CT or MRI imaging is recommended at this time
E. She should not be restricted from weight lifting

57. You follow a patient in clinic with Marfan syndrome and mitral valve prolapse. A systolic murmur and a midsystolic click are heard on examination. Which of the following is true regarding these findings?

A. Squatting maneuvers will result in the click moving closer to S_1
B. Decreased left ventricular contractility will result in the click moving closer to S_1
C. Standing will result in the click moving closer to S_1
D. Increased afterload will result in the click moving closer to S_1
E. The click may be followed by a low-pitched late systolic murmur of MR

58. You are seeing a 4-year-old boy with history of tetralogy of Fallot and peripheral pulmonic stenoses. The patient has history of a Kasai procedure and has butterfly vertebrae noted on x-ray. On examination, the child has a broad forehead, deep-set eyes, and a small, pointed chin. Which of the following genes are associated with this patient's spectrum of defects?

A. 22q11

B. JAG1

C. Nkx2.5

D. FBN1

E. Not associated with a known syndrome

59. You are explaining the diagnosis of hypertrophic cardiomyopathy (HCM) to an adolescent and his family. Which of the following is true regarding HCM?

A. Incidence is 1:1,000

B. Dissimilar patterns of LVH occur with the same genetic substrate, including in identical twins

C. LVH is usually present at birth

D. ECG abnormalities manifest late in the disease

E. Disorganized myocytes are present in nonhypertrophied areas of the LV

60. You perform an echocardiogram on an elite collegiate athlete, who is seeking a second opinion following being restricted from sports due to diagnosis of possible HCM. Which of the following findings supports an alternative diagnosis of the athlete's heart?

A. Transmitral Doppler waveform consistent with abnormal LV filling

B. LV end-diastolic dimension >55 mm

C. Documentation of HCM in a relative

D. Documentation of positive genetic testing for HCM

E. Female gender

ANSWERS

1. (E) The supplemental laboratory criteria used in the diagnosis of suspected incomplete Kawasaki disease include albumin ≤3.0 g/dL, anemia for age, elevation of alanine aminotransferase, platelets after 7 days ≥450,000/mm³, white blood cell count ≥15,000/mm³, and urine ≥10 white blood cells/high-power field.

2. (C) A patient with an isolated small to medium (>3 mm but <6 mm) coronary artery aneurysm in *a major* coronary artery is classified as risk level III. Recommended follow-up includes the following:

- Aspirin therapy should be continued until the aneurysms regress.
- Patients <11 years of age should have no physical activity restrictions.
- Patients 11 to 20 years of age should have stress tests every other year with myocardial perfusion performed to guide physical activity recommendations.
- Patients should be seen annually by a pediatric cardiologist with an echocardiogram and electrocardiogram.
- If a stress test shows myocardial ischemia, then coronary angiography should be performed.

3. (E) Cholesterol screening should be performed on all children with a positive family history of dyslipidemia or premature coronary vascular disease. Screening should also be performed on all children with unknown family history or the following risk factors: overweight or obese, hypertension, cigarette smoking, or diabetes mellitus. This child was appropriately screened given his positive family history of premature coronary vascular disease. Pharmacotherapy should not be started until the child is 8 years of age. At this age, weight management should be the focus to lower the LDL level.

4. (B) More information is needed for a conclusive diagnosis, but the patient has history and physical examination findings consistent with Marfan syndrome, in addition to a family history of aortic aneurysm.

FBN1 has been identified as the causal gene in Marfan syndrome. It is also associated with Shprintzen–Goldberg syndrome, Weill–Marchesani syndrome, and ectopia lentis syndrome. *TGFBR1* is associated with Loeys–Dietz syndrome and familial thoracic aortic aneurysm syndrome. *COL3A1* is associated with Ehlers–Danlos syndrome. *ADAMTS10* is associated with Weill–Marchesani syndrome. *ACTA2* is associated with familial thoracic aortic aneurysm syndrome.

5. (C) β-Blockers are generally given to most patients with Marfan syndrome and aortic root dilation. Use of losartan has increased in recent years. ACE inhibitors, ARBs, and calcium channel blockers are also used in patients with β-blocker intolerance. Digoxin usually has no role in this disease process.

6. (A) To confirm a diagnosis of hypertension, three blood pressure measurements are needed. This patient has two blood pressures that place him >95%, and the concern is that he has stage 1 hypertension. A single third blood pressure measurement could be performed at a later date. Alternatively, ambulatory blood pressure monitoring could be used. This is especially useful if there is any concern of "white-coat" hypertension. In addition, a thorough history and physical examination should be performed to identify any possible causes. If the patient does have stage 1 hypertension, then he needs a diagnostic workup.

7. (D) Prehypertension is defined as average systolic or diastolic blood pressure levels that are ≥90th percentile but <95th percentile. A thorough history and physical examination should be performed, and further testing performed if indicated. It is reasonable to start with lifestyle changes, and blood pressure should be repeated in 6 months.

8. (B) The patient has auscultation findings consistent with aortic regurgitation. The systolic ejection murmur is secondary to increased stroke volume. The blowing diastolic murmur is the aortic regurgitation. Widened pulse pressure is often found in aortic regurgitation, especially if it is moderate or severe. Widened pulse pressure occurs because there is an increased stroke volume that causes distension of the peripheral arteries and elevation in systolic blood pressure. Diastolic blood pressure is reduced because the regurgitation into the left ventricle leads to a rapid fall in pressure. A systolic ejection click is typically associated with the presence of a bicuspid aortic valve, which would be expected in a patient with physical findings of aortic stenosis/regurgitation.

9. (E) Rheumatic fever is diagnosed based on the Jones criteria. The probability is high if there is group A streptococcal infection as well as two major criteria or one major and two minor criteria. The five major criteria are migratory arthritis, carditis and valvulitis, central nervous system involvement/Sydenham chorea, erythema marginatum, and subcutaneous nodules. The four minor criteria are arthralgia, fever, elevated ESR or CRP, and prolonged PR interval. The patient has one major criterion—valvulitis. To confirm the diagnosis, one more major criterion would need to be present. Otherwise, two minor criteria would be required to make the diagnosis.

10. (B) In a patient with penicillin allergy, amoxicillin should also be avoided. A narrow-spectrum cephalosporin, such as cephalexin, for 10 days would be appropriate. In patients with a severe hypersensitivity reaction to penicillin, other choices include azithromycin, but a 5-day course is recommended, and clindamycin for a 10-day course.

11. (A) According to the 2009 guidelines for the diagnosis and management of syncope, there are several high-risk criteria that require hospitalization or intense evaluation (Table 8.1).

12. (E) This patient is at high risk for major cardiovascular events based on her episodes happening with exercise and having palpitations prior to the syncope. Therefore, it is reasonable to admit her to the hospital and do inpatient monitoring while a thorough workup is performed.

13. (C) Endomyocardial biopsy is the gold standard for establishing the diagnosis of myocarditis, although it only yields diagnostic information in 10% to 20% of cases. Currently biopsy

TABLE 8.1 Risk Stratification

Short-term high-risk criteria that require prompt hospitalization or intensive evaluation:

Severe structural or coronary artery disease (heart failure, low LVEF, or previous myocardial infarction)

Clinical or ECG features suggesting arrhythmic syncope:
- Syncope during exertion or supine
- Palpitations at the time of syncope
- Family history of SCD
- Nonsustained VT
- Bifascicular block (LBBB or RBBB combined with left anterior or left posterior fascicular block) or other intraventricular conduction abnormalities with QRS duration ≥120 msec
- Inadequate sinus bradycardia (<50 bpm) or sinoatrial block in the absence of negative chronotropic medications or physical training
- Preexcited QRS complex
- Prolonged or short QT interval
- RBBB pattern with ST elevation in leads V1–V3 (Brugada pattern)
- Negative T waves in right precordial leads, epsilon waves, and ventricular late potentials suggestive of ARVC

Important comorbidities:
- Severe anemia
- Electrolyte disturbance

LVEF, left ventricular ejection fraction; SCD, sudden cardiac death; VT, ventricular tachycardia; LBBB, left bundle branch block; RBBB, right bundle branch block; bpm, beats per minute; ARVC, arrhythmogenic right ventricular cardiomyopathy.

is a class IIb recommendation in the current American College of Cardiology/American Heart Association guidelines for the treatment of heart failure.

14. (A) Patients with sickle cell anemia have chronic anemia and therefore have increased cardiac output. This causes the heart to become enlarged, as can be seen on chest x-ray. Increased cardiac output can cause a flow murmur heard over the left parasternal area. Thrombotic crisis will cause acute chest syndrome, but this is usually not cardiac in nature. A patient with sickle cell anemia may have prolonged PR interval and nonspecific ST changes seen on ECG, but it is rare for arrhythmias to develop. Iron overload causes the cardiac abnormalities seen with thalassemia major.

15. (A) The American Heart Association recommends using a blood pressure cuff with a bladder that is at least 80% of the arm circumference. Utilizing a blood pressure cuff with measurements less than this can lead to falsely elevated measurements. Given the recent increase in pediatric obesity rates, it is important to remember that a child-size blood pressure cuff may not be appropriate for all children. While he may have a coarctation, his blood pressure should be accurately measured before undertaking further evaluation. Whether or not this child's blood pressure is elevated, his obesity should be addressed. When taking an auscultatory blood pressure, patients should be positioned in a seated position with their back flat to a firm surface. The arm should be at the level of the heart. Positioning the arm below the heart may lead to venous congestion and falsely elevated

readings. There are a total of five Korotkoff sounds described. Phase 1 is considered to be the SBP and is the first appearance of faint clear tapping sounds that gradually increase and are heard for at least two consecutive beats. Phase 2 is the softening of sounds, which may have a swishing nature. During phase 3, the sounds become more sharp and crisp again compared to phase 2, but less intense than phase 1. There is no described clinical significance of phase 2 or phase 3. Phase 4 is the distinct abrupt muffling of sounds, which become soft and blowing. Phase 5 is the point at which all sounds disappear. There has been debate over the years as to whether phase 4 or 5 should be used for determining DBP. Currently the AHA recommends using phase 5.

16. (B) Patients with an isolated ASD typically will exhibit left-to-right shunting. Given that the difference in atrial pressures is relatively small, the velocity of shunting across the defect is not high enough to cause a murmur. The increased volume in the right atrium may cause a diastolic flow murmur across the tricuspid valve (if the Q_p:Q_s is >2:1). The systolic ejection murmur is caused by increased stroke volume across a normal pulmonary valve.

17. (C) The constellation of symptoms in this patient is consistent with a decrease in the left-to-right shunting. The prominent S_2 and paradoxical splitting indicate that the pulmonary pressures are high. As the child breathes in, RV outflow increases and the splitting resolves but with expiration the RV outflow decreases and the increased pulmonary pressures result in faster and louder closure of the pulmonary valve. If the decrease in left-to-right shunt was from the ASD becoming smaller then you would expect the splitting to be physiologic and the P2 to be of normal intensity. The diastolic murmur has resolved because the decreased left-to-right shunt has reduced the flow across the tricuspid valve.

18. (D) This infant has signs of pulmonary overcirculation: poor feeding, tachypnea, and poor weight gain. The appropriate dose of furosemide for this patient is 1 mg/kg/dose given twice daily. One can make the case that surgical repair should be entertained in the near future but that is not one of the options. In the "patient management" type of questions, always note patient age, vital signs, and lesion. Management questions will be fairly straightforward if one notes these details in the question stem.

19. (C) The murmur described in this vignette is consistent with that of a Stills murmur. It is a common innocent murmur of childhood and thought to be periodically found in 75% to 85% of school-aged children. It is classically described as being musical in nature and having the qualities listed in the question stem. The true cause of this murmur is unknown, but there are many theories including physiologic narrowing of the left ventricular outflow area, systolic/diastolic hypermobility of the mitral valve chordae, small aortic diameter, the presence of left ventricular false tendons, or increased aortic flow volume and velocity. Given its position, it is important to differentiate a Stills murmur from that of HCM or a VSD. The murmur of HCM would be expected to get louder with Valsalva or standing (maneuvers that decrease venous return). A VSD would not be affected by physiologic maneuvers and has a harsh quality.

20. (B) The murmur described in the vignette is most consistent with a neonatal transitional murmur of peripheral pulmonary stenosis. Infants born prematurely and of low birth weight are more likely to have this murmur. In about two-thirds of infants, this will disappear by 6 weeks of age. The location of this murmur with radiation to the axilla and back is the hallmark of peripheral pulmonary stenosis. Persistence beyond 6 to 9 months of age warrants further evaluation for branch pulmonary artery stenosis. A murmur of pulmonary valve stenosis would best be heard at the left upper sternal border. A right-to-left shunt at the ventricular level would result in systemic desaturation. A PDA has a continuous murmur as does an AV fistula.

21. (A) In 2007 the American Heart Association significantly revised the guidelines for infective endocarditis prophylaxis. Prior guidelines had included not only patients considered to be in the highest risk category but also those in the moderate risk category. The new guidelines are based on the evidence that in most patients prophylaxis provides little benefit and the risk of potential adverse outcome from the medication outweighs possible benefit for all except the most high-risk patients. The highest risk patients include:

1. Patients with prosthetic heart valves, including bioprosthetic and homograft valves.
2. Patients with prosthetic material used for cardiac valve repair.
3. Patients with a prior history of IE.
4. Patients with unrepaired cyanotic congenital heart disease, including palliative shunts and conduits.
5. Patients with completely repaired congenital heart defects with prosthetic material or device, whether placed by surgery or by catheter intervention, during the first 6 months after the procedure.
6. Patients with repaired congenital heart disease with residual defects at the site or adjacent to the site of the prosthetic device.
7. Patients with "valvulopathy" in a transplanted heart. Valvulopathy is defined as documentation of substantial leaflet pathology and regurgitation.

It is recommended that prophylaxis be given for procedures that will likely result in bacteremia. These include dental procures involving manipulation of gingival tissue or the periapical region of the teeth or perforation of the oral mucosa. In regard to respiratory procedures, there is little direct evidence that bacteremias caused during these procedures lead to IE. The AHA does not recommend routine prophylaxis for respiratory procedures unless they involve incision or biopsy of the respiratory tract mucosa. Procedures in which prophylaxis would be indicated include tonsillectomy, adenoidectomy, or bronchoscopy with biopsy. The new guidelines no longer recommend prophylaxis for any GI (including diagnostic colonoscopy or esophagogastroduodenoscopy) or GU procedures, even in those patients with the highest risk lesions unless there is an active or ongoing infection of the GI or GU tract. Routine prophylaxis for either vaginal or caesarian section is not indicated unless there is an active infection which may increase the risk of IE, such as chorioamnionitis. Additional high-risk procedures would be those involving infected skin or musculoskeletal structure.

22. (B) Gram-positive cocci, particularly viridans group streptococci, are responsible for the vast majority of IE. Antibiotics choice should be tailored and directed against these pathogens. The first-line therapy for high-risk patients undergoing high-risk procedures (see question 26 explanation) is amoxicillin. For patients with penicillin allergies who can take oral medications, cephalexin, clindamycin, azithromycin, and clarithromycin are appropriate. The medication is typically given as a single dose 30 to 60 minutes before beginning the procedure.

23. (B) There are three phases of anthracycline-related cardiotoxicity. The greatest risk factor for any of these phases is related to the total cumulative anthracycline dose. The *acute phase* occurs within 1 week of the infusion (with higher doses cardiac dysfunction may be more immediate). This is often a transient phenomenon and can have a wide spectrum of findings from minor ECG abnormalities and sinus tachycardia to severe ventricular dysfunction and fulminant heart failure. Acute toxicity occurs in 1% of pediatric patients. *Early onset chronic progressive cardiomyopathy* occurs within the first year of treatment. This is a nontransient depression in myocardial function that is due to damage or death of myocytes. It occurs in ~2% of patients. *Late onset toxicity* occurs at least 1 year after treatment. Within 6 years of treatment, 65% of children who received 228 to 550 mg/m^2 of anthracycline have some abnormality of cardiac structure or function. The risk of clinical heart failure 15 to 20 years following chemotherapy is 4% to 5%.

24. (C) Studies in children with idiopathic PAH (IPAH) and hereditary PAH (HPAH) have shown that the survival of those treated prior to the advent of targeted therapies (1950s to 1990s) was 66%, 52%, and 35% for 1, 3, and 5 years, respectively. Studies utilizing targeted therapies such as sildenafil, bosentan, and IV prostacyclin have shown considerable improvement in the mortality as well as the symptoms associated with PAH. The 1-, 3-, and 5-year mortality rates improved to 94%, 88%, and 81% from a number of studies. The most likely presenting symptoms in children with PAH are dyspnea and fatigue and they may present with syncope or near-syncope. Children are unlikely to present with right heart failure as an initial finding as they are often quite active and dyspnea on exertion is an early symptom. Children or adults who develop PAH as a result of unrepaired congenital heart disease such as a large VSD typically have a lower mortality than those with IPAH or HPAH as it takes more time for secondary PAH to develop.

25. (D) According to the 2008 AAP Committee on Nutrition guidelines, patients with diabetes mellitus are at particular risk of coronary complications from hyperlipidemia. The most appropriate next step would be to start a statin at this time since the LDL is markedly elevated. The ADA recommends starting a statin in children >10 years of age if the LDL is >160 after lifestyle changes. Goal LDL is <100 mg/dL.

26. (C) This patient's examination is most consistent with someone who has pulmonary vascular disease. After long-standing left-to-right shunting through a large VSD, the patient has now developed elevated pulmonary vascular resistance and elevated RV pressure. The shunt has reversed and is now right to left, hence the systemic desaturation. The right and left ventricular pressures are likely equal, and there is low velocity flow across the VSD that is inaudible. As a result of the increased pulmonary pressures, she has developed right ventricular hypertrophy (RVH) resulting in the parasternal lift. LVH would present as a lift or heave along the apex. As a result of the RVH and the increased pulmonary pressures, she has developed audible tricuspid regurgitation. As result of the RVH, the murmur is displaced more rightward than normal. If the murmur were from increased pulmonary flow, it would be expected along the upper left sternal border and would likely be ejection in quality.

27. (A) The sister with a long QT should be restricted to class IA activities. She is asymptomatic but has baseline QT prolongation (QTc >470 msec or more in males, >480 msec or more in females) so she should be restricted to class 1A sports. If she had genetically proven type 3 LQTS, the restriction limiting participation to class IA activities may be liberalized. But the sisters have LQT1.

The sister with genotype-positive/phenotype-negative LQTS (i.e., identification of an LQTS-associated mutation in an asymptomatic individual with a nondiagnostic QTc) may be allowed to participate in competitive sports. The risk of sudden cardiac death is not zero, but there are no compelling data available to justify restricting these individuals from competitive activities.

Because of the strong association between swimming and LQT1, both sisters should refrain from competitive swimming.

The presence of an ICD would restrict both sisters to class IA activities.

28. (A) DCRV is an acquired lesion that generally presents in older children and in adulthood. Narrowing of the RV outflow tract develops in patients with membranous VSDs due to hypertrophy of muscle in the right ventricular infundibulum. When anomalous bands of muscle divide the RV cavity into two chambers, DCRV can occur.

DCRV has been reported to be in association with VSD in 63% to 90% of patients.

29. (D) Neurocardiogenic (vasovagal) syncope is very common in the teenage population. The most cost-effective initial evaluation includes taking a detailed history to insure that there is no family history of sudden death. After the history and physical examination, the next appropriate test is an ECG if the patient has had no previous evaluation. The other tests listed may be considered if further evaluation is needed or the examination and history raise suspicion of specific pathology.

30. (A) Chest wall pain is the most common cause of chest pain in children. Types of chest wall pain include costochondritis, Tietze syndrome, nonspecific (idiopathic) chest wall pain, precordial catch syndrome, slipping rib syndrome, hypersensitive xiphoid syndrome, trauma and muscle strain, and sickle cell disease. Other, less common causes of chest pain include asthma, infection, pericarditis, gastrointestinal, and pneumothorax. Least common are cardiac causes of chest pain that include HCM, aortic stenosis, pericarditis, arrhythmias, coronary insufficiency, dissecting aortic aneurysm, and mitral valve prolapse. The most common causes of coronary insufficiency in children are Kawasaki disease, Williams syndrome, anomalous origin of the coronary arteries, and coronary arteriovenous and coronary cameral fistulae.

31. (B) Pulsus paradoxus is defined as an exaggeration of the normal variation during the inspiratory phase of respiration, in which the blood pressure declines as one inhales and increases as one exhales. It is one of the hallmarks of cardiac tamponade. It is also a sign that is indicative of several other conditions including pericarditis, chronic sleep apnea, croup, and obstructive lung disease such as asthma or COPD.

Normally, inspiration results in negative intrathoracic pressures which cause an increase in systemic venous return to the right heart; it increases the capacity of the pulmonary vascular bed to a greater degree. This ultimately leads to a decrease in left-sided output even though there is increased systemic venous return to the right. In cardiac tamponade, right ventricular filling causes restriction to

left ventricular filling. With inspiration, this decreased left ventricular filling, coupled with the increased capacity of the pulmonary vascular bed, results in a greater reduction in systemic output and therefore a greater decline in systolic pressure (>10 mm Hg). To measure pulsus paradoxus, one should listen for the difference between the first Korotkoff sound (intermittent and heard only during exhalation) and the second Korotkoff sound (a constant sound not dependent on respiratory cycle) as a reflection of the pulsus paradoxus; this is best accomplished by slow deflation of the BP cuff, but can also be observed by a difference in systolic BP recorded on an invasive arterial pressure monitoring line in relationship to respiration.

32. (B) Early diastolic murmurs begin immediately after S_2 and are decrescendo in nature. High-pitched early diastolic murmurs are due to aortic regurgitation with higher diastolic pressure in the aorta. They are heard best with the diaphragm at the left midsternal border. This murmur radiates to the apex and is decrescendo in nature due to a decrease in the intensity of the murmur as the diastolic pressure gradient equalizes. This is also why the murmur is accentuated when the patient leans forward and exhales.

Pulmonary valve regurgitation also produces an early diastolic murmur that is generally low pitched, but can be high pitched if pulmonary hypertension is present. It is also heard at the left midsternal border or at the left upper sternal border; however, radiation of this murmur is down the left sternal border. Patients with significant pulmonary regurgitation have murmurs with to-and-fro qualities due to increased forward volume load during ejection across the pulmonary valve.

Tricuspid and mitral valve stenosis cause middiastolic or late diastolic murmurs. These murmurs are produced during the early filling phase of diastole when blood crosses a narrow or thickened AV valve (middiastolic) or with atrial contraction (late diastolic). These murmurs are low pitched and are heard best with the bell of the stethoscope.

Mitral valve regurgitation results in a high-pitched holosystolic murmur at the apex with radiation to the back, left axilla, or clavicular area.

33. (E) All these entities have been implicated as a cause of sudden cardiac death in the young. Many studies have described hypertrophic cardiomyopathy as the most common cause of sudden cardiac death in young athletes.

34. (B) After birth, as pulmonary artery pressures fall below systemic pressures and the pulmonary artery contains desaturated blood, left ventricular perfusion is compromised. Collateral flow is initially low, as collaterals do not form in fetal life when the pressures in the aorta and pulmonary arteries are essentially equal. As the left ventricle's demand for oxygen is not met, the left ventricular myocardial vessels dilate to reduce resistance and increase flow. When coronary vascular reserve is exhausted, the result is myocardial ischemia. In response to ischemic stimuli, collateral vessels form and enlarge between the normal right and the abnormal left coronary arteries. However, with the left coronary artery connected to the low-pressure pulmonary artery, there is pulmonary–coronary steal as blood tends to flow into the pulmonary artery rather than into the high-resistance myocardial vessels. This results in a left-to-right shunt, which is not significant in terms of cardiac output but which can be critical in terms of coronary flow and creating a "steal" phenomenon and resultant myocardial ischemia.

Any lesion that increases pressure in the pulmonary artery will help to decrease the pulmonary–coronary steal. If there is pulmonary hypertension, as may result with a large VSD or PDA, there may be adequate pulmonary artery pressure to drive left ventricular perfusion and to prevent left ventricular ischemia. In these cases, closure of the VSD or PDA results in a decrease in pulmonary arterial pressure, an effect that may decrease perfusion of the anomalous left coronary artery.

35. (A) There are several metabolic disorders resulting from specific enzyme deficiencies that cause restrictive cardiomyopathy (RCM). These include Hurler syndrome, Gaucher disease, Fabry disease, and glycogen-storage diseases that can be lysosomal disorders or cytoplasmic enzyme deficiencies. Amyloidosis does result in RCM; however, this disease is seen almost exclusively in the adult population, with only one reported case to date in the pediatric literature. Thiamin deficiency, muscular dystrophy, and collagen vascular diseases all cause dilated cardiomyopathy (DCM), not RCM.

36. (B) The most important factor in determining prognosis and natural history of rheumatic carditis and RHD is the severity of the initial carditis and rheumatic fever recurrence. Severe initial carditis and/or patients with recurrent episodes of rheumatic fever are more likely to develop persistent RHD than those with mild carditis and no recurrence.

Of those patients with acute valvular involvement, the prognosis for resolution is more favorable for acute mitral regurgitation than it is for acute aortic regurgitation. This is in part because aortic regurgitation usually occurs in combination with mitral regurgitation. Isolated aortic regurgitation only occurs in ~5% of patients with acute rheumatic carditis. Aortic regurgitation with mitral regurgitation occurs in ~15% to 20%.

Age and gender also play a role in the natural history of rheumatic carditis and RHD. Acute rheumatic carditis resolves more frequently in boys. More severe cardiac involvement and RHD are seen in patients who present before the age of 5 years.

37. (C) Most people with this anomaly are completely asymptomatic. There is, however, a risk of sudden death with this anomaly, although the exact incidence is unknown. Basso et al. reported 27 deaths in young athletes whose autopsies showed anomalous origin of a coronary artery from the wrong sinus. Fifteen athletes had no prior cardiovascular symptoms. Of the remaining 12 patients, 10 had symptoms including 4 with syncope, 5 with chest pain, 2 with palpitations, and 1 with dizziness.

38. (A) See Answer 21.

39. (C) See guideline statement and Answer 21.

40. (D) According to the 2015 AHA/ACC guidelines regarding competitive athletic participation in patients with cardiovascular abnormalities, in children with a large, unrepaired ASD, only low-intensity 1A sports are recommended. See Figure 8.1 for sports intensity classification. After ASD repair (or 6 months after device closure), children can play in sports unrestricted.

41. (B) Several ECG changes can be commonly attributed to training, especially in higher level athletes. These include sinus bradycardia, first-degree AV block, incomplete RBB, early repolarization, and isolated QRS voltage criteria for LVH. These findings require no further investigation in an asymptomatic individual. Uncommon changes should warrant further investigation.

42. (B) Cardiovascular manifestations are common in SLE; 50% to 80% of patients report some cardiovascular complication in their lifetime. The most frequent clinically apparent cardiovascular complication is pericarditis with a frequency of ~25% and a pericardial effusion may be detected in as many as 50% of patients.

While necropsy studies have found evidence of myocarditis in as many as 40% of SLE cases, the rate of clinically evident

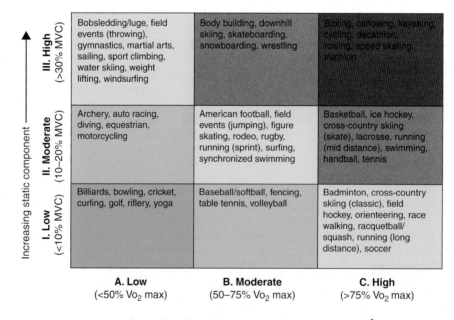

FIGURE 8.1 Classification is based on peak static and dynamic components acheived during exercise. Dynamic component is based on estimated percentage of maximal oxygen uptake (Vo₂ max), and static component is based on estimated percentage of maximal voluntary contraction (MVC). Sport classifications are consistent with 2015 AHA/ACC Eligibility and Disqualification Recommendations for Competitive Athletes with Cardiovascular Abnormalities.

myocarditis has been reported in <25% of patients. While less common, lupus myocarditis is an important cardiovascular complication because it has the potential to precipitate heart failure and arrhythmia and may contribute to the insidious development of cardiomyopathy. Libman–Sacks endocarditis is found in approximately 10% of SLE patients, usually on the mitral valve. It can also occur on the tricuspid or aortic valve. Angina is a complication of SLE, especially in the adult population, though not as common as pericarditis. Angina results from extramural and intramural coronary arteritis, accelerated atherosclerosis, embolism, thrombosis, spasm, or any combination thereof. These complications may be secondary to prolonged corticosteroid therapy and/or related to other lupus nonsteroid-related mechanisms such as lupus-induced lipid disturbances, lupus-related antiphospholipid antibodies, and lupus-related intimal damage.

43. (D) The brother's death during swimming last year is concerning for a possible fatal arrhythmia, and this may be an indication of an underlying inheritable abnormality such as long QT syndrome. This should be worked up further, with an ECG and additional family history at a minimum, and potentially with genetic testing as well.

The other answers are all explainable. The syncope is very consistent with vasovagal syncope and is not associated with exercise. The shortness of breath is attributable to asthma and is confirmed by the response to albuterol. The grandfather's heart attack would be concerning if it occurred at an age <50 years old. Finally, the heart murmur is consistent with a benign Stills murmur. It may still be worthwhile to work up if you're not completely sure that it is a benign murmur, but it is still not as concerning as the unexplained death in an immediate family member.

44. (B) ASDs found in infants between 3 and 5 mm in size have 80% to 90% chance of closing on their own, depending on the study. The chance of closing decreases with age. For example, if a 5-year-old patient was found to have the same size ASD (5 mm), it may actually be more likely to increase in size rather than close.

45. (B) Patients with coarctation of the aorta have a roughly 10% incidence of intracranial aneurysms, which is about 5 times greater than the general population. They can still occur after repair, and they are not always associated with hypertension (though uncontrolled hypertension may be a risk factor). Most patients that develop aneurysms do so in adulthood, but they can occur at younger ages as well. Screening for aneurysms with head imaging is still controversial, though it could be considered.

46. (C) Children with congenital heart disease have well-recognized deficits in neurodevelopmental outcomes. They have lower IQ scores, inferior achievement testing, and worse gross and fine motor functions. Children with cyanotic lesions have significantly more affected outcomes than those with acyanotic lesions. The duration of cyanosis is also associated with a greater decline in cognitive function. Visual–spatial skills are an area of specific weakness in children with congenital heart disease. Children with single ventricles are at highest risk of adverse developmental outcomes. Children with simple repaired lesions, such as those with an isolated ASD, often have normal neurodevelopmental outcomes.

47. (D) The dose of aspirin used to achieve an antiinflammatory effect during the acute phase of Kawasaki disease is relatively high, with a recommended range of 30 to 100 mg/kg per day

in four divided doses. Once fever has been absent for 48 hours, patients are generally switched to a low dose of aspirin, 3 to 5 mg/kg per day, for its antiplatelet effect. This low-dose aspirin regimen is continued until laboratory markers of acute inflammation (e.g., platelet count and CRP) return to normal, unless coronary artery abnormalities are detected by echocardiography.

48. (C) A patient with Wolff–Parkinson–White syndrome could have the potential EKG finding of LAD along with evidence of preexcitation. Other diagnoses to consider in patients with LAD include a primum ASD, tricuspid atresia, and an AV canal. Patients with hypertrophic cardiomyopathy are less likely to have evidence of LAD on EKG and instead will have findings consistent with LVH.

49. (B) The patient is likely being treated with flecainide, which is a sodium channel blocker. Flecainide levels increase once a patient stops breastfeeding or stops receiving formula. Given the patient's age of 12 months, it is likely that he is weaning off formula and one should be concerned about flecainide toxicity. Findings of toxicity include PR prolongation and possible signs of heart failure. The other answer options may all be normal findings on EKG in a 12-month-old patient.

50. (D) Vein of Galen malformations (VGAM) are rare embryonic arteriovenous shunts, seen in 1:25,000 live births and more common in males. Intracardiac anatomy may be normal, or VGAM can be associated with sinus venosus ASD or COA. Fetal presentation can range from mild cardiac failure to fetal hydrops, though VGAM is commonly diagnosed after birth with rapid deterioration and cardiac failure with large shunts. High-output cardiac failure is the primary clinical concern, and hemorrhage is uncommon. Smaller shunts may present later, most noticeably with macrocephaly and prominent facial veins. Initial assessment may include cranial US in an infant, followed by MRI or CT. Transcatheter chemical embolization approaches have been the most successful treatment method, though morbidity/mortality remains high.

51. (D) The patient outlined in the question stem has normal risk for an elevation of her cholesterol level. According to the 2011 NHLBI guidelines for cardiovascular health, all children should have a nonfasting lipid profile with a calculated non-HDL cholesterol performed once between the ages of 9 and 11. Children should be screened between the ages of 2 and 8 if:

- A parent, grandparent, aunt/uncle, or sibling has myocardial infarction (MI), angina, stroke, coronary artery bypass graft (CABG)/stent/angioplasty at <55 years in males and <65 years in females.
- Parent with TC >240 mg/dL or known dyslipidemia
- Child has diabetes, hypertension, or BMI >95th percentile, or smokes cigarettes
- Child has a moderate- or high-risk medical condition:

High risk:
- Diabetes mellitus type 1 and type 2.
- Chronic kidney disease/end-stage renal disease/postrenal transplant.
- Postorthotopic heart transplant.
- Kawasaki disease with current aneurysms.

Moderate risk:

- Kawasaki disease with regressed coronary aneurysms.
- Chronic inflammatory disease (systemic lupus erythematosus, juvenile rheumatoid arthritis).
- Human immunodeficiency virus infection.
- Nephrotic syndrome.

52. (C) This patient has a supracristal/subarterial/conal septal/infundibular ventricular septal defect. This type of defect does not warrant closure based solely on its location, although repair would be indicated if Q_p:Q_s on cardiac catheterization was 2:1 or greater. Closure would be indicated if there was an increase in the amount of aortic valve regurgitation, evidence of left heart volume overload, reversible pulmonary vascular resistance, or a history of infective endocarditis. This type of VSD is unlikely to close spontaneously.

53. (B) The most common indication for reoperation after repair of complete atrioventricular septal defect is left AV valve regurgitation; left AV valve stenosis is rare. Right AV valve regurgitation occurs less commonly, primarily in association with pulmonary hypertension or with tetralogy of Fallot. Late LVOT obstruction due to subaortic stenosis is more common with partial atrioventricular septal defect than with complete atrioventricular septal defect.

54. (D) The overall IQ in these patients is typically in the low range of normal, 86 to 90 in multiple studies. Important delays are seen in motor skills, visual–motor integration, and executive function, and there is a high incidence of behavioral problems including ADHD. Approximately one-third of children receive special education services. Lower full-scale IQ, verbal, and math scores are associated with longer hospital length of stay at the time of initial surgery. No differences have been seen in neurodevelopmental outcomes in HLHS patients in regard to the type of surgical approach: transplantation versus staged repair. Neurodevelopmental injury has been associated with hypoglycemia and hypoxia but not hypercarbia or acidosis. In one study of Fontan survivors 6 to 18 years of age, parents reported attentional problems in 46%, learning in 43%, development in 24%, and behavioral in 23%.

55. (E) Brugada is more common in men, and more arrhythmic events occur in men; higher testosterone levels are thought to have a significant role. Inheritance is autosomal dominant. ICD implantation is not indicated in asymptomatic Brugada patients with drug-induced type I ECG on the basis of family history of sudden cardiac death alone. Symptoms commonly occur during rest, sleep, febrile state, or vagotonic conditions, but rarely during exercise.

56. (C) Based on the Revised Ghent Nosology, she meets criteria for diagnosis of Marfan syndrome based on positive family history and aortic Z-score greater than or equal to 3 (below 20 years old). Following diagnosis, an echo should initially be performed at 6-month intervals to assess the progression of aortic involvement. Routine MRI or CT of the thoracic aorta is recommended if there is evidence of descending aortic dilation, type B dissection, or after repair of an ascending aortic aneurysm. β-Blocker therapy should be initiated at diagnosis or in the presence of significant aortic dilation.

57. (C) Squatting maneuvers will increase preload and delay prolapse, moving the click closer to S_2. Decreased left ventricular contractility and increased afterload will also delay the clinic, moving it closer to S_2.

58. (B) JAG1 is the gene for Alagille syndrome, a dominant disorder with bile duct paucity, CHD, skeletal and ocular abnormalities, and a characteristic face as described in the question stem. 22q11 deletion syndrome is highly variable and includes congenital heart disease, palatal anomalies, hypocalcemia, immunodeficiency, speech and learning disabilities, renal anomalies, psychiatric problems, and distinct facial features. Nkx2.5 is a transcription factor with multiple, varied associations to congenital heart disease, most commonly ASDs. FBN1 is associated with Marfan syndrome.

59. (E) The incidence of HCM is 1:500. Dissimilar patterns of LVH can occur in patients with the same genetic substrate, except in identical twins in which hearts have been shown to have the same patterns of LVH. Hypertrophy is usually not present at birth, and ECG abnormalities may be the initial clinical manifestation before LVH becomes evident.

60. (B) See Figure 8.2 regarding the differential diagnosis of HCM versus physiologic athlete's heart. Maximal LV wall thickness within the shaded gray area is consistent with both diagnoses. Clinical criteria used to distinguish nonobstructive HCM from athlete's heart are listed in the figure.

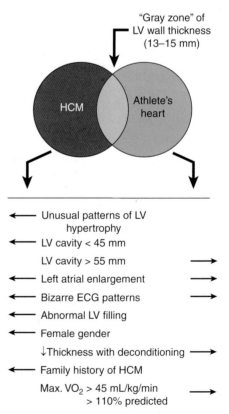

FIGURE 8.2 Differential diagnosis of hypertrophic cardiomyopathy (HCM) versus physiologic athlete's heart. (Adapted from Maron BJ, Pelliccia A. The heart of trained athletes: cardiac remodeling and the risks of sports, including sudden death. *Circulation.* 2006; 114:1633–1644.)

SUGGESTED READINGS

Allen HD, Driscoll DJ, Shaddy RE, et al., eds. *Moss and Adams' Heart Disease in Infants, Children and Adolescents.* 7th ed. Philadelphia, PA: Lippincott Williams & Wilkins; 2007:706–709.

Allen HD, Mendell JR, Hoffman TM. The heart in muscular dystrophies. In: Allen HD, Driscoll DJ, Shaddy RE, et al., eds. *Moss and Adams' Heart Disease in Infants, Children, and Adolescents.* Philadelphia, PA: Lippincott Williams & Wilkins; 2008:1514–1524.

American Heart Association. Dietary recommendations for children and adolescents. *Circulation.* 2005;112:2061–2075.

Barst RJ, Ertel SI, Beghetti M, et al. Pulmonary arterial hypertension: a comparison between children and adults. *Eur Res J.* 2011; 37(3):665–677.

Basso C, Maron BJ, Corrado D, et al. Clinical profile of congenital coronary artery anomalies with origin from the wrong aortic sinus leading to sudden death in young competitive athletes. *J Am Coll Cardiol.* 2000;35(6):1493–1501.

Borlaug BA. Pulsus paradoxus in pericardial disease. UpToDate. http://www.uptodate.com/contents/pulsus-paradoxus-in-pericardial-disease?source=search_result&search=pulsus+paradoxus-+in+pericardialdisease&selectedTitle=1%7E28

Godfrey M. Congenital Contractural Arachnodactyly. *Gene Reviews.* NCBI Bookshelf Online. 2011.

Corrigan JJ. Hematologic aspects of pediatric cardiology. In: Allen HD, Driscoll DJ, Shaddy RE, et al., eds. *Moss and Adams' Heart Disease in Infants, Children, and Adolescents.* Philadelphia, PA: Lippincott Williams & Wilkins; 2008:1514–1524.

Daniels SR, Greer FR, Committee on Nutrition. Lipid screening and cardiovascular health in childhood. *Pediatrics.* 2008;122: 198–208.

Gerber MA, Baltimore RS, Eaton CB, et al. Prevention of rheumatic fever and diagnosis and treatment of acute streptococcal pharyngitis. *Circulation.* 2009;119(11):1541.

Lipshultz SE, Colan SD, Gelber RD, et al. Late cardiac effects of doxorubicin therapy for acute lymphoblastic leukemia in childhood. *N Engl J Med.* 1991;324(12):808.

Loeys BL, Dietz HC, Braverman AC, et al. The Revised Ghent Nosology for the Marfan syndrome. *J Med Genet.* 2010;47:476–485.

Magnani JW, William G. Myocarditis: current trends in diagnosis and treatment. *Circulation.* 2006;113:876–890.

Mayosi, B. Natural history screening and management of rheumatic heart disease. UpToDate. http://www.uptodate.com/contents/natural-history-screening-and-management-of-rheumatic-heart-disease?source=see_link&anchor=H16376507#H16376507

McDaniel NL, Gutgesell HP. Ventricular septal defects. In: Allen HD, Driscoll DJ, Shaddy RE, et al., eds. *Moss and Adams' Heart Disease in Infants, Children, and Adolescents.* Philadelphia, PA: Lippincott Williams & Wilkins; 2008:667–672.

National High Blood Pressure Education Program Working Group on High Blood Pressure in Children and Adolescents. The fourth report on the diagnosis, evaluation, and treatment of high blood pressure in children and adolescents. *Pediatrics.* 2004;114:555.

Newburger JW, Takahashi M, Gerber MA, et al. Diagnosis, treatment and long-term management of Kawasaki disease: a statement for health professionals from the Committee on Rheumatic Fever, Endocarditis and Kawasaki Disease, Council on Cardiovascular Disease in the Young, American Heart Association. *Pediatrics.* 2004;114:1708–1733.

O'Brien ET, O'Malley K. ABC of blood pressure measurement: technique. *Br Med J.* 1979;2(6196):982–984.

Ogedegbe G, Pickering T. Principles and techniques of blood pressure measurement. *Cardiol Clin.* 2010;28(4):571–586.

Porter CJ, Edwards WD. Atrial septal defects. In: Allen HD, Driscoll DJ, Shaddy RE, et al., eds. *Moss and Adams' Heart Disease in Infants, Children, and Adolescents.* Philadelphia, PA: Lippincott Williams & Wilkins; 2008:632–634.

Rocchini AP. Sports screening and participation. In: Allen HD, Driscoll DJ, Shaddy RE, et al., eds. *Moss and Adams' Heart Disease in Infants, Children, and Adolescents.* Philadelphia, PA: Lippincott Williams & Wilkins; 2008:66–80.

Ruggiero A, Ridola V, Puma N, et al. Anthracycline cardiotoxicity in childhood. *Pediatr Hematol Oncol.* 2008;25(4):261–281.

Smith LA, Cornelius VR, Plummer CJ, et al. Cardiotoxicity of anthracycline agents for the treatment of cancer: systematic review and meta-analysis of randomized controlled trials. *BMC Cancer.* 2010;10:337.

The Task Force for the Diagnosis and Management of Syncope of the European Society of Cardiology, et al. Guidelines for the diagnosis and management of syncope (version 2009). *Eur Heart J.* 2009; 30(21):2631–2671.

Van Hare GF, Ackerman MJ, Evangelista JA, et al; American Heart Association Electrocardiography and Arrhythmias Committee of Council on Clinical Cardiology, Council on Cardiovascular Disease in Young, Council on Cardiovascular and Stroke Nursing, Council on Functional Genomics and Translational Biology, and American College of Cardiology. Eligibility and disqualification recommendations for competitive athletes with cardiovascular abnormalities: Task Force 4: congenital heart disease—a scientific statement from the American Heart Association and American College of Cardiology. *Circulation.* 2015;132(22):e281–e291.

Wilson W, Taubert KA, Gewitz M, et al. Prevention of infective endocarditis: guidelines from the American Heart Association: a guideline from the American Heart Association Rheumatic Fever, Endocarditis, and Kawasaki Disease Committee, Council on Cardiovascular Disease in the Young, and the Council on Clinical Cardiology, Council on Cardiovascular Surgery and Anesthesia, and the Quality of Care and Outcomes Research Interdisciplinary Working Group. *Circulation.* 2007;116:1736–1754.

Zipes DP, Ackerman MJ, Estes NA III, et al. Task Force 7: arrhythmias. *JACC.* 2005;45:1354–1363.

CHAPTER 9

Cardiac Intensive Care

Anthony C. Chang and Joseph T. Poterucha

QUESTIONS

1. In the relationship between total lung volume and pulmonary vascular resistance, the pulmonary vascular resistance is lowest at:

   A. Functional residual capacity
   B. Vital capacity
   C. Tidal volume
   D. Closing capacity
   E. Residual volume

2. A 5-month-old with single ventricle anatomy returns after a bidirectional cavopulmonary anastomosis. The saturation is 72% and the pressure in the superior vena cava is 22 mm Hg while the left atrial pressure is 4 mm Hg. Of the following conditions, the *most* likely explanation that would explain this hemodynamic profile is:

   A. Pericardial tamponade
   B. Junctional ectopic tachycardia
   C. Ventricular dysfunction
   D. Pulmonary artery thrombus
   E. Severe atrioventricular valve regurgitation

3. Of the following postoperative patients, which is the *least* likely to have junctional ectopic tachycardia?

   A. A 3-month-old after common atrioventricular canal repair
   B. A 4-month-old after bidirectional cavopulmonary anastomosis
   C. A 1-month-old with interrupted aortic arch and VSD after repair
   D. A 1-week-old after arterial switch and VSD repair
   E. A 4-month-old with tetralogy of Fallot after repair

4. A neonate with common atrioventricular canal and double outlet right ventricle with pulmonary atresia returns from the operating room after an aortopulmonary shunt and total anomalous pulmonary venous return repair. He is noted to have a heart rate (HR) range of 176 to 194 beats per minute (bpm) but stable blood pressure. The *most* likely tachydysrhythmia that he has is:

   A. Atrial ectopic tachycardia
   B. Junctional ectopic tachycardia
   C. Atrioventricular nodal reentrant tachycardia
   D. Permanent form of junctional reciprocating tachycardia (PJRT)
   E. Reentrant supraventricular tachycardia

5. Of the following patients, the *least* likely patient to have postoperative pulmonary hypertension after cardiac surgery is:

   A. A neonate with infracardiac total anomalous pulmonary venous return
   B. A 2-month-old with truncus arteriosus repair
   C. A 6-month-old with transposition of the great arteries and VSD
   D. A 5-month-old with common atrioventricular canal
   E. A 1-week-old with transposition of the great arteries

6. A 2-month-old infant returns after corrective surgery for a congenital heart defect on minimal inotropic support. The hemodynamic profile is as follows: CVP = 14 mm Hg; LA pressure = 5 mm Hg; and HR = 172 bpm. The blood pressure is stable. The *most* likely anatomic diagnosis is:

   A. Tetralogy of Fallot
   B. Total anomalous pulmonary venous return
   C. Transposition of the great arteries
   D. Anomalous left coronary artery from the pulmonary artery
   E. Coarctation of the aorta and VSD

7. A neonate returns after an arterial switch operation and VSD repair to the intensive care unit. The hemodynamic profile is as follows: HR = 162 bpm; CVP = 6 mm Hg; LA pressure = 14 mm Hg; and blood pressure = 88/64 mm Hg. Of the following conditions or diagnoses, the *least* likely is:

   A. Aortopulmonary collaterals
   B. Residual VSD
   C. LV dysfunction
   D. Coronary ischemia
   E. Pulmonary hypertension

8. The postoperative hypertension after coarctation repair in the first few hours is best characterized by:

   A. Increased diastolic pressure
   B. Mesenteric arteritis
   C. Elevation in norepinephrine
   D. Elevation in renin
   E. Response to therapy with ACE inhibition

9. A 3-year-old with single ventricle returns from the operating room after a Fontan operation. The PA pressure is 18 mm Hg and the left atrial pressure is 13 mm Hg. The *least* likely etiology for this hemodynamic profile is:

   A. Ventricular dysfunction
   B. AV valve regurgitation
   C. Pleural effusion
   D. Pericardial effusion
   E. Unfavorable mass/volume change

10. An infant is admitted to the cardiac intensive care unit for respiratory distress and is noted to have giant v waves on his CVP pressure tracing. Which of the following conditions is the most likely to be associated with this finding?

    A. Tricuspid stenosis
    B. Complete heart block
    C. Tricuspid regurgitation
    D. Right atrial myxoma
    E. Pulmonary hypertension

11. In a neonate with single ventricle anatomy and physiology and excellent ventricular function, the oxygen saturation (SaO_2) is 90% while the SvO_2 is 60%. What is the oxygen excess omega (Ω)?

    A. 0.3
    B. 0.5
    C. 2
    D. 3
    E. Cannot be calculated based on the available data

12. Of the following, the mediator that is *decreased* in pulmonary hypertension is:

    A. Prostacyclin
    B. Transforming growth factor β (TGF-β)
    C. Endothelin
    D. Serotonin
    E. Thromboxane A_2

13. A 3-month-old infant with double outlet right ventricle and a subaortic VSD is noted to have 75% systemic pressure in the pulmonary artery after corrective surgery. The surgeon calls you to the operating room to have input into the management of this problem as the blood pressure has been borderline. The first maneuver should be:

    A. Initiate inhaled nitric oxide at 20 ppm
    B. Initiate inhaled nitric oxide at 80 ppm
    C. Initiate intravenous milrinone at 0.5 μg/kg/min
    D. Hyperventilate to $PaCO_2$ <40 mm Hg and hyperoxygenate
    E. Perform a transesophageal echocardiogram

14. Amiodarone is now widely used in the treatment of postoperative junctional ectopic tachycardia. This important antiarrhythmic agent is classified as:

    A. Class IA
    B. Class IB
    C. Class IC
    D. Class II
    E. None of the above

15. A child who has a chronic indwelling central line developed an intracardiac thrombus. He is now admitted to the cardiac intensive care unit for tPA infusion. The correct mechanism of action for this medication is:

    A. It binds to fibrin
    B. It acetylates cyclo-oxygenase to inhibit production of thromboxane A_2, a platelet aggregator
    C. It is a mucopolysaccharide that increases the rate at which antithrombin III neutralizes thrombin, factor X, and also IX, XI, and XII
    D. It interacts with plasminogen to result in plasmin complex
    E. It interferes with posttranslational modification of the vitamin K-dependent coagulation factors (II, VII, IX, X, and proteins C and S)

16. An infant returns from the operating room after a VSD repair. The central venous pressure is 2 mm Hg with stable blood pressure and HR. The *least* likely etiology for this low CVP pressure is:

    A. Low intravascular volume
    B. Inadequate preload
    C. Catheter malfunction
    D. Pressure transducer below the level of the heart
    E. Pressure transducer improperly calibrated

17. A central venous line is placed in a child and the tip of the line is in the right atrium. An oxygen saturation of 47% is measured from a blood sample drawn from this line. The *least* likely explanation for this is:

    A. Increased oxygen extraction
    B. Catheter tip near the coronary sinus
    C. Anemia
    D. Decreased arterial oxygen saturation with a normal A–V O_2 difference
    E. Increased oxygen delivery

18. A child returns from the operating room after a VSD repair and was noted to be in complete heart block. Of the following types of VSD, which would be the *most* likely to result in heart block?

    A. Canal-type VSD with straddling tricuspid valve
    B. Apical muscular VSD
    C. Midmuscular VSD
    D. Subpulmonary VSD
    E. Anterior malalignment VSD

19. A neonate returns after cardiac surgery to the cardiac intensive care unit. The hemodynamics are as follows: HR = 183 bpm; right atrial pressure = 6 mm Hg; left atrial pressure = 15 mm Hg; and blood pressure = 76/52 mm Hg. The oxygen saturation is 98%. The most likely diagnosis is:

    A. Ventricular septal defect
    B. Truncus arteriosus
    C. Tetralogy of Fallot
    D. Total anomalous pulmonary venous connection
    E. Scimitar syndrome

20. Neosynephrine is occasionally used in the cardiac intensive care unit. Of the following situations (assuming no airway or lung issues), which is the *least* likely to benefit from an infusion of Neosynephrine?

    A. Infant with tetralogy of Fallot with hypercyanotic spell
    B. Infant with double outlet right ventricle/common atrioventricular canal and subpulmonary stenosis with saturation of 45%
    C. Infant with hypoplastic left heart syndrome and s/p Norwood with a narrowed aortopulmonary shunt and a saturation of 53%
    D. Infant with double outlet right ventricle and transposition physiology with a saturation of 56%
    E. Infant with tetralogy of Fallot s/p aortopulmonary shunt with narrowed shunt and a saturation of 48%

21. A neonate is born with severe respiratory distress minutes after birth. There is a loud to-and-fro murmur at the left sternal border. The management should be:

    A. CPAP with inspired oxygen
    B. Prone position and mechanical ventilation
    C. ECMO

    D. High-frequency ventilation
    E. Surfactant administration and mechanical ventilation

22. Of the following endogenous compounds with pulmonary vasoactivity, which is considered a pulmonary vasodilator?

    A. Angiotensin II
    B. Leukotriene C4
    C. Prostaglandin F2α
    D. Bradykinin
    E. Serotonin

23. A 3-year-old with tricuspid atresia returns after a Fontan operation. The HR is 146 bpm. The blood pressure is 84/54 mm Hg. The PA pressure is 18 mm Hg. Of the following interventions, which should be the first?

    A. An EKG
    B. Initiation of IV milrinone
    C. An echocardiogram
    D. Initiation of inhaled nitric oxide
    E. A cardiac catheterization

24. A neonate with pulmonary atresia and intact ventricular septum s/p an aortopulmonary shunt returns from OR. His blood pressure is 68/22 mm Hg, his HR is in the 150s, and his saturation is 87%. The hemoglobin is 8.8 g/dL. Which of the following interventions should *not* be performed?

    A. IV dopamine
    B. IV milrinone
    C. Transfusion of packed RBCs
    D. Decrease sedation
    E. Volume

25. A 3-year-old with valvar aortic stenosis and subvalvar obstruction of the LVOT now returns from the OR after a Ross–Konno operation. Which of the following postoperative residua is the *least* likely?

    A. Pulmonary hypertension
    B. Residual VSD
    C. Left ventricular dysfunction
    D. Right ventricular outflow tract obstruction
    E. Neoaortic insufficiency

26. A 4-week-old infant with transposition of the great arteries and a small ventricular septal defect returns after an arterial switch operation and ventricular septal defect closure. The HR is 185 bpm and the left atrial pressure is elevated at 17 mm Hg. Of the following, which is the *least* likely?

    A. Pericardial tamponade
    B. Junctional ectopic tachycardia
    C. Unprepared left ventricle
    D. Aortopulmonary collaterals
    E. Myocardial depression

27. An infant with asplenia returns after a palliative procedure that included an aortopulmonary shunt and repair of total anomalous pulmonary venous connection. The HR gradually increased to 184 bpm despite adequate volume resuscitation. Adenosine failed to convert the tachycardia. The *most* likely diagnosis is:

   A. Ectopic atrial tachycardia
   B. Reentrant type of supraventricular tachycardia
   C. Junctional ectopic tachycardia
   D. Ventricular tachycardia
   E. Junctional ectopic tachycardia with aberrancy

28. An infant with a known congenital heart disease arrives in the cardiac intensive care unit with grossly bloody stools consistent with ischemic bowel syndrome. Of the following diagnoses, which is the *least* likely?

   A. Hypoplastic left syndrome after a Norwood operation
   B. Tetralogy of Fallot with no surgical palliation or correction
   C. Truncus arteriosus with moderate truncal regurgitation awaiting surgery
   D. Coarctation of the aorta with a 80 mm Hg arch gradient
   E. Aortic stenosis with a 75 mm Hg stenotic gradient and poor ventricular function

29. Of the following inotropic agents and associated dosages, which would increase myocardial consumption the *least*?

   A. Epinephrine @ 0.4 mcg/kg/min
   B. Dopamine @ 12 mcg/kg/min
   C. Milrinone @ 0.4 mcg/kg/min
   D. Dobutamine @ 15 mcg/kg/min
   E. Isoproterenol @ 0.7 mcg/kg/min

30. An infant returns after a Norwood operation that included the traditional aortopulmonary shunt. The pulse oximetry is reading 83%. The chest roentgenogram showed clear lungs. Assuming that the cardiac output is adequate, the ratio of pulmonary to systemic blood flow is approximately:

   A. 5:1
   B. 4:1
   C. 2:1
   D. 1:1
   E. 0.7:1

31. A child with tricuspid atresia and prior aortopulmonary shunt now returns from the operating room after a bidirectional cavopulmonary anastomosis. The oxygen saturation is adequate at 85%. The SVC pressure is 18 mm Hg and the left atrial pressure reads 4 mm Hg. The *least* likely diagnosis is:

   A. Poor ventricular compliance
   B. Elevated pulmonary vascular resistance

   C. Undiagnosed pulmonary venous obstruction
   D. Large bilateral pleural effusion
   E. Thrombosis at the site of the anastomosis

32. Of the following children with their accompanying lesions, which is *most* likely to have pulmonary hypertension that will persist after surgical correction?

   A. A 6-year-old with a large secundum-type atrial septal defect
   B. A 9-month-old with a moderate-sized ventricular septal defect with mild aortic insufficiency
   C. A 4-month-old with Down syndrome and common atrioventricular canal
   D. A 9-month-old with transposition of the great arteries and unrestrictive ventricular septal defect
   E. A 3-month-old with truncus arteriosus and mild truncal insufficiency

33. A 3-month-old with tetralogy of Fallot and severe subpulmonary stenosis is admitted to the cardiac intensive care unit with an oxygen saturation of 53%. Of the following therapeutic measures, which is *not* the accepted therapy in this situation?

   A. Esmolol IV infusion
   B. Neosynephrine IV
   C. Oxygen 4 L by face mask
   D. Isoproterenol IV infusion
   E. Isotonic fluid IV bolus

34. A 2-month-old child returns after surgery. The HR is 152 bpm and the right and left atrial pressures are 5 and 15 mm Hg, respectively. Assuming that the surgical procedure is without technical problems or significant postoperative residua, this child is *least* likely to have:

   A. Anomalous left coronary artery from the pulmonary artery
   B. Tetralogy of Fallot with hypoplastic pulmonary arteries
   C. Transposition of the great arteries
   D. Aortic stenosis, valvar and subvalvar
   E. Total anomalous pulmonary venous return of the supracardiac type

35. A 5-month-old infant returns after repair of tetralogy of Fallot. The HR is 162 bpm and the right atrial pressure is 8 mm Hg. Blood pressure is borderline at 76/48 mm Hg. Of the following, which is *not* an appropriate intervention?

   A. Administer volume of 10 cc/kg
   B. Initiate an isoproterenol infusion
   C. Obtain an electrocardiogram
   D. Obtain an echocardiogram
   E. Initiate a milrinone infusion

36. The correct relationship between pericardial volume (*x*-axis) and pericardial pressure (*y*-axis) is (see Fig. 9.1):

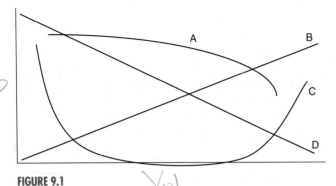

FIGURE 9.1

A. A
B. B
C. C
D. D
E. None of the above

37. A 6-month-old with coarctation of the aorta returns after end-to-end anastomosis repair of the coarctation. The blood pressure is 136/70 mm Hg. Of the following, which pharmacologic agent is not an accepted therapy for hypertension after coarctation repair?

A. Esmolol IV
B. Labetolol IV
C. Nitroprusside IV
D. Hydralazine IV
E. Isoproterenol IV

38. A 6-month-old with single ventricle who was previously palliated with an aortopulmonary shunt is now back from the operating room after a bidirectional cavopulmonary anastomosis. His oxygen saturation is 65%. Of the following, which is the *least* likely etiology for the systemic desaturation?

A. Pleural effusion
B. A decompression vein
C. Low arterial $paCO_2$
D. Atrioventricular valve regurgitation
E. Elevated pulmonary vascular resistance

39. The therapeutic options for the treatment of junctional ectopic tachycardia includes all of the following *except*:

A. Amiodarone IV
B. Hypothermia
C. Procainamide IV
D. Adenosine IV
E. Digoxin IV

40. The curve in Figure 9.2 depicts (*x*- and *y*-axes) the relationship:

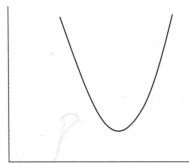

FIGURE 9.2

A. Lung volume vs. pulmonary vascular resistance
B. Pericardial volume and pericardial pressure
C. Pericardial fluid and HR
D. Hematocrit and viscosity
E. Viscosity and pulmonary vascular resistance

41. Of the following pediatric patients, which would be the *least* likely to have an elevated right atrial pressure of 14 mm Hg?

A. A 5-year-old with restrictive cardiomyopathy
B. A 3-year-old after an atrial septal defect repair with a large pericardial effusion
C. A 3-month-old with Ebstein anomaly and moderate tricuspid valve regurgitation
D. A 4-month-old after tetralogy of Fallot repair with a residual RVOT gradient of 60 mm Hg
E. A 12-year-old with chronic dilated cardiomyopathy

42. A neonate with the diagnosis of infracardiac total anomalous pulmonary venous drainage returns after corrective surgery. A pulmonary artery catheter is left in place and the pulmonary artery pressure is ¾ systemic. The left atrial pressure is 8 mm Hg. What is the appropriate first step in managing this patient?

A. Echocardiogram and if needed, catheterization
B. Inhaled nitric oxide
C. Inhaled nitric oxide and sildenafil, IV
D. Milrinone IV
E. Milrinone and sildenafil IV

43. All of the following therapies have been utilized for catecholamine-resistant shock after cardiopulmonary bypass *except*:

A. Vasopressin
B. Steroids
C. Phenoxybenzamine
D. Thyroxine
E. ECMO

44. The following are expected findings on an electrocardiogram for the lesions and/or repairs listed *except*:

   A. Tetralogy of Fallot repair and complete right bundle branch block

   B. Anomalous left coronary artery from the pulmonary artery and Q waves in leads I and avL

   C. Subaortic resection and left bundle branch block

   D. Transposition of the great arteries after arterial switch and Q waves in leads II, III, and avF

   E. Truncus arteriosus repair and complete right bundle branch block

45. A 3-year-old child with single left ventricle and who has had a "fenestrated" Fontan operation returns from the cardiac catheterization laboratory. The following data are reported: pulmonary artery pressure 18 mm Hg, left atrial pressure 5 mm Hg, and oxygen saturation 99%. There is no pressure gradient between a simultaneous pulmonary artery wedge pressure and an end-diastolic pressure of the ventricle of 4 mm Hg. Which of the following statements is the *least* likely to be true?

   A. The transpulmonary gradient is 13 mm Hg

   B. The fenestration is patent

   C. The patient has elevated pulmonary vascular resistance

   D. The patient has normal end-diastolic pressure for a Fontan surgery patient

   E. There is no evidence for atrioventricular valve or pulmonary venous stenosis

46. The LV pressure–volume curve is shown for a patient at times A and B (see Fig. 9.3). The increase in stroke volume shown at time B is due to:

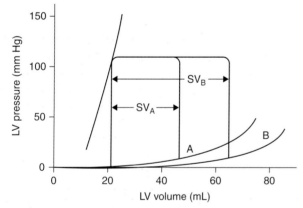

FIGURE 9.3

A. Increase in contractility

B. Afterload reduction

C. Improved lusitropy

D. Increased preload

E. Increased HR

47. A 4-year-old child is admitted to the cardiac intensive care unit with a history of a cerebrovascular accident. The electrocardiogram shows biatrial enlargement and intermittent atrial flutter. The echocardiogram shows dilated atria, LV ejection fraction of 62%, normal LV end-diastolic dimension, and an RV pressure estimated at 55% systemic pressure. The *most* likely diagnosis is:

   A. Dilated cardiomyopathy

   B. Restrictive cardiomyopathy

   C. Acute myocarditis

   D. Hypertrophic cardiomyopathy

   E. Pulmonary hypertension and RV failure

48. The following are vasoconstrictors that are part of the group of mediators that comprise the neurohumoral response in heart failure *except*:

   A. Angiotensin II

   B. Arginine vasopressin

   C. Norepinephrine

   D. B-type natriuretic peptide

   E. Endothelin

49. The EKG in Figure 9.4m is obtained in a 3-year-old who was admitted with cardiovascular collapse. The *most* likely diagnosis is:

   A. Anomalous left coronary artery from the pulmonary artery

   B. Ectopic atrial tachycardia

   C. Myocarditis

   D. Kawasaki disease and coronary thrombosis

   E. Congenitally corrected transposition of the great arteries

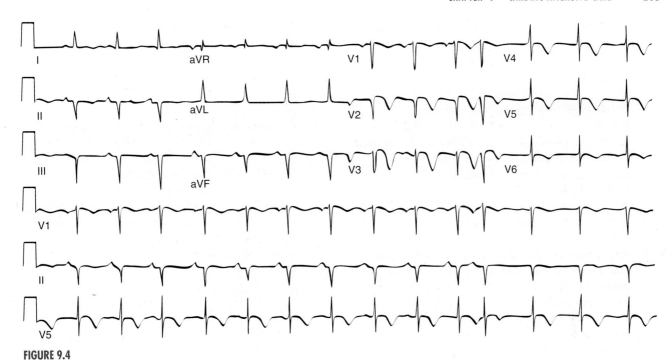

FIGURE 9.4

50. A patient after corrective surgery is admitted with borderline LV function and milrinone is initiated. If LV pressure–volume curves are plotted before and after milrinone was started (see Fig. 9.5), which of the following would best characterize its effects:

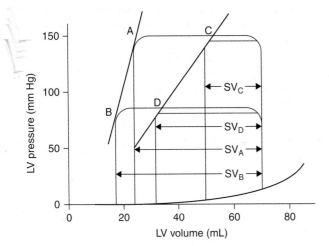

FIGURE 9.5

  A. C to B
  B. B to A
  C. C to A
  D. B to D
  E. C to D

51. A patient is sent for surgical repair of a large inferior secundum ASD. Immediately postoperatively the patient is persistently desaturated and cyanotic. The patient is sent for cardiac catheterization, but the interventionalist is unable to advance the catheter into the right ventricle or superior vena cava by femoral approach, but easily engages the left atrium. What explains the desaturation?

  A. Small residual patch leak
  B. Large patch dehiscence
  C. Anomalous pulmonary vein
  D. Pulmonary embolism
  E. Inferior vena cava baffle

52. You are called to the bedside to evaluate a 2-year-old boy postoperative day 0, for unresponsiveness. He underwent a primum ASD closure 12 hours prior. Exam reveals a blood pressure of 50/30 mm Hg, pulse 140 bpm, with distant heart sounds, severe jugular venous pressure elevation, and poor peripheral perfusion. Code is initiated and you perform a bedside echo. Which of the echo findings is most specific for cardiac tamponade?

  A. Diastolic collapse of the right atrium
  B. Diastolic collapse of the right ventricle
  C. Diastolic collapse of both the right atrium and the right ventricle
  D. Dilated inferior vena cava
  E. Left atrial collapse

53. You are assisting with postoperative management of a 2-day-old boy immediately after Norwood and modified Blalock–Taussig–Thomas shunt placement. You observe the following saturations: $SaO_2 = 60\%$, $SvO_2 = 40\%$. What is the estimated $Q_p{:}Q_s$ and what is the most appropriate management strategy to restore balanced hemodynamics?

 A. 2.0—Administer systemic vasodilators and sedate
 B. 1.0—Do nothing, wean support as tolerated
 C. 3.6—Consider surgical shunt restriction
 D. 1.5—Raise hemoglobin
 E. 0.5—Raise systemic vascular resistance, consider inhaled nitric oxide

54. A 2-year-old girl presents to the emergency department with 3 weeks of cough, myalgias, and malaise. An echocardiogram is obtained (Fig. 9.6). Viral myocarditis is suspected. The patient is admitted to the cardiac intensive care unit and started on carvedilol, enalapril, and milrinone. She remains hemodynamically stable on this regimen and infusion of intravenous immunoglobulin G (IVIG) is subsequently initiated. Three hours after infusion, she develops significant hypotension and suffers a seizure. MRI brain shows global diffuse severe white matter and cortical gray matter abnormalities on T1- and T2-weighted imaging.

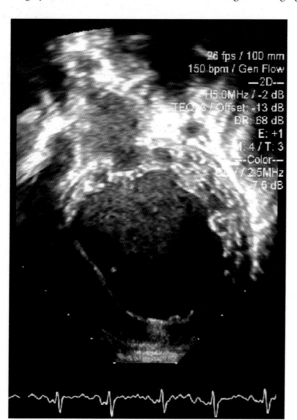

FIGURE 9.6

What intervention could have potentially prevented this unwanted outcome (best answer)?

 A. Bolus of milrinone
 B. Antiplatelet therapy
 C. Intravenous fluids in conjunction with IVIG infusion
 D. Antibiotic therapy
 E. Tissue plasminogen activator administration

55. An echocardiogram is performed for hypotension on a 2-day-old ex-32-week premature neonate born via cesarian section. Amniotic fluid was noted to be meconium stained upon birth. Chest x-ray shows diffuse interstitial opacities. Intracardiac anatomy is normal, although a large PDA is identified (Fig. 9.7). What is your recommendation to the neonatologist?

 A. Observation
 B. Indomethacin
 C. Surgical ligation
 D. Cath interventional ductal closure
 E. Mechanical ventilation, antibiotics, and nitric oxide

56. A 5-day-old boy with D-transposition of the great arteries postoperative day 0 after arterial switch operation develops progressive hypotension the night of surgery requiring significant vasoactive support. Central venous pressure has climbed to 20 mm Hg; however, there is no pressure variation with respiration. The infant remains mechanically ventilated without significant chest tube output and his hemoglobin and saturations are optimal. A few runs of nonsustained ventricular tachycardia are noted, but the baseline rhythm appears to be sinus tachycardia. A 4/6 systolic murmur is noted at the left lower sternal border with an S_3 gallop. Electrocardiogram is pending. What diagnosis should be at the top of your differential?

 A. Low cardiac output syndrome
 B. Severe neoaortic insufficiency
 C. Pulmonary vasospasm
 D. Tamponade
 E. Coronary ischemia

57. You are contacted by the transport team about accepting a term newborn boy born via repeat c-section who developed respiratory distress and lives 2 hours away. Chest x-ray is reported to show "RDS." Meconium aspiration is suspected. An echo has been obtained to evaluate for persistent fetal circulation. The echo (performed by the adult sonographer) shows normal ventricular size and function and a pulmonary venous confluence posterior to the left atrium—not all veins are visualized. You suspect obstructed infracardiac total anomalous pulmonary venous drainage. The baby has been intubated and given sodium bicarbonate boluses. The local neonatal

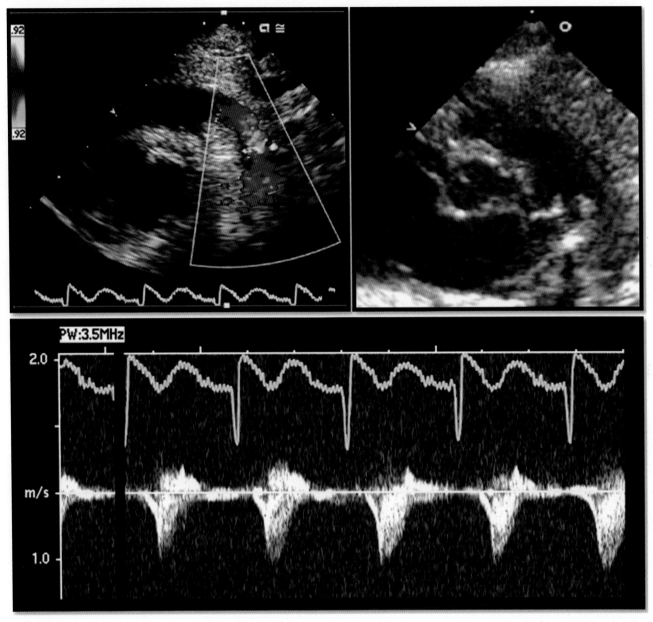

FIGURE 9.7

intensivist reports that a local pediatric cardiologist is available to perform a bedside septostomy if necessary. What do you recommend?

A. Start prostaglandin
B. Bedside septostomy
C. Transfer to your institution for cath-based septostomy
D. Transfer for corrective surgery
E. Prepare for extracorporeal mechanical support

58. You are managing a 4-month-old male infant with complete atrioventricular canal defect type C. On postoperative day 3, the resident remarks that the temporary pacing wires no longer work. Telemetry demonstrates complete atrioventricular dissociation with accelerated ventricular rhythm at 80 bpm. You inform the surgeon who reassures you that the rhythm will return in a few weeks. On postoperative day 10, the rhythm is unchanged. How long a waiting period is recommended before sending this patient for an epicardial pacemaker system?

A. 4 to 6 days
B. 7 to 10 days
C. 2 weeks
D. 3 weeks
E. 1 month

59. A 5-month-old boy with recurrent respiratory infection returns from the operative room after ligation of a small patent ductus arteriosus via left lateral thoracotomy. The patient is extubated in the operating room; however, he continues to exhibit respiratory distress and systemic desaturation (SaO_2 ~80%). Chest x-ray demonstrates a hypolucent left hemithorax. What is the etiology of this patient's clinical presentation?

A. Pneumothorax
B. Pulmonary hemorrhage
C. Left hemi-diaphragm paresis
D. Atelectasis
E. Inadvertent vessel ligation

60. Which of the following is a physiologic consequence of sternal closure?

A. Decreased intrathoracic pressure
B. Increased total lung compliance
C. Increased mean blood pressure
D. Decreased stroke volume
E. Increased cerebral oxygenation

61. A 2-week-old infant develops atrial flutter at a ventricular rate of 260 bpm 3 days after membranous ventricular septal defect patch closure. Atrial pacing wires are available. Adenosine and vagal maneuvers fail to break the arrhythmia. The patient is hemodynamically stable. You elect to attempt atrial overdrive pacing. How fast will you attempt to burst pace the patient?

A. 70% faster than the atrial rate
B. 70% faster than the ventricular
C. 70% faster than the atrial cycle length
D. 70% of atrial cycle length
E. Overdrive pacing is contraindicated

62. Inhaled nitric oxide is initiated on a 2-month-old boy with AV canal repair postoperative day 2 for pulmonary hypertensive crisis. Initial maximal therapeutic pulmonary vasodilatory effect is appreciated at what dose?

A. 5 ppm
B. 20 ppm
C. 40 ppm
D. 60 ppm
E. 80 ppm

63. Which of the pressure–volume loops in Figure 9.8 correctly depicts changes one would expect with systemic hypertension and decreased stroke volume?

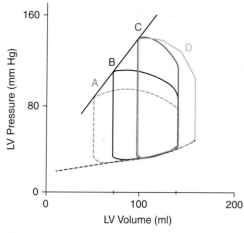

FIGURE 9.8

A. A
B. B
C. C
D. D
E. None of the above

64. What medication might you administer to improve cardiac output in Question 63?

A. Isoproterenol
B. Phenylephrine
C. Vasopressin
D. Epinephrine
E. Sodium nitroprusside

ANSWERS

1. (A) The effect of lung inflation on pulmonary vascular resistance (see U-shaped curve in Fig. 9.9) is such that resistance is at its nadir when the lung volume is at functional residual capacity (FRC). Any volume below FRC results in *underinflation* and thus atelectasis and alveolar hypoxia (reactive vasoconstriction), while any volume above the FRC results in *overinflation* and thus increased airway pressure and vascular stretch (secondary vasoconstriction).[1]

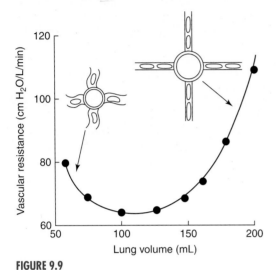

FIGURE 9.9

2. (D) Any *distortion of the pulmonary artery* (e.g., in situ thrombus, stenosis, external compression) would impede pulmonary blood flow and result in an elevated SVC pressure. This elevation in SVC pressure could result in the opening of vestigial veins that would then drain venous blood into the heart, thus leading to systemic desaturation. In this case, there was insufficient decompression of these veins as the SVC pressure was still very elevated.[2]

Other conditions that would result in similar hemodynamic profile (increased SVC pressure but without a concomitant increase in left atrial pressure) would be etiologic factors such as elevated pulmonary vascular resistance, pleural effusion, atelectasis, hyperinflation, pulmonary vein stenosis, and so on. The other conditions listed in the answer section would result in not just an elevated SVC pressure, but also an elevated left atrial pressure.

3. (B) *Junctional ectopic tachycardia* (JET) can be common after cardiac surgery in infants after surgery for tetralogy of Fallot, VSD, or common atrioventricular canal. This postoperative dysrhythmia would be extremely uncommon after a bidirectional cavopulmonary anastomosis. Management includes hypothermia, diminution of catecholamines, sedation, and antidysrhythmic agents such as amiodarone or procainamide with establishment of atrioventricular synchrony.[3]

4. (A) The anatomy is consistent with asplenia (double outlet right ventricle and common atrioventricular canal with pulmonary outlet obstruction as well as total anomalous pulmonary venous connection). These neonates can have *ectopic atrial tachycardia*, and this is often underdiagnosed.[4]

Junctional ectopic tachycardia is more commonly associated with infants after VSD surgery (tetralogy of Fallot or common

atrioventricular canal). The other types of SVT are not commonly associated with postoperative situations.

5. (E) After the first few days of life, a neonate with transposition of the great arteries is not likely to have elevated pulmonary vascular resistance. The other lesions at the listed ages are well known to have *elevated pulmonary vascular resistance* before surgery and can therefore have exacerbation of pulmonary vascular resistance after cardiopulmonary bypass.[5]

6. (A) *Tetralogy of Fallot* after cardiac surgery is characterized by a restrictive right ventricular physiology with an elevated CVP while the left atrial pressure remains normal. The other cardiac defects will usually have a higher left atrial pressure than CVP for different reasons. In *total anomalous pulmonary venous return*, the left atrium and ventricle are relatively noncompliant and borderline hypoplastic, so a higher filling pressure is required. In *transposition of the great arteries*, it is not uncommon to have some degree of LV dysfunction (depending on age) and a higher left atrial pressure is often noted especially in older infants with this diagnosis. In infants with *anomalous left coronary artery from the pulmonary artery*, the left ventricle is usually dilated and with significant dysfunction so that the filling pressure after surgery will be elevated. Lastly, an infant with *coarctation of the aorta and VSD* is more likely to have a higher left atrial pressure than CVP.[6]

7. (E) *Pulmonary hypertension* would lead to an elevated CVP with a normal or slightly elevated left atrial pressure. An *elevated left atrial pressure* will be seen with the other answers: aortopulmonary collaterals and residual VSD will lead to increased pulmonary venous return while LV dysfunction and/or coronary ischemia will lead to higher filling pressures.[6]

8. (C) Postcoarctectomy hypertension has a biphasic pattern. The *first phase* is most likely secondary to surgical stimulation of the sympathetic nerve fibers in the tissue of the aortic isthmus. This process leads to release of norepinephrine (as well as epinephrine) and can be effectively neutralized with preoperative treatment with propranolol. The *second phase* of postcoarctectomy hypertension occurs after the initial 24 hours and is characterized by an increase in renin and an elevated diastolic pressure. This phase is also associated with mesenteric arteritis.[7]

9. (C) Elevated PA pressure after the Fontan operation can be categorized into: (1) *abnormal transpulmonary gradient* (>5 mm Hg): etiologies include elevated pulmonary vascular resistance, pulmonary artery distortion, pulmonary issues (e.g., pleural effusion, pneumothorax, atelectasis), and pulmonary venous obstruction; and (2) *normal transpulmonary gradient* (but abnormal LA pressure): etiologies include ventricular dysfunction, unfavorable mass/volume changes (diastolic dysfunction), AV valve regurgitation, subaortic stenosis, AV dyssynchrony, and pericardial effusion.[8]

10. (C) In a *CVP pressure tracing*, the *a wave* is produced by atrial contraction and the *c wave* is caused by ventricular contraction against a closed tricuspid valve (with the valve bulging into the right atrium). The *v wave* is secondary to atrial filling. The *x descent* follows the *c wave* and is due to the tricuspid valve being pulled away from the right atrium during ventricular systole and the *y descent* occurs due to the blood filling the right ventricle. *Cannon a waves* have a myriad of etiologic factors, including (1) right atrium contracting against an obstructed tricuspid valve (tricuspid stenosis, right atrial masses, right atrial myxoma, complete heart block, and atrioventricular dyssynchrony) and resistance to right ventricular filling (pulmonary hypertension or pulmonary stenosis).[9]

11. (D) The *oxygen excess omega* (Ω) can be calculated with the formula:

$$\text{Oxygen excess omega } (\Omega) = \frac{\text{Oxygen delivery}}{\text{Oxygen consumption}}$$
$$= \frac{SaO_2}{SaO_2 - SvO_2}$$

This neonate with an oxygen saturation of 90% and a SvO_2 of 60% will have a calculated omega (Ω) of 3. Thus, the same neonate with poor ventricular function and SvO_2 of 30% will have a calculated omega (Ω) of 1.5, which is much lower than the neonate described in the question.[10]

12. (A) The mediators that are decreased in *pulmonary hypertension* include prostacyclin, matrix metalloproteinases, nitric oxide, and thrombomodulin. The other mediators listed above are all elevated in pulmonary hypertension, and these also include von Willebrand factor, P-selectin, plasminogen activating inhibitor, fibrinopeptide A, tissue plasminogen activator, angiotensin II, epinephrine, insulin-like growth factor, basic fibroblast growth factor, and platelet-derived growth factor A.[11]

13. (E) While it is possible to have a pulmonary hypertensive crisis after surgery for a VSD in an infant, a transesophageal echocardiogram is necessary to rule out the possibility of a significant residual VSD as the etiology for the elevated pulmonary artery pressure. Treatment for pulmonary hypertension should not be initiated until this possibility is ruled out. Otherwise, the measures to reduce pulmonary vascular resistance may actually further exacerbate hemodynamic instability if a significant residual VSD is present.

14. (E) The *Vaughn Williams classification* for *antiarrhythmic agents*[12] is as follows:

- *Class I*—local membrane-stabilizing activity: blocks fast sodium channel
    - IA—Moderate sodium blockade
    - Moderate phase 0 depression/intermediate slowing of conduction/prolongation of repolarization/prolongation of action potential and effective refractory period (quinidine, procainamide, disopyramide)
    - IB—Weak sodium blockade
    - Minimal phase 0 depression/little slowing of conduction/shortening of repolarization/shortening of action potential and effective refractory period (lidocaine, mexiletine, and phenytoin)
    - IC—Strong sodium blockade
    - Marked phase 0 depression/marked slowing of conduction/little effect on repolarization/little effect on action potential and effective refractory period (flecainide, encainide, propafenone)

- *Class II*—blocks β-adrenergic receptors (β-blockers)
- *Class III*—prolongs duration of cardiac action potential and repolarization but not conduction; blocks potassium channel (amiodarone, sotalol, bretylium)
- *Class IV*—blocks slow calcium channel and increasing effective refractory period of the AV node and slows conduction and reduces automaticity of sinus and AV nodes (verapamil)

15. (A) The *anticoagulants* commonly used in the cardiac intensive care setting with their mechanisms of action are:

- *Aspirin*—acetylation of cyclo-oxygenase to inhibit production of thromboxane A_2, a platelet aggregator
- *Heparin*—a mucopolysaccharide that increases the rate at which antithrombin III neutralizes thrombin, factor X, and also IX, XI, and XII
- *Streptokinase*—interacts with plasminogen to result in plasmin complex
- *Tissue plasminogen activator* (tPA)—binds to fibrin
- *Warfarin* (*coumadin*)—interferes with posttranslational modification of the vitamin K-dependent coagulation factors (II, VII, IX, X, and proteins C and S)

16. (C) A low *CVP* reading can be due to the pressure transducer above, not below, the level of the heart. The other answers are other causes of a reduced right atrial pressure.[6]

17. (E) A *reduced* oxygen saturation from the right atrium includes all the answers above except increased oxygen delivery, which increases oxygen saturation in the right atrium. An *increased* oxygen saturation in the right atrium can be due to an atrial level left-to-right shunt, an anomalous pulmonary venous vein, a left ventricular-to-right atrial shunt, increased oxygen delivery, decreased oxygen extraction, increased dissolved oxygen content, or catheter tip position near the renal vein.[6]

18. (A) A canal-type VSD with straddling tricuspid valve is a high-risk anatomic substrate for heart block. In addition, a perimembranous VSD is also at some risk for heart block as the bundle of His courses posterior-inferiorly to the defect. The other types of VSD, especially muscular and subpulmonary types, have much less risk for heart block.[13]

19. (D) In total anomalous pulmonary venous connection, the left-sided structures are borderline hypoplastic and noncompliant, resulting in relatively *high left atrial pressure* and tachycardia (although atrial flutter or atrial ectopic tachycardia will need to be ruled out). The other lesions usually do not lead to the left atrial pressure being higher than the right atrial pressure.[14]

20. (D) *Neosynephrine* is a pure α-agonist and is useful in the clinical situation of decreased pulmonary blood flow in the presence of an unrestrictive VSD or single ventricle as any increase in systemic vascular resistance will result in an increase in pulmonary blood flow. An infant with double outlet right ventricle and transposition physiology would be the least likely to respond favorably to neosynephrine.[15]

21. (B) The diagnosis with the distinctive murmur is *tetralogy of Fallot* with *absent pulmonary valve*. This lesion is associated with an enlarged main and branch pulmonary arteries that compress the proximal airways. In addition, there is distal airway disease as the serpigenous pulmonary arterioles encircle the distal bronchioles. The prone position can often decrease the proximal airway obstruction due to the massively dilated pulmonary arteries.[16]

22. (D) *Pulmonary vasoconstrictors* include angiotensin II, leukotrienes C4, D4, and E4, prostaglandin F2α, thromboxane A2, and serotonin. Pulmonary vasodilators include acetylcholine, bradykinin, prostaglandins E1, E2, and I2, and nitric oxide. Epinephrine, norepinephrine, endothelins, histamine, and prostaglandin D2 can have variable effect on the pulmonary circulation.[17]

23. (C) The first intervention in a Fontan patient with an elevated PA pressure should be an *echocardiogram* to rule out pericardial tamponade and to assess myocardial function. A *CXR* can also be very useful to assess pulmonary parenchyma. An *EKG* is of secondary importance as the HR is not exceedingly high to suggest intraatrial reentrant tachycardia. A *cardiac catheterization* can be performed if both the echocardiogram and the CXR are normal to rule out thrombosis and stenosis of the pulmonary arteries. *Initiation of IV milrinone* and *inhaled nitric oxide* should be reserved after a diagnosis is made.[8]

24. (B) The pathophysiology is excessive pulmonary blood flow and resultant *wide pulse pressure* and low diastolic pressure. IV dopamine can increase the diastolic pressure as can transfusion of packed RBCs and volume. Decreasing the sedation can also increase the blood pressure. IV milrinone would be very risky given the low diastolic pressure.[18]

25. (A) *Ross–Konno operation* involves enlargement of the LVOT via a patch so there is the possibility of a residual VSD or RVOT narrowing. LV function with valvar aortic stenosis is often impaired as a result of concentric hypertrophy and suboptimal myocardial protection during bypass. In addition, coronary ischemia can occur with the coronary implantation. Occasionally, the neoaortic valve can have some degree of insufficiency. Pulmonary hypertension would be uncommon and unexpected (see Fig. 9.10).[19]

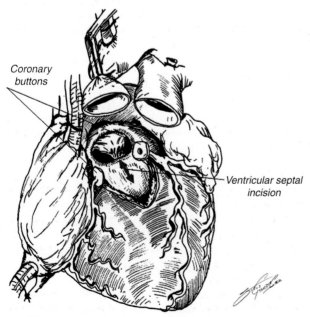

Coronary buttons

Ventricular septal incision

FIGURE 9.10

26. (D) A *pericardial tamponade* can lead to elevated right and left atrial pressures with concomitant tachycardia. *Junctional ectopic tachycardia,* usually more common in infants with corrective surgeries that involve a ventricular septal defect, can result in elevated filling pressures due to atrioventricular dyssynchrony. At 4 weeks of age, an infant with transposition of the great arteries could have an unprepared left ventricle and thus higher filling pressures. Myocardial depression from either cardiopulmonary bypass or a coronary transfer complication can both result in myocardial depression. While aortopulmonary collaterals can exist in the transposition of the great arteries and result in some left ventricular volume load, it is highly unlikely that the collaterals will lead to an elevated left atrial pressure.[6]

27. (A) Infants with asplenia and infants who had repair of total anomalous pulmonary venous return can have increased likelihood of *ectopic atrial tachycardia. Reentrant type of supraventricular tachycardia* mostly likely would have a sudden onset and would have responded to adenosine, which is very effective in converting reentrant type of supraventricular tachycardia. *Junctional ectopic tachycardia* is usually observed in infants who had corrective surgery that involved VSD closure (such as tetralogy of Fallot or truncus arteriosus). Lastly, *ventricular tachycardia* in a postoperative setting is usually associated with myocardial ischemia.[12]

28. (B) *Ischemic bowel syndrome* is usually associated with left-sided obstructive lesions such as hypoplastic left heart syndrome, coarctation, and aortic stenosis. Truncus arteriosus, with runoff into the pulmonary arteries and with truncal regurgitation, has a low diastolic pressure and therefore suboptimal perfusion to the mesenteric tract. Tetralogy of Fallot, particularly in the absence of excessive pulmonary blood flow from numerous aortopulmonary collaterals, is unlikely to be associated with ischemic bowel syndrome.[20]

29. (C) Milrinone usually does not increase HR or blood pressure, the components of rate pressure index, an indirect determinant of myocardial oxygen consumption. The other agents all increase HR and therefore the rate pressure index or myocardial oxygen consumption.

30. (C) The ratio of pulmonary to systemic blood flow can be easily calculated in *single ventricle physiology* patients by first making several assumptions. First, the a–v O_2 difference between the aorta and the mixed venous source is 25%. Second, there is no significant pulmonary venous desaturation so that the pulmonary venous saturation is 95% to 100%. Third, the aortic and pulmonary artery saturations are equal (the former measured by pulse oximetry). The equation is [Ao – mixed venous saturation]/[pulmonary venous – pulmonary artery saturation].[21] In this case, the equation is [25%]/[95% – 83%] or about 2:1.

31. (A) After a bidirectional cavopulmonary anastomosis, a myriad of issues can lead to an elevated SVC pressure with a large transpulmonary gradient. In this case, the transpulmonary gradient is 14 mm Hg, which is elevated. Among reasons for this finding would be elevated pulmonary vascular resistance, pulmonary venous obstruction, pulmonary problems such as pleural effusion or pneumothorax, and thrombosis within the cavopulmonary circuit. Poor ventricular compliance would also result in an elevated SVC pressure, but with an increased left atrial pressure.[2]

32. (D) The three common risk factors for irreversible pulmonary hypertension include *increased pulmonary blood flow, increased pulmonary artery pressure,* and *cyanosis.* Additional risk factors include pulmonary hypoplasia and pulmonary venous hypertension.

Of the choices, the 9-month-old with transposition of the great arteries is the oldest with all three risk factors (the other lesions with all three risk factors being common atrioventricular canal and truncus arteriosus) and therefore at highest risk for significant pulmonary hypertension after surgery. Children with atrial septal defect are at minimal risk for pulmonary hypertension, as they have only one of the three risk factors. Children with ventricular septal defects have more risk if the defect is unrestrictive.

33. (D) A *hypercyanotic spell* in tetralogy of Fallot is thought to be a decrease in systemic vascular resistance leading to increased right-to-left shunting and cyanosis. A β-blocker such as esmolol can be utilized to decrease HR and possibly decrease the right ventricular outflow tract narrowing. Neosynephrine, an α-agonist, will increase systemic vascular resistance and thereby force more flow to the pulmonary circulation via the right ventricular outflow tract. Oxygen, albeit of limited benefit, can improve oxygenation particularly if the etiology for the cyanosis is partly from pulmonary disease. Isoproterenol, a pulmonary and systemic vasodilator, can potentially exacerbate the cyanosis by inducing tachycardia and further narrowing of the right ventricular outflow tract. Lastly, fluids and packed red blood cells can increase the flow out the narrowed right ventricular outflow tract and improve systemic oxygenation; packed red blood cells can also increase systemic vascular resistance.

34. (B) The hemodynamic profile reveals left atrial hypertension while the right atrial pressure remains normal.

The etiologic factors for elevated left atrial pressure include left atrial outlet obstruction (e.g., mitral stenosis), left ventricular dysfunction (systolic or diastolic), hypoplasia of the left ventricle, pericardial tamponade, and atrioventricular dyssynchrony. Anomalous left coronary artery from the pulmonary artery is associated with left ventricular dysfunction which will persist months after surgery. A 2-month-old with transposition of the great arteries could have a left ventricle that has muscle regression and what is termed an "unprepared left ventricle." Left-sided obstructive lesions often will have left ventricle hypertrophy, therefore a less compliant left ventricle. Lastly, total anomalous pulmonary venous return has a small and noncompliant left ventricle as a result of the dilated right ventricle. Tetralogy of Fallot patients usually have an elevated right atrial pressure due to restrictive physiology of the hypertrophied right ventricle.

35. (B) A patient after tetralogy of Fallot repair has *restrictive right ventricular pathophysiology.* The right ventricle is noncompliant and has significant diastolic dysfunction. Judicious volume resuscitation will improve cardiac output as the right ventricle often requires a filling pressure >10 mm Hg. An electrocardiogram can be obtained to assess the possibility of junctional ectopic tachycardia. An echocardiogram at this point, while not critical, can be used to assess right ventricular volume status and rule out a significant pericardial fluid collection. Lastly, a milrinone infusion is efficacious as it has lusitropic properties. An isoproterenol infusion will have deleterious hemodynamic consequences of further tachycardia and lower systemic blood pressure.

36. (E) The relationship between the pericardial volume and pressure is curvilinear, so choices B and D are incorrect. The curves A and C are also incorrect. The pericardial pressure does not increase with volume until a certain volume threshold is reached, and then the pressure rapidly increases with further increase in volume. The curve C is only partially correct as only the right half of the curve accurately reflects the pericardial volume–pressure relationship.

37. (E) Hypertension occurring after coarctation repair is secondary to excess of endogenous catecholamines and can be treated with β-*blockade* (such as esmolol and labetolol). *Vasodilators* such as nitroprusside and hydralazine can also be used to lower systemic hypertension. Isoproterenol, a synthetic catecholamine, will increase HR and catecholamine state and is not indicated for this situation.

38. (D) In the bidirectional cavopulmonary circulation, any increase in pulmonary vascular resistance can open decompressing veins to result in a shunt of venous blood into the heart (often demonstrable with a contrast echocardiogram). A pleural effusion or any reason for an elevated pulmonary vascular resistance can result in this phenomenon. Low arterial paCO$_2$ can reduce cerebral blood flow, thus indirectly reducing pulmonary blood flow and thus oxygen saturation. Of the choices, atrioventricular valve regurgitation is the least likely to affect systemic oxygenation.[2]

39. (D) The pharmacologic agents that have been demonstrated to have efficacy for *junctional ectopic tachycardia* include amiodarone, procainamide, and digoxin. Hypothermia has also been shown to reduce the ectopic rate. As this is an ectopic tachycardia, adenosine can be a diagnostic agent but not a therapy for this tachydysrhythmia.[12]

40. (A) While the relationships B through E are curvilinear, only the relationship between lung volume and pulmonary vascular resistance is a "U"-shaped curve.[1]

41. (C) *Restrictive cardiomyopathy* patients have characteristically elevated right and left atrial pressures and pulmonary hypertension. A child with a large *pericardial effusion* will have elevated right atrial pressures. A child with *tetralogy of Fallot* will have right ventricular hypertrophy and a stiff right ventricle, and this is exacerbated by any residual right ventricular outflow tract obstruction. Finally, a child with chronic *dilated cardiomyopathy* will have elevated right and left atrial pressures. An infant with moderate tricuspid valve regurgitation, due to a relatively compliant right atrium, can have regurgitation and an enlarged right atrium but without significantly elevated right atrial pressure.

42. (A) In patients after repair for total anomalous pulmonary venous drainage, pulmonary hypertension occurs often but any residual pulmonary venous obstruction should be ruled out first by echocardiogram or, if necessary, cardiac catheterization. Any therapy (inhaled nitric oxide, IV sildenafil, or milrinone) should take place after significant residual pulmonary venous obstruction has been ruled out.

43. (C) In *catecholamine-resistant shock* after cardiopulmonary bypass, vasopressin, steroids, and even thyroxine have been studied and used to ameliorate hemodynamic profile.

Extracorporeal membrane oxygenation is used as a last resort in selected cases. Phenoxybenzamine is an α-antagonist and leads to vasodilation.

44. (D) Both tetralogy of Fallot and truncus arteriosus surgeries involve significant incisions into right ventricular muscle, resulting in a *complete right bundle branch block*. Similarly, subaortic muscle resection can result in a *left bundle branch block*. Q waves in leads I and avL is the classic EKG finding for anomalous left coronary artery from the pulmonary artery. After a successful arterial switch operation, there should not be any Q waves on a 12-lead EKG.

45. (B) The catheterization data show transpulmonary gradient of 13 mm Hg (pulmonary artery pressure − left atrial pressure). The patient therefore is likely to have an elevated pulmonary vascular resistance as the transpulmonary gradient is elevated. The end-diastolic pressure of 4 mm Hg is good for a single ventricle. Lastly, the simultaneous pulmonary artery wedge and end-diastolic pressure show no gradient, thus supporting evidence for no stenosis of the atrioventricular valve or pulmonary venous anatomy. With an oxygen saturation of 99% despite a pulmonary artery pressure of 18 mm Hg, it is not likely that the fenestration is still patent.

46. (C) The *LV pressure–volume curves* show an increase in stroke volume at time B compared to time A. The curves labeled A and B depict the end-diastolic pressure–volume relationship. Curve B shows improved diastolic function as the curve is more flat; this results in an increase in stroke volume.

47. (B) The history and noninvasive findings are most consistent with *restrictive cardiomyopathy*, which is a cardiomyopathy characterized by abnormal diastolic function and very dilated atria. The systolic function is often intact. The atrial pressures are elevated, thus affecting pulmonary artery pressures so that there is often pulmonary hypertension. Lastly, children succumb to cerebrovascular accidents, atrial tachydysrhythmias, and sudden death. Acute myocarditis and dilated cardiomyopathy would have decreased LV ejection fraction and increased LV end-diastolic dimension. Children with *hypertrophic cardiomyopathy* do not have dilated atria but hypertrophied ventricles. Pulmonary hypertension patients sometimes have dilated right atrium from tricuspid regurgitation but left atrium is usually not dilated.

48. (D) In heart failure, *angiotensin II* and *arginine vasopressin* as well as *endothelin* are known vasoconstrictors that result in cardiac stimulation and fluid retention. In addition, *norepinephrine* also stimulates the heart as part of the neurohumoral response in heart failure. B-type natriuretic peptide is a vasodilator and a natriuretic.

49. (C) The 12-lead EKG is most consistent with *myocarditis*. The voltages are diminished and there are T-wave flattening and inversions. *Anomalous left coronary artery from the pulmonary artery* would have Q waves in leads I and avL. *Ectopic atrial tachycardia* usually has an abnormal P-wave axis, although it can be in the sinus region (thus mimicking sinus tachycardia). There is no evidence for *myocardial infarction* as seen with coronary aneurysm and thrombosis. The EKG has no suggested findings consistent with congenitally corrected transposition of the great arteries.

50. (A) The *LV pressure–volume curves* show effects of both afterload reduction (A to B and C to D) as well as increase in inotropic state (line CD to line AB). Milrinone has both afterload reduction and inotropic state properties, so would most likely change the pressure–volume curve from C (high SVR and poor contractile function) to B (lower SVR and improved contractile function).

51. (E) The surgeon has inadvertently closed the atrial septal defect by sewing the patch onto the eustachian valve. This case highlights an *"IVC-confluent" secundum atrial septal defect*. In such cases the posterior rim of the septum primum is often absent and the defect may be contiguous with the IVC. The patient will develop profound desaturation and cyanosis.

52. (C) Both the right atrium (RA) and right ventricle (RV) are compliant structures and increased intrapericardial pressure leads to their collapse when intracavitary pressures are only slightly exceeded by those in the pericardium. *RV and RA diastolic collapse is the most specific echo finding demonstrated in severe tamponade*. See Figure 9.11.

- *Diastolic collapse of the right atrium (RA)*: At end-diastole (during atrial relaxation), the RA volume is minimal, but pericardial pressure is maximal, causing the RA to buckle (*lower left*).
- *Diastolic collapse of the right ventricle (RV)*: RV diastolic collapse occurs in early diastole when the RV volume is still low. RV collapse is more specific than RA collapse. However, RV collapse may not occur when the RV is hypertrophied or its diastolic pressure is greatly elevated (*upper and lower left*).
- *Left atrial collapse*: This condition occurs in only about 25% of patients with hemodynamic compromise (*upper right*).
- *Left ventricular collapse*: This condition is less common since the wall of the left ventricle is more muscular, but it can be seen in cases of regional cardiac tamponade.
- *IVC plethora*: Dilatation and less than a 50% reduction in the diameter of the dilated inferior vena cava (IVC) during inspiration, reflecting a marked elevation in central venous pressure, is frequently seen in patients with cardiac tamponade though not very specific (lower right).

See Reference 22 for further information.

53. (E)

$$\frac{Qp}{Qs} = \frac{SaO_2 - SvO_2}{SpvO_2 - SpaO_2}$$

After Norwood, $SaO_2 = SpaO_2$
Assume $SpvO_2 = 100\%$

$$0.5 = \frac{60 - 40}{100 - 60}$$

This patient has low systemic vascular resistance (SVR) and is cyanotic from poor pulmonary blood flow through the shunt. The patient would benefit from agents that increase afterload (α-agonist) and shift the balance of blood into the pulmonary bed (improved shunt flow). Inhaled nitric oxide may lower pulmonary vascular resistance and also improve pulmonary blood flow.

With excessive pulmonary blood flow, efforts should be made to decrease SVR and augment blood flow to the systemic bed.

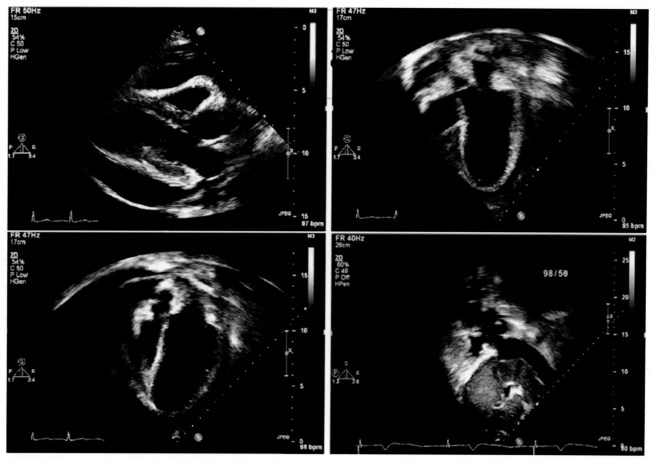

FIGURE 9.11

54. (C) This patient suffered a significant hypotensive event leading to cerebral hypoperfusion-related hypoxic ischemic encephalopathy (HIE) findings on MRI and clinical symptoms of seizure. This was to secondary to IVIG. After fever, chills, and rash, hypotension is the next most common infusion reaction related to IVIG. Hypotension can be attenuated in this case by the burden of other afterload-reducing heart failure medications. Hypotension can develop within 1 to 6 hours from onset of IVIG infusion.

Embolic stroke from apical or left atrial thrombus is a plausible cause of stroke in some patients and may be prevented by antiplatelet/anticoagulation therapy (answer B). This echo shows no evidence of thrombus and no evidence of endocarditis necessitating antibiotic therapy (answer D). However, a localized lesion of cerebral ischemia would have been evident on MRI. Lastly, a bolus of milrinone would have been inappropriate in this scenario because it may potentiate severe hypotension related to its peripheral vasodilatory effects (answer A).

55. (E) Echo findings demonstrate right-to-left shunting through patent ductus arteriosus (PDA) due to elevated pulmonary vascular resistance (PVR). In this scenario, elevated PVR is secondary to lung disease (immature lungs and infant RDS from meconium aspiration). This can lead to a physiology of *persistent fetal circulation* also known as *"persistent pulmonary hypertension."* (See Fig. 9.12.) Treatment of *mechanical ventilation, antibiotics, and nitric oxide* worked to decrease pulmonary vascular resistance and improve retrograde diastolic filling through the PDA. This resulted in improved PVR, pulmonary artery flow, systemic saturations,

cardiac function, and resolution of hypotension. Many infants refractory to such medical therapy may require extracorporeal mechanical support. Ductal closure in this scenario is *absolutely contraindicated.*

56. (E) *Coronary ischemia* after arterial switch and coronary reimplantation should be of high suspicion in a patient with signs of ventricular dysfunction and ventricular ectopy in the absence of tamponade physiology. Echocardiography may be useful to look for ventricular dysfunction or new valvular regurgitation consistent with papillary muscle ischemia and also to rule out tamponade. However, coronary origins are extremely difficult to visualize after

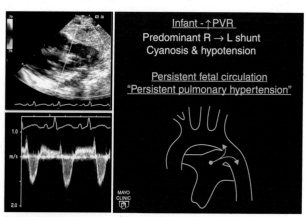

Infant - ↑PVR
Predominant R → L shunt
Cyanosis & hypotension

Persistent fetal circulation
"Persistent pulmonary hypertension"

FIGURE 9.12

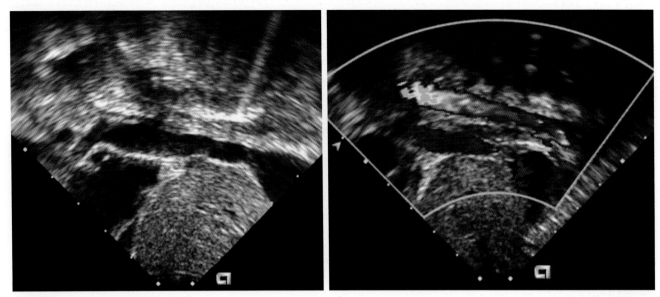

FIGURE 9.13

reimplantation. Electrocardiography may demonstrate a regional ischemic pattern. Definitive diagnosis may be ascertained with catheterization or computerized tomography-based coronary angiography.

57. (D) *Infracardiac TAPVR* (Fig. 9.13) is a surgical emergency. Corrective surgery should be performed as soon as possible, especially in patients with progressive acidosis. It can masquerade as RDS/pneumonia. Septostomy is no longer recommended because it delays surgery and is only palliative. Additionally, balloon dilatation of obstructed venous channels has been shown to be an unsuccessful approach. Before starting extracorporeal mechanical support in this child, confirmation of anomalous veins is critical because once on mechanical support, the intracardiac anatomy will be very difficult to visualize. Prostaglandin infusion is not helpful in this case, even harmful. It leads to increase pulmonary blood flow and reduces the pulmonary vascular resistance and may exacerbate the pulmonary venous congestion.

58. (B) Transient atrioventricular (AV) block is seen in about 2% of patients and nearly half will have return of conduction around 3 days while the remaining 1% will require pacemakers. Incidence of permanent complete AV block is highest with repair of lesions near the atrioventricular node (membranous and inlet ventricular septal defects) and in patients with congenital corrected transposition, AV canal defects, and tetralogy of Fallot. Studies suggest that if sinus rhythm does not return after 7 days, it will never return. Therein, the guidelines recommend *pacemaker implantation for postoperative AV block that persists for at least 7 days* following surgery.[23–27]

59. (E) Chest film demonstrates left lung oligemia. Computerized tomography of the chest showed a poorly vascularized left lung, a residual patent ductus arteriosus, and a ligated left pulmonary artery. Angiogram demonstrated paucity of flow to the left lung (Fig. 9.14). *Inadvertent ligation of the left pulmonary artery* is a rare complication of surgical closure of the patent ductus arteriosus. Asymmetric pulmonary blood flow should raise index of suspicion. Delayed recognition may negate surgical correction.[28]

60. (D) Sternal closure has several important hemodynamic consequences. The concept of "open chest" was developed to facilitate decompression of the heart and minimize tamponade physiology. Sternal closure acts to decrease stroke volume and subsequently cardiac output which yields secondary effects of decreased mean blood pressure and cerebral oxygenation. Pulmonary hemodynamics are also affected as there is an increase in intrathoracic pressure and decrease in total lung compliance. All clinical details must be assessed to determine the adequate timing of chest closure. All patients must be closely monitored for hemodynamic instability following closure.

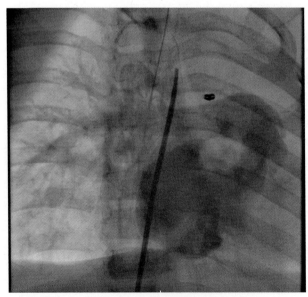

FIGURE 9.14

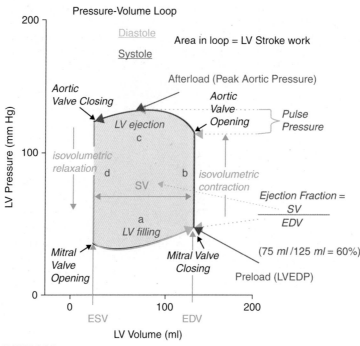

FIGURE 9.15

61. (D) Atrial overdrive burst pacing (3 to 4 seconds) can suc-cessfully convert atrial flutter. To avoid risk of deterioration into atrial fibrillation, utilizing burst rate of 70% of the atrial cycle length will successfully convert atrial flutter. If pacing wires are nonfunctional or not present, pacing may be instituted from esophageal leads. Electrical cardioversion (not listed here as an answer) would also be an acceptable option for elimination of atrial flutter.[29]

62. (B) Studies have demonstrated maximal therapeutic effects of nitric oxide at 20 ppm, with higher doses associated with increased risk of side effects and no improvement in outcome. Side effects include systemic hypotension, methemoglobinemia, rebound pulmonary hypertension upon weaning, and elevated nitrous oxide.[30,31]

63. (C) Systemic hypertension (↑ aortic pressure) will increase afterload. This increases the left ventricular pressure required to open aortic valve.

The aortic valve closes at a higher end-systolic pressure, which (without a change in inotropic state) yields reduced stroke volume (↓ width of pressure–volume loop). The end-systolic pres-sure–volume relationship (contractility slope) remains unchanged.

64. (E) Agents that increase systemic vascular resistance increase afterload and decrease stroke volume (phenylephrine, vaso-pressin, and epinephrine). Sodium nitroprusside will decrease afterload and improve stroke volume and cardiac output. β-Blockade may also be useful to slow HR and improve diastol-ic ventricular filling and coronary artery flow. (See Fig. 9.15.)

REFERENCES

1. Nelson DP, Wessel DL. Chapter 6: Normal physiology of the respiratory system. In: Chang AC, Hanley FL, Wernovsky G, et al., eds. *Pediatric Cardiac Intensive Care.* Philadelphia, PA: Lippincott Williams & Wilkins; 1998:76.
2. Wernovsky G, Bove EL. Chapter 18: Single ventricle lesions. In: Chang AC, Hanley FL, Wernovsky G, et al., eds. *Pediatric Cardiac Intensive Care.* Philadelphia, PA: Lippincott Williams & Wilkins; 1998:278–281.
3. Wernovsky G, Chang AC, Wessel DL, et al., Chapter 20: Cardiac intensive care. In: *Moss and Adams' Heart Disease in Infants, Children, and Adolescents.* 7th ed. Philadelphia, PA: Lippincott Williams & Wilkins; 2008:473–475.
4. Perry JC, Walsh EP. Chapter 30: Diagnosis and management of cardiac arrhythmia. In: Chang AC, Hanley FL, Wernovsky G, et al., eds. *Pediatric Cardiac Intensive Care.* Philadelphia, PA: Lippincott Williams & Wilkins; 1998:473–475.
5. Kulik TJ. Chapter 32: Pulmonary hypertension. In: Chang AC, et al., eds. *Pediatric Cardiac Intensive Care.* Philadelphia, PA: Lippincott Williams & Wilkins; 1998:500–501.
6. Roth S. Chapter 13: Postoperative care. In: Chang AC, Hanley FL, Wernovsky G, et al., eds. *Pediatric Cardiac Intensive Care.* Philadelphia, PA: Lippincott Williams & Wilkins; 1998: 168–170.
7. Chang AC, Burke RP. Chapter 16: Left ventricular outflow tract obstruction. In: Chang AC, Hanley FL, Wernovsky G, et al., eds. *Pediatric Cardiac Intensive Care.* Philadelphia, PA: Lippincott Williams & Wilkins; 1998:251–254.
8. Wernovsky G, Bove EL. Chapter 18: Single ventricle lesions. In: Chang AC, Hanley FL, Wernovsky G, et al., eds. *Pediatric Cardiac Intensive Care.* Philadelphia, PA: Lippincott Williams & Wilkins; 1998:281–284.
9. Hastings LA, Heitmiller ES, Nyham D. Chapter 19: Perioperative monitoring. In: Nichols DG, Underleider RM, Spevak PJ, et al.,

eds. *Critical Heart Disease in Infants and Children*. Philadelphia, PA: Mosby; 2006:490–491, Table 19-4.

10. Marino BS. Chapter 38: Single-ventricle lesions. In: Nichols DG, Underleider RM, Spevak PJ, et al., eds. *Critical Heart Disease in Infants and Children*. Philadelphia, PA: Mosby; 2006:790–791.

11. Smerling AJ, Schleien CL, Barst RJ, et al. Chapter 43: Pulmonary hypertension. In: Nichols DG, Underleider RM, Spevak PJ, et al., eds. *Critical Heart Disease in Infants and Children*. Philadelphia, PA: Mosby; 2006:890, Table 43-4.

12. Perry JC, Walsh EP. Chapter 30: Diagnosis and management of cardiac arrhythmia. In: Chang AC, Hanley FL, Wernovsky G, et al., eds. *Pediatric Cardiac Intensive Care*. Philadelphia, PA: Lippincott Williams & Wilkins; 1998:475–480.

13. Chang AC, Jacobs J. Chapter 15: Shunt lesions. In: Chang AC, Hanley FL, Wernovsky G, et al., eds. *Pediatric Cardiac Intensive Care*. Philadelphia, PA: Lippincott Williams & Wilkins; 1998:216.

14. Chang AC, Burke RP. Chapter 15: Shunt lesions. In: Chang AC, Hanley FL, Wernovsky G, et al., eds. *Pediatric Cardiac Intensive Care*. Philadelphia, PA: Lippincott Williams & Wilkins; 1998:227.

15. Spray TL, Wernovsky G. Chapter 17: Right ventricular outflow tract obstruction. In: Chang AC, Hanley FL, Wernovsky G, et al., eds. *Pediatric Cardiac Intensive Care*. Philadelphia, PA: Lippincott Williams & Wilkins; 1998:257.

16. Spray TL, Wernovsky G. Chapter 17: Right ventricular outflow tract obstruction. In: Chang AC, Hanley FL, Wernovsky G, et al., eds. *Pediatric Cardiac Intensive Care*. Philadelphia, PA: Lippincott Williams & Wilkins; 1998:263–264.

17. Kulik TJ. Chapter 32: Pulmonary hypertension. In: Chang AC, Hanley FL, Wernovsky G, et al., eds. *Pediatric Cardiac Intensive Care*. Philadelphia, PA: Lippincott Williams & Wilkins; 1998:499, Table 32.1.

18. Wernovsky G, Bove EL. Chapter 18: Single-ventricle lesions. In: Chang AC, Hanley FL, Wernovsky G, et al., eds. *Pediatric Cardiac Intensive Care*. Philadelphia, PA: Lippincott Williams and Wilkins; 1998:274–277.

19. Chang AC, Burke RP. Chapter 16: Left ventricular outflow tract obstruction. In: Chang AC, Hanley FL, Wernovsky G, et al., eds. *Pediatric Cardiac Intensive Care*. Philadelphia, PA: Lippincott Williams and Wilkins; 1998: 234–240.

20. Markowitz RI, Fellows KE. Chapter 27: Perioperative radiographic studies. In: Chang AC, Hanley FL, Wernovsky G, et al., eds. *Pediatric Cardiac Intensive Care*. Philadelphia, PA: Lippincott Williams and Wilkins; 1998:415–417.

21. Wernovsky G, Bove EL. Chapter 18: Single-ventricle lesions. In: Chang AC, Hanley FL, Wernovsky G, et al., eds. *Pediatric Cardiac Intensive Care*. Philadelphia, PA: Lippincott Williams & Wilkins; 1998:271–274.

22. Mercé J, Sagristà-Sauleda J, Permanyer-Miralda G, et al. Correlation between clinical and Doppler echocardiographic findings in patients with moderate and large pericardial effusion: implications for the diagnosis of cardiac tamponade. *Am Heart J*. 1999;138(4 Pt 1):759–764.

23. Epstein AE, Dimarco JP, Ellenbogen KA, et al. ACC/AHA/HRS 2008 guidelines for device-based therapy of cardiac rhythm abnormalities: executive summary. *Heart Rhythm*. 2008;5(6):934–955.

24. Ayyildiz P, Kasar T, Ozturk E, et al. Evaluation of permanent or transient complete heart block after open heart surgery for congenital heart disease. *Pacing Clin Electrophysiol*. 2016;39(2):160–165.

25. Lin A, Mahle WT, Frias PA, et al. Early and delayed atrioventricular conduction block after routine surgery for congenital heart disease. *J Thorac Cardiovasc Surg*. 2010;140(1):158–160.

26. Gross GJ, Chiu CC, Hamilton RM, et al. Natural history of postoperative heart block in congenital heart disease: implications for pacing intervention. *Heart Rhythm*. 2006;3(5):601–604.

27. Weindling SN, Saul JP, Gamble WJ, et al. Duration of complete atrioventricular block after congenital heart disease surgery. *Am J Cardiol*. 1998;82(4):525–527.

28. da Costa e Silva EJ, de Albuquerque SC. Left pulmonary artery ligation. *Pediatr Radiol*. 2010;40(Suppl 1):S86. Doi: 10.1007/s00247-010-1879-0.

29. Campbell RM, Dick M 2nd, Jenkins JM, et al. Atrial overdrive pacing for conversion of atrial flutter in children. *Pediatrics*. 1985; 75(4):730–736.

30. Cannon BC, Feltes TF, Fraley JK, et al. Nitric oxide in the evaluation of congenital heart disease with pulmonary hypertension: factors related to nitric oxide response. *Pediatr Cardiol*. 2005; 26(5):565–569.

31. Kinsella JP, Neish SR, Shaffer E, et al. Low-dose inhalation nitric oxide in persistent pulmonary hypertension of the newborn. *Lancet*. 1992;340(8823):819–820.

CHAPTER 10

Heart Failure, Pulmonary Hypertension, and Transplant

Sonja Dahl and Jonathan N. Johnson

QUESTIONS

1. Which of the following is a contraindication to heart transplantation to a pediatric patient?

   A. History of Fontan operation
   B. Elevated PVR = 12 Woods units on nitric oxide
   C. History of protein-losing enteropathy
   D. Prior alcohol addiction, has been sober for 1 year
   E. History of pulmonary embolism, resolved

2. A 14-year-old girl is referred for evaluation for cardiac transplantation. In the teenage years, which of the following is the most common indication for heart transplantation?

   A. Cardiomyopathy
   B. Congenital heart disease
   C. Retransplantation
   D. Malignancy
   E. Intractable arrhythmias

3. A 15-month-old male infant is 4 weeks post orthotopic heart transplantation. His parents bring him in with new-onset fussiness over the past day. He has been refusing to eat or drink for the last 4 hours. Of the following new physical examination findings, which one is most concerning for allograft rejection?

   A. Petechiae on his right foot
   B. Splitting of the first heart sound
   C. Dry mucous membranes
   D. Gallop rhythm
   E. Soft 1/6 systolic murmur at the left upper sternal border

4. A 14-year-old patient, 2 years post orthotopic heart transplant for dilated cardiomyopathy, presents with new-onset shortness of breath. An echocardiogram is performed as part of the workup. Which of the following echo findings is most concerning for rejection?

   A. Increase in the descending aorta flow velocity from 1.2 to 1.4 m/s
   B. Decrease in the left ventricular ejection fraction from 68% to 62%
   C. Increase in the lateral mitral valve e' velocity from 0.08 to 0.12 m/s
   D. Decrease in the IVC diameter from 2.3 to 1.8 cm.
   E. Increase in the degree of mitral regurgitation from trivial to moderate

5. A 14-year-old girl presents for routine follow-up. She had a heart transplant at age 7 months for hypoplastic left heart syndrome and ventricular dysfunction. On examination, she has a blood pressure in her right arm of 150/85 mm Hg. Echocardiography reveals the following abdominal aortic Doppler signal (see Figure 10.1). Which of the following is the next best step?

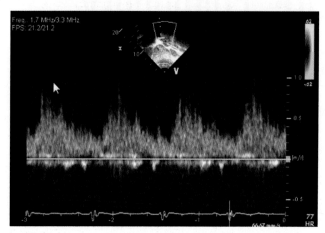

FIGURE 10.1

    A. ICU for administration of a steroid bolus (10 mg/kg/dose q24 hours × 3)
    B. Operating room for tricuspid valve repair
    C. Cardiac cath lab for balloon angioplasty or stenting
    D. Operating room for revision of IVC anastomosis
    E. Cardiac cath lab for coronary angiography with IVUS (intravascular ultrasound)

6. Which of the following is a contraindication to combined heart–lung transplant for a pediatric patient?

    A. Cystic fibrosis
    B. Active tuberculosis
    C. Idiopathic pulmonary hypertension
    D. Eisenmenger syndrome
    E. History of recurrent otitis media

7. A 7-year-old girl with a history of heart transplantation 2 years ago presents with new-onset seizures. The seizures are controlled successfully with benzodiazepine administration. Laboratory evaluation reveals that the patient's tacrolimus level is 31.2 (goal range 6 to 8). Two weeks ago, the child's tacrolimus level was 7.9. The family reports that the child was started on a new medication 1 week ago by their primary care pediatrician. Which of the following is the most likely medication that was started?

    A. Trimethoprim/sulfamethoxazole
    B. Phenytoin
    C. Loratadine
    D. Fluconazole
    E. Metoprolol

8. A 17-year-old boy, post heart–lung transplantation 7 years ago, presents with exertional dyspnea. He reports that his daily incentive spirometry values have decreased progressively in recent weeks, though otherwise he has felt well. He is noted to have elevated exhaled nitric oxide levels, and there is a decrease in midexpiration flow rates (FEF 25 to 75). Echocardiography reveals normal left and right ventricular systolic function. Which of the following is the most likely cause of his symptoms?

    A. Posttransplant lymphoproliferative disorder
    B. Cytomegalovirus viremia
    C. Bronchiolitis obliterans
    D. Congestive heart failure
    E. Tuberculosis

9. An 8-year-old boy with restrictive cardiomyopathy is admitted to the hospital with shortness of breath. Which of the following examination or test findings portends a poor prognosis for this child?

    A. Pulmonary venous congestion on chest radiography
    B. Increased medial mitral valve annular E′ velocity on echo
    C. 2/6 low-pitched systolic murmur heard at the left lower sternal border
    D. Right atrial enlargement on echo
    E. Isolated PACs on 24-hour Holter monitoring

10. You are seeing a 2-year-old patient in clinic who is now 4 months post orthotopic heart transplantation. His mother recently has gone back to work, and the patient is cared for by maternal grandmother. For the past two weeks, the child's mother reports that he has been more irritable and has a poor appetite. The child's pediatrician saw him the day prior and noted no significant examination findings other than a potential gallop rhythm. There have been several recent ill contacts for the patient, all of whom have been diagnosed with upper respiratory viral illnesses.

In this patient, the gold standard test to rule out rejection is:

    A. Chest radiography
    B. Plasma BNP
    C. Cardiac MRI
    D. Electrocardiogram
    E. Myocardial biopsy

11. A 14-year-old girl is admitted to the intensive care unit for monitoring after elective surgery. She has a history of hypoplastic left heart syndrome and underwent heart transplantation as a neonate. She has had a relatively uncomplicated course, with no arrhythmias or other complications. During monitoring overnight, her nurse noted intermittent premature ventricular contractions, with brief runs of ventricular tachycardia. Which of the following is the most likely cause of her new-onset arrhythmia?

   A. Myocarditis
   B. Coronary artery vasculopathy
   C. Posttransplant lymphoproliferative disorder (PTLD)
   D. EBV viremia
   E. Posterior reversible encephalopathy syndrome (PRES)

12. A 13-year-old boy sees you in clinic for routine follow-up. He is 2 years post orthotopic heart transplantation for dilated cardiomyopathy. He reports that he has felt "jittery" lately. When he lifts his hand, he is unable to keep it still. Which of the following medications likely is causing this degree of tremulousness in this patient?

   A. Prednisone
   B. Mycophenolate mofetil
   C. Azathioprine
   D. Tacrolimus
   E. Sirolimus

13. An 11-year-old girl with no significant past medical history is diagnosed with pulmonary hypertension. She has two other family members who also have been diagnosed with pulmonary hypertension. Mutations in which of the following genes have been implicated in patients with familial pulmonary hypertension?

   A. *MLL2*
   B. *TBX5*
   C. *BMPR2*
   D. *JAG1*
   E. *PTNP11*

14. Which of the following is the mechanism of action of sildenafil?

   A. Blocks the enzyme phosphodiesterase from degrading cyclic GMP in smooth muscle cells
   B. Blocks both endothelin A and B receptors
   C. Replaces the loss of endogenous prostaglandin I2
   D. Blocks calcium channels
   E. Suppresses production of prostaglandins and thromboxanes by irreversibly inactivating the cyclooxygenase enzyme

15. An 8-year-old boy with restrictive cardiomyopathy is admitted to the hospital with shortness of breath. He has pulmonary venous congestion on his chest radiogram. His echocardiogram is unchanged, but shows normal ventricular function, massively dilated atria, and an estimated right ventricular systolic pressure of 65 mm Hg (systemic systolic blood pressure 120 mm Hg). Which of the following is the next best step in management of this patient?

   A. Liver ultrasound
   B. Cardiac CT to rule out pulmonary vein stenosis
   C. Reassurance
   D. Begin ACE-inhibitor medication
   E. Begin evaluation for heart transplantation

16. A 7-year-old patient is diagnosed with dilated cardiomyopathy. Two months later, he is seen in heart failure clinic. At the time of his evaluation, the patient is on appropriate doses of enalapril, carvedilol, spironolactone, and furosemide. The patient's symptoms have improved since the initiation of the medications, though he does continue to have some dyspnea with exertion. He has been able to attend school full time. His echo reveals a left ventricular ejection fraction of 15% to 20%, unchanged compared to his echo at the time of diagnosis. Which of the following is the next best step in management?

   A. Wean the enalapril
   B. Start digoxin
   C. Start verapamil
   D. Start amlodipine
   E. Wean the carvedilol

17. Which of the following best describes the mechanism of action of spironolactone?

   A. Inhibits chloride–sodium–potassium cotransport in the thick ascending limb of the loop of Henle
   B. Inhibits carbonic anhydrase
   C. Inhibits sodium and chloride transplant in the distal convoluted tubule
   D. Acts on the distal tubule to inhibit the effects of aldosterone
   E. Blocks L-type calcium channels in the heart

18. Which of the following is the mechanism of action of bosentan?

   A. Blocks the enzyme phosphodiesterase from degrading cyclic GMP in smooth muscle cells
   B. Blocks both endothelin A and B receptors
   C. Replaces the loss of endogenous prostaglandin I2
   D. Blocks calcium channels
   E. Suppresses production of prostaglandins and thromboxanes by irreversibly inactivating the cyclooxygenase enzyme.

19. A 14-year-old girl with a history of orthotopic heart transplantation as a neonate presents to the emergency department with acute onset of nausea, vomiting, fever, and hypoxia. Yesterday she began taking levofloxacin for treatment of recurrent lower-lobe pneumonia. In clinic yesterday, her vitals were normal with an oxygen saturation of 97%. Today, however, her oxygen saturation is 92% while breathing 4 to 5 L of oxygen via nasal cannula. Her chest x-ray is unchanged. Her maintenance medications include tacrolimus and prednisone, as well as dapsone for pneumocystis prophylaxis. Her arterial blood gas shows a pO_2 of 262 mm Hg, pCO_2 of 25 mm Hg, pH of 7.38, base of −9, and HCO_3 of 15. Her hemoglobin is 8.9, and her methemoglobin is elevated at 10.7. Echocardiography is normal. Which of the following would explain her acute hypoxia in absence of new respiratory symptoms?

- **A.** Allograft rejection
- **B.** Rare complication of levofloxacin in transplant patients
- **C.** Methemolobinemia
- **D.** Systemic hypoxia due to long-term use of tacrolimus
- **E.** Lung fibrosis due to prednisone

20. A 19-year-old woman begins taking enalapril for mildly depressed left ventricular systolic function. Which of the following is true regarding this patient after starting this medication?

- **A.** Less angiotensin I will be converted to angiotensin II
- **B.** There will be increased production of aldosterone
- **C.** Heart rate will be increased
- **D.** There will be a reduction in circulating bradykinins
- **E.** The patient can be counseled that there are no concerns with pregnancy

21. A 16-year-old boy undergoes myocardial biopsy as part of a routine postheart transplant protocol. The pathologist reports that the biopsy samples have several areas of lymphocytic infiltration with associated myocyte damage. The next best step in management for this patient is:

- **A.** Administration of IVIG
- **B.** Administration of antibiotics
- **C.** List for retransplantation
- **D.** Renal dialysis
- **E.** Administration of steroids

22. A 15-year-old otherwise normal girl is diagnosed with dilated cardiomyopathy. The family asks whether other members of the family may develop dilated cardiomyopathy as well. You inform them that many cases are sporadic; however, in familial/inherited cases, the most common pattern of inheritance is:

- **A.** X-linked recessive
- **B.** X-linked dominant
- **C.** Autosomal recessive

- **D.** Autosomal dominant
- **E.** Mitochondrial

23. A 3-year-old boy sees you in clinic for routine follow-up. He is 1 year post orthotopic heart transplantation for congenital heart disease. On laboratory evaluation, he is found to have a white blood cell count of 1.2, with an absolute neutrophil count of 0.4. Which of the following medications is likely causing his leukopenia?

- **A.** Prednisone
- **B.** Mycophenolate mofetil
- **C.** Amlodipine
- **D.** Tacrolimus
- **E.** Aspirin

24. A 7-year-old girl undergoes orthotopic heart transplantation for restrictive cardiomyopathy. Her serologic testing shows:

Donor: CMV positive, EBV positive, toxoplasma positive

Recipient: CMV negative, EBV negative, toxoplasma negative

The patient received induction therapy with antithymocyte globulin in the operating room. Considering the results of the serologic testing, which of the following would be recommended to reduce the likelihood of the patient developing posttransplant lymphoproliferative disorder (PTLD)?

- **A.** Minimize immunosuppression therapy due to EBV mismatch
- **B.** Start antiviral therapy directed at CMV immediately posttransplant
- **C.** Identify and treat early rejection
- **D.** Close monitoring of CMV titers in the first year following transplant
- **E.** Early transition of the primary immunosuppressant medication from a calcineurin inhibitor to mTOR inhibitor

25. A newborn male infant is diagnosed with dilated cardiomyopathy via echocardiography. The neonatologist notes a mild degree of hypotonia as well as proximal muscle weakness. Genetic evaluation reveals increased levels of 3-methylglutaconic acid in the blood and urine. Laboratory evaluation reveals normal hemoglobin but low neutrophil count. Further genetic testing reveals a mutation in the *TAZ* gene. You counsel the family that the patient has a genetic syndrome with which of the following modes of inheritance?

- **A.** Autosomal recessive
- **B.** Autosomal dominant
- **C.** X-linked recessive
- **D.** Mitochondrial
- **E.** None of the above

26. A 16-year-old boy with dilated cardiomyopathy (DCM) presents for evaluation of new-onset cough. The patient had been diagnosed with DCM 2 months prior, and treatment was begun with enalapril, spironolactone, furosemide, and digoxin. He describes the cough as dry, hacking, and persistent. Which of the following is the most appropriate next step in management?

    A. Discontinue furosemide and initiate bumetanide

    B. Discontinue enalapril and initiate losartan

    C. Discontinue digoxin

    D. Evaluate for heart transplantation

    E. Make no changes to the medical regimen

27. An 11-year-old girl undergoes myocardial biopsy and coronary angiography as part of a routine postheart transplant protocol. She is 10 years post orthotopic heart transplantation for congenital heart disease. The pathologist reports that the biopsy samples showed no evidence of rejection. On coronary angiography, areas of diffuse coronary luminal narrowing are noted in multiple branches. The left ventricular end diastolic pressure is measured at 25 mm Hg. The patient's current medications include tacrolimus and mycophenolate mofetil.

The most appropriate next step in management for this patient is:

    A. Administration of antibiotics

    B. Administration of pulsed steroids

    C. Conversion of tacrolimus to cyclosporine

    D. Plasmapheresis

    E. List the patient for cardiac retransplantation

28. An 18-month-old male infant with hypoplastic left heart syndrome (post Norwood and Glenn operations) undergoes orthotopic heart transplantation. Six months posttransplant, his family notes increased irritability. On examination, you note prominent veins in his neck and forehead. An echocardiogram is obtained (Fig. 10.2). Which of the following is the most appropriate next step in management?

    A. Admission to the intensive care unit for pulsed steroids

    B. Cardiac catheterization with stenting of the aorta

    C. Operating room for revision of the biatrial anastomosis

    D. Cardiac catheterization with stenting of his superior vena cava

    E. Cardiac catheterization for myocardial biopsy to rule out rejection

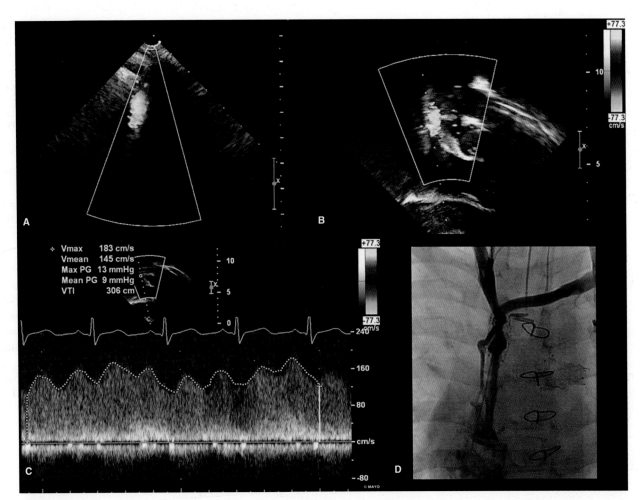

FIGURE 10.2

29. Which of the following best describes the mechanism of action of furosemide?

    A. Inhibits chloride–sodium–potassium cotransport in the ascending limb of the loop of Henle

    B. Inhibits sodium and chloride transport in the distal convoluted tubule

    C. Inhibits carbonic anhydrase

    D. Acts on the distal tubule to inhibit the effects of aldosterone

    E. Blocks L-type calcium channels in the heart

30. A 4-year-old girl presents with poor left ventricular function, estimated ejection fraction of 20%. There is a positive family history of cardiomyopathy, including her father who required cardiac transplantation at the age of 27. You decide to begin a heart failure regimen including carvedilol, enalapril, spironolactone, and furosemide. Which of the following best describes the mechanism of action of carvedilol in this patient?

    A. Selective blockade of β-1 adrenergic receptors, little or no effect on β-2 receptors

    B. Inhibition of angiotensin-converting enzyme, preventing conversion of angiotensin I to angiotensin II

    C. Direct vasodilation of arterioles with subsequent decrease in systemic resistance

    D. Nonselective β-adrenergic receptor blockade (β-1 and β-2) and α-adrenergic receptor blockade

    E. Blocks epithelial sodium channels in the late distal convoluted tubule and collecting duct, inhibiting sodium reabsorption from the lumen

ANSWERS

1. (B) An elevated pulmonary vascular resistance is a contraindication for transplantation, primarily due to the inability of the donor right ventricle to tolerate pumping against the elevated pressure and resistance. If the pulmonary hypertension is somewhat reversible with pulmonary vasodilators, transplantation might be considered, recognizing that significant right ventricular support may be needed postoperatively. A history of Fontan operation, protein-losing enteropathy, or plastic bronchitis are not contraindications to transplant; however, they do increase the risk of transplant due to multiple factors (extracardiac organ dysfunction, poor nutrition and wound healing, increased infection risk, increased risk of antibody-mediated rejection, and difficulty assessing for presensitization). Drug or alcohol addiction is a contraindication, unless the patient is able to fulfill a predetermined period of time of sobriety—the exact length of time is institution dependent. A history of resolved pulmonary embolism is not a contraindication, though an active pulmonary embolism is.

2. (A) For patients over the age of 1, especially in teenagers, the most common underlying diagnosis in patients having heart transplantation is cardiomyopathy (including dilated, restrictive, hypertrophic, and noncompaction cardiomyopathies). For infants, congenital heart disease is the most common indication, though this has been decreasing in the last several years. In the 1990s, almost 75% of infants having transplants had congenital heart disease; this has decreased to 53% in the most recent 5 years. The reasons behind this are multifactorial, but are at least in part indicative of improved Norwood outcomes for patients with hypoplastic left heart syndrome.

3. (D) Of all examination findings listed above, the presence of a new gallop rhythm is the most sensitive for rejection, though there typically are a constellation of findings. There may also be tachycardia, new murmurs of mitral regurgitation or tricuspid regurgitation, or evidence of congestion (hepatomegaly, jugular venous distension, abnormal chest x-ray, etc). Early after transplant, the patient may be anemic resulting in the soft flow murmur as in answer (E).

4. (E) There is no single echocardiographic finding that, by itself, has been shown to have perfect sensitivity or specificity for rejection in transplant patients. With this being said, the most common findings seen in patients with active rejection include new effusions, increased wall thickness and ventricular mass, and increased mitral or tricuspid valve regurgitation. Recent studies have shown that *decreases* in mitral valve tissue Doppler velocities may be very sensitive at detecting potential rejection episodes. The remainder of the findings listed are unlikely to be associated with rejection.

5. (C) The patient has evidence of diastolic continuation of forward flow in the abdominal aorta, consistent with upstream obstruction, most likely recoarctation. Patients with a history of hypoplastic left heart syndrome are at a particular risk for this complication after heart transplant.

6. (B) Contraindications to offering combined heart and lung transplants to pediatric patients include active tuberculosis, active malignancies, sepsis, severe systemic or neuromuscular diseases, multiorgan dysfunction, and any social concerns (involving the lack of social support networks). Patients on ECMO at the time of listing is controversial, with some centers listing and transplanting patients and others not listing patients on ECMO. Cystic fibrosis, pulmonary hypertension, and Eisenmenger syndrome are common indications for lung or heart–lung transplantation.

7. (D) Antifungal medications are a consistent cause of increased calcineurin inhibitor levels in transplant patients. As such, any time any of these medications are considered being started, close monitoring of tacrolimus/cyclosporine is required. Other medications that may increase tacrolimus/cyclosporine levels include amiodarone, macrolide antibiotics, calcium channel blockers, and metoclopramide. Medications that may decease tacrolimus/cyclosporine levels include octreotide, some anticonvulsants (phenytoin, phenobarbital, carbamazepine), and some antibiotics (nafcillin, IV bactrim). β-Blockers have little effect on tacrolimus/cyclosporine levels. Patients who have tacrolimus toxicity have irritability and tremulousness and may have seizures if levels are high enough.

8. (C) Bronchiolitis obliterans is chronic inflammation of the bronchioles that results in fibrous deposition, ultimately obstructing airways. It is considered a form of chronic rejection in lung transplant recipients. Clinical presentation can be nonspecific and subtle and may resemble a upper respiratory infection at first. An increase in exertional dyspnea may be common, as well as noted decreases in daily spirometry values. While this may not seem relevant to a pediatric cardiology board review, the ABP lists knowledge of bronchiolitis obliterans as a complication of heart–lung transplant in their content specifications for the cardiology examination.

9. (A) In patients with restrictive cardiomyopathy, the presence of significant cardiomegaly and pulmonary venous congestion on chest x-ray are poor prognostic indicators. Authors have also reported that the actual cath-measured left ventricular end diastolic pressure and the degree of left atrial dilatation are also predictive of poor survival. Patients with restrictive cardiomyopathy have low tissue Doppler parameters, including the medial mitral valve annular E′ velocity. Right atrial enlargement on echo and a murmur consistent with tricuspid regurgitation have not been shown in studies to predict poor outcomes, though may be indicative of the degree of right ventricular dysfunction.

10. (E) Despite advances in other imaging technologies in recent years, the gold standard test to "rule out" rejection in a patient remains a myocardial biopsy obtained in the cardiac catheterization laboratory. Cardiac MRI may be useful in certain situations; however, the lack of tissue diagnosis, the relative lack of availability in the acute setting, and lack of data in pediatric patients do not yet support its use. Electrocardiographic changes may be seen in patients with rejection, including low-voltage QRS signals, though this is rarely diagnostic in isolation. Plasma BNP has been shown in several studies to be indicative of potential rejection when compared to baseline, though this is more an adjunctive test than a diagnostic one. Echocardiography is used at many centers on an intermittent basis to rule out rejection and can be very useful at limiting the number of biopsies performed. However, the biopsy remains the gold standard.

11. (B) New-onset arrhythmia in a cardiac transplant recipient should raise concern for either rejection or coronary artery vasculopathy. In this patient 14 years out from transplant, the most likely diagnosis is coronary artery vasculopathy. Early after transplant, arrhythmias or ectopy may be a sign of rejection, though is relatively nonspecific.

12. (D) Irritability and tremulousness are common side effects of tacrolimus which tend to happen when serum levels are high. At high enough levels, tacrolimus toxicity can cause seizures to occur. The most common complication of azathioprine and mycophenolate is leukopenia, though many patients may have gastrointestinal side effects as well (constipation, diarrhea, nausea). The most common side effects of sirolimus are diarrhea and the development of mouth sores. The side effects of prednisone are well documented, including mood changes, increased appetite, increased blood glucose, weight gain, and a Cushingoid appearance. Long-term use is associated with the development of osteoporosis.

13. (C) Mutations in the *BMPR2* gene (chromosome 2) have been identified in both pediatric and adult patients with pulmonary hypertension. The mode of inheritance is autosomal dominant, though there is low overall penetrance (~20% of patients with known *BMPR2* mutations will develop pulmonary hypertension). Mutations in *TBX5* cause Holt–Oram syndrome, with associated large atrial septal defects and radial anomalies. Mutations in *MLL2* have been implicated in Kabuki syndrome. Mutations in *JAG1* cause Alagille syndrome. *PTNP11* is one of several genes which have been implicated in Noonan syndrome.

14. (A) Sildenafil is a phosphodiesterase type 5 inhibitor, which blocks the degradation of cyclic GMP in smooth muscle cells and promotes vasodilation. Bosentan, ambrisentan, and macitentan are endothelin receptor antagonists (ERAs), which block endothelin receptors. Ambrisentan is a selective endothelin A receptor antagonist, while bosentan and macitentan are dual antagonist, blocking both A and B. Prostacyclin (also known as prostaglandin I2) was used classically in an intravenous fashion to restore the balance of endogenous thromboxanes and prostacyclins and induce vasodilation. Aspirin suppressed the production of prostaglandins and thromboxanes by irreversibly inactivating the cyclooxygenase enzyme.

15. (E) In patients with restrictive cardiomyopathy, the presence of significant cardiomegaly and pulmonary venous congestion on chest x-ray are poor prognostic indicators. Current medical therapy options are ineffective, and thus cardiac transplantation is considered the definitive therapy. Without transplantation, some authors have reported up to 50% mortality within 2 to 3 years of diagnosis of restrictive cardiomyopathy. Outside of transplant, the only medical therapy that has been reported to be useful is limited diuresis, to help improve symptoms. Caution has to be used in this situation however; these patients are very sensitive to preload, and over-diuresis can be problematic. ACE-inhibition has not been shown to be of benefit in pediatric patients with restrictive cardiomyopathy. Ultrasound of the liver

will likely be performed as part of a transplant evaluation, as there is a risk of long-term hepatic congestion; however, this is very unlikely to change the ultimate course in a pediatric patient. Pulmonary vein stenosis should be ruled out in a patient with elevated right ventricular systolic pressure; however, the massive left atrial enlargement points to the ventricles being the problem rather than the pulmonary veins.

16. (B) In both recent sets of guidelines for pediatric heart failure (International Society of Heart and Lung Transplantation 2004 and 2014), digoxin is considered reasonable to add to a heart failure regimen in the presence of heart failure symptoms. Digoxin has not been advocated for patients who are otherwise asymptomatic. The guidelines do note that special attention may be needed for patients who are at risk of renal dysfunction and that lower doses may be needed in those patients concurrently on carvedilol or amiodarone. In the absence of improvement in ventricular function, none of the medications should be weaned at this point—if anything, care should be made to ensure doses are appropriately weight based, as the patients grow older and increase in size. Milrinone may be considered in the presence of ongoing symptoms, though the guidelines are careful to point out that use in the outpatient setting should be limited to bridging to transplant.

17. (D) Spironolactone acts to inhibit aldosterone at the distal tubule, reducing potassium loss in the urine. The diuretic effect is relatively mild, and it is most commonly used concurrently with the loop or thiazide diuretics. Carbonic anhydrase inhibitors include acetazolamide and act in the proximal convoluted tubule. Thiazide diuretics act to inhibit sodium and chloride transplant in the distal convoluted tubule. Loop diuretics such as furosemide act to inhibit chloride–sodium–potassium cotransport in the thick ascending limb of the loop of Henle. Calcium channel blockers block L-type calcium channels in the heart.

18. (B) Bosentan, ambrisentan, and macitentan are endothelin receptor antagonists (ERAs), which block endothelin receptors. Ambrisentan is a selective endothelin A receptor antagonist, while bosentan and macitentan are dual antagonist, blocking both A and B. Sildenafil is a phosphodiesterase type 5 inhibitor, which blocks the degradation of cyclic GMP in smooth muscle cells and promotes vasodilation. Prostacyclin (also known as prostaglandin I2) was used classically in an intravenous fashion to restore the balance of endogenous thromboxanes and prostacyclins and induce vasodilation. Aspirin suppressed the production of prostaglandins and thromboxanes by irreversibly inactivating the cyclooxygenase enzyme.

19. (C) While topical anesthesia agents such as lidocaine, benzocaine, and prilocaine are more common causes, dapsone has also been reported as a potential cause of methemoglobinemia. Dapsone is used in patients with any contraindication to using trimethoprim-sulfamethoxazole, as a second-line agent for prevention of pneumocystis. Treatment includes removal of the offending agent and administration of methylene blue.

20. (A) Enalapril, an angiotensin-converting enzyme (ACE) inhibitor, acts to decrease the amount of angiotensin I that is converted to angiotensin II. Angiotensin II is a potent vasoconstrictor, and as such, ACE-inhibitors thus promote vasodilation by blocking production of angiotensin II. ACE-inhibitors also decrease the degradation of circulating bradykinins and reduce the production of aldosterone. Patients should be counseled to avoid pregnancy if on ACE-inhibitor medications, due to the high risk of major congenital malformations.

21. (E) The biopsy findings are consistent with an International Society of Heart and Lung Transplantation (ISHLT) grade 2R rejection (cellular mediated). A finding of 2R rejection and greater should be treated, initially with pulsed steroids and further therapies as indicated. Treatment of grade 1R rejection is controversial; decisions on whether to treat a patient with 1R rejection include many factors including prior biopsy results, institutional protocols, and other comorbidities.

The ABP content specifications for the pediatric cardiology board examination include a section on knowledge of histologic findings of rejection. While it is unlikely that specific pathologic specimens will be presented on an examination, it may be worthwhile to understand the grading system used for cellular mediated rejection.

Grade 1R (mild) = interstitial and/or perivascular infiltrates with up to one focus of myocyte damage.

Grade 2R (moderate) = two or more foci of infiltrate with associated myocyte damage

Grade 3R (severe) = diffuse infiltrate with multifocal myocyte damage, with or without edema, hemorrhage, or vasculitis.

22. (D) In cases with identifiable familial origin, the pattern of inheritance is most commonly autosomal dominant. This confers a 50% risk of developing dilated cardiomyopathy for children of an individual who has dilated cardiomyopathy. There are rare forms of inherited cardiomyopathies inherited in an X-linked or autosomal recessive pattern, though these are often associated with neuromuscular disease or metabolic derangements.

23. (B) The most common complication of azathioprine and mycophenolate is leukopenia, though many patients may have gastrointestinal side effects as well (constipation, diarrhea, nausea). Irritability and tremulousness are common side effects of tacrolimus that tend to happen when serum levels are high. The side effects of prednisone are well documented, including mood changes, increased appetite, increased blood glucose, weight gain, and a Cushingoid appearance. Long-term use is associated with the development of osteoporosis.

24. (A) Posttransplant lymphoproliferative disorder is a significant cause of graft loss and death after transplant. Reduction in immunosuppression early after transplant has been recommended and led to improved survival. The majority of lymphomas after heart transplant have been found to be related to EBV. Retransplantation for survivors of PTLD continues to be controversial and institution dependent.

25. (C) The patient has Barth syndrome, an X-linked condition characterized by dilated or noncompaction cardiomyopathy, hypotonia, and proximal muscle weakness, all of which may be evident in early neonatal life. Though many present in neonatal life, the age and severity of presentation can vary widely. Neutropenia is common and may contribute to the patients developing recurrent infections. Short stature is common. Barth syndrome is one of a group of metabolic disorders which present with 3-methylglutaconic aciduria. The specific gene implicated in Barth syndrome is the *TAZ* gene, which encodes a protein called tafazzin. Barth syndrome is inherited in an X-linked recessive pattern.

26. (B) The patient is presenting with a dry, hacking cough after initiation of heart failure medication, most likely due to the ACE-inhibitor enalapril. ACE-inhibitor-induced cough is well described in adults, but relatively rare in children. The mechanism is not fully determined, but thought to be related to increased local concentration of kinins and substance P, which may induce bronchial irritation. It may also be related to arachidonic acid pathway activation, leading to elevated levels of thromboxane and subsequent bronchoconstriction. Treatment involves discontinuation of the ACE-inhibitor, after which the cough typically improves within a week. There is a high rate of recurrence, up to 67%, if a second challenge of medication is given. In a patient with dilated cardiomyopathy, afterload reduction is highly desirable, and an angiotensin-receptor blocker (ARB) such as losartan should be considered to replace the ACE-inhibitor.

27. (E) The patient is presenting with severe coronary artery vasculopathy. Options for management of the patient after this diagnosis are limited, but may include using aspirin, a statin drug such as pravastatin, and/or switching the patient from a calcineurin inhibitor (CNI) to an mTOR inhibitor such as sirolimus or everolimus. Stenting can be considered in certain situations, but typically does not have long-term benefit due to a very high incidence of restenosis. As such, listing the patient for retransplantation is the best option. Steroids or plasmapheresis are treatments for rejection, and in the absence of pathological findings or other evidence of acute rejection they are not indicated. This being said, many patients will often receive presumptive treatment for rejection in this setting, in the hope of clinical improvement, though it should not be done in lieu of listing for retransplantation.

28. (D) The patient is presenting with signs of superior vena cava (SVC) obstruction, including irritability and prominent venous distension in the head and neck. This may be seen acutely in patients with SVC thrombus or chronically in patients with obstruction at the SVC anastomosis. The risk of SVC obstruction increases in patients with prior intervention on their SVC, particularly the Glenn operation/bidirectional cavopulmonary anastomosis, and in those who have had a bicaval anastomosis for their transplant. Up to 10% of pediatric heart transplant recipients may require further interventions on their SVC. The first line of treatment is angioplasty with or without stenting.

29. (A) Loop diuretics such as furosemide act to inhibit chloride–sodium–potassium cotransport in the thick ascending limb of the loop of Henle. They are traditionally preferred as primary diuretic therapy in systolic heart failure. Thiazide diuretics act to inhibit sodium and chloride transplant in the distal convoluted tubule. Carbonic anhydrase inhibitors include acetazolamide and act in the proximal convoluted tubule. Potassium sparing diuretics such as spironolactone act to inhibit aldosterone at the distal tubule, reducing potassium loss in the urine. The diuretic effect is relatively mild, and it is most commonly used concurrently with the loop or thiazide diuretics. Calcium channel blockers block L-type calcium channels in the heart.

30. (D) Carvedilol has both β-receptor and α-receptor activity. In adult patients with heart failure, carvedilol has been shown to improve left ventricular performance and clinical status. Limited studies in children (including one large randomized trial) have shown varied results; however, it is still used widely in pediatric patients with systemic left ventricular dysfunction. Answer A describes metoprolol, an effective β-blocker which is selectively active on β-1 receptors. Answer B describes ACE-inhibitors including lisinopril, enalapril, and captopril. Answer C describes hydralazine, which effectively dilates peripheral arteries and decreases afterload, increases cardiac output, and may decrease filling pressures. Answer E describes amiloride, which blocks epithelial sodium channels in the late distal convoluted tubule and collecting duct, inhibiting sodium reabsorption from the lumen. This reduces the net negative potential of the lumen of the tubule, reducing both potassium and hydrogen excretion.

CHAPTER 11

Cardiac Pharmacology

Nathaniel W. Taggart, Sheri C. Crow, and Philip L. Wackel

QUESTIONS

1. An 11-year-old girl is admitted to the hospital after cardiac arrest from which she was successfully defibrillated. Her baseline electrocardiogram (ECG) from 1 month earlier when she was not on any medication is shown in Figure 11.1.

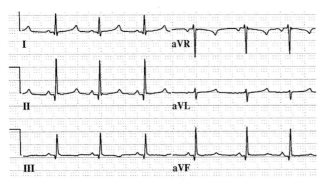

FIGURE 11.1

   Later that evening she develops recurrent nonsustained polymorphic ventricular tachycardia. Which of the following intravenous medications may be useful in treating this patient's dysrhythmia?

   A. Procainamide
   B. Magnesium sulfate
   C. Sotalol
   D. Quinidine
   E. Dofetilide

2. An 8-year-old boy is diagnosed with long QT syndrome (LQTS) associated with a mutation in sodium channel gene *SCN5A* following an evaluation for unexplained syncope. His baseline QTc interval is 490 msec. He undergoes placement of an ICD/pacemaker. While in the ICU, he has frequent episodes of nonsustained polymorphic

ventricular tachycardia, which are suppressed by intravenous lidocaine administration. Which of the following oral medications would be the best outpatient treatment for this patient?

   A. Quinidine
   B. Sotalol
   C. Dofetilide
   D. Procainamide
   E. Mexiletine

3. An 18-year-old man with a bileaflet aortic valve mechanical prosthesis that was placed 2 years ago is scheduled for an elective urological operation. He has no previous history of clots, arrhythmia, stroke, or transient ischemic attacks. On a recent echocardiogram, his left ventricular ejection fraction was 55%. Which of the following statements is most consistent with the 2008 recommendations from the American College of Cardiology for perioperative anticoagulation in this setting?

   A. Warfarin should be stopped 48 hours prior to procedure, and he should be bridged with unfractionated heparin
   B. Warfarin should be stopped 48 hours prior to procedure, and he should be bridged with subcutaneous heparin
   C. Warfarin should be stopped 48 hours prior to procedure, and he should be started on clopidogrel
   D. Warfarin should be stopped 72 hours prior to procedure, and no heparin bridging is necessary
   E. Warfarin should be stopped 72 hours prior to procedure, and he should be bridged with unfractionated heparin. Heparin should be stopped 4 to 6 hours prior to surgery.

4. A 16-year-old boy with a previously repaired partial AV canal defect and cleft mitral valve undergoes mechanical bileaflet mitral valve prosthesis placement for symptomatic severe mitral valve regurgitation. His discharge echocardiogram shows a left ventricular ejection fraction of 60%. He has no history of thromboembolic events or thrombophilia. Based on the 2008 American College of Cardiology recommendations for postoperative anticoagulation, which of the following is the best long-term anticoagulation strategy for this patient?

   A. Warfarin only (goal INR between 2 and 3)
   B. Warfarin only (goal INR between 2.5 and 3.5)
   C. Warfarin (goal INR between 2 and 3) and aspirin 81 mg
   D. Warfarin (goal INR between 2.5 and 3.5) and aspirin 81 mg
   E. Warfarin (goal INR between 2 and 3) and aspirin 325 mg

5. An 18-year-old woman with a history of parachute mitral valve and mechanical mitral prosthesis placement takes warfarin 4 mg/day. She has just learned that she is 14 weeks pregnant and wishes to continue with her pregnancy. Which of the following treatment options would you advise?

   A. Strongly recommend elective termination of the pregnancy
   B. Discontinue warfarin for the remainder of the pregnancy, then restart in the postpartum period
   C. Continue warfarin for the remainder of the pregnancy
   D. Discontinue warfarin now and restart at 25 to 30 weeks gestation, treating with subcutaneous heparin in the interim
   E. Continue warfarin till 36 weeks gestation, then treat with continuous intravenous heparin and deliver in 2 to 3 weeks

6. A 9-year-old patient with myocarditis, cardiomegaly, and reduced left ventricular systolic function develops a dry cough without other respiratory symptoms after starting oral heart failure therapy. Which of the following is the most likely mechanism of cough?

   A. Increased bradykinin
   B. Inhibition of Na^+–K^+ ATPase pump
   C. Inhibition of calcium entry into vascular smooth muscle cells
   D. Inhibition of activation of angiotensin II receptors
   E. Increased production of angiotensin II

7. A 7-year-old well child with a recent history of palpitations is admitted to the ED with shortness of breath and tachyarrhythmia. He has no previous history of syncope or exercise-induced symptoms. His ECG is shown in Figure 11.2. Vagal maneuvers have failed. His blood pressure (BP) is 100/60 mm Hg. The patient has undergone electrical cardioversion three times, with transient

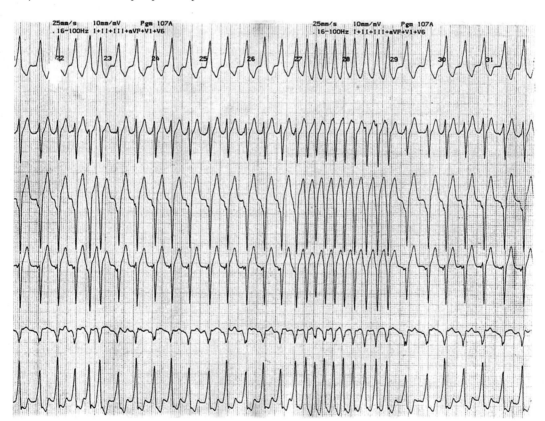

FIGURE 11.2

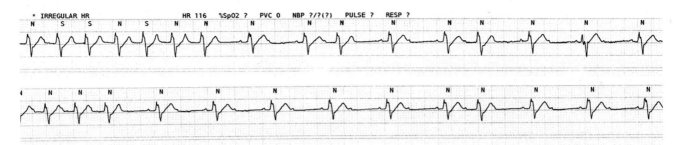

FIGURE 11.3

return to sinus rhythm, after which the tachycardia recurs. Which of the following medications would be most likely to treat this patient's arrhythmia?

A. IV adenosine
B. IV digitalis
C. IV amiodarone
D. IV β-blocker
E. IV diltiazem

8. A 10-month-old female infant presents 1 week after hospital discharge following repair of tetralogy of Fallot (TOF). Her parents describe a 3-day history of vomiting without diarrhea. She has not had a fever. Cardiac monitoring reveals the rhythm shown in Figure 11.3.

Which of the following medications is most likely to cause this patient's symptoms and electrocardiographic findings?

A. Digoxin
B. Propranolol
C. Furosemide
D. Amiodarone
E. Chlorothiazide

9. A 13-year-old boy with a history of catecholaminergic polymorphic ventricular tachycardia (CPVT) is admitted to the ICU after an episode of syncope with exertion. In the ICU, he is noted to have frequent episodes of polymorphic ventricular tachycardia associated with hypotension. Which of the following is the best antiarrhythmic therapy for this child?

A. Amiodarone
B. Lidocaine
C. β-Blocker
D. Calcium channel blocker (CCB)
E. Digoxin

10. A 13-month-old male infant referred to you for a heart murmur is diagnosed with a secundum atrial septal defect (ASD) measuring 6 mm. He was born at 38 weeks of gestation and has been thriving well without any symptoms. There is mild right heart enlargement on echocardiogram, and right ventricular systolic pressure is estimated

to be 30 mm Hg. His mom, who is a pediatric nurse, is concerned about RSV and wants to know whether her son needs any palivizumab prophylaxis for the RSV season. Which of the following is the most appropriate answer?

A. RSV prophylaxis is not indicated, because he is over 1 year old
B. RSV prophylaxis is recommended for him until he is 2 years old
C. His heart disease does not qualify him for RSV prophylaxis
D. RSV prophylaxis would only be recommended if he had a prior history of RSV infection
E. RSV prophylaxis would be recommended for him if he were exposed to cigarette smoke at home

11. You are evaluating a 14-month-old female infant in the outpatient pediatric cardiology clinic. She was diagnosed with hypoplastic left heart syndrome after a full-term delivery. She underwent a stage I Norwood procedure and a stage II superior cavopulmonary anastomosis (Glenn procedure) at 6 months of age. She is currently doing well. Her only medication is aspirin. Her resting oxygen saturation is 80%. Echocardiogram shows normal right ventricular size and function and a patent Glenn shunt with appropriate flow in the pulmonary arteries. She received palivizumab prophylaxis last RSV season. Her mother wants to know whether palivizumab would be helpful during the current RSV season. Which of the following is the most appropriate response to her question?

A. Palivizumab prophylaxis has been shown to reduce the risk of RSV infection and is therefore beneficial
B. Palivizumab prophylaxis has been shown to reduce mortality rate from RSV in patients with congenital heart disease and therefore is recommended
C. Palivizumab would protect her from most viral infections including influenza A and B
D. Palivizumab would likely decrease her need for hospitalization if she contracted RSV and therefore is recommended
E. Palivizumab is not recommended after 1 year of age

12. A 5-month-old female infant with dilated cardiomyopathy is started on furosemide. This medication acts by inhibiting which of the following ion channels?

   A. Na^+–$2Cl^-$–K^+ cotransporter in the loop of Henle
   B. Na^+–Cl^- cotransporter in the proximal tubule
   C. Na^+–K^+ ATPase pump in the distal tubule
   D. Na^+–H^+ cotransporter in the loop of Henle
   E. Na^+–Ca^{2+} cotransporter in the proximal tubule

13. A 17-year-old previously healthy girl presents to the ED with a 2-day history of chest pain. Her ECG shows diffuse ST segment elevation and PR segment depression suggestive of pericarditis. Echocardiogram shows normal biventricular size and function with a small pericardial effusion. There is no history of recent fever, rash, sore throat, or joint pains. Which of the following is the best treatment option for this patient?

   A. Aspirin 325 mg 4 times/day for 4 weeks
   B. Prednisone 1 mg/kg/day followed by tapering after 2 weeks once patient is asymptomatic
   C. Colchicine therapy for 4 to 6 days
   D. Ibuprofen 600 to 800 mg 3 times a day
   E. Clopidogrel 75 mg daily for 2 weeks

14. A 5-day-old neonate with hypoplastic left heart syndrome is being cared for in the cardiac ICU 2 days after a Norwood operation with right modified Blalock–Taussig shunt. Arterial blood gas (on $FiO_2 = 21\%$) shows a pH of 7.2. PO_2 is 42 mm Hg, PCO_2 is 45 mm Hg, SpO_2 is 80%, and hemoglobin is 14 g/dL. Near infrared spectroscopy (NIRS) probes consistently show saturations in the 40% range. ECG shows sinus tachycardia with a heart rate of 180 bpm. Arterial BP is 78/58 mm Hg. Chest x-ray shows no evidence of pulmonary congestion or significant infiltrates and lung fields are well expanded. The patient is on milrinone 0.4 mcg/kg/min and norepinephrine 1 mcg/kg/min. Urine output over the past 6 hours has averaged 1 cc/kg/hour. Limited bedside echo shows no significant pericardial effusion. The patient just received two 10 ml/kg boluses of normal saline. Which of the following interventions is most likely to benefit this patient?

   A. IV furosemide
   B. Decrease in norepinephrine infusion rate
   C. IV β-blocker therapy
   D. Decrease in milrinone infusion rate
   E. Increasing the inspired FiO_2 concentration

15. A 10-month-old infant is treated for Kawasaki disease (KD) with intravenous immunoglobulin (IVIG) and aspirin. Which of the following statements regarding use of steroids in KD is most accurate?

   A. A 24-hour continuous IV steroid infusion may be considered in addition to IVIG as primary therapy

   B. Oral steroids may be used instead of aspirin if the patient remains afebrile but shows persistent elevation of acute inflammatory markers (ESR, CRP)
   C. Steroids are contraindicated in Kawasaki patients
   D. IV steroids may be considered for primary therapy in this infant patient
   E. IV steroids may be considered if the patient has persistent or recrudescent fever after two doses of IVIG

16. A 7-year-old girl whose parents recently emigrated from Mexico is diagnosed with acute rheumatic fever (RF). She complains of mild chest pain, but no shortness of breath. Cardiac examination reveals normal S_1 and S_2, with a soft holosystolic murmur at the apex. Neck veins do not appear to be distended. Abdominal examination shows no organomegaly. Echocardiogram shows small pericardial effusion, mild-to-moderate mitral valve regurgitation, mild aortic valve regurgitation, mildly dilated left ventricle with an ejection fraction of 60%. Which of following treatment regimens should be initiated in the above patient?

   A. IV steroids
   B. Oral steroids
   C. High-dose aspirin
   D. β-Blocker therapy
   E. IVIG + aspirin

17. Which of the following statements is true regarding immunosuppressive medications used in patients following heart transplantation?

   A. Sirolimus is a calcineurin inhibitor
   B. Tacrolimus is not available for intravenous use
   C. Sirolimus acts by blocking gene transcription
   D. Tacrolimus has been associated with improved survival over cyclosporine
   E. Sirolimus is less nephrotoxic than cyclosporine

18. A 7-year-old girl who was appropriately treated for her first episode of RF with mild carditis is followed up at 3 months, 6 months, and then at 1 year. Serial follow-up echocardiograms show no residual pericardial effusion, trivial mitral valve regurgitation, no aortic valve regurgitation, normal left ventricular chamber size, and function. She is maintained on RF antibiotic prophylaxis and continues to remain asymptomatic without any recurrence of streptococcal sore throat. If there is no echocardiographic evidence of worsening ventricular or valvular function, which of the following is the best recommendation for ongoing antibiotic prophylaxis?

   A. Antibiotic prophylaxis should be continued for 5 years
   B. Antibiotic prophylaxis should be continued for 10 years
   C. Antibiotic prophylaxis should be continued until she is 21 years of age
   D. Antibiotic prophylaxis should be continued until she is 40 years of age
   E. She will need lifelong antibiotic prophylaxis

19. According to the 2007 AHA/ACC guidelines, infective endocarditis (IE) prophylaxis is recommended in which of the following clinical scenarios?

A. 7-year-old patient who has undergone cardiac transplantation 18 months ago with trivial tricuspid valve regurgitation prior to dental extraction

B. 8-year-old patient who has undergone device closure of ASD 4 months ago with residual shunt at the site of prosthetic device who is scheduled to undergo an upper gastrointestinal endoscopy

C. 9-year-old patient with TOF who underwent complete repair at 6 months of age and has an RV to PA conduit and is scheduled to have dental brace placement

D. 8-year-old patient with prosthetic mitral valve with previous history of IE who is scheduled for an outpatient cystoscopy

E. 12-year-old patient who has undergone percutaneous PDA closure 4 months ago who needs a root canal

20. A 14-year-old boy is referred to your clinic for management of elevated LDL cholesterol. Twelve months ago his LDL level was 196 mg/dL, and he was advised appropriate dietary intervention and weight reduction regimen. At present his LDL level is 202 mg/dL, HDL is 28 mg/dL, and triglycerides are 150 mg/dL. His BMI is 31 kg/m^2 and his TSH level is normal. He has been compliant with his diet and exercise program and has lost 3 kg over the past year. He was adopted and therefore family history is not well known. Which of the following statements is most accurate?

A. Continued dietary intervention alone will likely significantly reduce his LDL level over the next 6 months

B. Oral statin therapy should be strongly considered

C. Oral niacin therapy is the best first-line option due to its side effect profile

D. Fibric acid derivatives should be considered

E. If drug therapy is considered, bile acid-binding resins would be first-line therapy given their favorable safety and side effect profile

21. A 16-year-old boy recently diagnosed with hypertrophic cardiomyopathy (HCM) presents for evaluation. No other associated medical conditions are present. Medications include multivitamins. He is asymptomatic at rest, but complains of shortness of breath with exertion. There is no history of syncope/pre-syncope or family history of HCM or sudden death. His resting HR is 80 bpm and BP is 130/80 mm Hg. His echocardiogram shows a septal thickness of 26 mm, ejection fraction = 70%, left ventricular outflow tract maximum instantaneous gradient is 60 mm Hg. Cardiac MRI shows minimal late gadolinium enhancement. Recent Holter report showed frequent single PVCs, but no sustained tachycardia. On the basis of the above information, which of the following is the best initial treatment for this patient?

A. ICD placement
B. Digoxin
C. Furosemide
D. β-Blocker
E. Nifedipine

22. Which of the following medications used in heart transplant recipients can inhibit smooth muscle proliferation and may have the advantage of inhibiting coronary allograft vasculopathy?

A. Methylprednisolone
B. Sirolimus
C. Antithymocyte globulin (ATG)
D. Cyclosporine
E. Tacrolimus

23. A 3-day-old term neonate with hypoplastic left heart syndrome is initiated on cardiopulmonary bypass for Norwood palliation. Which of the following medications would be most likely to increase systemic perfusion in this patient following cardiopulmonary bypass?

A. Phenoxybenzamine
B. Epinephrine
C. Milrinone
D. Dopamine
E. Norepinephrine

24. A 5-year-old girl with idiopathic dilated cardiomyopathy undergoes induction with rabbit antithymocyte globulin (ATG) prior to orthotopic cardiac transplantation. Which of the following side effects of ATG is most common?

A. Fever
B. Rash
C. Abdominal pain
D. Hyperkalemia
E. Myalgia

25. A 15-year-old boy presents to the ER with fast heart rate (HR) and some shortness of breath. His ECG shows a regular narrow QRS tachycardia (HR 235 bpm) without discernible P waves. He was discharged 24 hours ago from the hospital following management of asthma exacerbation and received treatment in the intensive care unit. Vagal maneuvers have failed to bring down his HR. Which of the following statements regarding adenosine is true?

A. Adenosine should be slowly pushed to avoid bronchospasm

B. If bronchospasm results, it will only last several seconds, then resolve

C. Patients who have undergone orthotopic heart transplant are less responsive to adenosine

D. Transient hypertension may result from adenosine administration

E. Flushing of the face is a common side effect

26. A 13-year-old girl is newly diagnosed with idiopathic pulmonary arterial hypertension. She experiences shortness of breath at rest and has severe right ventricular enlargement with severe dysfunction. She is started on IV epoprostenol, oral sildenafil, and ambrisentan. Which of the following is the correct statement among the following regarding her pharmacological treatment?

   A. Ambrisentan is an endothelin A receptor agonist
   B. Epoprostenol is a prostaglandin (PGE2) analogue
   C. Ambrisentan does not affect cytochrome P450 enzyme activity
   D. Sildenafil is phosphodiesterase 3 inhibitor
   E. Multi-drug combination therapy has been shown to improve survival in children with idiopathic pulmonary hypertension

27. A 16-year-old boy is evaluated by his cardiologist following a recent episode of unexplained syncope. His resting ECG and echocardiogram are normal, and the history is not typical for vasovagal syncope. His father is an immigrant from Southeast Asia and was diagnosed with Brugada syndrome 1 year ago. Which of the following tests would be helpful in making a definitive diagnosis in this patient?

   A. Epinephrine challenge test
   B. Cardiac MRI
   C. Isoproterenol provocative test
   D. Provocative testing with procainamide
   E. Exercise test

28. A 10-year-old girl with known LQTS type 1 presents with status epilepticus to the emergency department. She is on oral nadolol therapy. Her ECG shows sinus rhythm (120 bpm) and her resting QT interval is 500 msec. The ER doctor prepares to administer IV phenytoin and consults the cardiologist regarding the safety of phenytoin use in the patient. Which of the following statements is accurate with regard to the current patient scenario?

   A. Phenytoin can prolong the QT interval and is therefore not safe in the patient
   B. Patient should be started on IV amiodarone before starting phenytoin
   C. Intravenous β-blocker can be administered concurrently with phenytoin drip
   D. Phenytoin has cardiac effects similar to mexiletine
   E. Phenytoin blocks cardiac potassium channels

29. An 18-year-old female patient with a history of repaired Ebstein anomaly is admitted to the ER with shortness of breath and a tachycardia (HR of 150 bpm). She is found to be in atrial flutter with variable conduction on ECG evaluation. She is hemodynamically stable. An echocardiogram done 1 year ago showed normal left ventricular function with mild right ventricular dysfunction. Which of the following options is most appropriate in the immediate management of the patient?

   A. Flecainide
   B. Diltiazem
   C. Disopyramide
   D. Heparin, transesophageal echocardiogram, and preparation for urgent electrical cardioversion
   E. Labetalol

30. Which of the following drugs is a calcium-sensitizing agent?

   A. Verapamil
   B. Digoxin
   C. Levosimendan
   D. Milrinone
   E. Nesiritide

31. A newborn baby is noted to be bradycardic with a HR of 40 bpm. An ECG shows complete AV block. Infusion of which of the following medications would be most useful to increase the HR in this scenario?

   A. Milrinone
   B. Atropine
   C. Digoxin
   D. Isoproterenol
   E. Dobutamine

32. A 15-year-old girl with Marfan syndrome is admitted to the intensive care unit with acute severe mitral valve regurgitation in the setting of a flail mitral valve leaflet. She is felt to be in a low cardiac output state with pulmonary edema. Heart rate is 120 bpm; blood pressure is 123/78 mm Hg. Her distal extremities are cool. Ejection fraction by echocardiogram is 70%. Which of the following medications would be most helpful in improving her cardiac output acutely prior to surgery?

   A. Nitroprusside infusion
   B. Intravenous Lasix
   C. Vasopressin infusion
   D. Intravenous digoxin
   E. Dopamine infusion

33. A 3-month-old child with unrepaired TOF is referred to the ER by his pediatrician because his oxygen saturation during a well-child visit was only 62%. On examination, the patient is cyanotic but alert. His parents note that he has been less active for the past few days. His HR is 180 bpm, SpO$_2$ is 55% to 60%, respiratory rate is 40/min, and BP is 88/50 mm Hg. The lungs are clear on auscultation and a grade 3/6 harsh systolic ejection murmur is heard over the precordium. He is not on any medications. His lab work done at his pediatrician's office is available: Na 142, K 3.8, chloride 105, bicarbonate 26, BUN 15, creatinine 0.6, hematocrit 26, WBC 9000, platelet count is 350,000. Which of the following therapies can be expected to improve the patient's condition?

   A. Intravenous propranolol
   B. Phenylephrine infusion
   C. Packed red blood cell transfusion
   D. Morphine administration
   E. Intravenous furosemide

34. A 2-day-old child with hypoplastic left heart syndrome is started on prostaglandin E1 (PGE1). The parents have opted for a cardiac transplantation for the child and the cardiology team has decided to maintain him on PGE1 until a donor heart becomes available for transplantation. Which of the following statements is true with regard to the side effects of PGE1?

   A. Assisted ventilation may be necessary because of primary hypoxia
   B. Hypothermia is a potential side effect
   C. Patient needs to be monitored for hypertension
   D. Seizures are not associated with administration of PGE1
   E. Cutaneous vasodilation and edema can develop as a side effect

35. Which of the following drugs used in the treatment of Marfan syndrome blocks TGF-β signaling?

   A. Losartan
   B. Propranolol
   C. Enalapril
   D. Verapamil
   E. Spironolactone

36. An 18-year-old man with dilated cardiomyopathy and LVEF of 30% comes for a follow-up outpatient evaluation. He has a chronically elevated potassium. Which of the following medications would be indicated considering his hyperkalemia?

   A. Eplerenone
   B. Spironolactone
   C. Captopril
   D. Metoprolol
   E. Enalapril

37. A 16-year-old patient who received a cardiac transplantation 10 years ago is managed as an outpatient. His LVEF has been in the 25% range for the past 1 year, and he is thought to have advanced coronary allograft vasculopathy. A 24-hour ECG monitoring shows repeated episodes of atrial flutter. He is currently on the following oral medications: carvedilol, atenolol, spironolactone, digoxin, enalapril, warfarin, cyclosporine, oral steroids. The treating cardiologist elects to start him on amiodarone. Which of the following statements is correct with respect to drug interactions in the setting of amiodarone therapy?

   A. Digoxin dose does not need to be adjusted when adding amiodarone
   B. Enhanced AV nodal conduction can occur and can result in rapid ventricular response in the setting of atrial arrhythmias
   C. Cyclosporine levels may be elevated after beginning amiodarone
   D. INR should be checked periodically as it may become subtherapeutic
   E. Steroid dose should be decreased after adding amiodarone

38. Which of the following statements is true regarding the antiarrhythmic action of amiodarone?

   A. It shortens the QTc interval
   B. It produces some degree of calcium channel blockade
   C. It activates cardiac sodium channel
   D. It has vagolytic effects
   E. Presence of hypokalemia reduces its pro-arrhythmic potential

39. A 11-year-old girl who received a heart transplant 10 years ago is maintained on tacrolimus, prednisone, and sirolimus. Which of the following statements is true with regard to associated side effects?

   A. The use of sirolimus is not associated with bone marrow suppression
   B. Lipid abnormalities typically do not develop until adolescence
   C. Tacrolimus is more commonly associated with the development of diabetes mellitus than cyclosporine
   D. Thiazides are the first-line antihypertensive agents in heart transplant recipients
   E. Sirolimus is more nephrotoxic than cyclosporine and tacrolimus

40. Which of the following drugs lowers pulmonary vascular resistance (PVR)?

   A. Nitrous oxide
   B. Ketamine
   C. Prostacyclin
   D. Dopamine
   E. Norepinephrine

41. A 4-year-old girl who underwent a non-fenestrated Fontan procedure 6 days ago develops acute arterial thrombosis of her right great toe. An emergency echocardiogram shows normal systemic ventricular function without any thrombus and a patent Fontan pathway. She is receiving heparin 10 units/kg/h through a central catheter in her internal jugular vein. She is currently on aspirin 81 mg/day, milrinone, and furosemide. She has been receiving frequent doses of fentanyl for severe pain. CBC today shows a hemoglobin of 12.8, white blood cell count of 12,000, and a platelet count of 60,000. Two days prior, her platelet count was 300,000. There is no evidence of any bleeding. The intensivist orders additional tests to clarify the diagnosis. Which of the following is most likely responsible for her drop in platelets?

    A. Milrinone
    B. Furosemide
    C. Aspirin
    D. Heparin
    E. Fentanyl

42. Which of the following medications is correctly listed with its teratogenic effect?

    A. Lithium: left-sided obstructive lesions
    B. Amiodarone: permanent fetal complete heart block
    C. Warfarin: defects in central nervous system
    D. ACE inhibitors: right-sided obstructive lesions
    E. High-dose folic acid: neural tube defects

43. An 18-year-old male patient with a history of TOF that was repaired 13 years ago presents to the emergency room with vomiting and complaints of visual disturbances (flashing lights and halos) and feeling dizzy. He has a history of underlying mild renal dysfunction. He was recently diagnosed with infectious mononucleosis. His oral intake has been reduced for the past few days, but he has been taking his digoxin, furosemide, and aspirin regularly. His HR is 40 bpm, respiratory rate is 18 breaths per minute, SpO_2 is 98%, and BP is 85/40 mm Hg. ECG shows underlying sinus rhythm, right bundle branch block with no evidence of peaked T waves, 3:1 AV block, ventricular bigeminy, and frequent three to four beat runs of premature ventricular contractions. Which of the following is the most likely to reveal the source of his symptoms?

    A. Serum potassium level
    B. Liver function tests
    C. Beta natriuretic peptide (BNP) level
    D. Aspirin level
    E. Digoxin level

44. A 6-year-old girl is 2 days post repair of coarctation of aorta and subaortic membrane resection. She is intubated and appears comfortable on the ventilator (FiO_2 40%). She is noted to have persistently elevated BP (190–200/100–110 mm Hg) despite use of intravenous fentanyl and furosemide. Her HR is 100 bpm and SpO_2 is 90%. Chest x-ray shows some atelectasis in both lung fields. Her morning labs are as follows: hemoglobin 8.5, WBC 9,000, platelets 150,000, BUN 38, creatinine 1.9, ALT 250, AST 300. Her outpatient medications include the following: methylphenidate, albuterol prn, fluticasone/salmeterol twice daily, and montelukast daily. Which of the following treatment options would be best for this patient?

    A. Inhaled nitric oxide therapy
    B. Intravenous nicardipine
    C. Intravenous labetalol
    D. Sodium nitroprusside infusion
    E. Dexmedetomidine infusion

45. A 6-year-old boy undergoes percutaneous pulmonary valvotomy for valvular pulmonary stenosis. His baseline SpO_2 is 98% on room air. His pre-procedure echocardiogram had demonstrated a mean gradient of 55 mm Hg across the valve, right ventricular hypertrophy with normal systolic function, patent foramen ovale, normal branch pulmonary arteries, and normal left ventricular chamber size/systolic function. Following his procedure in the catheterization laboratory, his peak to peak gradient decreased from 80 to 30 mm Hg and SpO_2 was 95% (room air). Three hours later he is noted to be desaturating with SpO_2 in the 80s on room air and with poor peripheral perfusion. Which of the following treatment options would be most helpful in this patient?

    A. Inhaled nitric oxide therapy
    B. Milrinone therapy
    C. Phenylephrine therapy
    D. Intravenous β-blocker
    E. Intravenous furosemide

46. A 14-year-old patient on a statin to lower his cholesterol presents with fatigue, back pain, and soreness in the arms and legs. Which of the following lab values is most likely to reveal the etiology?

    A. Serum potassium level
    B. Creatine kinase level
    C. Serum creatinine
    D. Serum cholesterol level
    E. Complete blood count

Please refer to the following case scenario for Questions 47 and 48:

A 1-week-old female infant is in the neonatal intensive care unit awaiting surgical palliation for tricuspid atresia with normally related great arteries and pulmonary stenosis. She is on prostaglandin to maintain ductal patency. Her oxygen saturations are 88% on room air and her lactate level is 0.6. The child is transported to the interventional radiology suite to have a percutaneous intravenous central (PICC) line placed.

47. Which of the following anesthetic induction regimens carries highest risk of cardiopulmonary compromise in this patient?

    A. Inhalational anesthetic agent and ketamine
    B. Inhalational anesthetic agent and midazolam
    C. Ketamine and midazolam
    D. Midazolam and fentanyl
    E. Fentanyl and ketamine

48. Mask induction is initiated with isoflurane and fentanyl. After several minutes of isoflurane delivery, the child is still awake and moving with stimulation. The anesthesiologist rechecks the IV and the isoflurane delivery system and confirms that the gas is flowing freely into the mask. Which of the following is the most likely explanation for the delay in achieving sedation?

    A. Isoflurane and fentanyl are not an effective approach for inducing general anesthesia
    B. Isoflurane uptake is reduced as a result of right-to-left shunting
    C. Isoflurane uptake is reduced as a result of left-to-right shunting
    D. The child is experiencing severe bronchospasm that is resulting in suboptimal inhalational anesthetic delivery
    E. *V*/*Q* mismatch

49. A 17-year-old boy with a history of coarctation of the aorta status post repair at 12 years of age presents to the emergency department via ambulance after overdosing his blood pressure medications at home. His heart rate is 35 bpm, blood pressure is 92/60 mm Hg. Blood glucose concentration is 65 mg/dL. Which of the following medications should be administered first?

    A. Glucagon
    B. Epinephrine
    C. Hydralazine
    D. Atropine
    E. Vasopressin

50. An 18-year-old woman with a history of mitral arcade and a remote history of atrial flutter has a tilting-disk mechanical prosthesis. She is being treated with warfarin, and her INR level had been therapeutic (2.5 to 3.5) over the previous 2 years with minimal medication adjustment. More recently, she has required a 50% increase in her weekly warfarin dose to maintain similar INR levels. Initiation of which of the following would be most likely to produce this effect?

    A. Amiodarone
    B. Levothyroxine
    C. Propranolol
    D. Sertraline
    E. St. John's wort

51. A 3-month-old male infant presents to cardiology clinic for evaluation of a small ASD. He was prescribed a proton pump inhibitor for several episodes of reflux that were noted in the first week of life. Since that time he has had normal growth and development despite occasional emesis around the time of feeding. Parents are asking whether they should continue to treat him for gastroesophageal reflux. How would you advise this family?

    A. Continue the proton pump inhibitor
    B. Refer the patient to a gastroenterology specialist
    C. Discontinue the proton pump inhibitor
    D. Change the medication from a proton pump inhibitor to an H2 antagonist
    E. Perform a barium swallow study to evaluate for resolution of the reflux.

52. A 3-year-old child underwent a Fontan procedure 5 days ago. Her postoperative course was complicated by bleeding and high venous pressures that warranted a return to the operating room on postop day 3 for fenestration and revision of her Fontan. She was intubated and sedated for five consecutive days beginning with the initial operation. After extubation, she is noticeably uncomfortable and agitated while taking shallow breaths. Which of the following would be the best approach to managing this patient's symptoms?

    A. Begin a dexmedetomidine infusion to manage her agitation and withdrawal
    B. Administer additional doses of midazolam and fentanyl to treat withdrawal
    C. Initiate fentanyl and midazolam infusions at a lower rate than that utilized while intubated
    D. Provide the patient with a hydromorphone patient-controlled analgesia (PCA) setup so that she can treat her own pain
    E. Emergent re-intubation

53. An intubated 2-week-old infant post Norwood/Sano procedure for hypoplastic left heart syndrome has an aspiration event during suctioning of his endotracheal tube. His oxygen saturations precipitously decline from 85% to 40%, following which he becomes profoundly hypotensive. Which of the following medications would be immediately helpful in this situation?

A. Vecuronium
B. Midazolam
C. Epinephrine 0.1 mcg/kg IV push
D. Lidocaine 1 mg/kg
E. Sevoflurane

54. A 5-year-old child presents with a pleural effusion 1 week after surgical intervention for Ebstein anomaly. He will require sedation for chest tube placement. Procedural sedation is planned with ketamine and midazolam. Which of the following agents is most important to have available during this procedural sedation?

A. Propofol
B. Fentanyl
C. Muscle relaxant and glycopyrrolate
D. Diazepam
E. Epinephrine

55. A 15-year-old girl with a history of moderately controlled asthma undergoes primary repair of coarctation of the aorta. On postoperative day 3 she remains hypertensive despite being on sodium nitroprusside at 8 mcg/kg/min. Her creatinine is 2.0 mg/dL and she is on a furosemide infusion to achieve adequate urine output in the setting of acute on chronic renal failure. Laboratory analysis reveals a metabolic acidosis. The patient is becoming agitated and is no longer oriented to person or place. Which of the following is the most likely cause of her metabolic acidosis and altered mental status?

A. Hypovolemia
B. Narcotic-induced delirium
C. Uremia
D. Cyanide toxicity
E. Ketoacidosis

56. A 5-day-old male infant is being treated as an inpatient for postnatal onset of AV reentrant tachycardia with propranolol. He has had a normal echocardiogram, a normal resting ECG, and is otherwise doing well. He continues to have frequent episodes of breakthrough supraventricular tachycardia and the decision is made to discontinue his propranolol and initiate flecainide therapy. Which of the following ECG changes are you most likely to observe on the day following initiation of flecainide?

A. ST depression
B. QT prolongation
C. PR shortening

D. T wave inversion
E. QRS prolongation

57. An 18-year-old woman with a history of surgical repair of a secundum atrial septal defect at 3 years of age presents now with palpitations that began 3 days ago. Her BP is 112/78. On examination her rhythm is regular, she has no murmur or gallop, her lungs are clear, and she has no edema. Her ECG shows atrial flutter with 2:1 AV conduction at a ventricular rate of 150 bpm. She is then given a medication after which her ventricular rate suddenly increases to 220 bpm, and she feels lightheaded and fatigued. Which of the following medications was most likely given?

A. Diltiazem
B. Procainamide
C. Lidocaine
D. Esmolol
E. Mexilitine

58. A 35-year-old man with D-transposition of the great arteries who underwent an atrial switch procedure as a child now presents with recurrent episodes of symptomatic intraatrial reentrant tachycardia despite attempted catheter ablation and an adequate trial of sotalol therapy. His most recent labs include normal TSH and free T4, mildly elevated AST and ALT, BUN of 18 mg/dL, and creatinine of 0.9 mg/dL. On physical examination his rhythm is regular, there is no murmur. He has mild hepatomegaly and no peripheral edema. Echocardiogram demonstrates moderately decreased systemic right ventricular function, no significant valve dysfunction, and no evidence of baffle obstruction. Which of the following would be the best medical therapy for this patient at this time?

A. Dofetilide
B. Flecainide
C. Amiodarone
D. Metoprolol
E. Dronaderone

59. You are considering starting dofetilide on a 25-year-old man with double inlet left ventricle who continues to have recurrent intraatrial reentrant tachycardia despite a surgical maze procedure and a Fontan revision. Which of the following is a contraindication to initiating dofetilide?

A. Thyroid dysfunction
B. Creatinine clearance of 45 mL/min
C. Serum potassium level of 2.9 mmol/L
D. QTc >440 msec in the presence of ventricular conduction delay
E. Moderate systemic ventricular dysfunction

60. A 3-year-old girl with ectopic atrial tachycardia has been treated with several antiarrhythmic medication combinations without sufficient control. She has been well controlled on amiodarone for the last 6 months and presents for follow-up. Which of the following adverse effects is most likely related to amiodarone therapy?

A. Low parathyroid hormone level
B. A rise in serum creatinine to twice normal
C. Nonproductive cough, fever, and dyspnea
D. Elevated amylase and lipase
E. Conjunctivitis

61. A 15-year-old girl with a history of moderately controlled asthma undergoes primary repair of coarctation of the aorta. She has persistent hypertension after surgery. Which of the following antihypertensive agents would you avoid?

A. Esmolol
B. Nicardipine
C. Clevidipine
D. Hydralazine
E. Lisinopril

ANSWERS

1. (B) Prolonged QT interval is noted on the given ECG. The patient probably has LQTS in the clinical scenario.

Class IIa recommendation: Management with intravenous magnesium sulfate is reasonable for patients who present with LQTS and few episodes of torsades de pointes. Magnesium is unlikely to be effective in patients with a normal QT interval (level of evidence: B). The other agents in the scenario tend to prolong QT interval and therefore are not recommended. [*J Am Coll Cardiol*. 2006;48(5):e247–e346.]

2. (E) The patient in this scenario likely has type-3 LQTS.

Class IIb recommendation: Intravenous lidocaine or oral mexiletine may be considered in patients who present LQT3 and torsades de pointes (level of evidence: C). The other agents in the given scenario tend to prolong QT interval and therefore are not recommended. [*Circulation*. 2010;121:1047–1060 (p. 1052).]

3. (D) In the given scenario, the patient has a bileaflet mechanical aortic valve without any additional risk factors for thromboembolism (see below). The recommendation as per the ACC/AHA 2008 guideline is to stop warfarin 72 hours prior to the procedure without any need for heparin bridging. Class I recommendations for perioperative anticoagulation strategy as per ACC/AHA 2008 guidelines is quoted below.

Class I recommendation:

1. In patients at low risk of thrombosis, defined as those with a bileaflet mechanical AVR with no risk factors,* it is recommended that warfarin be stopped 48 to 72 hours before the procedure (so the INR falls to less than 1.5) and restarted within 24 hours after the procedure. Heparin is usually unnecessary *(level of evidence: B)*.
2. In patients at high risk of thrombosis, defined as those with any mechanical MV replacement or a mechanical AVR with any risk factor, therapeutic doses of intravenous UFH should be started when the INR falls below 2.0 (typically 48 hours before surgery), stopped 4 to 6 hours before the procedure, restarted as early after surgery as bleeding stability allows, and continued until the INR is again therapeutic with warfarin therapy *(level of evidence: B)*.

*Risk factors: atrial fibrillation, previous thromboembolism, LV dysfunction, hypercoagulable conditions, older-generation thrombogenic valves, mechanical tricuspid valves, or more than one mechanical valve. [*J Am Coll Cardiol*. 2008;52:e1–e142 (p. e104).]

4. (D) Please refer to class I recommendations from ACC/AHA 2008 guidelines quoted below for postoperative anticoagulation management following mechanical valve placement.

Class I recommendation:

1. After MV replacement with any mechanical valve, warfarin is indicated to achieve an INR of 2.5 to 3.5 (level of evidence: C).
2. The addition of aspirin 75 to 100 mg once daily to therapeutic warfarin is recommended for all patients with mechanical heart valves and those patients with biological valves who have risk factors* (level of evidence: B).

*Risk factors: atrial fibrillation, previous thromboembolism, LV dysfunction, hypercoagulable conditions, older-generation thrombogenic valves, mechanical tricuspid valves, or more than one mechanical valve. [*J Am Coll Cardiol*. 2008;52:e1–e142 (p. e104).]

5. (E) Continuing warfarin till 36 weeks gestation, then treating with continuous intravenous heparin and delivering in 2 to 3 weeks is the most consistent with the guidelines and is also practical. Class I recommendations are quoted below.

Class I recommendations:

1. Pregnant patients with mechanical prosthetic valves who elect to stop warfarin between weeks 6 and 12 of gestation should receive continuous intravenous unfractionated heparin [UFH], dose-adjusted UFH, or dose-adjusted subcutaneous low molecular weight heparin [LMWH] (level of evidence: C).
2. For pregnant patients with mechanical prosthetic valves, up to 36 weeks of gestation, the therapeutic choice of continuous intravenous or dose-adjusted subcutaneous UFH, dose-adjusted LMWH, or warfarin should be discussed fully. If continuous intravenous UFH is used, the fetal risk is lower, but the maternal risks of prosthetic valve thrombosis, systemic embolization, infection, osteoporosis, and heparin-induced thrombocytopenia (HIT) are relatively higher (level of evidence: C).
3. In pregnant patients with mechanical prosthetic valves who receive dose-adjusted LMWH, the LMWH should be administered twice daily subcutaneously to maintain the anti-Xa level between 0.7 and 1.2 U per mL 4 hours after administration (level of evidence: C).
4. In pregnant patients with mechanical prosthetic valves who receive dose-adjusted UFH, the aPTT should be at least twice control (level of evidence: C).
5. In pregnant patients with mechanical prosthetic valves who receive warfarin, the INR goal should be 3.0 (range 2.5 to 3.5) (level of evidence: C).
6. In pregnant patients with mechanical prosthetic valves, warfarin should be discontinued and continuous intravenous UFH given starting 2 to 3 weeks before planned delivery (level of evidence: C). [*J Am Coll Cardiol*. 2008;52:e1–e142 (p. e82).]

6. (A) The patient was started on ACE inhibitor (captopril, enalapril, etc.). ACE converts angiotensin I to angiotensin II. It also inactivates bradykinin. ACE inhibitors therefore increase bradykinin levels and decrease angiotensin II levels. Increased bradykinin levels are thought to be responsible for dry cough symptoms in patients taking ACE inhibitors. Digoxin inhibits Na+–K+ ATPase pump. CCBs inhibit calcium entry into vascular smooth muscle cells. Angiotensin II receptor blockers (ARBs) inhibit the activation of angiotensin II receptors. Dry cough is not a recognized side effect of digoxin, CCBs, or ARBs.

7. (C) In the given scenario, atrial fibrillation with pre-excitation is the diagnosis. This is the most likely rhythm with an irregularly irregular wide complex tachycardia in an otherwise healthy patient. In atrial fibrillation with pre-excitation, the patient would be conducting antegrade to the ventricle through both AV node and accessory pathway, and some beats are likely to be fusion beats. Any AV nodal blocking agent (adenosine, digitalis, diltiazem, β-blocker) is likely to result in unopposed ventricular activation through accessory pathway and can result in ventricular fibrillation. Thus, AV nodal blocking agents are best avoided in this scenario. Amiodarone is a class III antiarrhythmic agent that slows cardiac conduction (including accessory pathway conduction). Direct current cardioversion is the treatment of choice. If this is not possible, amiodarone may be given in this situation as it can restore atrial fibrillation to sinus rhythm as well as decrease accessory pathway conduction.

8. (A) The ECG shows sinus rhythm with some conducted P waves as well as frequent nonconducted P waves. Accelerated junctional rhythm is also seen in the first part of the tracing. Of the medications given above, digoxin is the most likely culprit to produce nausea/vomiting and high-grade AV block with activation of ectopic pacemakers (junctional, ventricular, etc.).

9. (C) In CPVT patients with VT/VF storm, intravenous β-blocker therapy is considered to be the first line of treatment. General anesthesia can be used as a last resort if β-blocker therapy is ineffective.

10. (C) Since he does not have hemodynamically significant ASD, patient is unlikely to benefit from RSV prophylaxis. He does not meet other criteria for prophylaxis (prematurity or coexistent chronic lung condition).

Children who are 24 months of age or younger with hemodynamically significant cyanotic and acyanotic congenital heart disease will benefit from palivizumab prophylaxis.

Children younger than 24 months of age with congenital heart disease who are most likely to benefit from immunoprophylaxis include

- Infants who are receiving medication to control congestive heart failure.
- Infants with moderate to severe pulmonary hypertension.
- Infants with cyanotic heart disease. [*Pediatrics.* 2006;118: 1774–1793 (pp. 1784–1785).]

11. (D) This patient is a candidate for RSV prophylaxis until she is 2 years old. However, the primary benefit of immunoprophylaxis with palivizumab is a decrease in the rate of RSV-associated hospitalization. Results from double-blinded, randomized, placebo-controlled trials with palivizumab involving 2789 infants and children with prematurity, chronic lung disease, or congenital heart disease demonstrated a reduction in RSV hospitalization rates of 39% to 78% in different groups. None of the clinical trials have demonstrated a significant decrease in rate of mortality attributable to RSV infection in infants who receive prophylaxis. [*Pediatrics.* 2006;118:1774–1793 (pp. 1784–1785).]

12. (A) Furosemide inhibits $Na^+-2Cl^--K^+$ cotransporter in the loop of Henle and is therefore termed a loop diuretic. Thiazide diuretics inhibit Na^+-Cl^- cotransporter. Digoxin inhibits Na^+-K^+ ATPase pump.

13. (D) The patient in the given scenario most likely has idiopathic/viral pericarditis. Ibuprofen and aspirin have been most commonly used and provide prompt relief of pain in most patients but they do not alter the natural history of the disease. High-dose aspirin (800 mg orally every 6 to 8 hours for 7 to 10 days followed by gradual tapering of the dose by 800 mg per week for three additional weeks) is usually recommended if aspirin is used. Although acute pericarditis appears to respond dramatically to corticosteroids, early use of corticosteroids has been associated with an increased risk of relapsing pericarditis in multiple studies.

Routine use of colchicine in the treatment of acute pericarditis has been supported by the Colchicine for Acute Pericarditis (COPE) trial that randomized patients into receiving aspirin alone versus aspirin + colchicine. A 4-to-6-week colchicine therapy may be considered in patients with acute pericarditis, especially in those who have not benefitted from NSAID therapy after 1 week. In this given scenario, ibuprofen is the best option given the side effect profile of colchicines, and colchicine would require a longer course than listed. [*Mayo Clin Proc.* 2010;85(6):572–593 (pp. 577–578).]

14. (B) NIRS saturation is a good surrogate for tissue level saturation/oxygenation. NIRS saturation can be substituted for a mixed venous saturation (MVO_2). The difference between SaO_2 and MVO_2 is a surrogate for cardiac output that is likely to be low given the difference of 40 (80 − 40) in this scenario, which would explain the pH of 7.2 (acidosis).

The pulmonary venous O_2 can be assumed to be close to 100% given the FiO_2 of 21% and clear lungs. The Q_p/Q_s in this scenario is 20.

$$Q_p/Q_s = (SaO_2 - MVO_2)/(\text{pulmonary venous } O_2 - SaO_2)$$
$$= (80 - 40)/(100 - 80) = 40/20 = 2.$$

Thus, patient has a low systemic cardiac output state and his lungs are getting at least two times the systemic blood flow. Norepinephrine is a potent vasoconstrictor. Weaning norepinephrine would lower systemic vascular resistance (SVR) and improve cardiac output, making the Q_p/Q_s more balanced. This should be the first line of management in addition to giving fluids that has already been tried in this patient. IV furosemide would decrease the intravascular volume and be detrimental for the patient. IV β-blocker therapy may decrease cardiac inotropy and worsen the low output state. Decreasing the milrinone would reduce the systemic cardiac output by increasing the SVR and by decreasing the cardiac inotropy. Increasing the FiO_2 would lower the PVR and lead to more pulmonary blood flow at the expense of systemic blood flow (increase in Q_p/Q_s).

15. (E) Initial therapy for KD during the acute phase is IVIG and high-dose aspirin. In case of persistence or recurrence of fever despite one dose of IVIG, another dose should be repeated. For children who defervesce with a second IVIG infusion, but in whom fever recurs, a third dose of IVIG or alternately intravenous steroids (methylprednisolone) may be considered. Oral steroids would not be appropriate therapy for KD.

16. (C) The patient has mild-to-moderate carditis that needs therapy with high-dose aspirin (80 to 100 mg/kg/day in four divided doses in children). Oral prednisone is indicated for more severe carditis associated with a sicker patient in the setting of heart failure, severe valvular regurgitation, significant pericarditis/myocarditis, or reduced cardiac function. There is no recommendation for combining oral steroids with aspirin for treatment of acute RF. IVIG + aspirin is used in the treatment of KD. There is no indication for a β-blocker in pericarditis.

17. (C) Sirolimus acts at a more distal site in the lymphocyte activation cascade by blocking transcription of activation genes. Sirolimus (also known as rapamycin) is not a calcineurin inhibitor, but tacrolimus and cyclosporine are. Cyclosporine and tacrolimus are calcineurin inhibitors. Cyclosporine and tacrolimus are available for intravenous use. Tacrolimus offers no survival advantage over cyclosporine in heart transplant recipients. Sirolimus may be less nephrotoxic over the long term.

18. (C) The patient had mild carditis during RF, but is free of residual heart disease now. Per guidelines, she will need RF antibiotic prophylaxis for at least 10 years or until 21 years of age, whichever is longer.
As per the current guidelines,

1. RF patients with carditis and residual heart disease (persistent valvular disease) should receive treatment for a duration of 10 years or until 40 years of age (whichever is longer, sometimes lifelong) after the last attack of RF.
2. RF patients with carditis but without residual heart disease (no valvular disease) should receive treatment for a duration of 10 years or until 21 years of age (whichever is longer) after the last attack of RF.
3. RF patients without carditis should receive treatment for a duration of 5 years or until 21 years of age (whichever is longer) after the last attack of RF. [*Circulation.* 2009;119:1541–1551 (p. 1547).]

19. (E) Please refer to guidelines as quoted below.
Class IIa recommendations:

Prophylaxis against IE is reasonable for the following patients at highest risk for adverse outcomes from IE who undergo dental procedures that involve manipulation of either gingival tissue or the periapical region of teeth or perforation of the oral mucosa:

1. Patients with prosthetic cardiac valves or prosthetic material used for cardiac valve repair (level of evidence: B).
2. Patients with previous IE (level of evidence: B).
3. Patients with CHD (level of evidence: B).
   a. Unrepaired cyanotic CHD, including palliative shunts and conduits (level of evidence: B).
   b. Completely repaired congenital heart defect repaired with prosthetic material or device, whether placed by surgery or by catheter intervention, during the first 6 months after the procedure (level of evidence: B).
   c. Repaired CHD with residual defects at the site or adjacent to the site of a prosthetic patch or prosthetic device (both of which inhibit endothelialization) (level of evidence: B).
4. Cardiac transplant recipients with valve regurgitation due to a structurally abnormal valve (level of evidence: C).

IE prophylaxis is no longer recommended for the following dental procedures: routine anesthetic injections through noninfected tissue, dental radiographs, placement/removal of orthodontic/prosthodontic appliances, shedding of deciduous teeth, and bleeding

from trauma to lips/oral mucosa. [*Circulation.* 2008;118:887–896 (pp. 892, 893).]

20. (B) The child is ≥10 years old and meets criteria for pharmacological lipid-lowering therapy as per guidelines quoted below. His risk factors include male sex, obesity, low HDL, and high triglycerides. For children meeting criteria for starting lipid-lowering drug therapy, a statin is recommended as first-line treatment.
Recommendations of the NCEP Expert Panel:

1. Consider drug therapy in children ≥10 years of age (usually wait until menarche for females) and after a 6- to-12-month trial of fat- and cholesterol-restricted dietary management.
2. Consider drug therapy if LDL level remains ≥4.90 mmol/L (190 mg/dL) or LDL remains ≥4.10 mmol/L (160 mg/dL) and
   a. there is a positive family history of premature cardiovascular disease.
   b. ≥2 other risk factors are present in the child or adolescent after vigorous attempts to control these risk factors.

Risk factors and high-risk conditions include male gender, family history of premature cardiovascular disease or events, presence of associated low HDL, high triglycerides, obesity and aspects of the metabolic syndrome, diabetes, HIV infection, systemic lupus erythematosus, organ transplantation, survivors of childhood cancer, presence of hypertension, smoking, and elevated lipoprotein(a), homocysteine, and C-reactive protein.
Given the high prevalence of gastrointestinal complaints, poor palatability, low compliance, and limited effectiveness, it is unlikely that the bile acid-binding resins will be sufficient to achieve target LDL cholesterol levels in children who meet the criteria for lipid-lowering drug therapy.
Fibric acid derivatives should be used preferentially for children with severe elevations in triglyceride levels who are at risk for pancreatitis.
Given the reported poor tolerance, the potential for very serious adverse effects, and the limited available data, niacin cannot be routinely recommended for children who need treatment for hypercholesterolemia but may be considered for selected patients. [*Circulation.* 2007;115:1948–1967 (p. 1962).]

21. (D) The traditional therapeutic medication for HCM is β-blocker. If CCBs are used, then preferred medications would be diltiazem and verapamil. Dihydropyridine CCBs like nifedipine would cause peripheral vasodilatation and reflex tachycardia that are both detrimental in a HCM patient with obstruction. Furosemide by reducing preload and therefore left ventricular filling (through its diuretic effect) could worsen the degree of obstruction in a HCM patient. ICD is not indicated at present as the patient has no clear sudden death risk factors. [*Circulation.* 2011;124:37–85 (p. 54).]

22. (B) Sirolimus can inhibit smooth muscle proliferation and may have the advantage of inhibiting coronary vasculopathy. Sirolimus is not a calcineurin inhibitor and is most often used in combination with a calcineurin inhibitor (cyclosporine, tacrolimus). It may also be considered in lieu of calcineurin inhibitors. Sirolimus may be less nephrotoxic over the long term.

23. (A) Anesthetic drugs alone cannot fully eliminate the stress response associated with profound hypothermia. Phenoxybenzamine is a long-acting irreversible α-adrenergic blocker that reduces systemic vascular resistance (SVR) and may be useful in this setting, although hypotension and hypoperfusion may result. SVR is elevated and results in an unfavorable Q_p/Q_s ratio with reduced systemic blood flow and low cardiac output state. Phenoxybenzamine is useful to ameliorate this stress-induced SVR response. Milrinone, nitroprusside, and dobutamine have vasodilatory properties and can be useful adjuncts in reducing SVR. Norepinephrine on the other hand causes systemic vasoconstriction and elevates SVR. Milrinone and epinephrine would not be very useful in reducing the elevated SVR in this setting.

24. (A) All of the signs and symptoms listed can result from rabbit antithymocyte globulin infusion. The most common reported side effect is fever (over 60%). Other common side effects include rash (<25%), hyperkalemia (25% to 30%), abdominal pain (35% to 40%), myalgia (up to 40%), and shivering (55% to 60%).

25. (E) Both adenosine and β-blockers have the potential to exacerbate bronchospasm in this patient. Although the electrophysiologic effects of adenosine are temporary, the bronchospasm may persist for a long period of time. Heart transplant recipients are particularly sensitive to adenosine, and one-quarter to one-half the dose should be used initially as long periods of AV block may be noted with higher doses. Adenosine has a half-life of <2 seconds and is metabolized quickly in the blood. It therefore must be given as rapidly as possible in a large-bore IV as close to the heart as possible. Flushing and hypotension are common side effects. The bradycardia caused by adenosine may precipitate other arrhythmias including atrial fibrillation or ventricular tachycardia, so an external defibrillator should be readily available. The typical dose is 100 to 400 μg/kg in children.

26. (C) Ambrisentan is a newer, selective endothelin A receptor antagonist. It does not induce or inhibit cytochrome P450 enzymes and is metabolized through glucuronidation. Therefore it is much less hepatotoxic than bosentan. Epoprostenol is a prostacyclin (PGI2) analogue and is not a prostaglandin (PGE2) analogue. Sildenafil works through nitric oxide–cyclic GMP cascade, but it is a phosphodiesterase 5 inhibitor and not a phosphodiesterase 3 inhibitor. Milrinone is a phosphodiesterase 3 inhibitor. Combination therapy is increasingly used in children to treat severe pulmonary arterial hypertension despite the lack of published evidence. However, there are studies published on combination therapy in adult patients with pulmonary arterial hypertension.

27. (D) The ECG changes in Brugada syndrome can be dynamic and thus missed on a single ECG screening. Since the characteristic ECG hallmark may be concealed, drug challenge with sodium channel blockers (which may exacerbate the sodium channel dysfunction) to bring out the typical ECG changes has been proposed as a useful tool for the diagnosis of Brugada syndrome. Drugs employed for this purpose have included ajmaline, flecainide, procainamide, pilsicainide, disopyramide, and propafenone although the specific diagnostic value for all of them has not yet been systematically studied. Epinephrine challenge is helpful in identifying concealed LQTS. Cardiac MRI may

be used in the diagnosis of patients with arrhythmogenic right ventricular cardiomyopathy. Isoproterenol testing is commonly used in the EP lab to bring out arrhythmias. Exercise testing may be helpful in the diagnosis of CPVT.

28. (D) Phenytoin, lidocaine, and mexiletine are all class IB antiarrhythmic sodium channel blocking drugs characterized by rapid recovery of the blocked sodium channel. QT intervals may be slightly shortened by these drugs. There is no contraindication to phenytoin use in LQTS patients. There is at present no role for IV β-blocker or amiodarone in the absence of any significant ventricular ectopy. Class III agents like amiodarone, sotalol, and ibutilide block the potassium channels and prolong the QTc interval.

29. (B) The patient is symptomatic with atrial flutter but is hemodynamically stable. Therefore, the priority of the physician is to treat her symptoms using medication(s). Electrical cardioversion is not the first-line treatment for a stable patient. Of the medications given, IV diltiazem is the best option as it would slow down the rapid ventricular response and can produce symptomatic relief. IV β-blockers and sotalol are other options. Class IC antiarrhythmic agent flecainide can slow down the atrial conduction within the flutter circuit and therefore slow down flutter rate. Thus it can convert fast flutter with AV block into slow flutter with 1:1 AV conduction if administered alone. Class I antiarrhythmic agent disopyramide has anticholinergic activity and may enhance AV node conduction and worsen the situation when administered alone. Therefore flecainide and disopyramide are best administered in conjunction with an AV nodal blocking agent. IV labetalol is a nonselective β-blocker and is primarily used in hypertensive emergencies.

30. (C) Levosimendan is a calcium-sensitizing agent that binds to troponin C and improves contractile efficiency as well as reduces afterload. Verapamil is an "L"-type CCB and reduces intracellular calcium by reducing calcium-induced calcium release. Digoxin is a Na–K ATPase inhibitor and indirectly increases intracellular calcium. Milrinone is a phosphodiesterase 3 inhibitor. Nesiritide is a synthetic BNP used to treat decompensated heart failure patients.

31. (D) Isoproterenol stimulates myocardial β-1 receptors resulting in positive chronotropy and inotropy. It can result in the generation of a stable junctional/ventricular escape rhythm that is helpful in this setting allowing for additional time to pursue temporary pacemaker if necessary. Atropine is anticholinergic/vagolytic agent and only works in reversing AV block to excessive vagal effect. It would not be helpful in this situation. Milrinone and dobutamine do not have the same effect as isoproterenol and therefore are not indicated. Digoxin may slow the junctional rate and therefore is not indicated.

32. (A) The patient has low cardiac output despite a EF of 70% because a significant fraction of the left ventricular stroke volume can be expected to leak into the left atrium (LA) resulting in reduced forward systemic stroke volume. Elevated left atrial pressure can be expected and would result in pulmonary edema. She would benefit the most from a systemic vasodilator like nitroprusside that would increase her forward stroke volume and improve her cardiac output. IV furosemide would help by reducing pulmonary edema, but not primarily by improving forward stroke volume. Vasopressin is a vasoconstrictor and would be detrimental in this situation. Digoxin would not helpful as the patient does not have myocardial dysfunction or reduced EF. Dopamine is not a systemic vasodilator and would not improve the patient's hemodynamics.

33. (C) The given clinical scenario does not suggest a TOF spell. Since the RVOT murmur is still loud and the patient is alert, he is unlikely to be in any acute RVOT obstructive crisis. The patient's hematocrit is only 26, which is low for an unrepaired TOF patient. The low oxygen-carrying capacity in the setting of an underlying cyanotic heart disease could result in reduced activity levels.

Anemia could cause a drop in the SpO_2 in the following ways. Systemic vasodilation associated with anemia may shift blood flow from the lungs to the systemic circulation. Thus, there would be more right-to-left shunting as SVR drops causing a drop in SpO_2. Also in the setting of a low hemoglobin, tissue oxygen extraction would result in a much lower mixed venous saturation than compared to somebody with higher hemoglobin levels. In the absence of any right-to-left shunt, blood would be fully oxygenated in the lungs. But in the presence of a right-to-left shunt, a proportion of this blood (with lower mixed venous SpO_2) would mix with the oxygenated blood resulting in a much lower systemic SpO_2.

Since the patient is hypoxic and symptomatic treatment is indicated. Of the following options, blood transfusion would benefit the patient in the ER setting. It would increase his oxygen-carrying capacity and could also improve his SpO_2 for the above-mentioned reasons. Intravenous propranolol, phenylephrine infusion, and morphine administration are useful in patients who have a TOF spell that is not the case here. Furosemide therapy would not be helpful as pulmonary overcirculation is rare in TOF.

34. (E) Acute side effects of PGE1 include apnea (needing intubation), fever/hyperthermia, hypotension, and seizures. Cutaneous vasodilation and edema can develop. In patients who have been kept on long-term PGE1 therapy (beyond 2 weeks), various side effects including cortical hyperostosis has been described.

35. (A) Losartan is an angiotensin receptor 1 (AT1R) antagonist and has been shown to antagonize TGF-β signaling. The exact mechanism of action is uncertain, but activation of angiotensin type 1 receptors increases the expression of TGF-β ligands and receptors and induces the activation of thrombospondin, a powerful TGF-β activator. Propranolol, enalapril, verapamil, or spironolactone does not have the above effect.

36. (D) Eplerenone is a newer mineralocorticoid receptor (aldosterone receptor) antagonist. Most of its effects are similar to spironolactone (including hyperkalemia). Enalapril and captopril both increase potassium levels. Metoprolol has no effect on potassium levels.

37. (C) Amiodarone increases the levels of cyclosporine, digoxin, and warfarin (increased anticoagulant effect) by inhibiting the activity of cytochrome P450. In the setting of preexistent β-blocker therapy as in this patient there is potential for heart block (not enhanced AV nodal conduction) due to the AV nodal blocking effect of amiodarone. There is no interaction requiring dose adjustment with steroids and amiodarone.

38. (B) Amiodarone (class III antiarrhythmic agent) is primarily a cardiac potassium channel blocker. It prolongs repolarization and therefore QTc interval. However, it is also a broad-spectrum antiarrhythmic agent and blocks cardiac sodium and sodium channels as well. It produces β-blockade, causes reduced AV nodal conduction, and is not a vagolytic agent. Hypokalemia exacerbates the pro-arrhythmic potential of amiodarone and can precipitate torsades de pointes.

39. (C) It is true that tacrolimus recipients (8%) more often develop diabetes mellitus than cyclosporine recipients (2%). Higher tacrolimus levels, HLA-DR mismatch, and older age at transplantation may predispose to posttransplant diabetes. Sirolimus use is associated with bone marrow suppression, especially when used in conjunction with tacrolimus. Lipid abnormalities are common even in younger children who are heart transplant recipients, and lipid-lowering therapy is often instituted in this subgroup. CCB and ACE inhibitors are typically used for managing hypertension in pediatric heart transplant recipients. Sirolimus is less nephrotoxic than cyclosporine or tacrolimus.

40. (C) Drugs that lower PVR include tolazoline (a nonselective competitive α-adrenergic receptor antagonist), nitric oxide (not nitrous oxide), dobutamine (not dopamine), milrinone, prostaglandins, prostacyclins, sodium nitroprusside, and sildenafil. Ketamine may increase PVR. Norepinephrine is a systemic vasoconstrictor and is not a pulmonary vasodilator.

41. (D) The patient in the given scenario is likely to have heparin-induced thrombocytopenia with thrombosis (HITT) that develops in a subset of patients with HIT. Heparin combines with platelet factor 4 (PF-4) complex and makes it immunogenic. The resulting antibodies to this complex may result in the formation of platelet aggregates (which can cause vaso-occlusion) and cause immune-mediated platelet destruction resulting in thrombocytopenia (usually a >50% drop in platelet count). Diagnosis is made using specific antibody assay. However, once a thrombotic complication is noted in the setting of suspected HIT, urgent medical therapy is indicated. The best course of action is to completely stop heparin and provide immediate alternative anticoagulation medications.

The degree of platelet drop in HIT patients is not enough to cause clinically significant bleeding and therefore platelet transfusion is not indicated. Low molecular weight heparins (enoxaparin) may not provoke HIT, may still cross-react with heparin antibodies, and are not used in HIT patients.

42. (C) Use of warfarin during pregnancy is associated with various teratogenic side effects including defects in calcification of the epiphyses (chondrodysplasia punctata), retarded intrauterine growth, psychomotor deficit, hypotonia, convulsions, nasal hypoplasia, ocular and CNS anomalies. Risk is higher during the first trimester (~10%), and the critical period is between the sixth and ninth week of gestation. The risk is estimated ~3% to 5% for administration during the second and third trimesters. Lithium has been associated with Ebstein anomaly and not left-sided obstructive lesions. Amiodarone can cause hypothyroidism or hyperthyroidism, but complete heart block is not a typical finding and it is not permanent. ACE inhibitors can cause renal damage, cranial ossification defects, oligohydramnios, and delayed intrauterine growth, but right-sided obstructive lesions have not been described. They are contraindicated during pregnancy, especially the second and third trimesters. High-dose folic acid therapy is known to be protective against neural tube defects.

43. (E) The patient has serious digoxin toxicity and is symptomatic (dizziness and mild hypotension) with high-grade AV block. He also has significant ventricular ectopy including nonsustained VT.

Intravenous atropine and temporary pacing are recommended in such patients with high-degree symptomatic AV block. Digoxin antibody Fab should be administered in patients showing serious signs of digoxin toxicity (symptomatic AV block, serious ventricular arrhythmias), and this patient would be a candidate.

Concomitant therapy with agents such as activated charcoal and cholestyramine has also been recommended in patients showing serious digoxin toxicity in an attempt to bind digoxin in the gut. Such agents facilitate gastrointestinal elimination as well as increase the systemic clearance of digoxin. Through both passive diffusion and enterohepatic recycling of digoxin, the intestine acts as a dialysis membrane, and the binding of the charcoal resin aids in the elimination of digoxin.

Digoxin is 50% to 70% eliminated through the kidneys unmetabolized without significant hepatic contribution, and therefore, liver dysfunction (due to recent infectious mononucleosis) is not the direct reason for elevated digoxin levels. In the setting of preexisting renal dysfunction, reduced oral intake following the viral illness could have contributed to exacerbated renal dysfunction (prerenal etiology) and associated hyperkalemia. This could result in reduced renal excretion of digoxin and precipitate digoxin toxicity. Hyperkalemia exacerbates digoxin toxicity, and concurrent treatment of hyperkalemia would be beneficial, although the potassium level would not give the definitive cause of the AV block, and the QRS is not widened and the T waves are not peaked so the level is likely not severely elevated.

This patient needs the following management: IV fluids to improve renal perfusion and hypotension, treatment of hyperkalemia, IV atropine acutely (temporary pacing is also indicated), digoxin antibody therapy, and management of renal dysfunction. Intravenous lidocaine can be administered if the patient develops symptomatic ventricular arrhythmias before digoxin antibody becomes available.

44. (B) The patient has persistent postoperative hypertension that is significant, and in an intubated patient, it is not easy to evaluate symptoms. She should be treated for hypertension. She has a history of persistent asthma as judged by her medication list, and intravenous labetalol (β-blocker) can exacerbate bronchoconstriction and worsen her hypoxia. In the setting of concurrent renal and hepatic dysfunction, sodium nitroprusside is not safe due to potential buildup of cyanide. Nicardipine is a CCB and can be used in situations where β-blocker and sodium nitroprusside are contraindicated. It does not have any adverse effects on the myocardium.

The patient's hypoxia is most likely due to atelectasis, and since there is no mention of pulmonary hypertension, there is no role for nitric oxide therapy. Dexmedetomidine is a highly selective α-2 receptor agonist and is used for sedation. It can produce dose-dependent decreases in BP and HR as a result of its α-2 agonist effect on the sympathetic ganglia with resulting sympatholytic effects. However, it is not indicated in the current scenario as the patient seems to be well sedated already.

45. (D) The clinical scenario is consistent with a "suicidal right ventricle" due to persistent dynamic infundibular/subpulmonary obstruction that can follow acute relief of a distal fixed pulmonary valve obstruction. The severe subvalvular obstruction in the absence of a distal fixed obstruction can result in complete/near complete RVOT obstruction. This can lead to acute right ventricular failure with poor RV filling and right-to-left shunt through the patent foramen ovale. Intravenous β-blockers would be the drug of choice as they can relieve the dynamic RVOT obstruction and improve the hemodynamics. There is no role for pulmonary vasodilators like nitric oxide in this setting. Milrinone is an inotrope and can worsen the dynamic obstruction. Phenylephrine is a vasoconstrictor and is unlikely to produce any beneficial hemodynamic effects in this scenario. Intravenous diuretics like furosemide have no specific role in this situation. In fact it may reduce right ventricular preload and worsen the condition.

46. (B) Very rarely, statins can cause life-threatening rhabdomyolysis. The most common symptom is muscle pain. Creatine kinase levels should be checked to rule out this condition. Rhabdomyolysis can cause severe muscle pain, liver damage, kidney failure, and death. Other side effects include diarrhea, liver damage, gastrointestinal problems such as diarrhea or nausea, rash and flushing, and neurological side effects.

47. (B) Both the inhalational anesthetic agent and midazolam will cause a drop in systemic vascular resistance and unfavorably alter the $Q_p:Q_s$ for this patient. Ketamine increases systemic vascular resistance and fentanyl has minimal hemodynamic effects. The combination of ketamine and an inhalational anesthetic or midazolam would be preferred to offset the vasodilatory effects of these agents.

Anesthetic induction requires an individual approach to each congenital heart disease patient. A careful pre-sedation assessment is essential to determine the child's baseline cardiac reserve, cardiac physiology, and any noncardiac medical conditions that may impact sedation tolerance. Adequate sedation must be accomplished while simultaneously minimizing any anesthetic-/sedation-related disruption in cardiopulmonary stability. Inhalational anesthetic agents have variable impact on the cardiopulmonary system. However, they all pose significant risk for hemodynamic compromise in the child with limited cardiac reserve. Decreases in systemic blood pressure due to vasodilatation can occur with all inhalational anesthetics to some degree (halothane, isoflurane, and sevoflurane). Sevoflurane has the least impact on systemic blood pressure when compared with isoflurane and halothane.

48. (B) Isoflurane and fentanyl are effective approaches for achieving anesthesia but this is not the best combination of agents for this patient because of her intracardiac shunt. Isoflurane causes a decrease in blood pressure due to vasodilation. The decrease in systemic vascular resistance increases right-to-left shunting through this child's PDA. A significant right-to-left shunt reduces uptake of isoflurane from the lungs and lengthens the time required to achieve the desired level of sedation. Bronchospasm does not typically reduce uptake of inhalational anesthetic. In fact, isoflurane is a powerful bronchodilator and can even be used to break bronchospasm in life-threatening status asthmaticus.

49. (D) This patient has overdosed on β-blocker. β-Blocker toxicity manifests as bradycardia and hypotension and may involve hypoglycemia. Evidence of each of these signs are present, although the heart rate effect of β-blocker toxicity is most significant in this patient. Bradycardia can be counteracted by administering atropine, an anticholinergic. Hypotension may improve as the heart rate increases. Severe or recalcitrant hypotension should be managed with IV fluids and vasoconstrictive agents (e.g., epinephrine, vasopressin, dopamine) if necessary. This patient's hypoglycemia is mild and does not require urgent treatment with glucagon. Hydralazine is a systemic vasodilator and is not indicated in the treatment of this patient.

50. (E) Amiodarone, levothyroxine, propranolol, and sertraline all have the potential to increase warfarin effect, leading to higher INR levels and a need to decrease warfarin dosage. St. John's wort, an herbal supplement that has been promoted to improve mood and treat depression, has been shown to decrease the efficacy of warfarin.

51. (C) This child is most likely experiencing "uncomplicated gastroesophageal reflux" (GER) and therefore does not need to continue his medication. All infants have some degree of reflux. Babies that feed well despite regurgitation episodes, maintain weight gain and hydration, and do not experience significant irritability will typically not require treatment. Research that includes placebo-controlled randomized clinical trials and systematic reviews have demonstrated that acid suppression is not effective for alleviating the reflux-related symptoms of regurgitation and irritability in infants. Furthermore, recent evidence suggests that treatment of GER with proton pump inhibitors (PPI) and H2 receptor antagonists may increase susceptibility to enteric infections and pneumonia. Detailed information regarding current recommendations for referral, diagnosis, and treatment of GER and GERD can be found in the official consensus statement and systematic review issued by the North American Society of Pediatric Gastroenterology, Hepatology, and Nutrition (NASPGHAN) and European Society of Pediatric Gastroenterology, Hepatology, and Nutrition (ESPGHAN), and the American Academy of Pediatrics (AAP). Changing from a PPI to an H2 antagonist and increased dosing frequency have not been shown to improve the efficacy of these agents for reducing GER symptoms.

52. (A) A hydropmorphone PCA would treat pain but not agitation. If the patient is having benzodiazepine withdrawal the hydromorphone would not address this problem. Administration of fentanyl and versed intermittently or as an infusion would treat withdrawal but might worsen the situation if the patient is actually experiencing delirium. Withdrawal can occur following prolonged use of narcotics and benzodiazepines. Signs of withdrawal can include anxiety, insomnia, restlessness, yawning, stomach cramps, rhinorrhea, diaphoresis, mydriasis, vomiting, diarrhea, fever, muscle spasms, tremor, tachycardia, hypertension, and even seizures. Delirium on the other hand is a common complication observed in critically ill adults and children. Delirium can occur even after a short period of sedation. In adults, benzodiazepines appear to increase the risk for delirium. Some studies suggest that dexmedetomidine may reduce narcotic/benzodiazepine requirements and shorten duration of mechanical ventilation for ICU patients. Dexmedetomidine infusions are also used to manage anxiety and alleviate withdrawal

symptoms when narcotic/benzodiazepine weans are initiated. Dexmedetomidine is a centrally acting α-2-agonist. The drug has anxiolytic, sedative, and analgesic effects and does not interfere with respiratory drive. Dexmedetomidine can cause hypotension, hypertension, bradycardia, and atrial fibrillation but is generally well tolerated. [Barr J, Fraser GL, Puntillo K, et al. Clinical Practice Guidelines for the Management of Pain, Agitation, and Delirium in Adult Patients in the Intensive Care Unit. *Crit Care Med.* 2013;41:263.]

53. (A) This child is most likely having a pulmonary hypertensive crisis brought on by the aspiration event. Paralysis with vecuronium in combination with 100% oxygen can be administered immediately to try and reduce pulmonary vascular resistance (PVR) in the acute crisis. Sedation is an important component of treatment but midazolam does not have immediate onset of action. Vecuronium or the shorter acting rocuronium will take effect within 120 seconds of administration. Epinephrine administration is not warranted in pulmonary hypertensive crisis because it will actually increase PVR at high doses. Lidocaine can be used prior to suctioning or intubation to prevent laryngospasm but does not have a role in the acute management of pulmonary hypertension.

54. (C) Chest tube placement is painful and ketamine will provide both analgesia and sedation. Ketamine is also desirable because it will not interfere with this child's respiratory drive in case the pleural effusion is compromising the child's respiratory stability. Fentanyl and propofol will both cause respiratory depression, which increases the risk for further respiratory compromise. Fentanyl alone would provide good analgesia but inadequate sedation for this procedure. Diazepam is long acting and used to acutely treat seizures, which are unlikely during chest tube placement. The correct answer is C because ketamine poses a risk for laryngospasm and bronchorrhea. Glycopyrrolate (or atropine) can be used to manage increased secretions and a muscle relaxant may be necessary if laryngospasm were to occur.

55. (D) This patient is demonstrating metabolic acidosis and alterations in her mental status. These are symptoms of cyanide toxicity. Sodium nitroprusside can cause cyanide toxicity and the risk is increased in patients with renal insufficiency. The US Boxed Warning for the drug states the following:

Except when used briefly or at low (<2 mcg/kg/minute) infusion rates, nitroprusside gives rise to large cyanide quantities. Do not use the maximum dose for more than 10 minutes; if blood pressure is not controlled by the maximum rate (i.e., 10 mcg/kg/minute) after 10 minutes, discontinue infusion. Monitor for cyanide toxicity via acid–base balance and venous oxygen concentration; however, clinicians should note that these indicators may not always reliably indicate cyanide toxicity. The following conditions increase the risk for cyanide toxicity when sodium nitroprusside is used: hepatic impairment, cardiopulmonary bypass, and therapeutic hypothermia. Sodium thiosulfate can be administered with nitroprusside to prevent cyanide toxicity, but thiocyanate toxicity remains a risk especially in patients with renal dysfunction. Avoidance of prolonged high doses and monitoring for metabolic acidosis, bradycardia, confusion, and convulsions are critical to prevent and detect cyanide toxicity during nitroprusside infusion. Elevated cyanide levels have been observed in children at doses of 1.8 mcg/kg/min. Monitoring of cyanide levels every 72 hours is recommended with prolonged use. Treatment includes supporting airway, breathing, and circulation, while administering the antidote hydroxocobalamin and sodium thiosulfate. ["Sodium Nitroprusside: Pediatric Drug Information," Lexicomp, Inc.]

56. (E) Flecainide is a class IC antiarrhythmic. It is primarily a sodium channel blocker and therefore it prolongs phase 0 of the action potential in atrial myocardium, the His–Purkinje system, and the ventricular myocardium. This results primarily in an increase in the QRS duration. It can, however, also lengthen the PR interval. Generally there is very little effect on the QT interval, the ST segments, or the T waves unless toxic levels are reached.

57. (B) Procainamide is a class IA antiarrhythmic and primarily blocks sodium channels and also potassium channels. This results in slower conduction through the atrial myocardium, the His–Purkinje system, and the ventricular myocardium with little to no effect on the sinus and AV node. The above patient is in atrial flutter with 2:1 AV conduction. By giving procainamide, conduction through the atrial muscle can slow resulting in a slower atrial rate. The slower atrial rate can result in AV node conduction to going from 2:1 to 1:1 thereby increasing the ventricular rate resulting in her change in clinical status. Diltiazem is a calcium channel blocker often used to slow AV node conduction during macroreentrant atrial arrhythmias. Lidocaine and mexilitine are class IB antiarrhythmics that affect ventricular muscle and not AV node or atrial conduction. Esmolol is a β-blocker that would slow conduction through the AV node.

58. (A) According to the 2014 PACES/HRS expert consensus statement on the recognition and management of arrhythmias in adult congenital heart disease in patients with IART and complex congenital heart disease and concomitant ventricular dysfunction who have failed a catheter ablation attempt and have no treatable precipitating factors, the best choice of antiarrhythmic to maintain sinus rhythm is amiodarone or dofetilide. In this case, this patient has evidence of possible hepatic disease making amiodarone a less attractive choice as it can be hepatotoxic in addition to having several other potential long-term side effects. Dofetilide is excreted by the kidneys and dosing adjustments must be made in the face of renal dysfunction; however, this patient has a normal BUN and creatinine. Flecainide has been associated with an increased risk of mortality in those with depressed ventricular dysfunction and is generally avoided in

patients with complex congenital heart disease and ventricular dysfunction. Dronaderone is not recommended in patients with a history of heart failure, moderate or severe systolic ventricular dysfunction, or moderate or complex congenital heart disease because of potential concerns over worsening heart failure and increased mortality. Metoprolol may be useful in this patient to prevent a rapid ventricular response in the setting of IART but is not likely to maintain long-term sinus rhythm. [PACES/HRS Expert Consensus Statement on the Recognition and Management of Arrhythmias in Adult Congenital Heart Disease. *Heart Rhythm.* 2014;11:e102–e165.]

59. (C) Dofetilide is a class III antiarrhythmic that selectively inhibits the rapid component of the delayed rectifier potassium current which can prolong the QT interval. Patients should be admitted and observed for QT prolongation and arrhythmia during initiation due to the risk of torsades de pointes. Dofetilide is excreted by the kidneys and the dose must be adjusted for impaired creatinine clearance. Dofetilide does not affect thyroid function. Contraindications to dofetilide treatment include creatinine clearance <20 mL/min, hypokalemia, QTc >440 msec or ≥ 500 msec in the presence of ventricular conduction delay. [PACES/HRS Expert Consensus Statement on the Recognition and Management of Arrhythmias in Adult Congenital Heart Disease. *Heart Rhythm.* 2014;11:e102–e165.]

60. (C) Amiodarone has many potential side effects. The most common side effects include the following: hypothyroidism or hyperthyroidism; hepatitis resulting in a greater than twice normal AST and ALT level which can progress to hepatic failure in a small number; pulmonary toxicity commonly resulting in a cough, fever, dyspnea, opacities on chest x-ray, and a decreased DLCO on pulmonary function tests; dermatologic photosensitivity to UV light; rarely blue-gray skin discoloration; corneal microdeposits that are typically benign; and rarely optic neuropathy. Hypoparathyroid hormone, renal dysfunction, pancreatitis, and conjunctivitis are not known to be common side effects of amiodarone.

61. (A) This patient has moderately controlled asthma. Nonselective β-blockers can cause bronchospasm in asthmatics. Because esmolol is a selective beta-1-blocker it will theoretically only act on the beta-1 receptors in the heart. However, caution is still warranted when considering its use in asthmatics. The other three antihypertensive agents (nicardipine, clevidipine, and hydralazine) would be better choices for establishing blood pressure control in this patient with moderately controlled asthma.

SUGGESTED READINGS

American Academy of Pediatrics Subcommittee on Diagnosis and Management of Bronchiolitis. Diagnosis and management of bronchiolitis. *Pediatrics.* 2006;118:1774–1793 (pp. 1784–1785).

Bauman JL, Didomenico RJ, Galanter WL. Mechanisms, manifestations, and management of digoxin toxicity in the modern era. *Am J Cardiovasc Drugs.* 2006;6:77–86.

Beekman RH, Tuuri DT. Acute hemodynamic effects of increasing hemoglobin concentration in children with a right to left ventricular shunt and relative anemia. *J Am Coll Cardiol.* 1985;5(2 Pt 1): 357–362.

Bonow RO, Carabello BA, Chatterjee K, et al. 2008 focused update incorporated into the ACC/AHA 2006 Guidelines for the Management of Patients with Valvular Heart Disease.... *J Am Coll Cardiol.* 2008;52:e1–e142 (p. e104).

Botto LD, Goldmuntz E, Lin AE. Epidemiology and prevention of congenital heart defects (Chapter 25). In: *Moss and Adams Heart Disease in Infants, Children, and Adolescents.* 2013:524–545.

Bouck MM, Parisi F, Shaddy RE. Pediatric heart transplantation (Chapter 18). In: *Moss and Adams Heart Disease in Infants, Children, and Adolescents.* 2013:426–438 (p. 431).

Constantine E, Linakis J. The assessment and management of hypertensive emergencies and urgencies in children. *Pediatr Emerg Care.* 2005;21:391–396.

De Santis M, Straface G, Carducci B, et al. Risk of drug-induced congenital defects. *Eur J Obstet Gynecol Reprod Biol.* 2004;117: 10–19.

Drew BJ, Ackerman MJ, Funk M, et al. Prevention of torsades de pointes in hospital settings: a scientific statement from the American Heart Association and the American College of Cardiology Foundation. *Circulation.* 2010;121:1047–1060 (p. 1052).

Gerber MA, Baltimore RS, Eaton CB, et al. Prevention of rheumatic fever and diagnosis and treatment of acute Streptococcal pharyngitis: a scientific statement from the American Heart Association Rheumatic Fever.... *Circulation.* 2009;119:1541–1551 (p. 1547).

Gersh BJ, Maron BJ, Bonow RO, et al. 2011 ACCF/AHA Guideline for the Diagnosis and Treatment of Hypertrophic Cardiomyopathy. *Circulation.* 2011;124:37–85 (p. 54).

Kannankeril PJ, Fish FA. Disorders of cardiac rhythm and conduction (Chapter 14). In: *Moss and Adams Heart Disease in Infants, Children, and Adolescents.* 2013:293–342.

Khandaker MH, Espinosa RE, Nishimura RA, et al. Pericardial disease: diagnosis and management. *Mayo Clin Proc.* 2010;85(6):572–593 (pp. 577–578).

Lewis AB, Freed MD, Heymann MA, et al. Side effects of therapy with prostaglandin E1 in infants with critical congenital heart disease. *Circulation.* 1981;64:893–898.

Mason KP. Sedation trends in the 21st century: the transition to dexmedetomidine for radiological imaging studies. *Paediatr Anaesth.* 2010;20:265–272.

McCrindle BW, Urbina EM, Dennison BA, et al. Drug therapy of high-risk lipid abnormalities in children and adolescents: a scientific statement from the American Heart Association Atherosclerosis, Hypertension, and Obesity in Youth Committee, Council of Cardiovascular Disease in the Young, with the Council on Cardiovascular Nursing. *Circulation.* 2007;115:1948–1967 (p. 1962).

Nishimura RA, Carabello BA, Faxon DP, et al. ACC/AHA 2008 Guideline update on valvular heart disease: focused update on infective endocarditis: a report of the American College of Cardiology/American Heart Association Task Force on Practice Guidelines: endorsed by the Society of Cardiovascular Anesthesiologists, Society for Cardiovascular Angiography and Interventions, and Society of Thoracic Surgeons. *Circulation.* 2008;118:887–896 (pp. 892, 893).

Oishi P, Datar SA, Fineman JR. Pediatric pulmonary arterial hypertension: current and emerging therapeutic options. *Expert Opin Pharmacother.* 2011;12:1845–1864.

Olson TM, Hoffman TM, Chan DP. Dilated congestive cardiomyopathy (Chapter 57). In: *Moss and Adams: Heart Disease in Infants, Children, and Adolescents.* 2013:1195–1205 (p. 1204).

Prieto LR, Latson LA. Pulmonary stenosis (Chapter 40). In: *Moss and Adams Heart Disease in Infants, Children, and Adolescents.* 2013:835–859 (p. 845).

Prog Cardiovasc Dis. 2008;5:1–22.

Reddy SC, Saxena A. Prostaglandin E1: first stage palliation in neonates with congenital cardiac defects.*Indian J Pediatr.* 1998;65:211–216.

Siwik ES, Erenberg F, Zahka KG. Tetralogy of Fallot (Chapter 43). In: *Moss and Adams Heart Disease in Infants, Children, and Adolescents.* 2013:888–921.

Struthers A, Krum K, Williams GH. A comparison of the aldosterone-blocking agents eplerenone and spironolactone. *Clin Cardiol.* 2008;3:153–158.

Takahashi M, Newburger J. Kawasaki disease (Chapter 61). In: *Moss and Adams Heart Disease in Infants, Children, and Adolescents.* 2013:1242–1256 (p. 1251).

Tálosi G, Katona M, Túri S. Side-effects of long-term prostaglandin E(1) treatment in neonates. *Pediatr Int.* 2007;49:335–340.

Tani LY. Rheumatic fever and rheumatic heart disease (Chapter 62). In: *Moss and Adams Heart Disease in Infants, Children, and Adolescents.* 2013:1256–1280 (p. 1271).

Trujillo TC, Nolan PE. Antiarrhythmic agents: drug interactions of clinical significance. *Drug Saf.* 2000;23:509–532.

Tweddell JS, et al. Hypoplastic left heart syndrome (Chapter 50). In: *Moss and Adams Heart Disease in Infants, Children, and Adolescents.* 20-13:1005–1038 (pp. 1016, 1017, 1023).

Wernovsky G, Chang AC, Wessel, DL. Cardiac intensive care (Chapter 20). In: *Moss and Adams Heart Disease in Infants, Children, and Adolescents.* 2013:448–480 (p. 457).

Williams A, Davies S, Stuart AG, et al. Medical treatment of Marfan syndrome: a time for change. *Heart.* 2008;94:414–421.

Zipes DP, Camm A, Borggrefe M, et al. ACC/AHA/ESC 2006 Guidelines for management of patients with ventricular arrhythmias and the prevention of sudden cardiac death: a report of the American College of Cardiology/American Heart Association Task Force and the European Society of Cardiology Committee for Practice Guidelines (Writing Committee to develop guidelines for management of patients with ventricular arrhythmias and the prevention of sudden cardiac death). *J Am Coll Cardiol.* 2006;48(5):e247–e346.

CHAPTER 12

Surgical Palliation and Repair of Congenital Heart Disease

Nathaniel W. Taggart

QUESTIONS

1. A 4-month-old child with a large membranous ventricular septal defect (VSD) and large secundum atrial septal defect (ASD) develops complete heart block shortly after surgical repair. A suture "bite" placed too deep in which of the following sites is most likely responsible for the heart block?

   A. Posterior–inferior rim of the VSD
   B. Anterior-superior rim of the VSD
   C. Anterior rim of the ASD
   D. Posterior-superior rim of the ASD
   E. Posterior-inferior rim of the ASD

2. Which of the following surgical interventions carries the highest risk of pulmonary vascular obstructive disease among patients with tetralogy of Fallot and severe pulmonary stenosis?

   A. Central shunt
   B. Potts shunt
   C. Classic Blalock–Taussig (BT) shunt
   D. Modified BT shunt
   E. Late surgical repair

3. A 3-month-old female infant with Down syndrome undergoes successful repair of a balanced complete atrioventricular septal defect (AVSD). While discussing her long-term prognosis with her parents, you state that which of the following is the most common indication for reoperation after repair of AVSDs?

   A. Residual left-to-right shunt
   B. AV valve stenosis
   C. Left ventricular outflow tract (LVOT) obstruction
   D. Right AV valve regurgitation
   E. Left AV valve regurgitation

4. Which of the following is the strongest predictor for developing mitral valve regurgitation after the repair of AVSDs?

   A. Presence of a preoperative mitral valve cleft
   B. Preoperative severe mitral regurgitation
   C. Use of an annuloplasty ring on left atrioventricular (AV) valve annulus
   D. Postoperative left ventricular (LV) enlargement
   E. Postoperative LVOT obstruction

5. You perform a cardiac catheterization on a 12-month-old child with pulmonary atresia, VSD, and confluent pulmonary arteries status post placement of a 3.5 mm modified right-sided BT shunt at 1 week of age. His systemic arterial saturation is 62% on room air. Body surface area is 0.5 m^2. The RPA diameter is 8 mm and the LPA diameter is 9 mm just proximal to their first lobar branches. There is stenosis of the RPA proximal to the BT shunt insertion, measuring 6 mm in diameter. There are no significant aortopulmonary collateral arteries.

   On the basis of the calculated Nakata index, which of the following is the best intervention at this time?

   A. Revision of the BT shunt
   B. Placement of a left BT shunt
   C. Place an RV to PA conduit and leave VSD open
   D. VSD closure, placement of an RV to PA conduit, and RPA patch repair
   E. Takedown of BT shunt and placement of a bidirectional cavopulmonary anastomosis

6. A 3-year-old patient undergoes aortic valve replacement with a tissue bioprosthesis. Two days later, he develops complete heart block with no propagation of electrical activity through the AV node. Obstruction of which of the following would best explain this clinical scenario?

A. Posterior descending coronary artery
B. Right coronary artery
C. Left main coronary artery
D. Left anterior descending coronary artery
E. Left circumflex coronary artery

7. A 30-year-old woman with h/o tricuspid atresia s/p complete Fontan (nonfenestrated) at age 5 years presents with a 2-year history of dyspnea on exertion and cyanosis that is worse when in the standing position. What is the most likely cause of her symptoms?

A. Hepatic AVM
B. Vein of Galen malformation
C. Lower extremity AVM
D. Upper extremity AVM
E. Pulmonary AVM

8. Which of the following operations carries the highest risk of postoperative sinus node dysfunction?

A. Atrial switch (Mustard) procedure
B. Repair of truncus arteriosus
C. Repair of tetralogy of Fallot
D. Repair of a large muscular VSD
E. Mitral valve mechanical prosthesis replacement

9. You are meeting with the family of a 1-month-old infant with hypoplastic left heart syndrome prior to stage I of the hybrid Norwood procedure. Which of the following best describes the role of the interventional pediatric cardiologist in this procedure?

A. Balloon dilation of the pulmonary arteries
B. Stenting of the coarctation of the aorta
C. Endoluminal pulmonary artery banding
D. Stenting of the ductus arteriosus
E. Aortic balloon valvuloplasty

10. A 3-year-old patient is undergoing repair for tetralogy of Fallot and severe pulmonary stenosis. After initiation of cardiopulmonary bypass, using bicaval and aortic cannulation, the surgeon notes progressive left heart distention. This is most likely due to the presence of which of the following?

A. Persistent left superior vena cava
B. VSD
C. Patent foramen ovale
D. Aortic valve regurgitation
E. Aortopulmonary collaterals

11. A 17-year-old boy who had complete repair of a partial AVSD at 15 months of age presents with progressive shortness of breath. He has a 2/6 systolic crescendo–decrescendo murmur that is less prominent with Valsalva. Which of the following is the most likely cause of his symptoms?

A. Mitral regurgitation
B. Primary pulmonary hypertension
C. LVOT obstruction
D. Mitral stenosis
E. Residual ASD

12. A 14-year-old boy (100 kg) with a history of d-transposition of the great arteries s/p arterial switch with LeCompte maneuver undergoes neo-aortic valve replacement using a 23-mm bioprosthesis. Preoperative cardiac catheterization showed severe aortic regurgitation but no significant gradient from left ventricle to descending aorta. At follow-up 8 months later he has a harsh 4/6 systolic murmur at the upper sternal border and a palpable thrill over the left carotid artery. Transthoracic echocardiographic images were unable to define the etiology of the murmur, but Doppler interrogation from the suprasternal notch demonstrated a peak flow velocity of 4.5 m/s directed toward the transducer. MR angiography is performed (see Fig. 12.1). Which of the following is the most likely cause of this patient's findings?

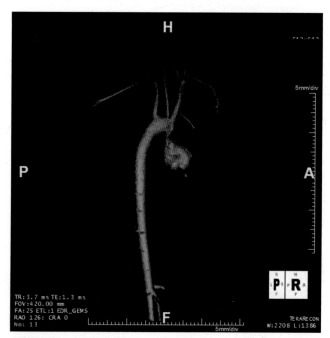

FIGURE 12.1

A. Aortic cannulation injury
B. Congenital supravalvar aortic stenosis
C. Patient–prosthesis mismatch
D. Aortic valve prosthesis endocarditis
E. Carotid artery stenosis

13. A 2-week-old infant is found to have anomalous left coronary artery from the pulmonary artery (ALCAPA). Which of the following preoperative findings is most closely associated with postoperative mortality and need for late reoperation?

  A. Mitral insufficiency
  B. Tricuspid insufficiency
  C. Aortic valve insufficiency
  D. Pulmonary valve insufficiency
  E. Pulmonary valve stenosis

14. What is the most common long-term complication in repaired Scimitar syndrome?

  A. Atrial arrhythmia
  B. Right ventricular systolic dysfunction
  C. Pulmonary vein obstruction
  D. IVC–RA junction stenosis
  E. Pulmonary vascular disease

15. A 5-year-old child has complex single ventricle, bilateral superior venae cavae, and interrupted IVC with azygous continuation to the right SVC. Initial palliation consisted of placement of bilateral bidirectional cavopulmonary anastomoses at 6 months of age. Postoperatively his oxygen saturation is 89%. Now his saturation is 75%. Which of the following is most likely to have contributed to his progressive desaturation?

  A. Erythrocytosis
  B. Intrapulmonary shunting
  C. Decreased chest wall compliance
  D. Increased coronary sinus drainage
  E. Increased pulmonary vascular resistance

16. You are asked to evaluate a 4-year-old child who recently moved to the United States from Russia. He has tricuspid atresia, normally related great arteries, and pulmonary stenosis. At 3 weeks of age, he had a modified BT shunt. His height and weight are in the 15th percentile. The left ventricular impulse is slightly overactive. S_1 is normal, S_2 is single, and there is a 2/6 continuous murmur at the base of the heart. The liver is 1 cm below the right costal margin. The hemoglobin is 17 g/dL. The data in Table 12.1 are

obtained at the time of cardiac catheterization. An angiogram reveals normal size and distributed pulmonary arteries. An echocardiogram reveals an LV ejection fraction of 60%. Which of the following would you recommend?

  A. Perform a bidirectional Glenn and takedown of the BT shunt
  B. Delay any operative intervention until the hemoglobin reaches 19 g/dL
  C. Perform an atriopulmonary connection and closure of the ASD and takedown of the BT shunt
  D. Perform an extracardiac fenestrated Fontan and takedown of the BT shunt
  E. Perform an extracardiac nonfenestrated Fontan and takedown of the BT shunt

17. You are asked to evaluate a 4-year-old child who recently moved from Russia. He has tricuspid atresia, normally related great arteries, and pulmonary stenosis. At 9 months of age, he had a classic Glenn anastomosis. An echocardiogram reveals normal left ventricular systolic function. The data in Table 12.2 are obtained at the time of cardiac catheterization. Which of the following is true?

TABLE 12.2 Cardiac Catheterization Data

	Saturation	Pressure (mm Hg)
SVC	60%	Mean = 10
Left atrium	90%	Mean = 6
Right lower pulmonary vein	65%	
Left lower pulmonary vein	98%	
Left ventricle	78%	110/0, 8
Aorta	78%	110/50
Pulmonary artery	78%	18/8

SVC, superior vena cava.

  A. The patient is not a candidate for a modified Fontan operation
  B. Fontan completion will include repair of an anomalous pulmonary vein
  C. Completion of a lateral tunnel nonfenestrated Fontan will result in complete separation of arterial (oxygenated) and venous (deoxygenated) circulations
  D. Perfusion of the right lung with hepatic effluent blood should improve systemic arterial oxygen saturation
  E. The Glenn anastomosis should be left intact and a modified BT shunt should be placed from the left subclavian artery to the right pulmonary artery

TABLE 12.1 Cardiac Catheterization Data

	Saturation	Pressure (mm Hg)
Right atrium	65%	Mean = 6
Left atrium	90%	Mean = 6
Pulmonary vein	99%	–
Left ventricle	82%	110/8
Aorta	82%	110/50
PA	82%	18/8, mean 11

PA, pulmonary artery.

18. A 1-day-old infant is diagnosed with tricuspid atresia, normally related great arteries, and a large ASD. Oxygen saturation is 60% to 65% on room air. On examination, the child is cyanotic but well perfused. Chest x-ray shows diminished pulmonary vascularity. Which of the following procedures will this patient most likely require as the first palliative intervention?

A. Balloon atrial septostomy
B. Modified BT shunt placement
C. Pulmonary artery banding
D. Damus–Kaye–Stansel (DKS) anastomosis
E. DKS anastomosis with pulmonary artery banding

19. A neonate is diagnosed with tricuspid atresia and d-transposition of the great arteries (d-TGA). On examination, you note poor perfusion and a loud, harsh ejection-type murmur. Oxygen saturation is 95% on room air. Which of the following is the best initial palliation for this patient?

A. Surgical enlargement of VSD
B. Modified BT shunt only
C. Pulmonary artery banding
D. DKS anastomosis with modified BT shunt
E. DKS anastomosis with pulmonary artery banding

20. A 2-year-old boy undergoes successful surgical valvotomy for a stenotic dysplastic pulmonary valve resistant to balloon dilation. Postoperative echocardiography documents mild valvular regurgitation with a predicted gradient across the valve of 10 mm Hg. What is the likelihood that this child will need reintervention on his pulmonary valve within the next 10 years?

A. 95%
B. 80%
C. 50%
D. 20%
E. 5%

21. A 4-year-old child has pulmonary atresia and intact ventricular septum. She had placement of a BT shunt as a neonate. Her pulmonary artery trunk diameter is 10 mm. Pulmonary arteriolar resistance is 2.5 WU × m^2. Her hemoglobin is now 20 g/dL. Tricuspid valve Z-score is -6 and there is evidence of right ventricular sinusoids. Which of the following is the best next step in this patient's management?

A. Partial exchange transfusion with a goal hemoglobin of 15 g/dL
B. Routine follow-up until symptoms develop
C. Bidirectional cavopulmonary anastomosis with takedown of the BT shunt
D. ASD closure, tricuspid valve repair or replacement, and RV outflow tract reconstruction
E. Modified (extracardiac) Fontan and BT shunt takedown

22. A 3-month-old infant has pulmonary atresia with intact ventricular septum and a right modified Blalock-Taussig shunt. His oxygen saturation is 70% on room air. An angiogram documents confluent pulmonary arteries with membranous atresia of the pulmonary valve. The right ventricle is tripartite but diminutive. The tricuspid valve is well developed with moderate regurgitation and an annulus Z-score of -2.3. There is no evidence of right ventricle-dependent coronary circulation. Which of the following is the best next treatment choice for this patient?

A. Left-sided modified BT shunt placement
B. Central shunt placement
C. RV outflow reconstruction
D. Unifocalization procedure with RV outflow reconstruction
E. Bidirectional cavopulmonary anastomosis with BT shunt takedown

23. The angiogram in Figure 12.2 is performed in a 4-day-old boy with pulmonary atresia with intact ventricular septum and a large patent ductus arteriosus. Which of the following operations is best for this patient at this time?

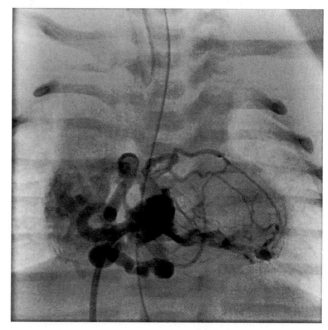

FIGURE 12.2

A. Radiofrequency perforation and dilation of the RV outflow tract
B. PDA ligation, modified BT shunt placement
C. PDA ligation, RV to PA conduit placement
D. PDA ligation, surgical pulmonary valvotomy
E. Continued prostaglandin infusion to allow for growth of right ventricle

24. A 3-year-old child has pulmonary atresia with VSD. He has a history of hypoplastic central pulmonary arteries and multiple noncommunicating major aortopulmonary collateral arteries (MAPCAs), with multiple surgeries including a central shunt and bilateral unifocalization procedures. He undergoes reconstruction of the central confluence, placement of RV–PA conduit, ligation of two MAPCAs, and VSD closure. When cardiopulmonary bypass is discontinued, his blood pressure is 84/60 mm Hg on multiple inotropic agents. Arterial blood oxygen saturation is 98% on 100% inhaled oxygen. Right ventricular systolic pressure is 69 mm Hg by direct measurement. TEE demonstrates patency of the conduit. Which of the following is the best next step?

A. Placement on ECMO until hemodynamics improve
B. Reopening the VSD
C. Takedown of RV–PA conduit and replacement of a central shunt
D. Replacement of the RV–PA conduit with a larger conduit
E. Treatment with nitric oxide to improve pulmonary vascular resistance

25. A neonate with prenatally diagnosed truncus arteriosus is born at 38 weeks gestation via uncomplicated vaginal delivery. On his postnatal echocardiogram, the pulmonary arteries arise from a common trunk and are unobstructed with increased, laminar flow. The aortic arch is right sided. The truncal valve is quadricuspid with mild regurgitation. There are no other complicating factors. Which of the following is the best treatment for this infant?

A. Truncal valve repair and BT shunt placement by 2 weeks of age
B. BT shunt placement only by 2 weeks of age
C. Complete repair within first month of life
D. Pulmonary artery banding by 4 months of age
E. Continue prostaglandin E1, surgery within 1 week

26. Which of the following is the most common indication for reoperation in a patient with a history of truncus arteriosus repair?

A. Neo-aortic valve regurgitation
B. Neo-aortic valve stenosis
C. RV–PA conduit failure
D. Residual VSD
E. Branch pulmonary artery stenosis

27. An asymptomatic 1-year-old female infant is referred for a murmur. Her blood pressure is 117/79 mm Hg (left arm) and 99/70 mm Hg (left leg). The echocardiogram confirms discrete coarctation of the aorta and bicuspid aortic valve with mild regurgitation. The midascending aorta is mildly dilated. Left ventricular function is normal

and wall thickness is at the upper limits of normal. Which of the following is the strongest reason to proceed with surgical intervention?

A. Blood pressure
B. Blood pressure gradient
C. Left ventricular wall thickness
D. Aortic valve regurgitation
E. Ascending aorta dilatation

28. You are discussing the mortality risks to parents of a newborn with hypoplastic left heart syndrome. They ask about the risk of dying during the various stages of the surgical Norwood procedure. You explain that current data suggest that the highest risk of mortality is during which of the following periods?

A. Prior to stage 1 palliation
B. Between stage 1 and stage 2 palliation
C. During stage 2 palliation
D. Between stage 2 and stage 3 palliation
E. During stage 3 palliation

29. One day after a hybrid Norwood palliation procedure, a 7-day-old term neonate with aortic and mitral valve atresia develops progressive cyanosis and mild metabolic acidosis. He is tachypneic with an oxygen saturation of 65% on room air. His heart rate is 160 per minute, blood pressure is 65/42 mm Hg. His chest x-ray demonstrates increased pulmonary vascular markings. Which of the following best explains his worsening clinical status?

A. Pulmonary hypertensive crisis
B. Retrograde aortic arch obstruction
C. Branch PA obstruction
D. Restrictive ASD
E. Hypovolemia

30. Which of the following is a goal of stage 1 surgical palliation (Norwood) for hypoplastic left heart syndrome?

A. Restriction of coronary artery blood flow
B. Creation of a nonrestrictive VSD
C. Establishment of an unrestricted source of pulmonary blood flow
D. Relief of ductal-dependent systemic blood flow
E. Unrestricted right-to-left atrial level shunt

31. Which of the following is the most common indication for reoperation in patients who have undergone arterial switch repair of d-TGA?

A. Supravalvular pulmonary stenosis
B. Supravalvular aortic stenosis
C. Neo-aortic root dilation
D. Neo-aortic valve regurgitation
E. Coronary artery occlusion

32. While being weaned off cardiopulmonary bypass following an arterial switch procedure for d-TGA, a neonate has persistent hypotension and decreased left ventricular function with posterior wall akinesis. Which of the following best explains this patient's clinical status?

A. Unrecognized coarctation of the aorta
B. Acidosis
C. Branch pulmonary artery obstruction
D. Coronary artery obstruction
E. Stress response to cardiopulmonary bypass

33. A neonate is found to have d-TGA with VSD and ASD. The VSD is nonrestrictive, but there is severe pulmonary valve stenosis. The patient's oxygen saturation is 68% on room air. What is the most appropriate initial intervention for this patient?

A. Jatene arterial switch with LeCompte maneuver
B. Mustard operation
C. Pulmonary balloon valvuloplasty
D. Balloon atrial septostomy
E. BT shunt

34. A 2-year-old child with L-TGA, large membranous VSD with outlet extension, and history of critical pulmonary stenosis has been palliated with a modified BT shunt in the neonatal period and a bidirectional cavopulmonary anastomosis at 6 months of age. His oxygen saturation is 70%. He has good biventricular size and function, and no AV valve straddling. He is presenting for surgical intervention. Which of the following is a reasonable alternative to a modified Fontan operation for this patient?

A. Arterial switch and baffling of the IVC to the tricuspid valve
B. Directing morphologic LV flow across the VSD to the aortic valve (Rastelli-type repair) and placement of a pulmonary conduit
C. Closing the VSD to direct LV flow to the pulmonary valve and baffling IVC to the tricuspid valve
D. Directing morphologic LV flow across the VSD to the aortic valve, placement of a pulmonary conduit, and baffling of IVC to the tricuspid valve
E. Directing morphologic LV flow across the VSD to the aortic valve, placement of a pulmonary conduit, and baffling of IVC to the mitral valve

35. You are performing an echocardiogram on a newborn infant in the neonatal ICU. You diagnose double outlet right ventricle with normally related great arteries and large doubly committed VSD, severe coarctation of the aorta, mild subaortic stenosis, and mitral valve which straddles the VSD. What is the most appropriate initial surgery for this patient?

A. Baffle VSD to aorta (Rastelli), repair coarctation
B. Repair coarctation, mitral valve annuloplasty, and chord lengthening

C. Repair coarctation only
D. Coarctation repair, aortopulmonary anastomosis, and nonvalved RV–PA conduit
E. Patch VSD to aorta, repair coarctation, resection of subaortic stenosis

36. What is the surgical procedure of choice for patients with Taussig–Bing anomaly?

A. Pulmonary artery banding with enlargement of the VSD
B. Arterial switch with baffle closure of the VSD to the neo-aorta
C. Systemic to pulmonary (BT) shunt
D. Patch closure of the VSD
E. Aortopulmonary anastomosis and pulmonary artery banding

37. A term neonate with a harsh systolic murmur at birth is found to have double inlet left ventricle with a hypoplastic subaortic right ventricle, a restrictive bulboventricular foramen, and severe subaortic stenosis. Prostaglandin E1 infusion is started. A subsequent echocardiogram documents a large ductus arteriosus. Which of the following is the most appropriate initial operation for this child?

A. Enlargement of the VSD
B. Pulmonary artery banding
C. Bidirectional cavopulmonary anastomosis
D. PDA stent placement and banding of the PAs (hybrid Norwood)
E. Aortopulmonary anastomosis (DKS) with BT shunt

38. A 5-year-old girl is found to have a murmur during a routine physical examination. Echocardiogram reveals a secundum ASD with continuous left-to-right shunt. Which of the following factors would be the strongest indication for surgical repair rather than percutaneous closure of the ASD?

A. Patient's age
B. Deficient anterior-superior septal rim
C. History of dyspnea on exertion
D. Severe tricuspid valve regurgitation
E. Estimated pulmonary artery pressure = 40 mm Hg

39. A child with tricuspid atresia has been palliated with a right-sided bidirectional cavopulmonary anastomosis. He is found to have an anomalous connection of the right lower pulmonary vein to the inferior vena cava. Placement of an extracardiac Fontan conduit at this time would most likely result in which of the following?

A. Thrombosis of the conduit
B. Infarction of the right lower lobe of the lung
C. Persistent cyanosis due to right-to-left shunt
D. Increased pulmonary blood flow due to right-to-left shunt
E. Pulmonary hypertension due to elevated left atrial pressure

40. A 31-year-old woman with a history of coarctation of the aorta has a chest x-ray performed for chronic cough (see Fig. 12.3).

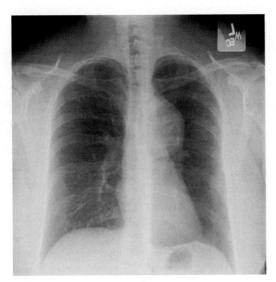

FIGURE 12.3

Which of the following interventions was she most likely to have previously undergone?

A. Percutaneous balloon dilation of coarctation
B. Percutaneous coarctation stent placement
C. Subclavian flap repair of coarctation
D. Synthetic patch repair of coarctation
E. Coarctation resection and end-to-end reanastomosis

41. A 17-year-old boy presents with a history of heart surgery, but he is uncertain about the specifics. As part of his evaluation, the electrocardiogram (ECG) in Figure 12.4 is obtained.

On the basis of these findings, which of the following interventions is he most likely to have undergone?

A. Left ventricular septal myectomy
B. Transannular patch of the RVOT
C. Pulmonary valvotomy
D. Surgical ASD repair
E. Arterial switch operation

42. Which of the following is the most frequently recognized postoperative complication after an atrial switch operation for d-TGA?

A. SVC baffle obstruction
B. IVC baffle obstruction
C. Tricuspid valve regurgitation
D. Mitral valve regurgitation
E. Tricuspid valve stenosis

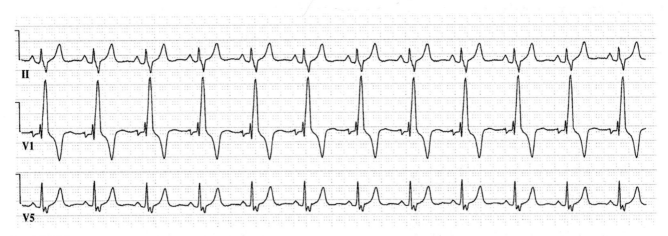

FIGURE 12.4

43. A 3-month-old child presents with congestive heart failure and is diagnosed with a large VSD in addition to the anomaly that is shown in Figure 12.5. In addition to repair of the VSD, which of the following interventions best addresses his coexisting anomaly?

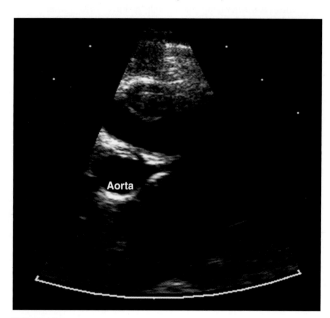

Aorta

FIGURE 12.5

    A. Dissection and reimplantation of the right coronary artery (RCA)

    B. Dissection and reimplantation of the left coronary artery (LCA)

    C. Unroofing of the proximal RCA

    D. Unroofing of the proximal LCA

    E. No additional intervention, as the risk of repair outweigh the benefits

44. A 5-year-old child has a sinus venosus ASD with anomalous pulmonary venous drainage. You explain the Warden repair of this defect with the parents. Which of the following maneuvers is incorporated into this procedure?

    A. Reimplantation of the anomalous vein into the posterior left atrium

    B. Reimplantation of the anomalous vein into the posterior right atrium, then baffling of the veins across the ASD

    C. Transection of the SVC above the anomalous vein insertion and anastomosis of the SVC to the right atrial appendage

    D. Baffling of the anomalous pulmonary veins from their IVC connection to the ASD

    E. Patch closure of the defect between the right upper pulmonary vein and the SVC

45. Which of the following findings in a neonate with d-TGA would be best addressed by a LeCompte maneuver as part of the surgical repair?

    A. Anterior–posterior relationship of the semilunar valves

    B. Large subarterial VSD

    C. Interarterial course of left coronary artery

    D. Pulmonary valve stenosis

    E. Right aortic arch

46. Among neonates who undergo the Ross procedure for aortic stenosis, which of the following is the most common indication for reoperation?

    A. Arrhythmia

    B. Subaortic stenosis

    C. Neo-aortic valve failure

    D. Coronary artery obstruction

    E. Pulmonary homograft failure

47. Which of the following modifications to repair of Ebstein anomaly is most beneficial in patients with a history of supraventricular tachyarrhythmia?

    A. MAZE procedure

    B. Right reduction atrioplasty

    C. Right ventricle plication

    D. Tricuspid valve annuloplasty

    E. Starnes procedure

48. An 8-day-old baby with d-transposition of the great arteries, intact ventricular septum, and atrial septal defect undergoes arterial switch operation with LeCompte maneuver and closure of the atrial septal defect. She is weaned from cardiopulmonary bypass and the chest is closed without complication. Over the course of 2 hours in the ICU, she becomes progressively more hypotensive despite multiple fluid boluses and increasing infusions of epinephrine and vasopressin. Blood pressure is 63/47 mm Hg. Central venous pressure is 18 mm Hg. Lactate level is 5.0 mmol/L (normal = 0.6 to 3.2 mmol/L). Emergent bedside echocardiogram shows underfilled ventricles with normal systolic function and no pericardial fluid or thrombus. Which of the following is the best next step?

    A. Emergent chest CT

    B. Coronary angiography

    C. Bedside pericardiocentesis

    D. Reopen the sternotomy

    E. Cannulation for ECMO support

49. An 8-month-old boy with a large patent ductus arteriosus (PDA) undergoes transcatheter device closure. Following device placement, review of the angiograms suggests diminished blood flow to the left pulmonary artery (LPA). A chest CT is performed (Fig. 12.6). Which of the following is the best next step?

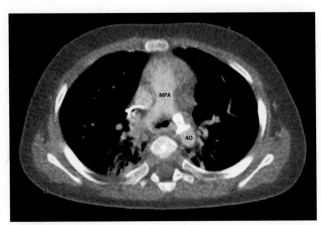

FIGURE 12.6 MPA, main pulmonary artery.

A. Stent placement in the LPA
B. Transcatheter removal of the PDA device
C. Surgical reimplantation of the LPA
D. Surgical removal of the PDA device and reconstruction of the LPA
E. Surgical patch angioplasty of the LPA

50. A 14-year-old otherwise healthy boy undergoes patch closure of a large secundum atrial septal defect. Three weeks after discharge from the hospital, he presents with low-grade fevers and chest pain that began about 4 days prior. His appearance is nontoxic with unlabored breathing. His heart rate is 89 bpm, blood pressure is 113/76 mm Hg. On examination he has crisp heart sounds, no murmur, and a pericardial friction rub. Chest x-ray shows clear lung fields and a cardiac silhouette unchanged from a chest x-ray obtained on day of discharge. Which of the following is the best next step?

A. Obtain blood cultures
B. Treat with high-dose aspirin
C. Treat with colchicine
D. Chest CT
E. Echo-guided pericardiocentesis

ANSWERS

1. (A) A significant concern during the repair of membranous VSDs, particularly when performed on young infants, is damaging the AV node when suturing the patch in place. The AV node courses along the posterior-inferior rim of membranous VSDs. Damage to the node could result in high-grade AV block immediately or shortly after surgical repair. AV block is not a significant risk of secundum ASD repair.

2. (B) Many adults with congenital heart disease have had surgical creation of direct aorta to pulmonary artery communication, either via an ascending aorta to right pulmonary artery connection (Waterston shunt) or via a descending aorta to left pulmonary artery connection (Potts shunt). These techniques have since been abandoned, due to difficulty regulating the size of the shunt and a high rate of branch pulmonary stenosis. Inappropriately large surgical shunts carry a high risk of pulmonary hypertension and, ultimately, pulmonary vascular obstructive disease. Central shunts and modified BT shunts utilize synthetic shunts of specific size, allowing for more predictable shunt volume. Classic BT shunts (direct connection of the left or right subclavian artery to the ipsilateral branch pulmonary artery) were frequently complicated by shunt obstruction and are no longer performed. In the presence of severe pulmonary valve stenosis, the pulmonary vascular bed would be reasonably protected and not at risk of pulmonary vascular disease, even with late repair.

3. (E) Modern surgical repair of AVSDs has resulted in tremendous improvement in life expectancy and quality of life for children (and now adults) with Down syndrome. The need for late reoperation after complete AVSD repair is approximately 15% to 20%. While small residual atrial or ventricular shunts may persist after repair and right AV valve (tricuspid) regurgitation may be present, they are uncommon indications for reoperation. Unlike in partial AV septal defects, LVOT obstruction is an infrequent indication for reoperation among patients with complete AV canal defects. Left AV valve (mitral) regurgitation, on the other hand, is the most common reason for late reoperation.

4. (B) Intuitively, severe preoperative AV valve regurgitation predicts postoperative AV valve regurgitation. A cleft in the left AV valve is universal in AV canal defects and does not predict postoperative regurgitation. While the use of an annuloplasty ring in repair of the left AV valve may reflect the degree of preoperative regurgitation, it does not independently predict postoperative regurgitation. Left ventricular size and hemodynamics may influence the degree of mitral regurgitation, but this association is not so strong.

5. (D) The Nakata index is commonly used to predict operability in patients with pulmonary atresia–VSD. Angiographic measurements of the central pulmonary arteries just proximal to the first lobar branches (and any MAPCAs that perfuse an entire pulmonary segment and can be unifocalized) are taken, and the cross-sectional area of each branch ($\pi \times radius^2$) is calculated. The sum of these areas is divided by body surface area:

$$\text{Nakata index} = \frac{\text{LPA area (mm}^2) + \text{RPA area (mm}^2) + \text{MAPCA area (mm}^2)}{\text{BSA (m}^2)}$$

The calculation for this patient is as follows:

$$\text{Nakata index} = \frac{64 \text{ mm}^2 + 50 \text{ mm}^2}{0.5 \text{ m}^2} = 228$$

Patients with a Nakata index >200 are generally considered good candidates for complete repair (including unifocalization, if necessary). Patients with an index <200 may be candidates as well, but are at higher risk of pulmonary hypertension and right heart failure. They may be better off without surgical intervention or with limited surgical palliation. For the patient in the scenario, RPA patch angioplasty or stent placement would be indicated as part of the repair.

6. (B) Postoperative heart block, ST segment changes, or ventricular dysfunction with regional wall motion abnormalities should raise concern of compromised coronary artery perfusion. This may result from mechanical compression or obstruction by a prosthetic valve, transection of a coronary artery, or tension and kinking with coronary artery reimplantation. The child in this vignette presents a history typical of coronary artery obstruction after a procedure (aortic valve replacement) that presents risk of the same. While definitive identification of the compromised artery requires angiography, the AV node is supplied by a branch of the right coronary artery in 90% of humans, making disruption of the RCA the most likely cause of AV node dysfunction in this patient.

7. (E) Pulmonary arteriovenous malformations occur commonly in patients following Fontan procedures. Dyspnea on exertion and orthostatic or exertional cyanosis in Fontan patients can occur due to right-to-left shunting at a widely patent fenestration or due to right-to-left shunting from pulmonary arteriovenous malformations. These most commonly occur in the basal region of the lung.

8. (A) The sinus node is located in the posterior right atrium along the superior-lateral aspect of the superior vena cava. As a result, surgical disruption of this area may result in damage to the sinus node. Of the choices available, only the atrial switch procedure affects the posterior aspect of the right atrium. In the Mustard/Senning atrial switch operations, systemic venous return is directed across the atrial septum to the left-sided, subpulmonary ventricle. This is done by suturing a patch baffle along the posterior (sinus venosus) wall of the right atrium, in close proximity to the sinus node.

9. (D) The hybrid Norwood procedure has been developed recently as an alternative to the traditional stage 1 Norwood procedure and reduces early-stage mortality in high-risk neonates. The goal of the hybrid procedure is the same as the traditional stage 1 procedure—to provide systemic blood flow from the right ventricle while maintaining adequate, but not excessive, pulmonary blood flow. During the hybrid Norwood procedure, the cardiac surgeon opens the sternum, exposing the heart and pulmonary arteries. The surgeon then bands the right and left pulmonary artery branches, to limit the amount of pulmonary blood flow. The role of the interventional cardiologist is to place a stent within the ductus arteriosus to maintain patency. This allows for the child to discontinue prostaglandin therapy in anticipation of dismissal from the hospital. The hybrid procedure takes place without the use of cardiopulmonary bypass and circulatory arrest, thus minimizing the associated risks.

10. (E) The role of the cardiologist in the operating room includes providing accurate echocardiographic description of cardiac anatomy, particularly the presence of shunts that may complicate cardiopulmonary bypass. In this scenario, the patient develops left heart distention after being placed on bypass, which suggests ongoing pulmonary venous return to the left atrium. This results from persistent pulmonary blood flow that is not accounted for in the bypass circuit. The most likely cause in this situation is a systemic to pulmonary shunt, such as aortopulmonary collateral arteries. If the aorta is not cross-clamped, significant aortic valve regurgitation may result in left ventricular distension, but this is less likely to be the case for this patient. The other options are important findings to note prior to bypass, but would not cause left heart distension. A persistent left SVC typically drains to the coronary sinus and would result in blood return to the right atrium.

11. (C) While the most common cause of reoperation in patients with partial AV canal defects is mitral valve regurgitation, LVOT obstruction is a common cause and much more common than in the complete form of AVSD. Shortness of breath, cardiomegaly, and increased pulmonary vascularity may be caused by mitral valve regurgitation or LVOT obstruction. However, the ejection-type systolic murmur that diminishes with Valsalva presented in this patient clearly suggests outflow tract obstruction as the underlying problem. Primary pulmonary hypertension is very rare in children, and one would expect to find diminished pulmonary vascularity on chest x-ray. Mitral stenosis may cause this patient's symptoms, but it is a less common late finding after partial AV canal defect repair and not suggested by the other findings in the vignette. A residual ASD could cause this patient's symptoms if it was large enough, but, again, LVOT obstruction is a more common postoperative complication.

12. (A) Echo and Doppler suggest a significant gradient at some point in the LVOT or ascending aorta. MRA shows supravalvar narrowing that would be consistent with the Doppler finding. This narrowing is in the region where the aorta would have been cannulated for cardiopulmonary bypass. This is a new finding, so congenital supravalvar stenosis is not likely. There may be some degree of patient–prosthesis mismatch, but the MRA clearly shows narrowing of the supravalvar aorta. Endocarditis is unlikely given the absence of fever or other symptoms. Carotid artery stenosis is not shown on the MRA.

13. (A) ALCAPA typically presents in the second or third month of life after pulmonary vascular resistance falls and the anomalous coronary artery loses perfusion pressure. Infants typically present with a dilated, poorly functioning left ventricle caused by myocardial ischemia. These children are at risk of ischemia and infarction of the mitral valve papillary muscles and resultant mitral valve regurgitation. The tricuspid valve papillary muscles are usually perfused by branches of the right coronary artery.

14. (C) Scimitar syndrome is the eponym for anomalous right pulmonary veins connecting to the inferior vena cava. Surgical repair typically depends on the proximity of the anomalous venous connection to the right atrium and the presence of an ASD. Typically the anomalous connection is transected and the right veins are reimplanted, either into the right or into the left atrium. If implanted into the right atrium, the right pulmonary venous return is then directed across an ASD into the left atrium by a patch baffle. The most common complication of this type of repair is obstruction of pulmonary venous return.

15. (B) The development of pulmonary arteriovenous fistulae has been identified as a risk of the classic cavopulmonary anastomosis (Glenn). Subsequently, it has been found to relate to the absence of hepatic effluent blood in the pulmonary circulation. While this patient had bilateral modified (bidirectional) Glenn anastomoses, the absence of hepatic venous return within the pulmonary circulation (due to IVC interruption) results in a similar lack of the hepatic factor that would otherwise prevent the development of the pulmonary AV fistulae. When surgically feasible, incorporation of hepatic venous return into the pulmonary circulation often results in diminution of the fistulae.

16. (E) The questions being posed by this scenario are whether this patient is a candidate for a Fontan-type palliation and how should the operation be performed. This patient's cardiac hemodynamics are favorable for single-ventricle palliation, specifically the PA pressure is low (mean 11 mm Hg) with a reasonable transpulmonary gradient (5 mm Hg). This is not surprising in the context of pulmonary stenosis, which protects the pulmonary vascular bed from systemic pressure. Infants presenting with single-ventricle physiology typically are repaired in a staged fashion, consisting of a BT shunt shortly after birth, Glenn anastomosis by 6 to 9 months, and Fontan completion in young childhood. As this child is 3 years old, there is no obvious need to perform a Glenn anastomosis prior to Fontan completion. The modified Fontan, using an extracardiac conduit or a lateral tunnel approach, is favored over a direct RA to PA anastomosis (classic Fontan). The question of when to fenestrate a Fontan connection is still debated, but it is clearly not indicated in children with optimal hemodynamics, such as in this patient.

17. (D) The development of pulmonary arteriovenous fistulae has been identified as a risk of the classic cavopulmonary anastomosis (Glenn), which consists of a direct, end-to-end anastomosis of the SVC to the right pulmonary artery. Subsequently, it has been found to relate to the absence of hepatic effluent blood from the pulmonary circulation, which contains a hepatic factor that prevents the development of these fistulae. Incorporation of hepatic venous return into the pulmonary circulation often results in diminution of the fistulae and improvement in systemic saturation as a result. This patient has desaturation of the right lower pulmonary vein, likely due to pulmonary arteriovenous malformations.

18. (D) The vignette above describes a neonate with single ventricle and inadequate pulmonary blood flow, as demonstrated by the child's oxygen saturation and paucity of pulmonary vascularity. This may result from valvular stenosis or obstruction at the VSD (bulboventricular foramen). The initial palliation, therefore, should be directed at increasing pulmonary blood flow. This is best accomplished by placing a modified BT shunt from the subclavian artery to the branch pulmonary artery. Balloon atrial septostomy may be necessary if the ASD is restrictive, but this is not the case with this patient. Pulmonary artery banding would decrease pulmonary blood flow. A DKS anastomosis consists of a direct ascending aorta to MPA (end-to-side) anastomosis. This is used in single-ventricle situations where there is left ventricular outflow obstruction (subaortic stenosis, valvular stenosis/atresia, coarctation) and allows for retrograde perfusion of the coronary arteries via a reconstructed "neo-aortic" arch.

19. (D) A DKS anastomosis consists of a direct ascending aorta to MPA (end-to-side) anastomosis. This is used in single-ventricle situations where there is systemic outflow obstruction (subaortic stenosis, valvular stenosis/atresia, coarctation) and allows for retrograde perfusion of the coronary arteries via a reconstructed "neo-aortic" arch. After a DKS anastomosis, the native pulmonary valve functions as the "neo-aortic" valve. The neonate in the vignette has tricuspid atresia with d-TGA—the aorta arises from the diminutive right ventricle. Since the tricuspid valve is atretic, systemic outflow is dependent on the size of the VSD (bulboventricular foramen). This patient presents with increased $Q_p:Q_s$, as evidenced by a systemic saturation of 95% and signs of poor systemic perfusion and a harsh ejection-type murmur. This may result from a restrictive VSD, subvalvular aortic stenosis, or aortic valve stenosis. In this situation, a DKS anastomosis allows for adequate systemic output and coronary artery perfusion. A BT shunt placed at the same time provides a stable source of pulmonary blood flow once the MPA is separated from the PA branches. Surgical enlargement of the VSD risks damage to the cardiac conduction system causing rhythm disturbances and ventricular dysfunction. A BT shunt alone does not address the problem of systemic outflow obstruction. PA banding would not be indicated as the primary problem is inadequate systemic output, not excessive pulmonary blood flow.

20. (E) Pulmonary valve stenosis can be managed initially with percutaneous pulmonary balloon valvuloplasty or surgical valvotomy. Percutaneous valvuloplasty tends to produce better relief of stenosis, but patients are often left with a greater degree of regurgitation than the surgical approach. A good initial surgical outcome, as described in this patient, carries a low risk of need for future operation, probably not more than 5% over the next 10 years.

21. (E) The type of surgical intervention indicated depends on a patient's age, hemodynamics, and underlying cardiac anatomy. The vignette describes a child with pulmonary atresia and intact ventricular septum. These patients may qualify for a two-ventricle–type repair with placement of a conduit from the right ventricle to the pulmonary arteries (which may be confluent or surgically unifocalized). If the right ventricle is not usable as a functional pumping chamber, either because of hypoplasia or because of coronary to RV fistulae, then the patient is not a candidate for complete repair and requires some form of palliation. This patient has a very diminutive RV, demonstrated by a tricuspid valve Z-score of −4. It has been shown that when the tricuspid annulus Z-score is less than −3, the outcome is very poor after attempted complete repair. As a result, this patient should undergo palliation. Her low pulmonary vascular resistance suggests that she is a good candidate for a Fontan operation. At 4 years of age, a complete Fontan can be performed as a single operation, rather than first performing a staged bidirectional cavopulmonary anastomosis.

22. (C) Patients with pulmonary atresia and intact ventricular septum may qualify for a two-ventricle–type repair with placement of a

conduit from the right ventricle to the pulmonary arteries (which may be confluent or surgically unifocalized). If the right ventricle is not usable as a functional pumping chamber, either because of hypoplasia or because of coronary to RV fistulae, then the patient is not a candidate for complete repair and requires some form of palliation. It has been shown that when the tricuspid annulus Z-score is less than −3, the outcome is very poor after attempted complete repair. Infants with a Z-score of −2 to −2.5 and a functional tricuspid valve may undergo placement of an RV to PA conduit. This patient has a small but usable RV, demonstrated by a tricuspid valve Z-score of −2.3 and the absence of coronary-cameral fistulae (RV-dependent coronary circulation). Low oxygen saturation suggests that he is outgrowing his BT shunt and should have the next stage operation, in his case a two-ventricle complete repair.

23. (B) The angiogram demonstrates a very small RV chamber with multiple sinusoids and coronary-cameral fistulae. These fistulae are common in pulmonary atresia with intact ventricular septum, where the RV is severely hypoplastic. Decompression of the RV by transcatheter or surgical means (e.g., pulmonary valvotomy or placement of a conduit) may decrease coronary perfusion pressure and cause diffuse myocardial ischemia. This patient should continue down a single-ventricle palliation pathway, with placement of a modified BT shunt as a first stage.

24. (B) Successful outcome after complete repair of pulmonary atresia and VSD has been shown to correlate with the postoperative right ventricular systolic pressure. Poor systemic blood pressure and near-systemic RV systolic pressure suggest limited cardiac output due to increased pulmonary arterial resistance. Under these circumstances, the surgeon should reopen the VSD to allow the left ventricle to contribute to pulmonary blood flow. If pulmonary resistance cannot be improved by surgical or transcatheter means, these patients may require surgical palliation rather than complete repair. The patient described is at high risk of pulmonary hypertension given the history of hypoplastic pulmonary arteries.

25. (C) Complete repair of truncus arteriosus has become the favorable approach in US congenital cardiac surgery centers. This patient will need intervention early in life to prevent irreversible pulmonary vascular obstructive disease. Historically, these children underwent pulmonary artery banding procedures within the first month of life. Now, complete repair within the first month of life—with VSD closure, repair of the truncal (neo-aortic) valve if needed, and placement of a conduit from the RV to the pulmonary arteries—is the operation of choice in most centers. This child has nonrestrictive pulmonary blood flow and does not need a BT shunt. The pulmonary arteries arise directly from the common arterial trunk and there is no aortic arch interruption, so prostaglandin is not needed.

26. (C) All of the choices listed are potential indications for reoperation after repair of truncus arteriosus. Homograft or synthetic conduits tend to last 10 to 15 years but almost universally become stenotic and/or regurgitant and are less durable in the youngest patients. Neo-aortic valve regurgitation is very common, but often can be managed without surgical intervention until it becomes moderate or severe. Stenosis of the neo-aortic valve is less common than regurgitation. Residual VSDs and branch PA stenosis are infrequently reasons for reoperation.

27. (A) Severity of coarctation of the aorta can be measured anatomically, via estimated Doppler gradient or by noninvasive blood pressure measurement. Whether to intervene and the timing of intervention depend primarily upon the blood pressure gradient. In the absence of systemic hypertension, LV dysfunction, or significant collateral arteries, a systolic blood pressure gradient of less than 20 mm Hg by itself is not an indication for surgical intervention. The patient has systemic hypertension in addition to a mild gradient and discrete coarctation, so surgical treatment is warranted.

28. (B) The classic Norwood procedure for hypoplastic left heart syndrome consists of three stages. Stage 1 consists of excision of any remaining atrial septal tissue, separation of the pulmonary arteries from the MPA trunk, placement of a BT shunt to the branch PAs, and construction of a neo-aortic arch using the MPA tissue. The right ventricle then serves as the systemic ventricle and the pulmonary valve functions as the systemic (neo-aortic) valve. This stage is usually performed within the first week of life in term neonates without comorbidities. Stage 2 consists of takedown of the BT shunt and placement of an SVC to PA anastomosis (bidirectional cavopulmonary anastomosis). This typically occurs around 6 to 9 months of age, depending on the patient growth and degree of cyanosis. The Norwood is completed in stage 3 with anastomosis of the IVC to the PAs via an extracardiac conduit or tunnel along the lateral wall of the right atrium (modified Fontan). This final stage may be performed as early as 2 years of age. As one would expect, the highest mortality occurs early during the Norwood stages. Specifically, it has been shown to be highest after stage 1 and prior to stage 2.

29. (D) This child is showing signs of poor perfusion and cyanosis. The presence of tachypnea and increased pulmonary vascularity suggest pulmonary congestion from pulmonary venous obstruction. In children with hypoplastic left heart syndrome, the only way for pulmonary venous return to reach the systemic circulation is through an ASD. A small, restrictive ASD would best explain the findings in this child. Pulmonary hypertensive crisis would present more acutely. Retrograde aortic arch obstruction from the PDA stent may manifest as coronary hypoperfusion and decreased ventricular function; desaturation would not be an initial sign. Obstruction of the branch PAs would result in decreased oxygenation, but lung fields would be clear on x-ray. Hypovolemia is unlikely to be the primary cause as evidenced by the pulmonary congestion on chest x-ray.

30. (D) Neonates with hypoplastic left heart syndrome have no left ventricular output, so systemic blood flow is derived from RV/pulmonary artery output via a patent ductus arteriosus. This circulation is adequate in utero, but is not a stable situation postnatally. As a result the goal of the first stage of the Norwood palliation is to provide a stable source of systemic blood flow. Surgically, this is done by separating the branch pulmonary arteries from the MPA trunk, placing a BT shunt to the branch PAs, and creating a neo-aortic arch by enlarging the native aortic arch using tissue from the MPA trunk. After this procedure, neonates do not require ongoing prostaglandin-E1 infusion and can be dismissed from the hospital.

31. (A) The arterial switch procedure has replaced the atrial switch (Mustard/Senning) as the repair of choice for d-TGA. It provides a more anatomic repair, with the left ventricle serving as

the systemic ventricle and the right ventricle as the pulmonary ventricle. Complications of the arterial switch are primarily related to the mobilization and relocation of the great arteries and coronary arteries. In d-TGA the aorta is located anterior to the pulmonary artery. Relocation of the pulmonary artery anteriorly introduces the risk of supravalvar stenosis as the artery is stretched behind the ascending aorta. For this reason, the LeCompte maneuver is sometimes used. This is performed by transecting the main pulmonary artery and relocating the entire PA trunk and bifurcation anterior to the aorta. Distortion of the coronary arteries carries a higher risk of mortality than supravalvular PS, but is less common overall.

32. (D) In addition to verifying the status of the surgical repair, the role of the pediatric cardiologist performing the TEE in the operating room is to assess ventricular function. Markedly diminished ventricular function after bypass should be investigated and explained. The patient in this scenario demonstrates poor function with regional dysfunction, concerning for myocardial ischemia. In addition, any procedures involving manipulation of the coronary arteries portend a risk of occlusion of the coronary arteries and myocardial ischemia. This patient clearly has evidence of inadequate coronary artery perfusion, likely related to mechanical obstruction.

33. (E) This patient's anatomy consists of a subpulmonary left ventricle with obstruction. This manifests clinically as severe hypoxemia due to inadequate pulmonary blood flow. The best intervention in this neonate to increase pulmonary blood flow is placement of a modified BT shunt. The arterial switch procedure may be part of this child's future treatment, but not in the context of LV outflow tract obstruction. The Mustard (atrial switch) operation is now usually performed only in patients with congenitally corrected TGA. Manipulation of the LVOT with a balloon is unlikely to relieve obstruction. PDA stenting as an alternative to BT shunt placement is advocated in some centers, but is not a widely accepted option.

34. (D) The patient in the vignette has complicated anatomy consisting of congenitally corrected TGA, pulmonary stenosis, and a large VSD. He has a bidirectional cavopulmonary anastomosis providing (presumably) the bulk of his pulmonary blood flow. His AV valve and the presence of two well-formed ventricles, however, are favorable for a two-ventricle, physiologic repair. This would be accomplished by directing the remainder of his systemic venous return across the atrial septum to the left-sided AV valve (tricuspid valve), baffle closure of the VSD to direct right ventricle output across the aortic valve, and placement of a pulmonary conduit from the morphologic left ventricle to the pulmonary arteries. Choice A would result in the stenotic pulmonary valve having to function as the neo-aortic valve. Choices B, C, and E would result in the IVC flow being directed to the systemic (subaortic) ventricle.

35. (D) The straddling of the mitral valve chordae precludes physiologic repair of this neonate's defect. As a result, the best option of the choices listed is a Norwood (aortopulmonary anastomosis) palliation with Sano (nonvalved RV–PA conduit). While the severe coarctation does not itself necessitate a single-ventricle repair, a Norwood-type aortic arch reconstruction is appropriate in this situation as the left AV valve morphology has already dictated a Fontan palliation. The Sano shunt is sometimes used as an alternative to a BT shunt to provide pulmonary blood flow from the right ventricle. Some advocate this approach rather than a BT shunt, as the pulsatile flow from a Sano shunt may promote better growth of the branch pulmonary arteries over time. Like the BT shunt, the Sano shunt is temporary and would be removed at the time of bidirectional cavopulmonary anastomosis. In the presence of a functionally normal left AV valve, this patient would likely be a candidate for repair of the VSD and coarctation and resection of the subaortic stenosis (choice E).

36. (B) Taussig–Bing anomaly is a form of double outlet right ventricle where the VSD is located below the pulmonary valve. The physiology of this anomaly resembles that of complete transposition of the great arteries. The pulmonary artery receives primarily saturated blood from the left ventricle through the subpulmonic VSD. The aorta, which is remote from the VSD, receives desaturated systemic venous blood from the right ventricle. Given the arrangement of the great arteries relative to the VSD, the left ventricle cannot be baffled to the distant aortic valve. Instead, the great arteries are surgically switched, as they are for d-TGA, and the VSD is closed to the pulmonic (neo-aortic) valve.

37. (E) This child's heart defect does not allow for complete (two-ventricle) repair. The aorta arises from a hypoplastic right ventricle which itself has no AV valve inflow. Thus, systemic outflow is dependent on the size of the VSD and the patency of the LVOT. With a restrictive VSD (bulboventricular foramen) and severe subaortic stenosis, systemic outflow is severely compromised and should be addressed surgically. The remainder of the aortic arch is presumably normal, so this child can have a direct anastomosis of the main pulmonary artery to the ascending aorta (DKS). Pulmonary blood flow is then accomplished by placement of a BT shunt. Later palliation would consist of a modified Glenn and, ultimately, a modified Fontan. Enlargement of the VSD may improve LVOT obstruction, but does not address the issue of ductal-dependent pulmonary blood flow. PA banding by itself does not address the issue of LVOT obstruction. Placement of a bidirectional Glenn is not indicated in this patient as pulmonary vascular resistance has not yet fallen. The hybrid Norwood procedure is reserved for neonates with hypoplastic left heart syndrome and not used in children with DILV and subaortic stenosis.

38. (D) Most centrally located secundum ASDs can be closed safely and effectively in the cardiac catheterization laboratory. Indications for surgical repair of a secundum ASD includes deficiency of the posterior-inferior septal rim and the presence of coexisting abnormalities that would benefit from surgical repair. Specific recommendations for surgical repair include moderate or severe tricuspid valve regurgitation, which would benefit from annuloplasty or repair of the valve.

39. (B) Completion of the Fontan in this patient would result in persistent connection of the anomalous pulmonary vein to the systemic venous (Fontan) circuit. While initially this may seem to cause persistent left-to-right shunt, in this patient, there is no driving pressure across the right lower pulmonary artery (RLPA pressure = Fontan pressure = RLPV pressure). As a result this lung segment would inevitably become ischemic and infarct.

40. (D) Of the interventions listed, synthetic patch repair of coarctation is known to carry a significant risk of pseudoaneurysm

at the site of repair. In this patient, this is clearly seen as a large mass in the area of the previous coarctation repair.

41. (B) The ECG shown demonstrates sinus rhythm with right bundle branch block. In the postoperative patient, this is most often due to incision of the right ventricular wall, such as from VSD repair or transannular patch. LV septal myectomy may produce left, not right, bundle branch block. The remaining choices are all accomplished without damage to the RV myocardium.

42. (A) Atrial switch operation (Mustard/Senning) is accomplished by baffling SVC and IVC flow to the left-sided AV valve and into the subpulmonic ventricle. Obstruction of either baffle can occur and produces symptoms of central venous obstruction. SVC obstruction is more common and results in jugular venous distension and facial edema and may cause increased head size in infants with an open fontanelle. IVC obstruction, which is less common, may cause hepatomegaly, ascites, and lower extremity edema. SVC and IVC baffle obstruction may be amenable to stent placement in the interventional catheterization laboratory, but may require surgical revision.

43. (C) The echocardiographic image demonstrates anomalous origin of the right coronary artery from the left sinus of Valsalva. The treatment of this lesion is unroofing the intramural segment of the RCA to enlarge the effective orifice. Some question whether any intervention is necessary when this anomaly is found incidentally in asymptomatic individuals. As this patient is going to have a VSD repair, unroofing the coronary artery does not add significant additional risk to the operation.

44. (C) The Warden repair for sinus venosus ASD with anomalous right upper pulmonary veins involves transection of the SVC above the insertion of the pulmonary veins, baffling of the anomalous pulmonary vein/SVC stump to the ASD, and reimplantation of the upper SVC to the right atrial appendage.

45. (A) The LeCompte maneuver is performed as part of the arterial switch operation when mobilization of the pulmonary artery is complicated by the arrangement of the great arteries. This is particularly problematic in cases where the pulmonary artery is directly posterior to the aorta, where simple "switch" of the great arteries would result in stenosis of the MPA or RPA. The LeCompte maneuver is performed by transecting the main pulmonary artery and relocating the entire PA trunk and bifurcation anterior to the aorta.

46. (E) The Ross procedure involves autograft replacement of the stenotic native aortic valve with the native pulmonary valve. A homograft is then placed in the pulmonary position. While all of the choices are risks associated with the Ross procedure, the most common indication for reoperation is failure of the pulmonary homograft.

47. (A) The MAZE ablative procedure involves intraoperative cryoablation or radiofrequency ablation across several segments of the right atrium. This procedure is very effective in treating supraventricular tachyarrhythmias, including atrial fibrillation and atrial flutter. The remaining choices may be performed during repair of Ebstein anomaly but has not been shown to significantly reduce the risk of atrial arrhythmias. The Starnes procedure is typically performed in cases of neonatal Ebstein anomaly with severe right ventricle hypoplasia and significant tricuspid valve regurgitation. It involves patch occlusion of the tricuspid valve at the annulus, removal of the atrial septum, and placement of a systemic to pulmonary artery shunt (e.g., BT shunt). This procedure is performed in anticipation of a single-ventricle (Fontan) palliation.

48. (D) With poor perfusion (manifest by elevated lactate levels) in the face of elevated central venous pressure and normal systolic ventricular function, restriction to ventricular function is very likely. Underfilled ventricles suggest external restriction to filling. The absence of pericardial fluid effectively rules out tamponade due to pericardial effusion, thus pericardiocentesis is not indicated. Perioperative swelling can increase intrathoracic pressure and restrict diastolic filling, particularly in small babies. The treatment would be emergent opening of the sternotomy to relieve increased intrathoracic pressure. The available data support this intervention; additional imaging, such as a chest CT, is not indicated. Coronary artery obstruction can occur in patients with d-TGA after repair, but is unlikely given normal ventricular systolic function.

49. (C) The CT demonstrates a left pulmonary artery arising from the right pulmonary artery and passing posterior to the bronchi, typically called a left pulmonary artery (LPA) sling. The treatment for this lesion is reimplantation of the LPA anterior to the bronchi. The vessel is hypoplastic and may require angioplasty or stent placement in the future. The PDA device appears quite large but is not impinging on the LPA and does not need to be removed.

50. (A) This patient's symptoms of fever and chest pain are most likely due to postpericardiotomy syndrome, which can occur following cardiac surgery, particularly repair of tetralogy of Fallot, atrial septal defects, and ventricular septal defects. While fever is often a presenting sign of postpericardiotomy syndrome, blood cultures should be drawn to evaluate for endocarditis. After appropriate workup, the initial treatment of postpericardiotomy syndrome is high-dose aspirin for 4 to 6 weeks. Steroids may benefit those who do not respond to aspirin alone. Colchicine is not used in the treatment of postpericardiotomy syndrome. Chest CT is not indicated as part of the initial workup. The presence of a friction rub indicates a pericardial effusion, but the patient's appearance and vital signs do not suggest a significant effusion or tamponade.

CHAPTER 13

Adult Congenital Heart Disease

Sabrina D. Phillips, Bryan C. Cannon, and Frank Cetta

QUESTIONS

1. A 24-year-old woman presents to the ACHD clinic at 12 weeks gestation of her first pregnancy. She was recently diagnosed with a bicuspid aortic valve. She has never had an intervention. Her echocardiogram was performed 6 months ago. It demonstrated mild eccentric aortic valve regurgitation, a bicuspid aortic valve with fusion between the right and left cusps. Mean gradient was 14 mm Hg. Left ventricular wall thickness, chamber dimensions, and ejection fraction were all within the normal range. Her ascending aorta measured 32 mm at the sinus, 37 mm at the midascending level. What would you recommend?

    A. Proceed with pregnancy, expect vaginal delivery
    B. Proceed with pregnancy, expect cesarean section for delivery
    C. Obtain an MRI of the thoracic aorta before giving an opinion
    D. Start an angiotensin receptor blocker
    E. Recommend immediate termination

2. A 24-year-old woman presents at 6 weeks gestation of her first pregnancy. She was born with a bicuspid aortic valve and eventually required aortic valve replacement with mechanical prosthesis. She tells you that she usually runs her INR "a bit high" at 3.0 to 3.5. Her average daily dose of warfarin is 4 mg daily. How would you manage her anticoagulation during this pregnancy?

    A. Discontinue warfarin immediately and begin low molecular weight heparin
    B. Continue warfarin at the present dose, discontinue at 36 weeks gestation, and switch to low molecular weight heparin

    C. Continue warfarin and aspirin throughout pregnancy
    D. Discontinue warfarin immediately and start low molecular weight heparin, resume warfarin therapy at 12 weeks gestation
    E. Terminate pregnancy

3. A 20-year-old woman with a history of surgical repair of a secundum atrial septal defect who has short arms with the thumbs that are displaced proximally along the length of the arm comes to clinic in anticipation of pregnancy. She asks about the risks of her baby inheriting her genetic syndrome. Assuming complete penetrance, what percent would you quote to her?

    A. 100%
    B. 75%
    C. 50%
    D. 25%
    E. 10%

4. In the same woman described in Question 3, what is the chance that her child will have congenital heart disease?

    A. 100%
    B. 75%
    C. 50%
    D. 35%
    E. 3% to 5%

5. A 30-year-old woman presents to the ACHD clinic complaining of shortness of breath, intermittent palpitations, and dyspnea with exertion. She notes that she was able to run 10 miles per day fairly briskly when she was 20 years old. Now she is barely able to cover a mile without feeling exhausted. A twelve-lead electrocardiogram (ECG) was performed and demonstrated sinus rhythm and an rSR′ pattern in lead V1. Physical examination demonstrates a right ventricular lift, a normal first sound, and widely fixed and split second sound; the intensity of the pulmonary component of the second heart sound was normal. There is a 2/6 systolic ejection murmur at the left upper sternal border and 2/4 low-pitched diastolic rumble at the lower sternal border. No third or fourth heart sounds. No rubs. The abdomen is soft and nontender. There is no hepatosplenomegaly. Jugular venous pulsations are normal. Transthoracic echocardiography demonstrated a centrally located secundum ASD with adequate rims. Pulmonary venous connections were normal and there was only mild tricuspid valve regurgitation. Based on this clinical scenario and imaging, what is the next most appropriate step?

   A. Cardiac catheterization to measure Q_P/Q_S and pulmonary vascular resistance
   B. Transesophageal echocardiography
   C. Cardiac MRI
   D. Either surgical closure or device closure based on patient preference
   E. No intervention, patient has irreversible pulmonary hypertension

6. In the patient from the previous question, the source of the diastolic murmur is:

   A. Flow through an ASD
   B. Flow across the pulmonary valve
   C. Flow across the tricuspid valve
   D. Flow across the mitral valve
   E. It is a normal murmur in children

7. A 48-year-old man with a history of d-transposition of the great arteries, status post a Senning operation, is being evaluated in the ACHD clinic. It is noted that total cholesterol is 260, LDL 190, and HDL 45. His pooled cohort risk assessment score is 12.5%. Which of the following medications would you recommend?

   A. Niacin
   B. Gemfibrozil
   C. Simvastatin
   D. Aspirin
   E. Losartan

8. A 25-year-old man with a history of tricuspid valve atresia who had an atriopulmonary Fontan connection performed at age 8 years was seen for a routine follow-up visit. He recently started feeling palpitations. A Holter monitor was performed. It demonstrated sinus bradycardia and brief (10-beat) runs of nonsustained supraventricular tachycardia. An echocardiogram demonstrated a left ventricular ejection fraction of 45%. There is trivial mitral valve regurgitation. The right atrium is dilated. There is spontaneous echo contract demonstrated in the inferior vena cava as it enters the right atrium. There is a patent fenestration. The mean gradient through the fenestration is 7 mm Hg.

   Which of the following is the best anticoagulation strategy in this patient?

   A. No anticoagulation
   B. Aspirin
   C. Warfarin
   D. Aspirin and warfarin
   E. Aspirin and clopidogrel

9. In the patient described in Question 8, the Fontan fenestration gradient correlates best with which of the following?

   A. Right atrial mean pressure
   B. Left atrial mean pressure
   C. Left ventricular end diastolic pressure
   D. Pulmonary capillary wedge pressure
   E. Transpulmonary gradient

10. A 25-year-old is referred for evaluation of a murmur that was recently heard during a general physical. On examination, there is a regular rate and rhythm. No lift or thrill. First heart sound is normal in intensity. Second heart sound is hard to distinguish. There is a 3/6 continuous murmur, heard best at the left sternal border. It peaks around the second heart sound. No third or fourth heart sounds. No rubs. Right radial, right carotid and femoral pulses are all easily palpable. Blood pressure is 120/40 mm Hg in both the right and left arms. Which test is most likely to define the source of the murmur?

   A. Twelve-lead ECG
   B. Transesophageal echocardiogram
   C. Transthoracic echocardiogram
   D. Exercise ECG
   E. Dobutamine stress echocardiogram

11. An 18-year-old with unrepaired pulmonary valve atresia/VSD (PA/VSD) comes to clinic for an annual evaluation. On examination, the patient has upper and lower extremity clubbing. There is a regular rate and rhythm. A parasternal lift is present but no thrill. First heart sound is normal. Second heart sound is single. There is a 3/6 continuous murmur which is heard best at the right scapula. No third or fourth heart sounds. Blood pressure is 120/40 mm Hg in both the right and left arms. The origin of the murmur is most likely the:

   A. Right coronary artery fistula
   B. Aortic valve regurgitation
   C. Mitral valve stenosis
   D. Patent ductus arteriosus
   E. Pulmonary valve regurgitation

12. A 25-year-old woman presents to clinic with a 3-month history of exercise intolerance. She also had palpitations recently. Holter monitor demonstrated sinus rhythm. She was wearing the Holter monitor when she had three episodes of palpitations. Echocardiogram demonstrated a 20-mm secundum atrial septal defect with adequate anterior/superior and posterior/inferior rims. Echocardiogram also demonstrated right atrial and right ventricular dilation with preserved function. Trivial pulmonary regurgitation, severe tricuspid regurgitation, right ventricular systolic pressure was 35 mm Hg.

   What is the next best step in this patient's management?

   A. Diagnostic cardiac catheterization to determine pulmonary vascular resistance
   B. Transcatheter closure of the ASD
   C. Annual follow-up
   D. Electrophysiology study
   E. Surgical repair of ASD with tricuspid valve repair

13. A 20-year-old man with a history of tricuspid valve atresia, status post a classic Glenn to the right pulmonary artery and subsequent lateral tunnel Fontan to the left pulmonary artery, presents with a history of progressive cyanosis and exercise intolerance. He undergoes cardiac catheterization, superior vena cava saturation is 75%, right pulmonary artery 75%, left pulmonary artery 78%, descending aorta 88%, right upper pulmonary vein 88%, and left upper pulmonary vein 98%.

   The ratio of pulmonary blood flow (Q_P) systemic blood flow (Q_S) is:

   A. 1.3:1
   B. 1.5:1
   C. 1.8:1
   D. 2:1
   E. Cannot be calculated

14. A 31-year-old with history of tricuspid valve atresia and an atriopulmonary Fontan connection performed in 1989 presents to the ACHD Clinic. The patient has progressive dyspnea on exertion. Physical examination is remarkable for oxygen saturation of 94%, elevated jugular veins, single first and second heart sounds, no murmurs. Liver edge is palpable 8 cm below the costal margin. No ascites, no edema. Liver function including transaminases, total bilirubin, and alkaline phosphatase are all normal. Hepatitis C screening is ordered. Which of the following is a true statement regarding hepatitis C?

   A. A positive antibody test indicates active hepatitis C infection
   B. 20% of patients who had cardiac surgery prior to 2000 have hepatitis C infection
   C. Hepatitis C virus polymerase chain reaction testing confirms presence of infection
   D. Hepatitis C cannot be transmitted from an infected mother to her neonate
   E. Normal liver function testing makes a diagnosis of hepatitis C unlikely

15. BNP levels have been shown to have prognostic value in which subset of patients with congenital heart disease?

   A. Eisenmenger syndrome
   B. Tetralogy of Fallot
   C. Ebstein anomaly
   D. Congenitally corrected transposition of the great arteries
   E. Shone syndrome

16. A 22-year-old woman presents for evaluation of a murmur. She has been asymptomatic. There is right atrial and right ventricular enlargement. Her tricuspid valve is normal with no tricuspid regurgitation. ECG shows right atrial enlargement and left axis deviation. Left ventricular size and function are normal. No shunt is evident at ventricular level.

   The next most appropriate step in the care of this patient would be

   A. Referral for surgical ASD closure
   B. Referral for ASD device closure in the cardiac cath lab
   C. Initiation of ACE inhibition
   D. Cardiac cath with coronary angiography
   E. Observation with follow-up in 2 years

17. A 26-year-old man with tetralogy of Fallot had an episode of syncope while playing basketball. He had no pulse and an AED was placed within 2 minutes of the episode of syncope. Tracings from the AED show ventricular tachycardia at a rate of 260 beats per minute (bpm) and an AED shock was delivered with conversion to sinus rhythm. An echocardiogram showed free pulmonary regurgitation, moderate right ventricular enlargement, and normal right ventricular systolic function.

Which of the following statements is true about implantable cardioverter defibrillator placement in this patient?

A. Catheter-based VT ablation is an alternative to ICD placement

B. Incidence of ICD-related complications is the same as the adult postmyocardial infarction population

C. Inappropriate ICD shocks occur in <10% of patients with tetralogy of Fallot

D. Amiodarone can be offered as an alternative to ICD placement

E. Transvenous ICD can be placed despite severe pulmonary regurgitation

18. You are seeing a 24-year-old woman with a history of a dysmorphic right thumb. She was recently diagnosed with a secundum atrial septal defect. Which of the following genetic mutations is most likely in this patient?

A. TGFBR2

B. FBN1

C. Trisomy 21

D. TBX5

E. NKX 2.5

19. A 16-year-old girl is being evaluated for a systolic murmur that was heard during a presports participation screening examination. She tells you that two of her family members had surgical repair of an ASD. Her ECG demonstrated second degree type II AV block. Which gene mutation is most likely in this patient?

A. NKX 2.5

B. BX5

C. GATA IV

D. NOTCH I

20. Which structure is associated with septum primum?

A. Valve of the fossa ovalis

B. Superior limbus of the atrial septum

C. Inferior limbus of the atrial septum

D. Right atrial appendage

E. Endocardial cushion

21. Which of the following patients has the highest risk of cardiac complication during pregnancy?

A. 32-year-old G2P1 with a large (15 mm) secundum atrial septal defect (ASD) with estimated RV pressure of 30 mm Hg, moderate right ventricular enlargement with normal right ventricular systolic function

B. 20-year-old G1P0 with tricuspid atresia status postextracardiac Fontan. No history of arrhythmia or thromboembolic event, NYHA functional class I. Systemic ventricular ejection fraction 55%

C. 25-year-old G1P0 with repaired tetralogy of Fallot. One prior episode of atrial fibrillation treated with sotalol, severe pulmonary valve regurgitation with moderate right heart dysfunction on echocardiogram. Peak VO_2 58% of predicted

D. 30-year-old G2P1 with bicuspid aortic valve with a mean systolic gradient across the aortic valve of 30 mm Hg. No history of syncope, chest pain, CHF, or arrhythmia. Peak VO_2 95% of predicted

22. A 22-year-old woman with a history of partial AV septal defect and cleft mitral valve presents for evaluation at 6 weeks gestation. Her partial AV canal defect was repaired at age 2 with no residual defect. She had severe mitral valve regurgitation from her cleft mitral valve repaired 3 years ago. Her left ventricular ejection fraction was reduced to 40% postoperatively, and she has been on a medical regimen of lisinopril, carvedilol, digoxin, and aspirin since surgery. Her ejection fraction was noted to be 60% on her last echocardiogram 9 months ago. Which of the following statements is true regarding her medical therapy?

A. Lisinopril should be continued until 24 weeks gestation. It should be discontinued then as fetal renal dysfunction can develop in the third trimester

B. Lisinopril should be discontinued and an angiotensin receptor blocker should be initiated

C. Lisinopril should be discontinued now and hydralazine plus a nitrate should be initiated

D. Lisinopril should be continued throughout pregnancy since it has already been used during a period of critical embryogenesis

23. In which of the following patients is pregnancy absolutely contraindicated?

A. 20-year-old with bicuspid aortic valve with a mean systolic gradient of 30 mm Hg

B. 20-year-old with Marfan syndrome with an ascending aorta diameter of 38 mm

C. 20-year-old with Ebstein anomaly, severe right heart enlargement, and tricuspid regurgitation

D. 20-year-old with an unrepaired VSD and pulmonary artery pressure of 80 mm Hg

24. A 23-year-old woman with a history of bicuspid aortic valve presents to your office at 6 weeks gestation. She has previously undergone aortic valve replacement with a 21-mm St. Jude mechanical valve. She is currently taking warfarin for anticoagulation with a target INR of 2.5 with an average daily dose of 7 mg. What is the best recommendation for further management?

   A. Continue warfarin but decrease daily dose to 5 mg daily
   B. Continue warfarin until 34 weeks gestation then discontinue warfarin and start unfractionated heparin until delivery
   C. Discontinue warfarin now, start Lovenox injection daily, continue at dose of 1 mg/kg daily
   D. Discontinue warfarin now, start Lovenox injection, and continue at dose to achieve therapeutic anti-Xa levels

25. A 19-year-old patient with tricuspid atresia status post RA-PA Fontan connection requests reversible contraception. She had a thrombus in her right atrium 2 years ago and she is taking warfarin anticoagulation. She is unmarried and has had 2 partners. Which of the following should you recommend?

   A. Essure fallopian tubal implant
   B. Mirena intrauterine device
   C. Diaphragm
   D. Low-dose estrogen cyclical oral contraception
   E. Depo-Provera intramuscular injection

26. A 19-year-old patient presents to your office for evaluation. His family history is notable for an aortic dissection in his mother (at an unknown aortic dimension). Physical examination is normal except for mild hypertelorism and a bifid uvula. He does not have ectopia lentis. Blood pressure: 110/50 mm Hg. Echocardiogram demonstrates a sinus of Valsalva dimension of 32 mm. Which of the following is most appropriate?

   A. Initiation of β-blocker and repeat imaging in 6 months
   B. Initiation of ARB and repeat imaging in 6 months
   C. No therapy and repeat imaging in 6 months
   D. Surgical referral for valve sparing aortic root replacement
   E. Initiation of calcium channel blocker and repeat imaging in 6 months

27. A 42-year-old man with trisomy 21 and an unrepaired AV canal defect presents to the office to establish care. His caregivers have noted that he is more short of breath during daily activities over the last year. His room air oxygen saturation is 80% and his hemoglobin is 17 g/dL and MCV 70. Which of the following is most appropriate?

   A. One unit phlebotomy with 500 cc saline replacement
   B. One unit phlebotomy without saline replacement

   C. Initiate oral iron therapy and recheck hemoglobin in 1 month
   D. Initiate IV iron therapy and recheck hemoglobin in 2 weeks
   E. Refer for hematology consultation

28. A 28-year-old woman presents at 24 weeks gestation with dyspnea on exertion, orthopnea, and paroxysmal nocturnal dyspnea. Physical examination is notable for a 4/6 late peaking systolic murmur heard at the upper sternal margins with radiation to the carotids. Echocardiogram demonstrates a heavily calcified bicuspid aortic valve with severe stenosis, systolic mean Doppler gradient: 80 mm Hg. What is the most appropriate management strategy?

   A. Advise bedrest and see the patient back in 4 weeks
   B. Balloon valvotomy
   C. Delivery of the fetus now with immediate replacement of the aortic valve
   D. Percutaneous aortic valve implantation
   E. Surgical replacement of the aortic valve and continuation of the pregnancy

29. A 32-year-old man with a history of coarctation of the aorta repaired at age 9 (end-to-end) presents for follow-up. Echocardiogram demonstrates a coarctation gradient of 7 mm Hg with a normal abdominal aorta Doppler signal. Blood pressure in the office is 160/92. Laboratory data reveal a total cholesterol of 354, LDL cholesterol of 200, HDL of 34, triglycerides of 130. What is the best therapy for his dyslipidemia?

   A. Low-fat, low cholesterol diet alone
   B. Diet plus Niaspan 500 mg daily
   C. Diet plus fish oil 3 g daily
   D. Diet plus simvastatin 40 mg daily
   E. Diet plus gemfibrozil

30. A 32-year-old man with a history of coarctation of the aorta repaired at age 9 (end-to-end) presents for follow-up. Echocardiogram demonstrates a coarctation gradient of 7 mm Hg with a normal abdominal aorta Doppler signal. Blood pressure in the right arm is 160/92, right leg 162/94 mm Hg, heart rate: 50 bpm. Laboratory data reveal total cholesterol of 354, LDL cholesterol of 200, HDL of 34, triglycerides of 130. What is the best therapy for his hypertension?

   A. Stent implantation to relieve the coarctation gradient
   B. Metoprolol 25 mg twice daily
   C. Diltiazem 120 mg daily
   D. Losartan 25 mg daily
   E. Lasix 20 mg daily

31. A 45-year-old man underwent stress echocardiography to evaluate chest pain. He has no other medical history. The stress echocardiogram was negative for ischemia, but views of the atrial septum demonstrated a patent foramen ovale with tiny bidirectional shunt by color Doppler imaging. Agitated saline injection was positive for small right-to-left shunt. The echocardiogram was otherwise normal. What should you recommend?

A. No further testing
B. Coumadin therapy with a target INR of 2 to 3
C. Device closure of the patent foramen ovale
D. Surgical closure of the patent foramen ovale
E. Cardiac MRI to evaluate right ventricular volumes

32. A 75-year-old woman presented to her primary care physician with complaints of exercise intolerance, worsening over the past year. She has extreme dyspnea on exertion and lightheadedness. This has progressed to the point that she is only comfortable while lying supine. She has no lower extremity edema and she denies chest pain. Transthoracic echocardiogram demonstrates normal chamber sizes and normal valvular function. There is a sigmoid ventricular septum of normal thickness. Exercise testing demonstrates poor exercise capacity with a low oxygen saturation of 90% at the start of the test and 82% at 2 minutes of exercise. What is the next best step for evaluation?

A. Pulmonary function tests with methacholine challenge
B. V/Q scan
C. Cardiac catheterization
D. Adenosine sestamibi cardiac perfusion scan
E. Measurement of oxygen saturation while supine

33. A 60-year-old woman presents for evaluation of a secundum ASD. Her past medical history is notable for systemic hypertension, now treated with three drugs. An echocardiogram was performed to evaluate a complaint of dyspnea on exertion. The transthoracic echocardiogram demonstrated a 7-mm secundum ASD with left-to-right shunt, normal left ventricular systolic function, moderately increased left ventricular wall thickness without regional wall motion abnormalities, and mild right ventricular enlargement with normal systolic function. There was no valvular dysfunction. What do you recommend?

A. Device closure of the ASD
B. Surgical closure of the ASD
C. Left and right heart catheterization
D. Aspirin therapy and return to clinic in 1 year
E. Sildenafil therapy and return for cardiac cath in 1 year

34. A 22-year-old woman with a history of bicuspid aortic valve presents to your office at 12 weeks of pregnancy. She is physically active with no symptoms. Her echocardiogram demonstrates a bicuspid aortic valve with a systolic peak Doppler gradient of 34 mm Hg. The left ventricular chamber size and function are normal. The aortic dimension is normal. There is no evidence for coarctation. What would you estimate is her risk of cardiac complication during the pregnancy?

A. 1%
B. 5%
C. 10%
D. 25%
E. 50%

35. A 29-year-old man with a history of coarctation of the aorta status post surgical repair at age 3 years presents for routine follow-up. A cardiologist has not seen him in 12 years. He has no complaints. On physical examination, blood pressure is 120/80 mm Hg in the right arm and unobtainable in the left arm. There is no radial femoral delay. Cardiac examination reveals a normal S_1 followed by a systolic ejection click and a 2/6 midpeaking systolic murmur. What imaging studies would you recommend?

A. Transthoracic echocardiogram
B. Transthoracic echocardiogram and CT scan of the aorta
C. Transthoracic echocardiogram and MRI scan of the aorta
D. Cardiac MRI
E. Transthoracic echocardiogram, MRI scan of the aorta, and MRA scan of the brain

36. A 27-year-old woman with Marfan syndrome presents for routine follow-up. Her echocardiogram demonstrates a sinus of Valsalva dimension of 42 mm with a midascending aorta dimension of 39 mm, mitral valve prolapse, and trivial mitral regurgitation. Her only complaint is of fatigue, which by description is daytime hypersomnolence rather than decline in stamina. She is currently taking metoprolol succinate 25 mg daily and losartan 25 mg daily. On examination, her blood pressure is 100/60 mm Hg, HR 60 bpm. What would you recommend?

A. Overnight oximetry
B. Discontinue metoprolol and increase losartan
C. Continue current medical regimen and return in 1 year
D. Discontinue losartan and increase metoprolol
E. Discontinue both losartan and metoprolol and initiate amlodipine

37. A 36-year-old man with a history of repaired tetralogy of Fallot is seeing a local psychiatrist for moderate depression. The psychiatrist would like to know which of the following medications would be safest for the patient given his cardiac history?

A. Sertraline
B. Citalopram
C. Venlafaxine
D. Bupropion
E. Amitriptyline

38. Dabigatran therapy would be most appropriate for which patient?

A. 23-year-old with Ebstein anomaly with persistent atrial fibrillation
B. 23-year-old man with bicuspid aortic valve status post mechanical aortic valve replacement who has difficulty checking his INR regularly
C. 23-year-old woman 10 weeks pregnant who has a mechanical mitral valve prosthesis
D. 23-year-old with atrial fibrillation who needs bridging anticoagulation for noncardiac surgery
E. 23-year-old man with atrial fibrillation who has had recent GI bleeding while taking warfarin

39. Simvastatin has an important drug–drug interaction with which antihypertensive agent?

A. Metoprolol
B. Lisinopril
C. Amlodipine
D. Hydrochlorothiazide
E. Losartan

40. Which drug has a class D pregnancy classification?

A. Metoprolol
B. Atenolol
C. Amlodipine
D. Verapamil
E. Diltiazem

41. A 38-year-old woman with a mechanical mitral valve and chronic atrial fibrillation presents with a complaint of menometrorrhagia. She is not interested in any future pregnancies. What would you recommend?

A. Ortho Tri-Cyclen
B. Depo-Provera
C. Essure implantation
D. Endometrial ablation
E. Hysterectomy

42. You elect to start a patient on flecainide for atrial fibrillation. How should the drug be initiated?

A. Outpatient initiation at full dose with ECG daily for 3 days to check QT interval
B. Outpatient initiation at full dose with ECG daily for 3 days to check QRS duration
C. Outpatient initiation at half dose for 1 day, increasing to full dose if no side effects reported
D. Inpatient initiation at full dose for five doses with daily ECG to check QT interval
E. Inpatient initiation at full dose for five doses with daily ECG to check QRS duration

43. A 30-year-old man with a history of repaired tetralogy of Fallot is treated with amiodarone for atrial fibrillation. What testing should you obtain at least annually?

A. TSH, AST, bilirubin, alkaline phosphatase, pulmonary function tests
B. TSH, BUN, creatinine, pulmonary function tests
C. Pulmonary function tests, AST, bilirubin, alkaline phosphatase, creatinine
D. AST, bilirubin, alkaline phosphatase, BUN, creatinine, lipid panel
E. TSH, pulmonary function tests, CPK

44. Which pulmonary vasodilator has the highest incidence of lower extremity edema?

A. Bosentan
B. Sildenafil
C. Tadalafil
D. Iloprost
E. Atenolol

45. Patients prescribed the "mini pill" progesterone-only oral contraceptive should be counseled to which of the following?

A. Use barrier contraception for the first 60 days after initiation
B. Avoid prolonged sun exposure
C. Expect cessation of all menstrual flow
D. Stop using SBE prophylaxis
E. Take the dose at the exact same time daily

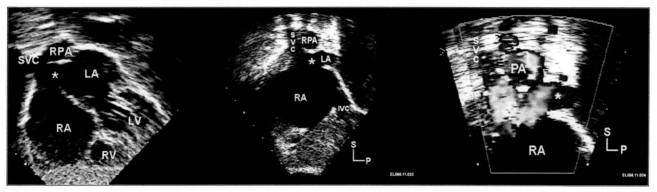

FIGURE 13.1

46. A 45-year-old woman is evaluated for exertional dyspnea and decreased exercise tolerance. On examination, a 2 to 3/6 systolic ejection murmur is appreciated at the left upper sternal border and the second heart sound is widely split and fixed. An ECG demonstrates right atrial enlargement and right ventricular hypertrophy. Echocardiography demonstrates the following (Fig. 13.1). Which of the following is the best course of action?

A. Observe the patient without intervention
B. Perform cardiopulmonary exercise testing to determine need for intervention
C. Recommend surgical ASD closure only
D. Recommend surgical ASD closure with pulmonary venous baffle
E. Recommend device closure of the ASD

47. A 52-year-old woman falls while snow skiing and injures her wrist. On seeking medical care, a systolic murmur is identified, and she is referred for cardiac evaluation. She is normotensive. Her physical examination demonstrates a holosystolic murmur heard best at the left sternal border. An ECG is normal. A transthoracic echocardiogram demonstrates a muscular ventricular septal defect in the midseptum with a peak systolic velocity of 5 m/s. There is no chamber enlargement. The right ventricular systolic pressure is estimated to be normal by tricuspid regurgitant velocity. Which of the following is the best initial management of this lesion?

A. No intervention
B. Surgical closure of the ventricular septal defect
C. Cardiac catheterization to quantify ventricular level shunting
D. Restriction of vigorous physical activity with no immediate intervention
E. Device closure of the ventricular septal defect

48. A 28-year-old man is found to have cardiomegaly on chest x-ray. An echocardiogram demonstrates flow acceleration at the level of the pulmonary valve (peak velocity 2.1 m/s) and moderate dilation of the right-sided chambers. Which of the following is the best next step?

A. Additional echocardiographic imaging to demonstrate PDA
B. Additional echocardiographic imaging to demonstrate ASD
C. Cardiac catheterization with pulmonary balloon valvuloplasty
D. Serial annual evaluation to assess for ventricular dysfunction
E. Cardiopulmonary exercise testing

49. An 18-year-old woman had neonatal arterial switch operation for dextro-transposition of the great arteries (d-TGA). She presents to a cardiology clinic after 4 years without medical care. She has slowly developed exertional dyspnea and now can only climb one flight of stairs without resting. Her physical examination reveals normal jugular venous pressure and pulsation. A grade 3/6 ejection systolic murmur is audible at the upper left sternal border with no diastolic murmur. Which of the following is the most likely explanation of the symptoms?

A. Supravalvar pulmonary stenosis
B. Atrial fibrillation
C. Pulmonary valve regurgitation
D. Aorto-pulmonary window
E. Subacute bacterial endocarditis

50. A 40-year-old woman with a membranous ventricular septal defect underwent prosthetic patch repair as a child. Subsequently, at age 18, she was successfully treated for *Streptococcal viridans* endocarditis involving her mitral valve. Regarding future endocarditis prevention at the time of dental work, which of the following includes the most appropriate counseling?

A. *S. viridans* is an unusual pathogen for endocarditis
B. Prophylactic antibiotics are not indicated in the absence of a residual shunt
C. Prophylactic antibiotics are indicated due to history of bacterial endocarditis
D. Prophylactic antibiotics are indicated daily due to her history of VSD repair
E. No prophylactic antibiotics are indicated

51. A 43-year-old man with d-TGA underwent a Mustard procedure in early childhood. His pulse oximetry reveals an oxygen saturation of 96% at rest. His family history includes colon cancer in his father at the age of 40, and the patient is scheduled for elective colonoscopy. Regarding endocarditis prevention at the time of colonoscopy, which of the following includes the most appropriate counseling?

A. Routine antibiotic prophylaxis should be administered

B. Broad-spectrum antibiotic prophylaxis with anaerobic coverage should be administered

C. No antibiotic prophylaxis is indicated

D. Full colonoscopy should be delayed due to endocarditis risk

E. Limited sigmoidoscopy should be performed

52. A 25-year-old man with Ebstein anomaly had a witnessed, transient loss of consciousness while walking down his apartment stairs immediately after eating dinner. He had brief upper extremity twitching as he regained consciousness. Evaluation in the emergency room reveals normal blood pressure and perfusion. The patient had no prodrome. His ECG demonstrates sinus rhythm, right atrial enlargement with prominent peaked P waves, first-degree atrioventricular block, and right bundle branch block. Which of the following is the most likely explanation for this patient's symptoms?

A. Neurocardiogenic (vasovagal) syncope

B. Seizure disorder

C. Ventricular tachycardia

D. Atrioventricular reentrant (accessory pathway) tachycardia

E. Complete heart block

53. A 32-year-old woman with tricuspid atresia underwent lateral tunnel Fontan palliation as a teenager. She has been followed since that intervention with minimal functional limitation. In the past 2 weeks, she has noted increasing abdominal girth and decreasing exercise tolerance. On examination, she is bradycardic and her liver edge is palpable 4 cm below the costal margin. Her ECG demonstrates junctional rhythm at 42 bpm. Which of the following is the most appropriate intervention?

A. Increased diuresis

B. Atrial pacemaker

C. Fontan revision surgery

D. Cardiopulmonary rehabilitation

E. Digoxin therapy

54. A 50-year-old man is undergoing right-sided diagnostic heart catheterization in the setting of biventricular systolic dysfunction. He acutely develops third-degree atrioventricular block and subsequent hypotension. A pacing catheter is placed emergently. An echocardiogram is performed in the catheterization suite, and chordal attachments are noted from the left-sided atrioventricular valve to the interventricular septum. Which of the following is the underlying congenital lesion that explains these events?

A. Partial atrioventricular septal defect (AVSD)

B. Congenital pulmonary stenosis

C. Congenitally corrected transposition

D. Double-chamber right ventricle (DCRV)

E. Parachute mitral valve

55. A 41-year-old man is new to your practice after living in remote Africa for the past 5 years. He was born with pulmonary atresia with an intact ventricular septum, and palliation was performed in early childhood with placement of a central shunt. He has routinely had therapeutic 300 mL phlebotomy. He denies symptoms including headaches, visual changes, or other neurologic symptoms before or after phlebotomy. He is euvolemic on examination. His initial laboratory results include hemoglobin 21 g/dL and hematocrit 70%. Which of the following is the next best step?

A. Administer 500 mL isotonic crystalloid intravenously

B. Initiate therapeutic heparinization

C. Initiate iron chelation

D. Therapeutic phlebotomy with crystalloid volume replacement

E. Order serum iron studies

56. A 38-year-old woman with tetralogy of Fallot had a right ventricle to pulmonary artery homograft connection. She requires pulmonary valve replacement. She is an active smoker and has a family history of premature coronary artery disease. Fasting cholesterol panel is normal. Prior to surgical intervention that is scheduled in 1 week, which of the following is most urgent?

A. Tobacco cessation

B. Routine preoperative laboratory evaluation only

C. Coronary angiography

D. Prophylactic statin therapy

E. Surveillance blood cultures

57. An 18-year-old man is referred to you after his primary provider hears an early systolic click at the apex. Echocardiogram confirms a bicuspid aortic valve with normal function. There is no family history of heart disease. He has two healthy siblings, and his parents accompany him. Your recommendations for the patient's first-degree relatives should include which of the following?

A. Physical examination of first-degree relatives to assess for aortic valve click

B. Echocardiographic screening of all first-degree relatives

C. Cardiac MRI of any first-degree relatives with abnormal physical examination findings

D. Cardiac MRI of the patient to determine need for family screening

E. No evaluation of first-degree family members is needed

58. A 20-year-old woman returns for routine follow-up after repair of coarctation of the aorta in early childhood. Physical examination demonstrates normal femoral pulses and no brachiofemoral delay. Her right upper extremity and lower extremity blood pressures are equivalent. She has had serial echocardiograms demonstrating no recoarctation of the aorta. At this time, ongoing evaluation should include which of the following?

A. Coronary angiography
B. Neurocognitive testing
C. MRI/MRA of the head and CT or MRI of the thoracic aorta
D. TEE
E. 24-hour Holter monitor

59. A 35-year-old patient with trisomy 21 and repaired partial AVSD is admitted for new onset atrial fibrillation with rapid ventricular conduction. The ventricular rate decreases appropriately with medical therapy and perfusion is normal. On physical examination, there is a prominent apical impulse, and a grade III/VI harsh systolic ejection murmur is heard at the upper sternal border. Echo reveals a mean left ventricular outflow tract (LVOT) gradient of 55 mm Hg at rest. Which of the following is the best choice for therapeutic intervention?

A. Chronic β-blockade therapy
B. Chronic amiodarone therapy
C. Chronic ACE inhibition
D. Aortic balloon valvuloplasty
E. Surgical outflow tract repair

60. A 35-year-old woman with trisomy 21 and repaired complete AVSD has routine follow-up evaluation. She is noncompliant with CPAP therapy for obstructive sleep apnea. Her echocardiogram reports mild tricuspid regurgitation with a velocity of 5 m/s. Cardiac catheterization is performed under general anesthesia to evaluate right ventricular hypertension. The right ventricle and pulmonary artery pressures are found to be normal. Which of the following is the most likely explanation for the discrepancy in echo and catheterization data?

A. Improved right ventricular pressure with adequate ventilation
B. Left ventricle to right atrial shunting
C. Doppler contamination with right ventricular outflow signal
D. Transient pulmonary vasospasm
E. No discrepancy is present

61. A 26-year-old man is prompted by his wife to return for cardiac care. His medical record describes a grade II/VI high-pitched holosystolic murmur consistent with known small membranous ventricular septal defect. On current examination, a right ventricular heave is present, and a prominent thrill is palpable at the left upper sternal margin. Which of the following is the most likely diagnosis?

A. Supravalvular pulmonary stenosis
B. Double-chamber right ventricle
C. Increase in left ventricular pressure
D. Decrease in ventricular septal defect size
E. Increase in ventricular septal defect size

62. A 52-year-old tow truck driver had repair of tetralogy of Fallot at 4 years of age. He presents to the emergency department due to syncope while loading a car onto his truck. He had no prodromal symptoms. He had only the one surgery in childhood. He had last sought cardiac care in 1970. His ECG shows sinus rhythm at 80 bpm, PR interval 100 msec. There is right bundle branch block and the QRS duration is 199 msec. An electrophysiology study is most appropriate to evaluate for which of the following?

A. Inducible ventricular arrhythmia
B. Inducible atrial arrhythmia
C. Sinus node dysfunction
D. Atrioventricular node dysfunction
E. Accessory pathway characteristics

63. A 40-year-old man with d-TGA underwent Mustard procedure in infancy. On examination, his heart rate is 40 bpm and regular. Resting oxygen saturation is 92%. Jugular venous pressure is elevated 10 cm above the angle of the sternum. ECG confirms junctional rhythm. Exercise testing elicits sinus rhythm with a peak heart rate of 65 bpm and with poor exercise capacity. Prior to transvenous pacemaker placement, evaluation should include which of the following?

A. Thrombophilia laboratory assessment
B. Computed tomography coronary angiography
C. Electrophysiology study to evaluate for inducible ventricular tachycardia
D. Cardiac catheterization to evaluate for SVC obstruction and baffle leak
E. Cardiac catheterization to evaluate for proximal coronary obstruction

64. A 25-year-old woman with d-TGA underwent arterial switch operation in infancy. Twice while shoveling snow, she developed a dull ache between her scapulae. Symptoms abated with rest. She walks up to 3 miles per day without symptoms. In addition to routine echocardiography, you would recommend which of the following?

   A. Coronary angiography
   B. Transesophageal echocardiogram
   C. Fasting lipid panel
   D. Cardiac MRI with gadolinium
   E. No additional evaluation

65. A 35-year-old man with congenitally corrected L-TGA and no previous surgery was found to have periods of complete heart block. Therefore, a dual-chamber transvenous pacemaker was placed. The echo immediately after the intervention demonstrated stable findings including mildly reduced systolic function of the systemic ventricle and minimal systemic atrioventricular valve regurgitation. Six months later, the patient returns with new onset of paroxysmal nocturnal dyspnea and decreased exercise tolerance. Pacemaker interrogation is unremarkable. Repeat echo demonstrates moderate systemic ventricular systolic dysfunction and moderate mitral valve regurgitation. Which of the following is the most likely explanation for these changes?

   A. Myocardial ischemia
   B. Pacemaker-induced dysfunction
   C. Paradoxical supraventricular tachycardia
   D. Obstructive sleep apnea
   E. Subacute bacterial endocarditis

66. A 32-year-old man with lateral tunnel Fontan palliation of tricuspid atresia presents to an emergency department with sinus tachycardia and tachypnea after a presyncopal event. There was concern for pulmonary embolism and after placing a right upper extremity IV, a ventilation perfusion scan (VQ scan) demonstrated no perfusion of the left lung with normal perfusion of the right lung. Prior to initiation of treatment for pulmonary embolus occluding the left pulmonary artery, what would you recommend that the treating team perform next?

   A. Repeat the study with a lower extremity IV
   B. Perform a transesophageal echocardiogram
   C. Place a central venous line
   D. Perform invasive pulmonary angiography
   E. Draw blood for thrombophilia assays

67. A 48-year-old man undergoes computed tomography angiogram in the setting of exertional chest discomfort. His right coronary artery arises from the left coronary cusp of the aorta with a proximal intramural course, subsequently passing between the pulmonary artery and the aorta that are normally positioned. Which of the following is the best intervention?

   A. Saphenous vein graft to the distal left main coronary artery
   B. Internal mammary artery anastomosis to the distal left main coronary artery
   C. Unroofing of intramural right coronary artery
   D. Coronary button translocation to the left coronary cusp
   E. No intervention is indicated

68. A 30-year-old man with congenital heart disease repaired in infancy undergoes right- and left-sided cardiac catheterization with this anterior–posterior image of catheter position (Fig. 13.2). The course of the cardiac catheter (not the wire) is best described as which of the following?

   A. IVC, systemic venous baffle, mitral valve, morphologic left ventricle, aorta

   B. IVC, systemic venous baffle, tricuspid valve, morphologic right ventricle, pulmonary artery

   C. IVC, systemic venous baffle, mitral valve, morphologic left ventricle, pulmonary artery

   D. IVC, systemic venous baffle, tricuspid valve, morphologic left ventricle, pulmonary artery

   E. IVC, pulmonary venous baffle, tricuspid valve, morphologic right ventricle, pulmonary artery

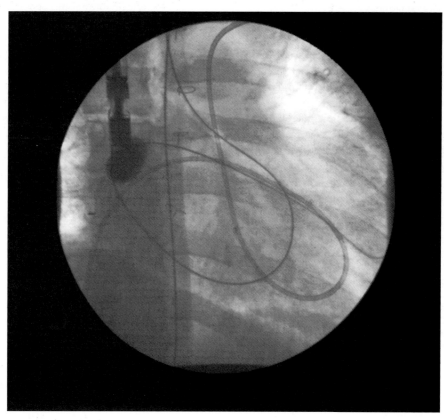

FIGURE 13.2

69. A 20 year old with a history of a bicuspid aortic valve, no cardiac murmur, and normal LA and LV sizes and function on a recent echocardiogram is referred for an chest MRI/MRA for surveillance of his aorta. Based on the MRA image in Figure 13.3, what would be the best course of action for this patient?

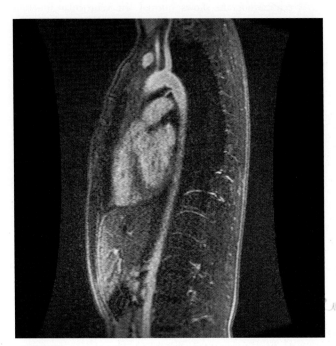

FIGURE 13.3

    A. Referral to surgery for aortic root replacement
    B. Referral for coronary angiography
    C. Referral for interventional cath procedure
    D. Follow-up echocardiography in 3 to 5 years

70. Figure 13.4 shows a chest radiograph of a patient who most likely has which of the following?

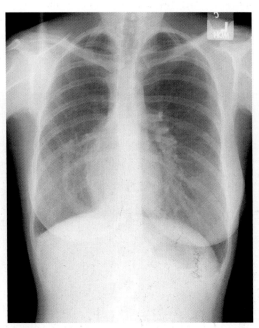

FIGURE 13.4

    A. VSD
    B. ASD
    C. Intact atrial septum
    D. Left SVC
    E. Anomalous coronary artery

71. A patient presents with congenitally corrected TGA. The ECG of this patient would likely show which of the following?

    A. Q waves in leads I and AVL
    B. Northwest QRS axis
    C. Left axis deviation
    D. Complete heart block
    E. Right bundle branch block

72. A teenager presents with progressive symptoms of stridor during exercise. In retrospect, he recalls having these symptoms for most of his life. His mother told him that periodically he was cyanotic as a baby. In the office today oxygen saturation in room air is 99%. The CT scan shown in Figure 13.5 was performed. Which of the following would be most likely?

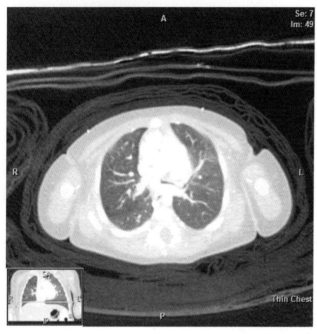

FIGURE 13.5

A. Anterior indentation of the esophagus on barium esophagram
B. Large VSD seen on echo
C. Left SVC seen on CT
D. Partial anomalous pulmonary venous connections
E. Short stature and webbed neck

73. A 19-year-old woman with congenital complete AV block presents for a routine follow-up evaluation. She has been doing well with no symptoms. Her baseline ECG and 24-hour cardioscan both show complex ventricular ectopy with frequent multiform premature ventricular contractions (PVCs). There is no evidence of AV conduction with an average ventricular rate of 64 bpm. Her echocardiogram shows mild ventricular dysfunction with an ejection fraction of 45%.

The next most appropriate step in the care of this patient would be:

A. Pacemaker implantation
B. Close follow-up for development of symptoms
C. Initiation of amiodarone therapy
D. Electrophysiology study
E. Institution of ACE inhibition

74. A 24-year-old man with a large unrepaired ventricular septal defect and pulmonary hypertension presents after an episode of syncope preceded by palpitations. A 24-hour cardioscan monitor shows a 10-minute episode of monomorphic ventricular tachycardia at a rate of 180 bpm during which time the patient reports symptoms of dizziness. His echocardiogram shows normal left ventricular function with an ejection fraction of 58%. There is a large ventricular septal defect with bidirectional shunting. An electrophysiology study reveals inducible ventricular tachycardia at a rate of 210 bpm with a blood pressure drop to 50/30 mm Hg which spontaneously converts to sinus rhythm after 1 minute. The patient is cyanotic with a resting saturation of 84% but otherwise doing well with minimal symptoms. The next most appropriate step in the care of this patient would be:

A. Implantation of a transvenous implantable cardioverter defibrillator (ICD)
B. Implantation of an epicardial ICD
C. Initiation of amiodarone therapy
D. Surgical closure of the ventricular septal defect
E. Initiation of bosentan and a β-blocker and repeat EP study

75. A 24 year old with tricuspid atresia who has undergone an atriopulmonary Fontan procedure presents complaining of fatigue. Echo shows good left ventricular function. An ECG is obtained (Fig. 13.6). The ECG is consistent with:

A. Ventricular tachycardia requiring lidocaine
B. Incisional atrial flutter requiring cardioversion
C. Normal sinus rhythm requiring evaluation for other sources of fatigue
D. Ventricular dyssynchrony requiring a biventricular pacemaker
E. Sinus node dysfunction requiring a pacemaker

76. A 20-year-old obese woman presents to the clinic complaining of shortness of breath with exertion for 9 months. She denies any other symptoms. She has no significant past medical or surgical history. On physical examination, she has a normal S_1 and a fixed split S_2 with a I/VI systolic ejection murmur at the upper left sternal border. The rest of her examination is unremarkable. An echocardiogram has very poor acoustic windows, but shows normal left ventricular function and a mildly dilated right ventricle. An ECG is obtained (Fig. 13.7). The additional test most likely to reveal the diagnosis in this patient is:

A. Coronary angiography
B. Thyroid function tests
C. Agitated saline contrast echocardiogram
D. Pulmonary function testing
E. Exercise treadmill test

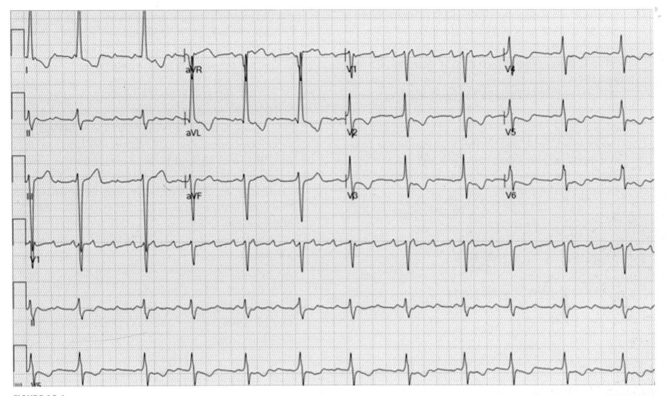

FIGURE 13.6

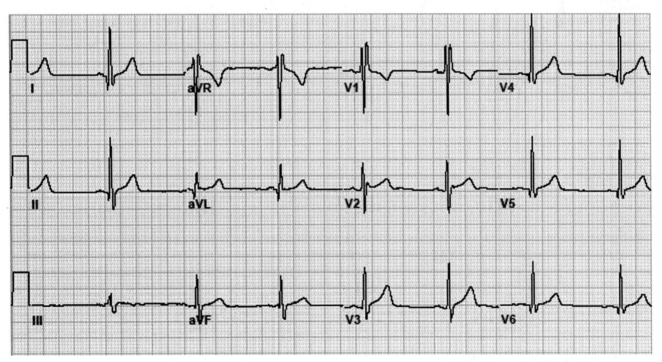

FIGURE 13.7

77. A 26-year-old woman with tetralogy of Fallot had an episode of syncope while playing a game of volleyball at her gym. She had no pulse and an AED was placed within 3 minutes of the episode of syncope. Tracings from the AED show ventricular tachycardia at a rate of 260 bpm and an AED shock was given which converted the patient into sinus rhythm. An echocardiogram shows free pulmonary regurgitation, but only mild right ventricular enlargement and normal right ventricular function as well as normal left ventricular size and function. Which of the following statements is true about ICD placement in this patient?

A. Ablation can be offered as an alternative to ICD placement

B. ICD complications are the same as the adult post-myocardial infarction population

C. Cardiac resynchronization therapy can be offered as an alternative to ICD placement

D. Amiodarone decreases the sudden cardiac death incidence as much as ICD placement

E. A transvenous ICD can be placed even in the presence of severe pulmonary regurgitation

78. A 26-year-old man with d-transposition of the great arteries had a Mustard operation at 3 years of age. He has been doing well with no symptoms and works full time as an accountant. On examination, his blood pressure is 110/65 mm Hg and he has no murmurs or gallops. An echocardiogram shows a dilated right ventricle with moderately depressed right (systemic) ventricular function and moderate tricuspid regurgitation. An ECG is obtained (Fig. 13.8).

Which of the following medications is indicated for his clinical situation?

A. Digoxin

B. Lisinopril

C. Amiodarone

D. Carvedilol

E. Rivaroxaban

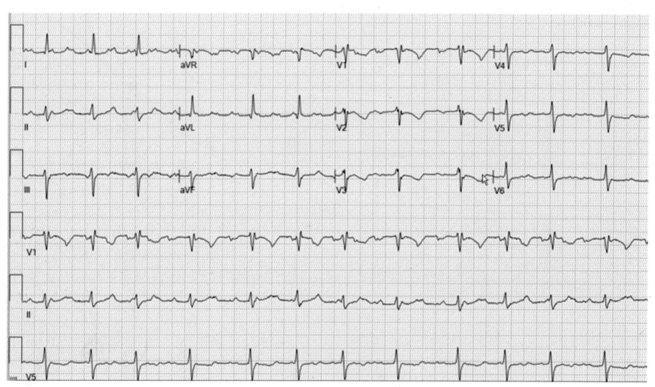

FIGURE 13.8

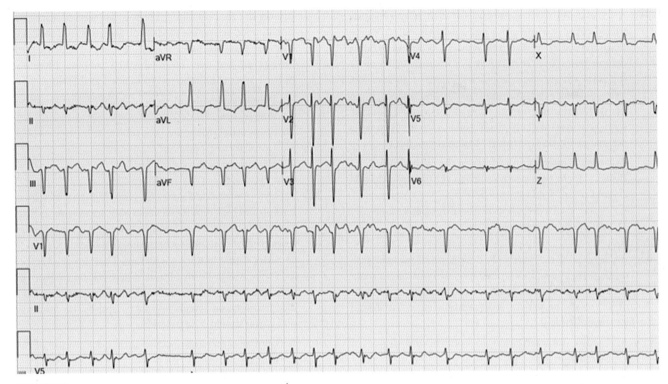

FIGURE 13.9

79. A 27-year-old woman with a history of a large primum atrial septal defect underwent repair at age 14 years. She has been doing well with normal biventricular function and no symptoms. Three days prior to her visit with you, she began feeling fatigued and short of breath. She presents to the ER after an episode of syncope while running to catch a bus. Her blood pressure is 94/62 mm Hg and she is alert. An echocardiogram shows a small residual atrial septal defect and a decrease in her left ventricular ejection fraction from 55% 2 months ago to 45% now. Her ECG is shown in Figure 13.9.

Which of the following is indicated for her clinical situation?

A. Coumadin for 3 weeks, then DC cardioversion
B. Emergent cardioversion in the emergency room
C. IV Amiodarone bolus
D. Transesophageal echocardiogram and DC cardioversion
E. Device closure of the residual ASD

80. Which of the following patients should be transferred to a regional center specializing in care for adults with congenital heart disease for cholecystecytomy?

A. 42-year-old woman with a bicuspid aortic valve and severe aortic valve regurgitation; echocardiogram demonstrates left ventricular end diastolic dimension of 60 mm with ejection fraction 62%
B. 36-year-old man with tricuspid atresia status post lateral tunnel Fontan. No history of heart failure or arrhythmia

C. 50-year-old woman with atrial septal defect and pulmonary valve stenosis; Echocardiogram demonstrates right ventricular systolic pressure of 50 mm Hg and peak velocity across the pulmonary valve of 3 m/s
D. 52-year-old woman with unrepaired membranous ventricular septal defect; echocardiogram demonstrates peak velocity across the defect of 5 m/s, left ventricular end diastolic dimension of 50 mm, end diastolic pulmonary valve regurgitation velocity of 1.4 m/s

81. A 32-year-old man with trisomy 21 and a history of complete AV canal defect status post surgical repair is referred by family medicine for evaluation of a murmur. Echocardiogram demonstrates turbulent flow in the left ventricular outflow tract related to anomalous chords. The maximal instantaneous gradient through the outflow tract is 50 mm Hg. There is mild aortic valve regurgitation and mild-moderate left AV valve regurgitation. Patient is asymptomatic according to caregivers and participates in all group home activities. What is the best recommendation for therapy at this time?

A. Start a β-blocker
B. Start an ACE inhibitor
C. Recommend surgery to relieve left ventricular outflow tract obstruction
D. Recommend continue current activities, start no medication, return to clinic in 1 year

82. A 24-year-old woman presents for evaluation of supra-valvar aortic stenosis. She has a known elastin mutation. She has never had intervention. Echocardiography demonstrates discrete narrowing of the proximal ascending aorta with a mean Doppler gradient of 40 mm Hg. Left ventricular size, ejection fraction, and wall thickness are within normal limits. The patient is asymptomatic with activities of daily living. She is contemplating a pregnancy in the near future. You recommend:

A. Surgical intervention to relieve the obstruction
B. Permanent contraception given the elastin mutation and risk of fetal transmission
C. Proceed with pregnancy without further testing
D. Initiate β-blockade

83. A 22-year-old is referred for evaluation of valvular pulmonary stenosis. Echocardiography demonstrates a maximal instantaneous velocity across the pulmonary valve of 3.2 m/s. The patient is asymptomatic. What should be recommended?

A. Cardiac catheterization to confirm the degree of obstruction
B. Referral for Melody valve implantation
C. Repeat echocardiogram in 1 year
D. Repeat echocardiogram in 3 years

84. A 20-year-old man with d-transposition of the great arteries, status post arterial switch presents to establish care in the ACHD clinic. He was last seen 5 years ago, but stopped seeing his cardiologist since he felt well and was "too busy" to make an appointment. He denies any symptoms, but has no established exercise program. What testing should be recommended at this time?

A. Pulmonary function tests to evaluate for restrictive lung disease
B. Stress echocardiogram
C. Coronary angiography
D. Six-minute walk

85. An asymptomatic, sedentary 62-year-old man with hypertension and hyperlipidemia underwent stress echocardiography for preoperative clearance before knee replacement surgery. The baseline echocardiogram demonstrated a coronary fistula to the right atrium. The cardiac chamber sizes were within normal limits. There was no evidence of ischemia during the test by ECG or imaging criteria. Cardiac examination reveals normal S_1 and S_2, no murmur, no S_3. You should recommend:

A. Cardiac catheterization for further delineation of the fistula
B. Cardiac CT for further delineation of the fistula
C. No further testing or intervention
D. Surgery for closure of the fistula

ANSWERS

1. (C) This young woman has never had alternative imaging of her aorta. Since she has dilation of the ascending aorta, it would be appropriate to perform more extensive imaging at least once early in adulthood and prior to pregnancy. She has mild aortic valve stenosis and regurgitation and likely would tolerate pregnancy well. Unless obstetrical complications occur, one would expect a normal spontaneous vaginal delivery. ACE inhibitors and angiotensin receptor blockers are contraindicated during pregnancy.

2. (B) It is considered safe to continue warfarin at a dose of 5 mg or less daily if an INR of 3.0 can be obtained during pregnancy. The risk of warfarin embryopathy at a dose of less than 5 mg daily is felt to be low enough that one could continue warfarin during pregnancy. Alternatively, if one cannot maintain an INR of 3.0 on this dose and need a higher dose, then warfarin should be discontinued by the sixth week of gestation and resumed after the twelfth week of gestation. Low molecular weight heparin 1 mg/kg twice daily should be administered. The patient should have her anti-Xa level checked weekly or twice weekly depending on the clinical situation. Anti-X levels of 0.7 to 1.3 should be obtained. If this is a mechanical AV valve, one would want to have a higher Anti-X level. Warfarin should be discontinued at 36 weeks gestation in anticipation of delivery. Patients should be switched to low molecular weight heparin at this time. The last dose of low molecular weight heparin should be 12 hours prior to planned delivery. Postpartum if there is no unexpected bleeding, warfarin therapy can be reinstituted while bridging with low molecular weight heparin until the INR is at least 2.0. Pregnancy is considered a hypercoaguable state due to the elevated estrogen levels. Patients remain in this state of hypercoagulability in the first several weeks postpartum.

3. (C) The woman likely has Holt–Oram syndrome (radial hypoplasia associated with secundum atrial septal defect). It is inherited on an autosomal dominant fashion; therefore, 50% of her offspring would be expected to inherit this syndrome assuming complete penetrance.

4. (D) The woman has Holt–Oram syndrome. It is inherited in an autosomal dominant fashion; 50% of her children would be expected to be effected with this syndrome. Of patients with Holt–Oram syndrome, 75% have congenital heart disease. Therefore, the risk of CHD in the child would be closest to 35%.

5. (D) This case scenario demonstrates a typical presentation of a young adult with a previously undiagnosed atrial septal defect. Transthoracic imaging prior to intervention demonstrates a centrally located defect that is amenable to device closure. This defect can also be closed surgically. If the pulmonary veins were adequately visualized entering the left atrium then no further imaging usually is required. Her clinical examination is consistent with a large left-to-right shunt from an atrial level defect (presence of diastolic rumble). There is no evidence on echocardiography or clinical examination for pulmonary hypertension; therefore, cardiac catheterization would not be needed.

6. (C) The diastolic flow rumble in a patient with an ASD is due to excess flow across a normal tricuspid valve. Presence of this

sound is associated with a $Q_p/Q_s > 1.5$ to 2.0. The systolic murmur, similarly, is due to excess flow across an otherwise normal pulmonary valve. Flow across the ASD is low velocity and inaudible. Young children with large VSDs will have a diastolic flow murmur due to flow across the mitral valve. Diastolic murmurs are not "normal."

7. (C) The 2013 ACC/AHA Guidelines recommend either high-intensity or moderate-intensity statin regimen for patients with an ASCVD risk score that is ≥7.5%. Gemfibrozil and niacin are not statins. Aspirin therapy is not contraindicated but would not address this issue directly. Losartan does not treat hyperlipidemia.

8. (C) The patient has a residual right-to-left shunt and atrial arrhythmia with spontaneous echo contrast in the right atrium. Risk of paradoxical embolus is important. Based on the adult congenital guidelines warfarin therapy is indicated.

9. (E) The fenestration gradient is equal to the transpulmonary gradient (RA or Fontan pressure minus LA pressure). Values of 5 to 8 mm Hg are usually expected. An increased gradient correlates with obstruction in the Fontan circuit, lungs, or pulmonary veins. It is primarily dependent on total pulmonary vascular resistance. Elevated LA or ventricular end diastolic pressures do not change the transpulmonary gradient. A low fenestration gradient is associated with hypovolemia. (Phillips SD, O'Leary PW. Echocardiographic evaluation of the functionally univentricular heart after Fontan operation. In: Eidem BW, O'Leary PW, Cetta F., eds. *Echocardiography in Pediatric and Adult Congenital Heart Disease*, 2nd edition. Alphen aan den Rijn, the Netherlands: Wolters Kluwer; 2015:677–696.)

10. (C) The murmur described in the examination is a continuous peaking around the second heart sound—typical of a patent ductus arteriosus. An audible patent ductus arteriosus usually can be visualized with transthoracic echocardiography. If that imaging is suboptimal, CT or MRI of the chest may be helpful. If the PDA is audible, especially in a patient with a wide pulse pressure, one would expect left ventricular and left atrial enlargement. This patient should undergo closure of the PDA, usually via a transcatheter procedure.

11. (D) The continuous murmur is typical of a patent ductus arteriosus or systemic arterial to pulmonary artery collateral vessels (common in patients with pulmonary atresia). Patients with PA/VSD frequently have a right-sided aortic arch and the ductus arteriosus may be best heard over the right back. A right coronary fistula may produce a continuous murmur but is unlikely to be heard best in the back. The other choices do not generate continuous murmurs.

12. (E) The patient has an ASD that technically would be amenable to device closure. But, other issues need to be addressed such as intervention for the tricuspid valve—dictating that the patient is best served with surgical management. Patients who may need additional cardiac surgery for coronary revascularization, valve repair, or arrhythmia surgery should be treated with surgery rather than sole transcatheter device closure of the ASD.

13. (E) The patient has two sources of pulmonary blood flow, superior vena cava exclusively supplies the right pulmonary artery, inferior vena cava flow via the Fontan conduit supplies the left pulmonary artery exclusively. In addition, the patient has substrate for right lung fistula due to the classic Glenn procedure. Pulmonary blood flow cannot be accurately quantitated nor can pulmonary vascular resistance be assessed.

14. (C) Polymerase chain reaction is needed to confirm presence of active infection. Antibody positivity indicates immunization or prior infection. Prior to 1992, no formal testing was available for what was formerly called "non A-non B hepatitis." It is estimated that 5% of patients with congenital heart disease who had cardiac surgery prior to 1992 are infected with hepatitis C.

15. (A) Serum BNP levels >140 pg/mL correlated with poor long-term outcome in patients with Eisenmenger syndrome. (Reardon LC, Williams RJ, Houser LS, et al. Usefulness of serum brain natriuretic peptide to predict adverse events in patients with the Eisenmenger syndrome. *Am J Cardiol.* 2012;110:1523–1526.)

16. (A) The patient in this scenario has a primum ASD. A primum ASD is located in the most anterior and inferior aspect of the atrial septum at the level of the mitral and tricuspid valves. It is associated with a cleft mitral valve. Any ASD with this amount of right ventricular volume overload should be closed. There is decreased mortality after surgical closure (compared to medical treatment), although nonfatal cardiovascular complications are similar. Unlike secundum ASDs, primum ASDs should not be closed using a device in the cath lab. Although there is right atrial enlargement, the patient is not hypertensive and there is no definitive role for ACE inhibition in shunt lesions. Patients with primum ASDs will frequently have left axis deviation on ECG that is related to the lesion rather than any coronary artery disease. There is no indication for a cardiac cath (unless there is concern for pulmonary hypertension). (Konstantinides S, Geibel A, Olschewski M, et al. A comparison of surgical and medical therapy for atrial septal defect in adults. *N Engl J Med.* 1995;333(8):469–473; Rigatelli G, Cardaioli P, Hijazi ZM. Contemporary clinical management of atrial septal defects in the adult. *Expert Rev Cardiovasc Ther.* 2007;5(6):1135–1146.)

17. (E) Any patient who survived a cardiac arrest due to nonreversible causes should have an ICD placed. There is no evidence of a reversible cause in this patient. Ablation may be offered as an alternative in a patient with a slow, stable, monomorphic ventricular tachycardia, but not the fast ventricular tachycardia resulting in cardiac arrest seen in this patient. The incidence of ICD complications was reported to be 30% in one study of patients with tetralogy of Fallot, compared to about 10% in the postmyocardial infarction population. The incidence of inappropriate shocks in tetralogy of Fallot is about 25%, which is similar to that seen in other congenital heart lesions. Antiarrhythmic medications are not as effective as an ICD in preventing recurrent arrhythmias. β-Blockers, amiodarone, and sotalol do not decrease the risk of appropriate ICD shocks in patients with tetralogy of Fallot. A transvenous system can be performed in a patient with free pulmonary regurgitation. Patients with residual intracardiac shunts should not have transvenous pacing/ICD leads. (Yap SC, Roos-Hesselink JW, Hoendermis ES, et al. Outcome of implantable cardioverter defibrillators in adults

with congenital heart disease: a multi-centre study. *Eur Heart J.* 2007;28(15): 1854–1861; Khairy P, Harris L, Landzberg MJ, et al. Implantable cardioverter-defibrillators in tetralogy of Fallot. *Circulation.* 2008; 117(3):363–370; Walsh EP. Arrhythmias in patients with congenital heart disease. *Card Electrophysiol Rev.* 2002;6(4):422–430; ACC/AHA/HRS 2008 Guidelines for Device-Based Therapy of Cardiac Rhythm Abnormalities: executive summary. *Circulation.* 2008;117:2820–2840.)

18. (D) TBX5 mutation is associated with Holt–Oram syndrome. It is inherited in an autosomal dominant fashion; TGFBR 1 and 2 with Loeys–Dietz; FBN1 with Marfan syndrome; trisomy 21 with down Syndrome; NKX 2.5 with ASD + heart block.

19. (A) NKX 2.5 mutation is associated with familial occurrence of ASDs and progressive AV block. The GATA IV mutation is associated with ASDs *without* AV block. TBX5 is associated with Holt–Oram syndrome; NOTCH mutations are associated with AVSD.

20. (A) The embryologic origin of the valve of the fossa ovalis is derived from septum primum. The superior and inferior limbus originate from the septum secundum. Atrial appendage morphology is not related to development of the atrial septum. The endocardial cushions are important in septation of the atrioventricular septum and delamination of the atrioventricular valves.

21. (C) The Cardiac Disease in Pregnancy (CARPREG) Investigators demonstrated in a prospective multicenter study that maternal cardiac risk could be predicted with the use of a risk index. Cardiac events were defined as pulmonary edema, arrhythmia, stroke, or cardiac death. The four predictors of primary cardiac events were (1) prior cardiac event; (2) baseline NYHA class II or cyanosis; (3) left heart obstruction (mitral valve area <2 cm^2, aortic valve area <1.5 cm^2, or *peak* LVOT gradient >30 mm Hg by echocardiography); and (4) reduced systemic ventricular systolic function (EF <40%). The risk of maternal cardiac complication with zero predictors was 5%, with one predictor it was 25%, and with greater than one predictor the risk was 75%. The risk score was further refined by the Boston Adult Congenital Heart Disease Group in a study that demonstrated that including decreased subpulmonary ventricular function and/or severe pulmonary regurgitation as a predictor in the risk index improved the accuracy of the risk assessment. Of the answers listed, the patient described in C has the highest predicted risk with a prior cardiac event (history of atrial fibrillation) and severe pulmonary valve regurgitation. Her poor peak VO$_2$ may be a further indication of poor outcome, even if she has no complaints clinically. The 32-year-old patient has no predictors. The 30-year-old patient has one predictor. The 20-year-old patient could be considered to have one predictor—poor subpulmonary ventricular function.

22. (C) ACE inhibitors can cause fetal renal dysfunction in the third trimester, but have also been demonstrated to be a teratogen. Therefore, ACE inhibitors should be avoided throughout pregnancy. ARBs should be considered to have the same risk profile and should be avoided. Hydralazine and nitrates are safe in pregnancy and together provide similar physiologic response to ACE inhibition.

23. (D) Women with Eisenmenger syndrome are at exceptionally high risk of complication and death during pregnancy and the peripartum period. Pregnancy should be avoided in these patients. The patient with bicuspid aortic valve with a mean systolic gradient of 30 mm Hg has one predictor of cardiac complication (predicted to have a complication risk of 25%) but has a low risk of death. Patients with Marfan syndrome can have dissection during pregnancy, but pregnancy is not absolutely contraindicated unless the aorta is larger than 40 mm. The patient with Ebstein anomaly with severe right heart enlargement and severe tricuspid regurgitation has a risk of cardiac complication, but no absolute contraindication.

24. (D) Patients with mechanical valve prostheses pose significant difficulties for anticoagulation management. Warfarin probably provides the optimum anticoagulation, but it is a teratogen and should be avoided if possible during the first trimester of pregnancy. Also, warfarin crosses the placenta, and a fetus of a mother anticoagulated with warfarin should not be delivered vaginally secondary to the risk of fetal intracranial bleeding. However, studies have shown that if *therapeutic* anticoagulation can be achieved with a daily dose of <5 mg daily, the risk of warfarin embryopathy is quite low. A currently accepted management strategy is to provide alternative anticoagulation during at least the first trimester.[4] Low molecular weight heparin is an attractive alternative to warfarin as it does not cross the placenta. However, weight-based dosing alone is not effective anticoagulation during pregnancy secondary to altered volume of distribution and drug metabolism. If low molecular weight heparins are used, anti-Xa levels must be followed closely (at least weekly) to ensure adequate anticoagulation.

25. (E) Depo-Provera injection provides the best option for this patient, though there is some risk of hematoma at the injection site. Essure tubal implants are an irreversible form of contraception. Mirena IUD is reversible and safe to implant, but is not the best option in patients who are not monogamous as the incidence of pelvic inflammatory disease may be increased. Barrier contraception such as a diaphragm does not have the same efficacy as Depo-Provera, but the patient should be encouraged to use condoms with a new partner to prevent sexually transmitted disease. Estrogen containing oral contraception would not be a good choice in a patient at risk for thrombus.

26. (B) This patient likely has Loeys–Dietz syndrome, a mutation of TGF-β receptor that results in arterial fragility. ARBs have been shown to reduce TGF-β signaling and reduce the risk of arterial complications in animal models. ARBs are the drug of choice in this situation. While patients with Loeys–Dietz can have aortic complication at this degree of dilatation, it is acceptable to follow closely with routine imaging at this aortic dimension.

27. (C) This patient had appropriate secondary erythrocytosis related to his cyanosis. This increase in hemoglobin is necessary to provide appropriate oxygen delivery and is not associated with stroke or other small vessel occlusion unless the patient is microcytic, as microcytotic red cells are less deformable as the traverse small capillary beds. This patient likely feels unwell because he has poor oxygen delivery. He should be treated with iron therapy for 1 month with a goal of normalizing the MCV and ferritin.

28. (E) This patient has symptomatic aortic stenosis. Bedrest may be advisable, but 4 weeks is too long of a follow-up interval. Balloon valvotomy is not a good choice since the valve is calcified. Delivery of the fetus now is not optimal since this degree of prematurity would provide a high risk of neonatal complication and death. Percutaneous valve implantation is currently not an option in this situation and would likely carry some risk to mother and fetus. Surgical replacement of the aortic valve can be done with low risk to mother and relatively low risk to the fetus and is the best option in this scenario.

29. (D) This patient is at higher risk of coronary artery disease given his history of coarctation. His LDL cholesterol goal should be 70 mg/dL or less. Diet can be helpful, but the patient will benefit from a statin drug to lower LDL. Niaspan, fish oil, and gemfibrozil do not have significant LDL-lowering effects.

30. (D) This patient does need treatment for hypertension. While a recurrent coarctation can cause residual hypertension, there is no evidence from the echocardiogram that the patient has any significant residual obstruction; hence, stent implantation is unlikely to provide much benefit. This patient likely has hypertension related to stiff arterial vasculature and a relatively late coarctation repair. All the drugs listed can treat hypertension, but metoprolol and diltiazem would not be favored given the low resting heart rate. Daily Lasix will probably not be effective in controlling the hypertension and would not be a first-line choice. Losartan has the most advantages with a low side effect profile, no heart rate changes, and possible protection against aortic dilatation (for which this patient is at risk).

31. (A) Patent foramen ovale is present in 25% to 30% of the adult population. Currently there are no data that treatment with medication or closure to prevent paradoxical emboli is indicated in an asymptomatic patient. Patent foramen ovale should not cause right ventricular volume overload; hence, MRI would not provide clinically useful information.

32. (E) The patient has symptoms of platypnea-orthodeoxia syndrome, related to positional right-to-left shunting across a patent foramen ovale. Elderly patients with patent foramen ovale are more prone to right-to-left shunting as the cardiac geometry changes with age.[8] A normal supine saturation would make this diagnosis more likely. Treatment would be closure of the patent foramen ovale. Pulmonary function test with methacholine challenge would be helpful for diagnosing asthma, but asthma would not explain the patient's decline in saturation. V/Q scan would be helpful to determine whether there had been pulmonary emboli, but the patient would potentially have right heart changes on echocardiography if emboli were so extensive to cause this degree of desaturation. Diastolic dysfunction or coronary artery disease can lead to dyspnea on exertion, but this degree of desaturation would be unlikely.

33. (C) ASDs can cause right heart enlargement secondary to left-to-right shunting, but at this age and with the history of hypertension, it is possible that the left-to-right shunt volume is increased secondary to left ventricular diastolic dysfunction. If the left ventricular filling pressures are extremely high, the patient may become more dyspneic with closure of the ASD since the left atrial pressure will increase after ASD closure. Therefore, the best initial step in this patient's evaluation is to perform left and right heart catheterization to determine filling pressures. If the pressures are elevated, an attempt at balloon occlusion of the ASD can be performed to ensure that left atrial pressures do not become excessively increased with ASD closure.

34. (D) This patient has one risk factor—left heart obstruction (mitral valve area <2 cm², aortic valve area <1.5 cm², or *peak* LVOT gradient >30 mm Hg by echocardiography). In the CARPREG model, one risk factor predicts a 25% risk of cardiac complication during pregnancy.

35. (E) This patient is best served by transthoracic echocardiogram to evaluate the function of the left ventricle and the bicuspid aortic valve, MRI scan of the aorta to evaluate for thoracic aorta dilation and complications at the coarctation repair site, as well as MRA scan of the brain to evaluate for intracranial aneurysms since patients with a history of coarctation have an increased risk of intracranial aneurysm. The other choices listed could evaluate the heart and the thoracic aorta, but would not evaluate the intracranial vasculature.

36. (A) Blood pressure medications can cause fatigue as a side effect, but this patient is complaining of hypersomnolence. Patients with Marfan syndrome should be screened for obstructive sleep apnea as they are at high risk for this condition, which can result in daytime hypersomnolence, hypertension, and aortic dilatation. Overnight oximetry is a simple, but effective, screening tool to evaluate possible obstructive sleep apnea.

37. (A) Sertraline has a low risk of cardiac complications. Citalopram and amitriptyline can cause prolonged QT that could be a problem in a patient with tetralogy of Fallot. Venlafaxine and Bupropion both inhibit the neuronal uptake of norepinephrine and can cause hypertension and tachycardia.

38. (A) Dabigatran is an oral direct thrombin inhibitor. Unlike warfarin, dabigatran therapy does not need to be monitored to ensure achievement of therapeutic anticoagulation. It is currently approved for use in patients with atrial fibrillation, but not for use with mechanical valves. There are no data currently regarding the use of this agent during pregnancy. Dabigatran is not useful for bridging anticoagulation as it is recommended that dabigatran should be discontinued 1 to 2 days prior to surgery (with abnormal creatine clearance, this recommendation increases to 3 to 5 days). Dabigatran should not be used in patients with significant bleeding issues as there is no direct reversal agent available.

39. (C) Concomitant use of amlodipine and simvastatin increases the risk of myopathy and rhabdomyolysis. If it is necessary to use both drugs, it is recommended that the dose of simvastatin not exceed 20 mg/day.

40. (B) Atenolol has an FDA pregnancy classification of class D—*There is positive evidence of human fetal risk, but the benefits from use in pregnant women may be acceptable despite the risk (e.g., if the drug is needed in a life-threatening situation or for a serious disease for which safer drugs cannot be used or are ineffective)*—because a study in hypertensive women taking atenolol demonstrated lower birthweight infants. The other drugs are labeled class C—*Either studies in animals have revealed adverse effects on the fetus (teratogenic or embryocidal or other) and there are no controlled studies in women or studies in women and animals are not available. Drugs should be given only if the potential benefit justifies the potential risk to the fetus.*

41. (D) Endometrial ablation is a safe minimally invasive procedure that can reduce menstrual bleeding significantly (especially in women >35 years of age) and can be performed without interruption of anticoagulation. Endometrial ablation should not be performed if interested in future pregnancies. Hysterectomy can provide the same relief of symptoms, but for this patient to have hysterectomy, she would have to interrupt her warfarin anticoagulation and undergo a surgical procedure. Oral estrogen containing contraception can be a good choice to treat menometrorrhagia in some patients, but is not favorable in this patient secondary to the increased risk of thrombosis. Depo-Provera can improve menometrorrhagia, but is not as effective as endometrial ablation. Essure tubal ligation effectively prevents pregnancy, but does not treat menometrorrhagia.

42. (E) Flecainide is a class IC antiarrhythmic agent. It can cause pro-arrhythmia and QRS prolongation, so is best initiated in hospital with continuous monitoring for five doses with a daily ECG to check the QRS duration.

43. (A) Amiodarone can cause liver, pulmonary, and thyroid toxicity. Therefore, TSH, liver function tests, and pulmonary function tests should be monitored routinely. Liver function tests ideally should be reviewed twice yearly and thyroid function tests every 3 to 6 months.

44. (A) One of the most common side effects of bosentan is lower extremity edema. This side effect is not significant in the other drugs listed. β-Blockers are not considered pulmonary vasodilators.

45. (E) It is very important that the drug be taken at the same time daily for optimum effectiveness. It does not take 60 days for the pill to become effective. Rash can occur, but not sun sensitivity. Amenorrhea can occur, but is not the norm. Antibiotics may reduce the effectiveness of contraception, but patients who need SBE prophylaxis should continue using antibiotics when appropriate and be counseled to use alternative contraception for that cycle.

46. (D) The physical examination and ECG are consistent with the echocardiographic image demonstrating a sinus venosus ASD with partial anomalous pulmonary venous return with the right superior pulmonary vein draining to the superior vena cava—right atrial junction. Given the cardiac chamber dilation with respiratory and exercise symptoms, it is appropriate to proceed with surgical intervention. ASD closure alone will allow persistent left-to-right shunting through the right superior pulmonary vein. To eliminate this shunt and volume load of the right heart, ASD closure and surgical pulmonary venous redirection to the left atrium are indicated. Device closure is reserved for secundum defects only.

47. (A) Small ventricular septal defects may be detected at any age, particularly in patients who have avoided medical care. Management of this newly discovered lesion is based on the hemodynamic effects of the lesion. Evidence that the ventricular level shunt is small and of no hemodynamic consequence includes the absence of left atrial and ventricular chamber enlargement, normal right ventricular systolic pressure, and a very high flow velocity across the ventricular septal defect, although the latter may be the least trustworthy of these findings. No intervention or additional evaluation is required. The patient should be reassured about the benign nature of this lesion. There is no need for SBE prophylaxis.

48. (B) The flow acceleration demonstrated by echocardiogram is mildly elevated. However, mild pulmonary stenosis should not result in right atrial and right ventricular chamber enlargement. Additional evaluation is needed to explain the chamber dilation. Patent ductus arteriosus with normal pulmonary vascular resistance would result in increased pulmonary venous return and enlarged left-sided chambers. A hemodynamically significant ASD would result in left-to-right shunting with right atrial and right ventricular dilation.

49. (A) Arterial switch operation for d-TGA has been the preferred surgical procedure since the early 1980s. The most common late postoperative complication after the arterial switch operation is supravalvar pulmonary stenosis. This may be amenable to stent implantation with care taken to avoid the pulmonary valve. Balloon valvuloplasty without stenting has a low success rate. Stenosis of the aorta is less common. Coronary ostial stenosis is a known complication but is not consistent with the physical examination. Atrial arrhythmias late after arterial switch operation are rare.

50. (C) The 2007 ACC/AHA guidelines continue to recommend prophylactic antibiotics prior to dental work for anyone with a prior history of bacterial endocarditis. For nonvalvular prosthetic patch material, antibiotic prophylaxis is recommended for only the first 6 months following surgery in the absence of a residual peripatch shunt. There is no indication for daily antibiotics. *S. viridans* remains a common pathogen for infective endocarditis.

51. (C) Antibiotic prophylaxis is not indicated for patients undergoing nondental interventions (colonoscopy or upper endoscopy) in the absence of active systemic infection. Comprehensive care of patients with congenital heart disease includes preventative screening procedures at recommended ages.

52. (C) While there is a clear association between Ebstein anomaly and atrioventricular reentrant accessory pathway tachycardia, patients with Ebstein anomaly are also at risk for life-threatening ventricular arrhythmias. This is particularly true for patients with deterioration in hemodynamic status. Atrioventricular reentrant accessory pathway tachycardia is less likely to cause a sudden loss of consciousness. The absence of prodromal symptoms also makes a ventricular tachycardia more likely. Myoclonus is common in any loss of consciousness. This patient requires additional arrhythmia monitoring and evaluation of hemodynamic status and cardiac function.

53. (B) The symptoms and physical examination findings are consistent with elevated IVC and central venous pressures in this Fontan patient's circulation. While these symptoms could be consistent with obstruction in the Fontan connection, the ECG

demonstrates junctional bradycardia. This is a common and often delayed finding in multiple forms of congenital heart disease after Mustard, Senning, and Fontan procedures. The onset of junctional rhythm may cause significant hemodynamic impact. This is a class I indication for atrial or dual-chamber pacemaker placement.

54. (C) In congenitally corrected TGA, the conduction system is abnormal in location and structure, making it vulnerable to physical trauma during catheterization in addition to spontaneous heart block associated with increasing age. The diagnosis of this congenital cardiac abnormality may be delayed into adulthood in individuals with adequate systemic ventricular function and no obvious murmur from a VSD or pulmonary/subpulmonary stenosis.

55. (E) Routine phlebotomy for erythrocytosis in cyanotic patients is not recommended in the absence of symptoms and often leads to *iron deficiency* anemia with resulting microcytosis. Microcytosis independently increases viscosity, perpetuating a cycle of phlebotomy and worsening microcytosis leading to symptoms. For euvolemic patients with hemoglobin >20 g/dL and hematocrit >65% *with symptoms of hyperviscosity*, therapeutic phlebotomy with equal volume crystalloid replacement is indicated.

56. (C) The 2008 ACC/AHA valvular heart disease updated guidelines recommend cardiac catheterization with coronary angiography for "men aged 35 years or older, premenopausal women aged 35 years or older who have coronary risk factors, and postmenopausal women" (class I, level of evidence: C). Tobacco cessation 1 week prior to surgery may increase respiratory secretions in the perioperative period. There is no indication for statin therapy at this time.

57. (B) Both bicuspid aortic valve anatomy and isolated ascending aortic dilation have been identified in first-degree family members of patients with bicuspid aortic valve. The abnormalities resulting in bicuspid aortic valves have clear association with abnormal aortic dilation and are not a process isolated to the aortic valve alone. For patients with bicuspid aortic valve, all first-degree relatives should be screened with transthoracic echocardiograms. Cardiac MRI is not recommended as first-line screening. Screening is recommended regardless of physical examination findings since ascending aortic dilation may be present in the setting of a normal physical examination.

58. (C) Patients with repaired coarctation of the aorta have associated risk for cerebral aneurysms and for pseudoaneurysm formation at the site of prior surgical repair. While there is no evidence of aortic recoarctation by physical examination or by echocardiographic evaluation of the aortic lumen and blood flow, this does not exclude pseudoaneurysm formation. CT or MRI imaging of the thoracic aorta should be performed. Cardiac catheterization is not required. Head MRI with MR angiography may be utilized for cerebral aneurysm screening. Neurocognitive testing may be appropriate for an individualized patient.

59. (E) Late postoperative complications following AVSD repair include LVOT obstruction, heart block, and left atrioventricular valve regurgitation. New onset of atrial arrhythmias should prompt a thorough anatomic and hemodynamic evaluation for postoperative complications resulting in atrial fibrillation. Treating the arrhythmia with medical therapy without additional evaluation is insufficient. Isolated LVOT obstruction with a mean gradient >50 mm Hg or a maximum instantaneous gradient >70 mm Hg is an indication for surgical intervention. Afterload reduction with ACE inhibition is relatively contraindicated in the presence of fixed LVOT obstruction and may result in hypotension and coronary hypoperfusion.

60. (B) Left ventricle to right atrial shunting in the setting of normal right-sided pressures results in a high-velocity left-to-right shunt. This Doppler signal may contaminate the tricuspid regurgitation signal. Initiation of pulmonary vasodilator therapy without additional investigation would be inappropriate. Patients with trisomy 21 are at increased risk of obstructive sleep apnea and pulmonary hypertension.

61. (B) Isolated membranous ventricular septal defect is associated with the development of DCRV that may occur in adulthood. DCRV is defined by a proximal, upstream portion of the right ventricle that is at high pressure, separated by abnormal muscular hypertrophy from a more distal low-pressure outflow portion. The pulmonary arterial pressure is distal to the obstruction and should be normal. The development of DCRV is often heralded by an increase in murmur intensity, onset of a thrill, and findings of right ventricular pressure loading including an increased right ventricular impulse and RVH by ECG. Surgical resection of the muscle bundles is needed.

62. (A) Risk factors for sudden death after repair of tetralogy of Fallot are QRS duration >180 msec, poor right ventricular hemodynamics, older age at repair, and prolonged palliative shunts. Invasive electrophysiology study is appropriate to provide additional risk stratification, but some would argue for internal defibrillator placement regardless of the outcome. Atrial arrhythmia and atrioventricular node dysfunction are both known complications following surgical repair, but are not the primary indication for additional electrophysiology study at this time.

63. (D) Mustard and Senning atrial switch procedures are associated with sinus node dysfunction and atrial arrhythmias. Other complications are baffle leaks and baffle obstruction. Placement of transvenous, intracardiac pacemaker leads may worsen baffle stenosis, and paradoxical embolus may occur across a baffle leak. Incorrect positioning of ventricular leads across the baffles is also observed. Pacemaker placement in this patient should be performed at a center with experience in adult congenital cardiac care. There is no history given for thrombophilia. While sudden death does occur in patients with repaired d-TGA, there is no history of atrial or ventricular tachycardia in this patient even with exercise.

64. (A) The arterial switch operation for d-TGA requires reimplantation of coronary artery buttons. There is risk of both early and late coronary obstruction. There is evidence that the risk may be greater with single coronary artery anatomy. Symptoms of coronary ischemia may present in atypical fashion. The history of exertional chest pain that resolved with rest warrants evaluation. Coronary angiography is the gold standard for coronary assessment, although computed tomography angiography may be appropriate.

65. (B) Progressive systemic ventricular dysfunction may occur following initiation of ventricular pacing. The ventricular lead crosses

the right-sided mitral valve (in L-TGA) and may cause mitral regurgitation. Following pacemaker placement, surveillance of the patient should be increased to detect these changes. Biventricular pacing may reverse these effects in some patients. Supraventricular tachycardia should be detected by pacemaker interrogation.

66. (A) Patients with Fontan palliation are at increased risk for systemic venous thromboembolic events. Pulmonary embolism may present with variable symptoms, and this presentation is consistent with a pulmonary embolism but is not specific for this diagnosis. Streaming of blood flow in the Fontan circulation may result in superior vena cava blood flowing preferentially to one lung with inferior vena cava flow to the other lung. Contrast or isotope may need to be injected into upper and lower extremities to accurately demonstrate bilateral pulmonary perfusion. Invasive pulmonary angiography remains the gold standard, but may not be required in this scenario.

67. (C) Anomalous coronary arteries are detected as incidental findings in the current era of advanced imaging. The intramural course of the anomalous artery in a long segment through the wall of the aorta is a risk factor for cardiac ischemia and death. The preferred intervention is an unroofing of this segment, opening the internal portion of the aortic wall to the aortic lumen. Bypass grafting a vessel that is not stenotic at baseline will typically result in a failed graft. Coronary button translocation is not required if unroofing is successful.

68. (C) The anatomy demonstrated is d-TGA after a Mustard procedure. The wire and small balloon catheter can be traced retrograde from the aorta to the right-sided, morphologic right ventricle, tricuspid valve, and pulmonary venous baffle with a balloon inflated in the pulmonary venous baffle adjacent to the TEE probe tip. The wire extends beyond the heart border in a left-sided pulmonary vein. The larger catheter can be followed antegrade through the inferior vena cava, systemic venous baffle, mitral valve, morphologic left ventricle, and proximal pulmonary artery. The pulmonary artery runs parallel to the aorta.

69. (D) The MRA (Fig. 13.3) demonstrates a normal thoracic aorta and a small PDA. The stem tells us that there is no murmur and no left-sided volume overload. The PDA likely will never need intervention. Need for lifelong SBE prophylaxis is controversial. Follow-up echo for surveillance of the bicuspid aortic valve in several years is the most reasonable option.

70. (C) This is a classic chest radiograph (CXR) (Fig. 13.4) of a patient with Scimitar syndrome. There is anomalous connection of right lower pulmonary vein to the IVC. This is evident on the CXR. Sometimes the right upper and middle pulmonary veins also connect to the IVC. In 25% of cases there is associated intracardiac congenital heart disease (usually an ASD). But in the majority of cases the atrial septum is intact. Scimitar patients also have right lower lobe hypoplasia, sequestration, and arterial supply from a vessel originating from the descending aorta. Due to right lung hypoplasia the cardiac silhouette is shifted rightward.

71. (D) By age 40 years complete heart block and need for pacemaker insertion is very common in patients with congenitally corrected TGA. Q waves in leads I and AVL are seen in anomalous left coronary artery from the pulmonary artery (ALCAPA).

Northwest and left QRS axes are seen in AVSD. RBBB is associated with Ebstein anomaly and patients after surgery for VSD and ToF repair.

72. (A) The CT (Fig. 13.5) demonstrates a patient with an LPA sling. There is origin of the LPA from the RPA, not at the level of the true PA bifurcation. The LPA crosses between the bronchus and the esophagus. On barium esophagram an anterior indentation occurs.

73. (A) Congenital complete AV block occurs in 1 per 14,000 to 20,000 live births and is thought to be the result of transplacental passage of autoantibodies against Ro and La intracellular ribonuclear proteins from the mother who may have a clinical autoimmune disease such as systemic lupus erythematosus or Sjögren syndrome. These patients may be completely asymptomatic throughout childhood and adolescence and require no active cardiology intervention, but there are certain findings that require intervention regardless of symptoms. According to the ACC/AHA/HRS 2008 Guidelines for Device-Based Therapy of Cardiac Rhythm Abnormalities, permanent pacemaker implantation is indicated for congenital third-degree AV block with a wide QRS escape rhythm, complex ventricular ectopy, *or* ventricular dysfunction (class I indication, level of evidence B). This is independent of the presence of symptoms as a wide complex escape rhythm may be unreliable and result in abrupt pauses that may result in cardiac arrest. Ventricular dysfunction is not common and when present is best treated with pacemaker implantation although ACE inhibition may be used in combination with device therapy. There is no indication for an electrophysiology study in patients with congenital complete AV block. There is no role for amiodarone, especially since it may slow the underlying junctional escape rhythm. (ACC/AHA/HRS 2008 Guidelines for Device-Based Therapy of Cardiac Rhythm Abnormalities: executive summary. *Circulation.* 2008;117:2820–2840; Michaelsson M, Jonzon A, Riesenfeld T. Isolated congenital complete atrioventricular block in adult life. A prospective study. *Circulation.* 1995;92:442–449.)

74. (B) An epicardial ICD system is the most appropriate step in this patient who is at risk for an arrhythmic sudden death. According to the ACC/AHA/HRS 2008 Guidelines for Device-Based Therapy of Cardiac Rhythm Abnormalities, in patients with congenital heart disease, spontaneous sustained VT or unexplained syncope with inducible sustained hypotensive VT are considered class I ICD indications when other remediable causes (hemodynamic or arrhythmic) have been excluded. The ACC/AHA 2008 Guidelines for the Management of Adults with Congenital Heart Disease state that epicardial pacemaker and device lead placement should be performed in all cyanotic patients with intracardiac shunts who require devices (class I indication). In a study by Khairy et al.,[20] transvenous leads incurred a greater than twofold increased risk of systemic thromboemboli in patients with any intracardiac shunt independent of the administration of coumadin or aspirin, so consideration for epicardial lead placement should be given to all patients with intracardiac shunts. An ICD is superior to amiodarone in the prevention of sudden cardiac death. As the patient has pulmonary hypertension, surgical repair would likely result in right ventricular failure and therefore would not be a viable option. Although bosentan is likely indicated with her pulmonary hypertension, she has a class I indication for an ICD. There is no reason to repeat her EP study.

(Connolly SJ, Gent M, Roberts RS, et al. Canadian Implantable Defibrillator Study (CIDS): a randomized trial of the implantable cardioverter defibrillator against amiodarone. *Circulation.* 2000;101:1297–1302; Khairy P, Landzberg MJ, Gatzoulis MA, et al. Transvenous pacing leads and systemic thromboemboli in patients with intracardiac shunts: a multicenter study. *Circulation.* 2006;113(20):2391–2397; Epstein AE, Dimarco JP, Ellenbogen KA, et al. ACC/AHA/HRS 2008 Guidelines for Device-Based Therapy of Cardiac Rhythm Abnormalities: executive summary. *Circulation.* 2008;117: 2820–2840; Warnes CA, Williams RG, Bashore TM, et al. ACC/AHA Task Force on Practice Guidelines (Writing Committee to Develop Guidelines on the Management of Adults with Congenital Heart Disease). *J Am Coll Cardiol.* 2008;52(23):e1–e121.)

75. (B) This patient is having an atrial arrhythmia called incisional atrial flutter or intra-atrial reentrant tachycardia (IART). This arrhythmia is a unique type of atrial flutter seen in patients who have had previous cardiac surgeries on their atria or have extensive scarring of the atria for other reasons. It is present in about 7% of patients following the Fontan operation. IART tends to have slower rates than atrial flutter. The ECG is different in that there frequently is an isoelectric baseline in between two consecutive P waves, unlike atrial flutter where there is typically constant activity creating the "saw-tooth" pattern (see Fig. 13.10 with arrows pointing to the IART P waves). Patients who have baseline bradycardia and present with faster heart rates or have no variation in their heart rate should have an ECG to evaluate for IART. The T wave must be closely examined for the presence of P waves and a P wave will often be obscured by the QRS complexes. This arrhythmia typically requires cardioversion, although evaluation for the presence of a thrombus and/or anticoagulation therapy is indicated prior to cardioversion to help prevent embolization of a thrombus which may have formed due to stasis in the atria from the arrhythmia. As the function on echocardiogram was normal, dyssynchrony is an unlikely cause of the patient's symptoms and a biventricular pacemaker would not likely be beneficial. The ventricular rate in this ECG is too slow for ventricular tachycardia. Although the P wave axis is relatively normal (between 0 degree and 90 degrees), this patient is not in sinus rhythm. The patient may have underlying sinus dysfunction, but there is no evidence based on this ECG. (Walsh EP. Arrhythmias in patients with congenital heart disease. *Card Electrophysiol Rev.* 2002;6(4):422–430; Stephenson EA, Lu M, Berul CI, et al. Pediatric Heart Network Investigators. Arrhythmias in a contemporary Fontan cohort: prevalence and clinical associations in a multicenter cross-sectional study. *J Am Coll Cardiol.* 2010;56(11):890–896.)

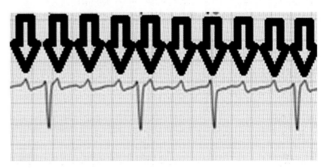

FIGURE 13.10

76. (C) The patient in the scenario most likely has an atrial septal defect. The most common presentation of a small to moderate defect is exercise intolerance typically in the second decade of life. The fixed split second heart sound and pulmonary flow murmur from left-to-right shunting at the atrial level are classic findings. The ECG will frequently show an incomplete right bundle branch block with an rSR' in lead V1 and may show right atrial enlargement. Imaging atrial septal defects may be challenging in adults, particularly in obese individuals. An agitated saline contrast echocardiogram (agitated saline is injected into a peripheral vein while imaging the right and left atrium) may show contrast in the left atrium, indicating a shunt at the atrial level. Alternatively, transesophageal imaging or cardiac magnetic resonance imaging may be performed to make the diagnosis. An exercise treadmill test is nonspecific and is unlikely to yield a diagnosis. Although she may have hypothyroidism, the murmur is not consistent with a thyroid problem and she is not bradycardic. She has no direct indication of pulmonary disease, so pulmonary function testing is unlikely to be helpful. Despite her obesity, coronary artery disease in an 18 year old would be very rare and does not explain the ECG or examination findings. (Soliman OI, Geleijnse ML, Meijboom FJ, et al. The use of contrast echocardiography for the detection of cardiac shunts. *Eur J Echocardiogr.* 2007;8(3):S2–S12.)

77. (E) Any patient who has survived a cardiac arrest due to nonreversible causes should have an ICD placed. There is no evidence of a reversible cause in this patient. Ablation may be offered as an alternative in a patient with a slow, stable, monomorphic ventricular tachycardia, but not the fast ventricular tachycardia resulting in cardiac arrest seen in this patient. The incidence of ICD complications was reported to be 30% in one study, compared to 10% in the postmyocardial infarction population. Antiarrhythmic medications are not as effective as an ICD in preventing recurrent arrhythmias and sudden cardiac death. β-Blockers, amiodarone, and sotalol do not significantly decrease the risk of appropriate ICD shocks in patients with ToF. A transvenous system is the preferred method of ICD placement in a patient who does not have a specific indication for surgery to replace the pulmonary valve. A transvenous system can be performed in a patient with free pulmonary regurgitation. Although cardiac resynchronization therapy (biventricular pacing) may improve hemodynamics and cardiac symptoms as well as decrease the QRS duration, it is not an alternative to ICD placement and there is no indication for resynchronization therapy in a patient with normal ventricular function. (Yap SC, Roos-Hesselink JW, Hoendermis ES, et al. Outcome of implantable cardioverter defibrillators in adults with congenital heart disease: a multi-centre study. *Eur Heart J.* 2007;28(15):1854–1861; Khairy P, Harris L, Landzberg MJ, et al. Implantable cardioverter-defibrillators in tetralogy of Fallot. *Circulation.* 2008;117(3):363–370; Walsh EP. Arrhythmias in patients with congenital heart disease. *Card Electrophysiol Rev.* 2002;6(4):422–430.)

78. (E) The ECG tracing shows intra-atrial reentrant tachycardia (IART) with variable conduction.

Clues to the IART are

- Heart rate above normal in a patient with sinus node dysfunction
- Marked variability of ventricular rate or no heart rate variability (i.e., heart rate 90 always)

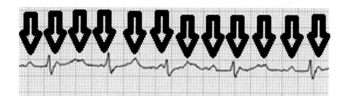

FIGURE 13.11

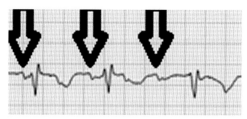

FIGURE 13.12 IART with arrows showing P waves marching through. Variability of PR interval.

- Abnormal P wave axis (Fig. 13.11)
- Prolongation of PR interval
- Variability of PR interval throughout the tracing (Fig. 13.12)

The ACCP Evidence-Based Clinical Practice Guidelines recommend that antithrombotic therapy be initiated for both atrial fibrillation and atrial flutter. As he is clinically stable, there is no indication for cardioversion and as long as he does not have a rapid ventricular response to his arrhythmia, he should be anticoagulated for 3 weeks and then undergo a cardioversion. Both coumadin and rivaroxaban are reasonable medications for anticoagulation. Rivaroxaban is a novel anticoagulation agent that has a similar efficacy and safety profile to coumadin, but has the advantage of not needing to check INR to adjust the dosage. Although digoxin and β-blockers may slow conduction in the AV node preventing rapid conduction of an atrial arrhythmia, there is no evidence of rapid conduction of the arrhythmia in this patient. Although it would be reasonable to start digoxin or β-blockers, anticoagulation is more important. ACE inhibition may be beneficial in patients with a systemic right ventricle, but would not have any effect on this acute arrhythmia. There is no indication to start amiodarone immediately. Amiodarone may have significant side effects, it is typically not the first choice for long-term therapy in young, otherwise healthy patients.

79. (D) The tracing shows an irregularly irregular rhythm characteristic of atrial fibrillation. There is chaotic atrial activity with no definitive P waves. The ventricular response is relatively fast with an average rate of 136 bpm, but a stretch in the middle of the tracing with a heart rate over 150 bpm. The episode of syncope that she had is likely due to a rapid ventricular response caused by a catecholamine surge when running for the bus. Her decreased function is also likely due to the arrhythmia. Although it would be ideal to anticoagulate for 3 weeks and then cardiovert, the acute nature of her syncope and depressed function as well as symptoms necessitate cardioversion. Although the ventricular response is relatively rapid, her vital signs are stable and there is no indication for emergent cardioversion. Performing a transesophageal echocardiogram to rule out a large thrombus that might be dislodged by the cardioversion is indicated in this situation. If a large thrombus is present, it is reasonable to anticoagulate for a period of time prior to performing the cardioversion. If there is no thrombus, a cardioversion can be performed immediately, although there is some risk of a small thrombus that cannot be seen on echocardiogram dislodging and causing a stroke. DC cardioversion is likely to be more effective and quicker than IV amiodarone at converting the atrial fibrillation. There is no indication for urgent device closure of the residual ASD and this will not acutely correct the current problem of atrial fibrillation.

80. (B) ACC guidelines suggest that patients with prior Fontan procedure, severe pulmonary arterial hypertension, cyanotic CHD, complex CHD or malignant arrhythmia be referred to regional ACHD centers for noncardiac surgery. A is not correct as the patient does not have complex CHD without evidence of heart failure; the patient described in C does not have pulmonary artery hypertension, but right ventricular hypertension, and the patient in D has no evidence of significant VSD.

81. (D) Patient s/p AVSD repair should have surgical intervention for LVOT obstruction if the maximal instantaneous gradient is >70 mm Hg or if there is a lower gradient in association with significant mitral or aortic valve regurgitation. Therefore, this patient does not have a surgical indication. There is no evidence that β-blockade improves outcome or symptoms in this situation. ACE inhibition is not indicated.

82. (A) Class I indications for surgical intervention of supravalvar AS include a mean gradient of 50 mm Hg or greater in asymptomatic patients. Patients with lesser degrees of obstruction should be considered for surgical intervention if they are symptomatic, have LVH, or are planning a pregnancy.

83. (D) Asymptomatic patients with maximum instantaneous pulmonary valve gradients gradient >30 mm Hg should have follow-up echocardiograms every 2 to 5 years. There is no indication for cardiac catheterization or intervention on this patient.

84. (B) Noninvasive testing for ischemia provocation is recommended every 3 to 5 years for patients after arterial switch procedures. Six-minute walk is not indicated for ischemia provocation. The patient has no pulmonary symptoms, so PFTs are not needed.

85. (C) Small coronary fistulae with no symptoms, no murmur, and no evidence of hemodynamic compromise do not need further evaluation or treatment.

SUGGESTED READINGS

Ammash N, Warnes CA. Cerebrovascular events in adult patients with cyanotic congenital heart disease. *J Am Coll Cardiol.* 1996; 28(3):768–772.

Bonow RO, Carabello BA, Chatterjee K, et al. 2008 Focused update incorporated into the ACC/AHA 2006 guidelines for the management of patients with valvular heart disease: a report of the American College of Cardiology/American Heart Association Task Force on Practice Guidelines. *Circulation.* 2008;118(15): e523–e661.

Hiratzka LF, Bakris GL, Beckman JA, et al. 2010 ACCF/AHA/AATS/ ACR/ASA/SCA/SCAI/SIR/STS/SVM guidelines for the diagnosis and management of patients with thoracic aortic disease. *Circulation.* 2010;121:e266–e369.

John AS, Gurley F, Schaff HV, et al. Cardiopulmonary bypass during pregnancy. *Ann Thorac Surg.* 2011;91(4):1191–1196.

Khairy P, Ouyang D, Fernandes SM, et al. Pregnancy outcomes in women with congenital heart disease. *Circulation.* 2006; 113(4):517–524.

Nishimura RA, Warnes CA. Anticoagulation during pregnancy in women with prosthetic valves; evidence, guidelines and unanswered questions. *Heart* 2015;101:430–435.

Sanikommu V, Lasorda D, Poornima I. Anatomical factors triggering platypnea-orthodeoxia in adults. *Clin Cardiol.* 2009; 32(11):e55–e57.

Singer DE, Albers GW, Dalen JE, et al. American College of Chest Physicians. Antithrombotic therapy in atrial fibrillation: American College of Chest Physicians Evidence-Based Clinical Practice Guidelines (8th Edition). *Chest.* 2008;133(6 Suppl):546S–592S.

Siu SC, Sermer M, Colman JM, et al. Prospective multicenter study of pregnancy outcomes in women with heart disease. *Circulation.* 2001;104(5):515–521.

Warnes CA, Williams RG, Bashore TM, et al. ACC/AHA 2008 Guidelines for the Management of Adults with Congenital Heart Disease: a reports of the American College of Cardiology/ American Heart Association Task Force on Practice Guidelines. *Circulation.* 2008;118(23):e714–e833.

CHAPTER 14

Statistics and Research Design

Anthony C. Chang and Heather Anderson

QUESTIONS

1. Of the following types of data-descriptive term pairs, which is the pair that incorrectly matches the data with the type of data?

   A. Blood groups—nominal data
   B. American Heart Association (AHA) class—ordinal data
   C. Number of surgical procedures—discrete data
   D. Pulmonary vascular resistance—categorical data
   E. Cardiac index—continuous data

2. A pediatric cardiology fellow is interested in studying the potential relationship between exposure to lithium and Ebstein anomaly with an observational study. He decided to use a case–control methodology for his study. Of the following observations of studies, which is a disadvantage for this case–control study?

   A. Information on exposure and past history is primarily based on interview and may be subject to recall bias
   B. Exposure patterns, for example, the composition of oral contraceptives, may change during the course of the study and make the results irrelevant
   C. Not suited for the study of rare diseases because a large number of subjects are required
   D. Expensive to carry out because a large number of subjects are usually required
   E. Baseline data may be sparse because the large number of subjects do not allow for long interviews

3. A new drug is available for the treatment of heart failure and is undergoing phase III trials in adults with heart failure. Of the following statements, which most closely describes a phase III trial for a medication?

   A. A small group (20 to 80 subjects) of volunteers to assess the safety and pharmacokinetic profile of the medication
   B. Randomized controlled multicenter trial on a relatively large group (300 to 3,000 or more subjects)

depending on the medical condition and is to assess the effectiveness of the drug in comparison with an accepted therapy
   C. A large group (20 to 300 subjects) to assess safety in a larger group of patients as well as effectiveness of the drug
   D. Administration of a single subtherapeutic dose of the drug to a small group (10 to 15 subjects) to gather preliminary data on pharmacokinetics and pharmacodynamics
   E. Involves safety surveillance and ongoing technical support of a drug after permission for it to be distributed

4. A pediatric cardiologist would like to compare atrioventricular (AV) valve regurgitation severity data from two unpaired groups of children that are relatively small in number (<5). Of the following statistical methods, which should he select?

   A. Chi-squared (χ^2) test
   B. Fisher exact test
   C. McNemar test
   D. Mantel–Haenszel test
   E. Student t-test

5. An investigator in pediatric cardiology would like to use a statistical method to compare groups that have clinical data with normal distributions. Of the following, which statistical test should be used to analyze such parametric data?

   A. Wilcoxon signed-rank test
   B. Mann–Whitney U-test
   C. Wilcoxon rank sum test
   D. Kruskal–Wallis test
   E. Analysis of variance (ANOVA) test

6. A pediatric cardiologist wishes to study the prevalence and incidence of congenital heart disease in his home city. Which of the following is the relationship between prevalence (P) and the incidence (I) with duration of disease (D)?

  A. $P = I - D$
  B. $P/I = D$
  C. $P \times I = D$
  D. $P = I/D$
  E. None of the above

7. The graph in Figure 14.1 depicts which of the following?

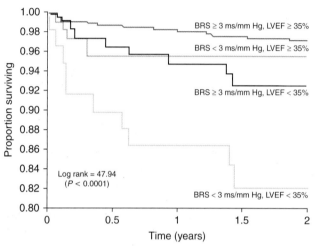

FIGURE 14.1 Used with permission from La Rovere MT, Bigger Jr JT, Marcus FI, et al., on behalf of the ATRAMI Investigators. Baroreflex sensitivity and heart rate variability in prediction of total cardiac mortality after myocardial infarction. *Lancet.* 1998;351:478–484.

  A. Kaplan–Meier survival curve
  B. Linear regression curve
  C. Logistic regression curve
  D. Poisson regression curve
  E. Correlation curve with Spearman coefficient

8. Figure 14.2 depicts normal and disease populations with frequency on the *y*-axis and the diagnostic test value on the *x*-axis. The cutpoint is indicated by the vertical black line, above which we consider the test to be abnormal and below which we consider the test to be normal. TN is true negatives and TP is true positives. The arrow is pointing at the area that is which of the following?

  A. False negatives
  B. True negatives
  C. Positive predictive value (PPV)
  D. Negative predictive value (NPV)
  E. Sensitivity/specificity

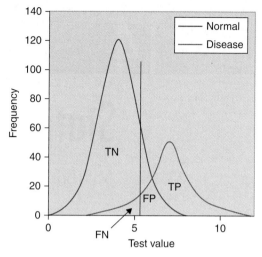

FIGURE 14.2 From gim.unmc.edu/dxtests/ROC1.htm.

9. A normal or Gaussian distribution is a well-recognized curve that reflects a continuous probability distribution that is bell-shaped (unimodal) and symmetrical about the mean with two parameters, the mean (μ) and the variance (σ^2). Which of the following continuous probability distributions most closely resembles the normal or Gaussian distribution?

  A. *t*-distribution
  B. χ^2-distribution
  C. *F*-distribution
  D. Binomial distribution
  E. Poisson distribution

10. The mean systolic blood pressure before an antihypertensive medication was given for a group of 50 patients was 165 mm Hg. The mean decrease in blood pressure after the medication was administered was 20 mm Hg. The 95% confidence interval (CI) was −5 to 45 mm Hg. Which of the following statements is ***correct***?

  A. The CI can be decreased with a smaller sample of patients
  B. One can be 95% confident that the treatment can lower the blood pressure in all patients by at least 20 mm Hg
  C. There is a >5% chance that there would be no true change in blood pressure in the entire population
  D. The standard deviation (SD) in this study is the same as the CI
  E. There is 95% chance that the study sample accurately reflects the general population

11. Of the following, which is a type of inferential statistical method?

  A. Arithmetic mean
  B. Mode
  C. Student *t*-test
  D. Median
  E. Histogram

12. Which of the following statements regarding hypothesis testing is **true**?
    A. A type I error (α error) occurs when a null hypothesis that is correct is accepted
    B. A type II error (β error) occurs when a hypothesis that is incorrect is rejected
    C. A type III error is a study design that produces the wrong answer to the right question
    D. The *P* (probability) value is the probability that defines how likely it is that the null hypothesis is false
    E. The *P*-value is the probability of an observed difference occurring solely by chance

13. Which of the following would **increase** the power of a study?
    A. Smaller significance level
    B. Larger effects
    C. Increased variability of the observations
    D. Smaller sample size
    E. None of the above

14. An economic assessment method is utilized in which the costs and consequences of alternative cardiac interventions are expressed in costs per unit of health outcome. This commonly used methodology is applicable to health programs as well as health services to help determine the preferred action that requires the least cost to produce a given level of effectiveness. Which of the following is this assessment tool?
    A. Cost-effectiveness analysis (CEA)
    B. Cost–utility analysis (CUA)
    C. Cost–benefit analysis (CBA)
    D. Cost-minimization analysis (CMA)
    E. Cost–value analysis (CVA)

15. A meta-analysis is a technique where results from a number of studies that are similar in nature are gathered to give one overall estimate of the effect. Which of the following is a disadvantage of this technique?
    A. Refinement and reduction of large amount of information
    B. Efficiency relative to a new study
    C. Publication bias for statistically significant studies
    D. Power to detect effects of interest
    E. Precision greater than a single study

16. In a prospective study of a new antiarrhythmic agent, the investigators found that 16 of 465 children (3.4%) in the treatment group had arrhythmias while in the placebo group, 23 of 465 children (4.9%) had arrhythmias. What is the risk ratio?
    A. 1.44
    B. 0.44
    C. 0.69
    D. 0.31
    E. None of the above

17. Which of the following is the relative risk reduction (RRR) in this study?
    A. 44%
    B. 31%
    C. 69%
    D. 144%
    E. None of the above

18. What is the number of patients who need to be treated (NNT) for one to get benefit of the drug?
    A. 67
    B. 15
    C. 20
    D. 29
    E. None of the above

19. In a typical receiver operating characteristic (ROC) curve, what is the significance of the upper left corner or coordinate (0,1)?
    A. 100% sensitivity and specificity
    B. 0% sensitivity and 100% specificity
    C. 100% sensitivity or 0% specificity
    D. 0% sensitivity and specificity
    E. 50% sensitivity and 50% specificity

20. The measure of precision of the sample mean or how close the sample mean is likely to be to the population mean is termed as which of the following?
    A. Variance
    B. Coefficient of variation
    C. SD to the mean
    D. SD
    E. Standard error of the mean (SEM)

21. Figure 14.3 shows the relationship between accuracy and precision to be which of the following?

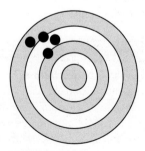

FIGURE 14.3

    A. Accurate and precise
    B. Not accurate but precise
    C. Accurate but not precise
    D. Neither accurate nor precise
    E. None of the above

22. Some children with supraventricular tachycardia were treated with digoxin while others were treated with propranolol. The results in a contingency table are shown in Table 14.1.

What additional information is necessary for the calculation of *P*-value?

TABLE 14.1 Digoxin versus Propranolol for SVT			
	Digoxin	**Propranolol**	**Total**
No SVT	30 (60%)	34 (67%)	64 (64%)
Some SVT	20 (40%)	16 (33%)	36 (36%)
Total	50 (100%)	50 (100%)	100 (100%)

$\chi^2 = 2.3$

    A. Degree of freedom (df)
    B. SEM
    C. Variance
    D. Power
    E. Covariance

23. Which of the following statements regarding the correlation coefficient *r* is **true**?

    A. It is dimensionless
    B. When $r = 0$, there is perfect correlation
    C. A correlation between *x* and *y* implies that there is a cause and effect relationship
    D. The correlation coefficient *r* can be calculated when there are several outliers
    E. A nonlinear relationship does not imply that a correlation coefficient cannot be calculated

24. A cardiologist reviews the database for elevated (>100 pg/mL) serum BNP in his practice and tabulated the data in Table 14.2 for the cardiac patients he follows. What is the PPV for BNP >100 pg/mL for cardiac disease in his patient population?

TABLE 14.2 Cardiac Disease and BNP			
	Cardiac Disease		
BNP >100 pg/mL	**+**	**−**	**Total**
+	50	5	55
−	25	100	125
Total	75	105	180

    A. 50/55
    B. 50/75
    C. 25/180
    D. 25/75
    E. 50/180

25. For the same database, what is the likelihood ratio (LR) (Table 14.2)?

    A. $(100/105)/[1 - (50/75)]$
    B. $[1 - (50/75)]/(100/105)$
    C. $(50/75)/[1 - (100/105)]$
    D. $[1 - (100/105)]/(50/75)$
    E. Cannot calculate as prevalence of disease is not stated

26. A randomized controlled trial (RCT) is a trial in which the patients are randomized to receive either the new or a control treatment. An ideal randomization involves equal group sizes, low selection bias, and low probability of confounding (accidental bias). Which of the following is **not** a refinement of simple randomization?

    A. Stratified randomization
    B. Blocked randomization
    C. Observational randomization
    D. Cluster randomization
    E. Response-adaptive randomization

27. Bias occurs when there is a systematic difference between the results of a study and the true results. A bias that occurs when a spurious association is noted due to a failure to adjust fully for factors leading to an erroneous conclusion is called:

    A. Observer bias
    B. Confounding bias
    C. Selection bias
    D. Information bias
    E. Allocation bias

28. An association is any relationship between two measured quantities that relates them to be statistically dependent. Which of the following is **not** a criterion for concluding causation in addition to an association in an observational study?

    A. Temporality
    B. Dose–response
    C. Repetition in a different population
    D. Consistency with other studies
    E. Expert consensus

29. A pediatric cardiologist is conducting a research project on the use of a new drug for heart failure in children. He is being very truthful to the parent regarding the possible side effect of hypotension with the use of this new drug. He is abiding by which principle of the Belmont report?

    A. Respect for persons
    B. Beneficence
    C. Justice
    D. Lack of conflict of interest
    E. Scientific reasoning

30. An independent group of experts that continuously monitors data from various aspects of a clinical trial to ensure patient safety as well as validity and scientific merit is which of the following?

   A. Institutional Review Board
   B. Ethics Committee
   C. Data Safety Monitoring Board (DSMB)
   D. Independent Ethics Committee
   E. Clinical Trials Safety Committee

31. Which of the following is a statistical term to describe the consistency of a set of measurements or a measurement tool or its repeatability and reproducibility?

   A. Precision
   B. Accuracy
   C. Reliability
   D. Validity
   E. Power

32. A pediatric cardiologist is studying the efficacy of a new antiarrhythmic agent in the treatment of junctional ectopic tachycardia. He is interested in a randomized, double-blind placebo-controlled trial. To calculate the number of patients needed for the study with a power of 0.80 and a statistical significance of 0.05, he needs which additional information?

   A. Standardized difference
   B. SEM
   C. CI
   D. Bias
   E. Expected mean

33. Which of the following statements is an advantage of a cohort study?

   A. Not suited for the study of rare diseases because a large number of subjects are required
   B. Not suited when the time between exposure and disease manifestation is very long, although this can be overcome in historical cohort studies
   C. Exposure patterns, for example, the composition of oral contraceptives, may change during the course of the study and make the results irrelevant
   D. Maintaining high rates of follow-up can be difficult
   E. Permit calculation of incidence rates (absolute risk) as well as relative risk

34. A cardiology researcher has a research project and needs to find a statistical method that allows paired comparisons of two nonnormal patient populations. Which of the following would be the **correct** choice?

   A. Wilcoxon signed-rank test
   B. Mann–Whitney U-test
   C. Wilcoxon rank sum test
   D. Kruskal–Wallis test
   E. ANOVA

35. Which of the following is a statistical test used for two large (>5) groups of unpaired categorical data?

   A. One-way ANOVA
   B. χ^2 test
   C. McNemar test
   D. Fisher exact test
   E. Wilcoxon rank sum test

36. Data can be categorized into categorical or numerical data. Which of the following data is an example of a categorical type of data called ordinal data?

   A. Severity of AV valve regurgitation
   B. Single ventricle and biventricular surgical strategies
   C. Blood pressure measurements before and after angiotensin-converting enzyme (ACE) inhibitors
   D. Number of reinterventions after Norwood procedure
   E. Antiarrhythmic agent for supraventricular tachycardia

37. A pediatric cardiologist is interested in prospectively studying the relationship between length of time of neonatal surgical cardiopulmonary bypass and fine motor development at ages 5 and 10 years. He will be enrolling neonates in this study. This type of study is which of the following?

   A. Case–control study
   B. Cohort study
   C. Case series
   D. Retrospective study
   E. Historical cohort study

38. A pediatric cardiologist is interested in studying intravenous milrinone in pediatric septic shock and is organizing a randomized controlled multicenter trial involving over 300 children with septic shock. He is primarily interested in assessing the benefit of milrinone compared to traditional inotropic agents. This phase of the clinical trial would be considered as which of the following?

   A. Phase 0
   B. Phase I
   C. Phase II
   D. Phase III
   E. Phase IV

39. A chi-squared (χ^2) test is most closely related to which of the following statistical tests?

   A. ANOVA
   B. Student t-test
   C. Kolmogorov–Smirnov test
   D. Wilcoxon signed-rank test
   E. Fisher exact test

40. The department of public health is interested in knowing the prevalence of congenital heart disease in the city. Which of the following is the correct definition for **prevalence** of congenital heart disease?

A. Number of new cases of the disease that occur in a population during a period of time/sum for each individual in the population of the length of time at risk of getting the disease

B. Number of individuals who get the disease during a certain period/number of individuals in the population at the beginning of the period X

C. Existing number of individuals having the disease at a specific time/number of individuals in the population at that point in time

D. Number of new cases of the disease that occur in a population during a period of time/number of individuals in the population at the beginning of the period X

E. Number of individuals who get the disease during a certain period/sum for each individual in the population of the length of time at risk of getting the disease

41. A public health officer asks a pediatric cardiologist to assess the CBA of an intervention. CBA is **best** defined as which of the following?

A. An economic assessment method in which the costs and consequences of alternative interventions are expressed in costs per unit of health outcome

B. A methodology that is applicable to health programs as well as health services to help determine the preferred action that requires the least cost to produce a given level of effectiveness

C. An economic tool which uses quality-of-life measurements expressed as utilities (such as quality adjusted-life year or QALY) in the value equation

D. An economic assessment methodology that seeks to translate all relevant healthcare considerations into monetary terms by analyzing economic and social costs of medical care and benefits of reduced loss of net earnings due to preventing premature death or disability

E. None of the above

42. A review article on the most current management of heart failure discussed a myriad of medical therapies. The use of a particular β-blocker is discussed and "level C" is included at the end of the discussion. This designation is interpreted as which of the following?

A. At least fair scientific evidence that risks outweigh the benefit

B. Scientific evidence is lacking, or poor quality, or conflicting

C. At least fair scientific evidence (benefit and risk too close)

D. Good scientific evidence (benefits substantially outweigh risk)

E. At least fair scientific evidence (benefits outweigh the risk)

43. An athlete in a high-school football game recently collapsed and died from hypertrophic cardiomyopathy. A screening program to identify hypertrophic cardiomyopathy in a local high school with electrocardiograms (ECGs) and echocardiograms for all student athletes yielded the following data in Table 14.3.

What is the **sensitivity** for the ECG?

TABLE 14.3 Hypertrophic Cardiomyopathy and ECG

ECG	Hypertrophic Cardiomyopathy		
	Present	Absent	Total
Positive	1	20	21
Negative	1	785	786
Total	2	805	807

A. 1/805
B. 1/21
C. 1/2
D. 1/786
E. 1/807

44. What is the **specificity** for the ECG (Table 14.3)?

A. 20/805
B. 785/805
C. 785/786
D. 20/807
E. 785/807

45. What is the **PPV** for the ECG (Table 14.3)?

A. 1/21
B. 1/805
C. 1/2
D. 20/805
E. 21/807

46. What is the **NPV** for the ECG (Table 14.3)?

A. 785/786
B. 1/786
C. 785/805
D. 1/805
E. 1/2

47. What is the *LR* (Table 14.3)?
    A. (785/805)/[1 – (1/2)]
    B. (1/2)/[1 – (785/805)]
    C. (785/786)/[1 – (1/2)]
    D. (1/21)/[1 – (785/805)]
    E. (1/2)/[1 – (785/786)]

48. The efficacy and safety of an angiotensin receptor blocker in Duchenne muscular dystrophy patients with severe heart failure is being studied in a multi-institutional study. In the treated group, 5 of 200 patients had hospital admission for exacerbations of heart failure while 25 of the 250 in the untreated group were hospitalized. What is the *risk ratio*?
    A. 2.5/10
    B. 5/200
    C. 5/250
    D. 25/200
    E. 25/450

49. What is the *RRR* for the treated group?
    A. 25%
    B. 75%
    C. 50%
    D. 7.5%
    E. None of the above

50. What is the *NNT* in this study for the treatment group?
    A. 13.3
    B. 7.5
    C. 4
    D. 2
    E. Cannot calculate based on the available data

51. You are investigating whether the use of thiazide diuretics plus angiotensin converting enzyme inhibitors in the treatment of children with hypertension results in higher rates of long-term blood pressure control compared to thiazide diuretics alone.

    The *most* reliable results would occur with which type of study?
    A. Interrupted time series study
    B. Double-blind, placebo-controlled trial
    C. Retrospective case–control study
    D. Observational prospective study
    E. Cross-sectional studies

52. You received a grant for research and wish to conduct a study to investigate the role of maternal diabetes as a risk factor for congenital heart disease. You must decide whether to do a case–control or a cohort study. After comparing the advantages of each type of study, you determine that a case–control study would be the better option.

    Which is *true* regarding a case–control study?
    A. Allows for the study of one potential risk factor at a time
    B. Allows for calculation of rates of disease in exposed and unexposed
    C. Well suited for conditions with a short latency
    D. Relies on recall or records of past events
    E. Well suited for rare conditions

53. You have a patient who presents to clinic with the chief complaint of chest pain. You review the current literature and find an article about the prevalence of chest pain in children and adolescents in your area. In this study an anonymous survey was sent out to families with children 5 to 18 years of age registered within the local school district. This survey included various demographic and clinical questions, one of which asked about the presence of chest pain within the last 6 months.

    Which of the following *best* describes the study design used above?
    A. Prospective cohort study
    B. Census
    C. Retrospective cohort study
    D. Cross-sectional study
    E. Observational prospective study

54. A child is referred to your practice for the diagnosis of aortic coarctation with a peak instantaneous pressure gradient of 30 mm Hg. The family has consented to participate in a multi-institutional study looking at the efficacy of surgical repair versus balloon angioplasty. The medical student working with you asks why it is important to accrue a large number of participants.

    Of the following, the *most* appropriate response would be that:
    A. Increasing the sample size improves the ability to detect adverse events
    B. The likelihood of a type II error increases with increased sample size
    C. The larger the sample size, the less likely a type I error is made
    D. A larger sample size decreases the power of a study
    E. The larger the detectable difference in effect, the larger the sample size required

55. The parents of a patient ask if treatment with an angiotensin II receptor blocker in addition to a β-blocker improves protection against progressive aortic root dilation in children with Marfan syndrome. You find a study where researchers investigated whether angiotensin II receptor blockers were a protective factor against progressive aortic root dilation 10 years after diagnosis in patients concurrently on β-blockers. Participants were identified as to whether they were on an angiotensin II receptor blocker plus β-blocker or β-blocker monotherapy and then followed at 1-year intervals for a total of 10 years.

Which of the following statements is **true** regarding this study?

A. The patients were studied retrospectively
B. The cohort was biased by the healthy entrant effect
C. This represents a type of prospective cohort study
D. The natural epidemiology of aortic root dilation in patients with Marfan syndrome could be studied in this cohort
E. None of the above

56. A 16-year-old girl presented to the emergency department 2 days ago with syncope. Her description of the syncopal episode was consistent with vasovagal syncope. An ECG obtained in the emergency department showed prolongation of the QTc interval to 460 msec. She was diagnosed with long QT syndrome and the ED provider recommended initiation of β-blocker therapy. Her mother requested an evaluation by Pediatric Cardiology prior to starting this treatment. In your office, the patient is appropriate with normal vital signs. Her repeat ECG is normal with QTc of 400 msec. You recommend no treatment for QT prolongation.

Of the following, which limitation of the testing performed in the emergency department **best** supports your action:

A. Generalizability
B. Negative predictive value
C. Sensitivity
D. Specificity
E. Validity

57. In your effort to help older adolescents with hyperlipidemia, you seek studies of effective nutrition strategies in college-age students. You find one where 336 subjects were studied. In this study, 154 were allocated to food intake recording, weekly weigh-ins, and weekly group education, while the remaining 182 were allocated to a wait-list control arm. At four months, the intervention group showed greater cholesterol management than the wait-listed group (mean 162 (95% CI 149 to 173) vs. 189 (95% CI 179 to 197)); $P = 0.007$. The authors concluded that, at least compared to the wait-list, a structured consultation program resulted in significantly greater short-term cholesterol management.

Which of the following statements **best** describes the information provided by the 95% confidence interval for cholesterol levels for the intervention group?

A. 95% of sample participants in the intervention group achieved a cholesterol level 149 to 173
B. There is a probability of 0.95 that the sample mean cholesterol level for the intervention group was between 149 and 173
C. 95% of the population would achieve a cholesterol level between 149 and 173 if they received the intervention
D. There is a probability of 0.95 that the population mean cholesterol level at 4 months with the intervention would be between 149 and 173
E. There is a 95% chance that the results of the study are accurate

58. You propose to your colleagues a study regarding risk factors for sudden death in patients with hypertrophic cardiomyopathy. Your plans include data collection with a survey of parents regarding the presence of chest pain in their child prior to their sudden death event.

This type of data collection is **most** vulnerable to:

A. Lead-time bias
B. Selection bias
C. Recall bias
D. Length bias
E. Referral bias

59. You are doing a preoperative evaluation of a patient with atrioventricular septal defect and note that the patient is anemic with a hemoglobin level of 9.7 gm/dl. You do a literature search to find the prevalence of anemia in children with AV canal defects and find a study looking at children with both ventricular septal defect (VSD) and AV canal defect and their rates of anemia. In this study they found an odds ratio of 0.21 (95% CI 0.07–0.68) for the risk of anemia in patients with AV canal defects.

Based on this information, which statement is **true**?

A. The P-value is likely to be >0.05
B. The risk of anemia is lower in children with AV canal defect
C. Children with anemia are more likely to have an AV canal defect than a VSD
D. The odds of having anemia are lower in a child with a VSD
E. 21% of patients in the study have an AV canal defect

60. A medical student rounding with the cardiology team asks about the use of sirolimus for immunosuppression in children after undergoing heart transplant. You present the student with a study showing the incidence of rejection in children both prior to and following sirolimus initiation. Thirty children were included in this study and all were 2 years status-post initial heart transplant. The average number of rejection episodes was found to be 3.2 +/– 0.7 prior to initiation of sirolimus. After initiation of sirolimus, the children were followed for another 2 years and the average number of rejections episodes was 2.7 +/– 0.4.

The type of statistical analysis most appropriate in this study is:

A. Paired Student *t*-test
B. Wilcoxon signed-rank test
C. Chi-squared
D. Odds ratio
E. Kaplan–Meier curve

61. A pediatric cardiology fellow performs a case–control study to evaluate the association between children with a history of prosthetic valve replacement surgery and subsequent endocarditis. He obtains the results presented in Table 14.4.

What is the odds ratio for the development of endocarditis in patients with a previous valve replacement?

TABLE 14.4 A Case–Control Study in Cardiology: Results

	Endocarditis Present	No Endocarditis Present
Prosthetic valve replacement	10	40
No prosthetic valve replacement	2	48

A. $(10 \times 48)/(40 \times 2)$
B. $(40 \times 2)/(10 \times 48)$
C. $(2 \times 48)/(40 \times 10)$
D. $(2 \times 10)/(40 \times 48)$
E. Unable to calculate with the information provided

62. A new antiarrhythmic medication has been developed and is going to be compared to standard treatment for neonatal supraventricular tachycardia. The research team anticipates using a χ^2 analysis to evaluate their findings.

Based on this information, which statement is *false*.

A. This study involves the collection of continuous data
B. Each group must be completely independent of the others for the intervention of interest
C. Expected values in each cell of a 2×2 table must be at least 5
D. The *P*-value calculated from the χ^2 analysis tells you how likely it is that the outcomes observed could have been found by chance

63. The pediatric resident rounding with the cardiology team is following a patient after Fontan surgery. The resident reports on rounds that she has found a study in

which patients who received sesame seeds every day had improved survival after Fontan surgery. However, she is concerned because this study utilized a parametric test for analysis, but has a very small number of patients in the study.

For comparison of survival between two nonnormally distributed groups, each with only 10 participants, which would be the *most* appropriate test?

A. Fischer exact test
B. Student *t*-test
C. Wilcoxon signed-rank test
D. χ^2 test
E. None of the above

64. When creating a Kaplan–Meier survival curve for patients with Down syndrome after AV canal repair, it is important to remember that censored patients will include all these *except*:

A. Patients who died
B. Patients who withdrew from the study
C. Patients lost to follow-up
D. Patients still alive at the end of the study period

65. You are evaluating a new medication for the treatment heart failure and would like to test its ability to improve cardiac function in patients with myocarditis. You have a study in which patients with newly diagnosed myocarditis are randomized to receive either placebo or the new medication. There are 52 patients in the treatment group and 47 in the placebo group. The ejection fraction (EF) is followed for each patient for 6 months. The average EF in patients on treatment at 6 months is 51% (±6%) versus 40% (±5%) in the placebo group.

What is the number needed to treat (NNT) with this new medication to maintain cardiac function in patients with myocarditis?

A. Unable to calculate
B. 9
C. 10
D. 50
E. 100

66. A pediatric cardiologist would like to evaluate how fellows self-evaluate their catheterization procedures. She has both pediatric cardiology staff and fellows score each catheterization procedure based on a standardized scoring system and then compares their evaluations.

What would be the best test to analyze these data?

A. Sensitivity
B. Kappa statistic
C. Regression analysis
D. Receiver operating curve
E. Beta factor

67. A study designed to look at mortality in children with interrupted aortic arch utilizes chi-squared analysis to describe mortality rates in children with interrupted arch as compared to those with coarctation of the aorta. As you review the results section of this study, you notice that there were only 10 patients in the interrupted aortic arch group with 3 deaths and 25 patients in the coarctation group with 4 deaths.

What would have been the most appropriate type of test to use for analysis of the data in this study?

A. Fischer exact test
B. The most appropriate test was already used
C. Kruskal–Wallis test
D. ANOVA
E. Student t-test

68. A multi-institutional study comparing the use of an angiotensin II receptor blocker, an angiotensin converting enzyme inhibitor, and a beta-blocker for the management of heart failure is conducted. The authors decide to analyze the data using ANOVA analysis.

What is a potential concern with the use of ANOVA analysis in this study?

A. If P is <0.05, this study demonstrates a difference among the groups, but not specifically between which groups the difference occurs or how big the difference is
B. ANOVA analysis requires four or more different groups
C. ANOVA will underestimate the difference between the groups
D. ANOVA analysis is very time consuming and does not provide clinically relevant data
E. There is a very high incidence of false-positive results using ANOVA

69. You are studying the mean blood pressure values in children with body mass index (BMI) >85th percentile randomized to treatment with lisinopril, weight management regimen, or placebo medication. This study

includes 30 participants with 10 patients in each group. The distribution of the data for the group of patients given lisinopril is shown in Figure 14.4.

What would be the best test to compare the mean blood pressures between the groups?

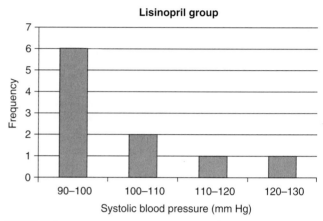

FIGURE 14.4

A. Kruskal–Wallis test
B. ANOVA
C. χ^2 test
D. Student t-test
C. None of the above

70. A pediatric cardiologist is studying the association between certain genetic markers and DiGeorge syndrome. Which of these statements would be ***false*** about the null hypothesis in this study?

A. The null hypothesis would be that none of the markers are associated with DiGeorge syndrome
B. The null hypothesis is what you would like to disprove
C. The null hypothesis is confirmed if P <0.05
D. Type I error is rejecting the null hypothesis when it is true
E. None aof the above

ANSWERS

1. (D) Data from variables can be categorical (qualitative) or numerical (quantitative).

Categorical data include (1) nominal data that describe data that can be in categories but have no particular order or magnitude differences (such as blood groups) and (2) ordinal data that are data that can be allocated to an ordered set of categories (such as AHA classes I to IV or severity of AV valve regurgitation from mild to severe).

Numerical data include (1) discrete data that can only be certain whole numbers (such as number of surgeries or catheterizations) and (2) continuous data that can be any numerical value (such as cardiac indices or pulmonary vascular resistances). Pulmonary vascular resistance, therefore, would be numerical data of a continuous nature.

2. (A)
Case–control studies:
Advantages:

1. Permit the study of rare diseases.
2. Permit the study of diseases with long latency between exposure and manifestation.
3. Can be launched and conducted over relatively short time periods.
4. Relatively inexpensive as compared to cohort studies.
5. Can study multiple potential causes of disease.

Disadvantages:

1. Information on exposure and past history is primarily based on interview and may be subject to recall bias.
2. Validation of information on exposure is difficult, incomplete, or even impossible.
3. By definition, concerned with one disease only.
4. Cannot usually provide information on incidence rates of disease.
5. Generally incomplete control of extraneous variables.
6. Choice of appropriate control group may be difficult.
7. Methodology may be hard to comprehend for nonepidemiologists and correct interpretation of results may be difficult.

Cohort studies:
Advantages:

1. Allow complete information on the subject's exposure, including quality control of data, and experience thereafter.
2. Provide a clear temporal sequence of exposure and disease.
3. Give an opportunity to study multiple outcomes related to a specific exposure.
4. Permit calculation of incidence rates (absolute risk) as well as relative risk.
5. Methodology and results are easily understood by nonepidemiologists.
6. Enable the study of relatively rare exposures.

Disadvantages:

1. Not suited for the study of rare diseases because a large number of subjects are required.

2. Not suited when the time between exposure and disease manifestation is very long, although this can be overcome in historical cohort studies.
3. Exposure patterns, for example, the composition of oral contraceptives, may change during the course of the study and make the results irrelevant.
4. Maintaining high rates of follow-up can be difficult.
5. Expensive to carry out because a large number of subjects are usually required.
6. Baseline data may be sparse because the large number of subjects does not allow for long interviews.

(From Metric O. Cohort and Case–Control Studies, WHO)

3. (B) A clinical trial is research involving administration of a test regimen to humans to evaluate both efficacy and safety. The several phases of a clinical trial are (1) phase I—safety and pharmacologic profiles; (2) phase II—pilot efficacy studies; (3) phase III—extensive clinical trial; and (4) phase IV—studies after FDA approval for distribution.

Phase 0—administration of a single subtherapeutic dose of the drug to a small group (10 to 15 subjects) to gather preliminary data on pharmacokinetics and pharmacodynamics; phase I—a small group (20 to 80 subjects) of volunteers to assess the safety and pharmacokinetic profile of the medication; phase II—a large group (20 to 300 of subjects) to assess safety in a larger group of patients as well as effectiveness of the drug; phase III—randomized controlled multicenter trial on a relatively large group (300 to 3,000 or more subjects) depending on the medical condition and is to assess the effectiveness of the drug in comparison with an accepted therapy; and phase IV—involves safety surveillance and ongoing technical support of a drug after permission for it to be distributed.

4. (B) The Fisher exact test is used when the numbers in the contingency table of categorical variables are relatively small while the McNemar test is used for two groups with paired data. The Mantel–Haenszel test is an extension of the χ^2 test used when comparing several two-way tables (such as for meta-analysis studies). χ^2 test is a measure of the difference between actual and expected frequencies with categorical variables.

5. (E) Parametric tests are used to compare samples of normally (or Gaussian) distributed data. These tests include (1) the Student *t*-test (used to compare two samples to test the probability that the samples come from a population with the same mean value) and (2) the ANOVA (used to compare the means of two or more samples to see whether they are derived from the same population). The analysis of covariance (ANCOVA) is an extension of ANOVA to accommodate continuous variables. *Note:* The Kolmogorov–Smirnov test is used to test the hypothesis that the collected data are from a normal distribution so that the parametric statistics can be used.

Nonparametric tests are used when the data are not normally distributed so that the above tests are not appropriate. These tests include (1) the Wilcoxon signed-rank test (for comparing the difference between paired groups, as in *t*-test for parametric data); (2) the Mann–Whitney *U*-test or the Wilcoxon rank sum test (for comparing two sets of data that are derived from two different sets of subjects); and (3) the Kruskal–Wallis test (for comparing two or more independent groups, as in ANOVA for parametric data).

6. (E) Incidence describes the frequency of occurrence of new cases during a time period, whereas prevalence describes what proportion of the population has the disease at a specific point in time. The prevalence P depends on both the incidence I and duration D of the disease $(P = I \times D)$.

Incidence is useful to explore causal theories or to evaluate effects of preventive measures, whereas prevalence is relevant to planning of health services or assessing need for medical care in a population. Lastly, while chronic diseases can have lower incidence than prevalence, acute illnesses can be the opposite.

Incidence:

Incidence (I) (also incidence rate or incidence density) (person-time units):

$$I = \frac{\text{Number of new cases of the disease that occur in a population during a period of time}}{\text{Sum for each individual in the population of the length of time at risk of getting the disease}}$$

whereas

Cumulative incidence (CI) (also cumulative incidence rate or incidence proportion) (0–1 or %):

$$CI = \frac{\text{Number of individuals who get the disease during a certain period}}{\text{Number of individuals in the population at the beginning of the period}}$$

Prevalence:

Prevalence (P) (also prevalence rate, point prevalence rate, or prevalence proportion) (0–1 or %):

$$P = \frac{\text{Existing number of individuals having the disease at a specific time}}{\text{Number of individuals in the population at that point in time}}$$

7. (A) Correlation is often confused with "regression," which quantifies the association between two variables. Regression analysis is used to delineate how one set of data relates to another through a best fit line, in which the regression coefficient is the slope of the line. While this describes a simple linear regression, other types of regression include (1) logistic regression (variation of linear regression when there are only two possible outcomes); (2) Poisson regression (variation of regression calculations to allow for frequency of rare events); and (3) Cox proportional hazards regression model (used in survival analysis to investigate the relationship between an event and several variables).

The most common survival curve method is the Kaplan–Meier curve, which graphically displays the survival of a cohort with calculation of survival estimates upon each death or event (as seen in Figure 14.1). This figure depicts Kaplan–Meier event-free survival curves for arrhythmic events according to the combination of left ventricular ejection fraction (LVEF) with nonsustained ventricular tachycardia and baroreflex sensitivity (BRS). The total population has been divided into four groups after dichotomization of LVEF according to <35% and >35% and BRS and SD of normal intervals according to the ATRAMI cutoff values of <3 msec/mm Hg and >3 msec/mm Hg. The probability

value refers to differences in events rate between subgroups. A nonparametric test to compare the survival between two potential Kaplan–Meier curves is the log rank test.

8. (A) The sensitivity and specificity of a diagnostic test depends on more than just the "quality" of the test; they also depend on the definition of what constitutes an abnormal test. Look at the idealized graph in Figure 14.2 showing the number of patients with and without a disease arranged according to the value of a diagnostic test. This distributions overlap; the test (like most) does not distinguish normal from disease with 100% accuracy. The area of overlap indicates where the test cannot distinguish normal from disease.

In practice, we choose a cutoff (indicated by the vertical black line) above which we consider the test to be abnormal and below which we consider the test to be normal. The position of the cutpoint will determine the number of true positive, true negatives, false positives, and false negatives. We may wish to use different cutoffs for different clinical situations if we wish to minimize one of the erroneous types of test results.

9. (A) A normal or Gaussian distribution is a well-recognized curve (Fig. 14.5). This reflects a continuous probability distribution that is bell-shaped (unimodal) and symmetrical about the mean with two parameters, the mean (μ) and the variance (σ^2). The SD is the measure of dispersion or variability in a sample. The SD is used for data that are normally distributed ($\pm 1SD = 68.2\%$, $\pm 2SD = 95.4\%$, and $\pm 3SD = 99.7\%$ of data). The mean and the median of a normal distribution are equal.

Note: A quick check to see whether a distribution is normally distributed is to see whether two SD away from the mean are still within the possible range for the variable.

The t-distribution is similar to the normal distribution but more spread out with longer tails.

Examples of continuous probability distributions that are not normal include the χ^2-distribution (a right skewed distribution characterized by degrees of freedom); the F-distribution (also skewed to the right and used for comparing two variances); and the lognormal distribution (highly skewed to the right as it is the probability distribution of a random variable whose log follows the normal distribution). The binomial and Poisson distributions are types of discrete probability distributions.

10. (C) CI is the range that is likely to contain the true population mean value that would be present (if the data for the whole population is obtained). A 95% CI means that there is 95% chance that the population value lies within the stated limits. The SD indicates the variability in a sample. In a normal distribution, 95% of the distribution of the sample means is within 1.96 SD of the population mean. The SD is the SEM and the 95% CI for the mean is calculated by

Sample mean − 1.96 × SEM to sample mean + 1.96 × SEM

The size of the CI would be related to the sample size of the study (the larger the study population, the narrower the CI).

11. (C) There are two types of applied statistics. Descriptive statistics (means, medians, modes, SD, quartiles, and histograms) describe the data in a sample. Inferential statistics are statistical methods that estimate whether the results suggest a real difference between populations (such as the Student t-test, ANOVA, and the χ^2 test).

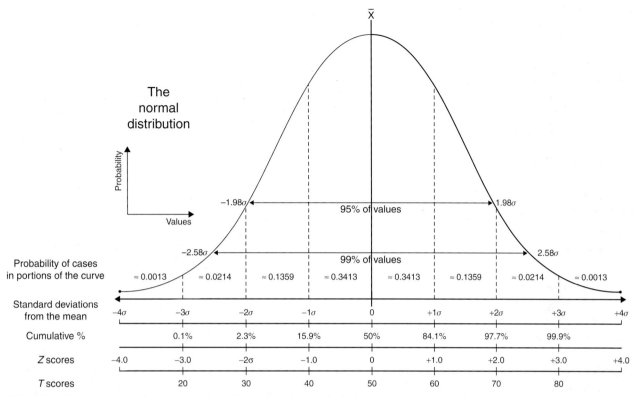

FIGURE 14.5 The normal distribution. From http://en.wikipedia.org/wiki/File:The_Normal_Distribution.svg.

12. (E) A type I error (α error) occurs when a null hypothesis that is correct is rejected (declaring that there is a difference when there is not). A type II error (β error) occurs when a hypothesis that is incorrect is accepted (declaring that a difference does not exist when in fact it does). The chance of making a type I error is the same as the *P*-value. *Note:* A type III error is a study design that produces the right answer to the wrong question.

The *P* (probability) value is the probability that defines how likely it is that a hypothesis (usually the null hypothesis) is true (that there is no difference between two treatments). The *P*-value is therefore the probability of an observed difference occurring solely by chance. The usual *P*-value at the significance level is 0.01 to 0.05. *Note:* A method used to adjust the *P*-value for multiple testing is the Bonferroni adjustment.

13. (B) The power of a study is the probability that it would detect a statistically significant difference. As the β value is the probability of accepting a hypothesis that is false, the power of the study ($1 - \beta$) is therefore the probability of rejecting the null hypothesis when it is false. The power of a study should be at least 80% and is increased by several factors including larger significance level, larger effects, decreased variability of the observations, and larger sample size.

14. (A) A CEA is an economic assessment method in which the costs and consequences of alternative interventions are expressed in costs per unit of health outcome. This commonly used methodology is applicable to health programs as well as health services to help determine the preferred action that requires the least cost to produce a given level of effectiveness.

Another economic tool is the CUA, which uses quality-of-life measurements expressed as utilities (such as QALY) in the value equation. A disability-adjusted life year (DALY) is also a measure used but is for the overall "burden of disease." It quantifies the impact of not only premature death as in QALY but also disability on a population by combining them into a single, comparable metric.

A third economic assessment methodology is the CBA, which seeks to translate all relevant healthcare considerations into monetary terms by analyzing economic and social costs of medical care and benefits of reduced loss of net earnings due to preventing premature death or disability.

Other less common methods of economic evaluation include cost-consequence analysis (CCA), CMA, and even CVA.

15. (C) A meta-analysis is a technique in which results from a number of studies that are similar in nature are gathered to give one overall estimate of the effect. The formal steps include the following: (1) decide on effect of interest, (2) check for statistical homogeneity, (3) estimate the average effect of interest with CIs, and (4) interpret the results and present the findings (forest plot). The advantages include refinement and reduction, efficiency, generalizability and consistency, reliability, and power and precision. The disadvantages include publication bias, clinical heterogeneity, quality differences, and lack of independence of study subjects.

A systemic review (such as the international network called the Cochrane collaboration with its Cochrane database of systematic reviews) often uses meta-analysis techniques to render well-informed clinical decisions; it is an essential part of evidence-based medicine. Major disease categories will often have sufficient number of randomized clinical trials for at the minimum a meta-analysis to determine the value of such an intervention.

16. (C) Risk ratio (also relative risk), used in prospective cohort studies, is calculated by dividing the risk in the treated or exposed group by the risk in the control or unexposed group (as in odds ratio, risk ratio can be <1, 1, or >1 and given with their 95% CI—if the CI includes 1, it is not statistically significant). In this case, the risk ratio is 3.4/4.9 = 0.69.

The RRR is the proportion by which the intervention reduces the event rate while the absolute risk reduction (ARR) is the difference between the event rates in the intervention versus control groups. The RRR in this study is 4.9 − 3.4/4.9 = 31%.

The NNT is the number of patients who need to be treated for one to get benefit and is the reciprocal of ARR (ARR = 100/NNT). The ARR in this case is 4.9 − 3.4 = 1.5%, so the NNT = 100/ARR = 100/1.5 = 67.

Odds ratio, used in retrospective case–control studies, is calculated by comparing odds (calculated by dividing the event occurrence by the number of times that the event does not happen) of the exposed versus control groups (odds ratio can be <1, 1, or >1 and given with their 95% CI—if the CI includes 1, it is not statistically significant).

17. (B) Risk ratio (also relative risk), used in prospective cohort studies, is calculated by dividing the risk in the treated or exposed group by the risk in the control or unexposed group (as in odds ratio, risk ratio can be <1, 1, or >1 and given with their 95% CI—if the CI includes 1, it is not statistically significant). In this case, the risk ratio is 3.4/4.9 = 0.69.

The RRR is the proportion by which the intervention reduces the event rate while the absolute risk reduction (ARR) is the difference between the event rates in the intervention versus control groups. The RRR in this study is 4.9 − 3.4/4.9 = 31%.

The NNT is the number of patients who need to be treated for one to get benefit and is the reciprocal of ARR (ARR = 100/NNT). The ARR in this case is 4.9 − 3.4 = 1.5%, so the NNT = 100/ARR = 100/1.5 = 67.

Odds ratio, used in retrospective case–control studies, is calculated by comparing odds (calculated by dividing the event occurrence by the number of times that the event does not happen) of the exposed versus control groups (odds ratio can be <1, 1, or >1 and given with their 95% CI—if the CI includes 1, it is not statistically significant).

18. (A) Risk ratio (also relative risk), used in prospective cohort studies, is calculated by dividing the risk in the treated or exposed group by the risk in the control or unexposed group (as in odds ratio, risk ratio can be <1, 1, or >1 and given with their 95% CI—if the CI includes 1, it is not statistically significant). In this case, the risk ratio is 3.4/4.9 = 0.69.

The RRR is the proportion by which the intervention reduces the event rate while the absolute risk reduction (ARR) is the difference between the event rates in the intervention versus control groups. The RRR in this study is 4.9 − 3.4/4.9 = 31%.

The NNT is the number of patients who need to be treated for one to get benefit and is the reciprocal of ARR (ARR = 100/NNT). The ARR in this case is 4.9 − 3.4 = 1.5%, so the NNT = 100/ARR = 100/1.5 = 67.

Odds ratio, used in retrospective case–control studies, is calculated by comparing odds (calculated by dividing the event

occurrence by the number of times that the event does not happen) of the exposed versus control groups (odds ratio can be <1, 1, or >1 and given with their 95% CI—if the CI includes 1, it is not statistically significant).

19. (A) The ROC curve is a two-way plot of the sensitivity (true-positive rate) against one minus the specificity (false-positive rate) for different cutoff values for a continuous variable in a diagnostic test (see excellent website with moving description of all the above at www.anaesthetist.com/mnm/stats/roc/Findex.htm). The upper left corner or coordinate (0,1) is called the perfect classification (100% sensitivity or no false negatives and 100% specificity or no false positives) (Fig. 14.6).

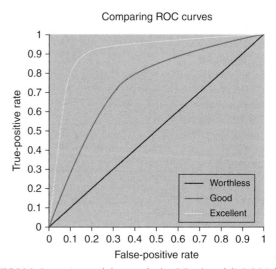

Comparing ROC curves

FIGURE 14.6 From www.mlahanas.de/MOEA/Med/ROC21.htm.

20. (E) The variance is the square of the SD while coefficient of variation is the ratio of the SD to the mean. While the SD is a measure of spread away from the mean and is equal to the square root of the variance, the SEM is a measure of precision of the sample mean or how close the sample mean is likely to be to the population mean.

21. (B) Accuracy is the degree of closeness of measurements to that quantity's true value while precision is the reproducibility of a study result with the study to be repeated under the same circumstances (measured by standard error of measurement) (Fig. 14.7).

22. (A) Chi-squared (χ^2) test is a measure of the difference between actual and expected frequencies with categorical variables; a contingency table is set up to calculate the χ^2 value. If there is no difference between actual and expected frequencies, then χ^2 would be 0. The larger the difference, the bigger the χ^2 value (but it is easier to note the P-value that accompanies the χ^2 value). The df is the number of independent comparisons that can be made between members of the sample and is used with χ^2 value to calculate the P-value. In this case, the df (of 1) is needed to calculate the P-value. The χ^2 test is sometimes used with Yates continuity correction to improve the accuracy of the P-value.

The Fisher exact test is used when the numbers in the contingency table of categorical variables are relatively small while

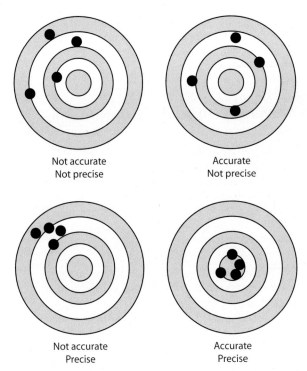

Not accurate
Not precise

Accurate
Not precise

Not accurate
Precise

Accurate
Precise

FIGURE 14.7 From http://celebrating200years.noaa.gov/magazine/tct/tct_side1.html.

the McNemar test is used for two groups with paired data. The Mantel–Haenszel test is an extension of the χ^2 test used when comparing several two-way tables (such as for meta-analysis studies).

23. (A) Correlation coefficient is the strength of the linear relationship between two variables, and this relationship is denoted by the letter r that ranges from −1 to +1 (R^2 is sometimes given to correct for negatively correlated relationships). The coefficient r cannot be calculated when there is neither a nonlinear relationship nor when there are outliers.

When the degree of linear relationship is extended to several variables, it is known as multiple correlation coefficient. The Pearson correlation coefficient "r" is used if the values are sampled from a normally distributed populations (if not, the Spearman correlation coefficient "rs" is used).

24. (A)

25. (C) Sensitivity is the probability that a diseased individual is correctly classified as sick, and specificity is the probability that a healthy individual is correctly classified as healthy. There is interdependence between sensitivity and specificity (see Fig. 14.6).

$$\text{Sensitivity} = \frac{\text{Number of sick people who are classified as sick}}{\text{Total number of sick people}}$$

$$\text{Specificity} = \frac{\text{Number of healthy people who are classified as healthy}}{\text{Total number of healthy people}}$$

Also, sensitivity/specificity and predictive values (positive and negative) relate to each other by the two-way (Table 14.5).

TABLE 14.5 Disease and Test Result

Test Result	Disease Present	Disease Absent	Total
Positive	A	B	A + B
Negative	C	D	C + D
Total	A + C	B + D	A + B + C + D

Sensitivity: A/A + C (how often the test is positive if the patient has the disease)

Specificity: D/D + B (how often the test is negative if the patient is healthy)

PPV: A/A + B (likelihood that patient has disease if test is positive)

NPV: D/D + C (likelihood that patient is healthy if test is negative)

The higher the calculated value, the more valuable the test as the perfect test will have a calculated value of 1.

An LR is the likelihood that a test result would be expected in a patient with the condition compared to the likelihood that the same result would be in a patient without the condition. To calculate this: LR = Sensitivity/(1 − Specificity).

For this case, the PPV is A/A + B or 50/55.

The LR is (A/A + C)/[1 − (D/D + B)] = (50/75)/[1 − (100/105)]. The latter implies that if the test is positive in a patient, that patient is many more times likely to have the disease than not have it.

26. (C) An RCT is a trial in which the patients are randomized to receive either the new or a control treatment. An ideal randomization involves equal group sizes, low selection bias, and low probability of confounding (accidental bias). Refinements of simple randomization include stratified randomization (controls for effects of factors), blocked randomization (assures treatment groups to be equal sized), and cluster randomization (allocates groups of patients). In addition, there is response-adaptive randomization (also termed outcome-adaptive randomization) in which the probability of being assigned to a group increases if the responses of the prior patients is deemed favorable. Allocation bias and confounding are avoided as much as possible to maximize efficiency of the study. A placebo-controlled study involves a control group that does not receive the treatment.

27. (B) Bias occurs when there is a systematic difference between the results of a study and the true results. The types of bias include observer bias (observer inaccurately assesses variable), confounding bias (spurious association), selection bias (selected study subjects not representative), information bias (measurements incorrectly recorded), publication bias (only positive results are published), and others (recall, assessment, and allocation bias).

28. (E) An association is any relationship between two measured quantities that relates them to be statistically dependent, whereas correlation defines a linear relationship between the two quantities. Causation in addition to association includes the following criteria: temporality, strength of causality, dose–response, repetition in a different population, consistency with other studies, and biologic plausibility.

29. (A) The Belmont report elucidates three principles of research ethics: (1) respect for persons: protecting the autonomy of all people and treating them with courtesy and respect and allowing for informed consent. Researchers must be truthful and conduct no deception; (2) beneficence: the philosophy of "do no harm" while maximizing benefits for the research project and minimizing risks for the research subjects; and (3) justice: ensuring reasonable, nonexploitative, and well-considered procedures are administered fairly and equally.

30. (C) The Internal Review Board (IRB), also known as the ethical review board, is a committee that is designated to approve and review research involving human subjects to protect the rights and welfare of human research subjects. The DSMB is an independent group of experts that continuously monitors the data from various aspects of a clinical trial to ensure patient safety as well as validity and scientific merit of the trial. The difference between the IRB and the DSMB is that the IRB is primarily responsible for the review of clinical protocols and related documents while the DSMB's main responsibility is to review the trial safety and efficacy data.

31. (C) Validity is the extent to which the study measures what it is intended to measure so that validity is a measurement of systematic error or bias (examples are confounding and selection bias). Reliability is the consistency of a set of measurements or a measurement tool, or the repeatability and reproducibility of such a methodology (inversely related to random error).

Accuracy is the degree of closeness of measurements to that quantity's true value while precision is the reproducibility of a study result with the study to be repeated under the same circumstances (measured by standard error of measurement).

32. (A) Sample size calculation involves the following parameters: power (usually 0.80); significance level (usually 0.01 or 0.05); variability of the observations (or the SD); and the smallest effect of interest (the standardized difference).

33. (E)
Case–control studies:
Advantages:

1. Permit the study of rare diseases.
2. Permit the study of diseases with long latency between exposure and manifestation.
3. Can be launched and conducted over relatively short time periods.
4. Relatively inexpensive as compared to cohort studies.
5. Can study multiple potential causes of disease.

Disadvantages:

1. Information on exposure and past history is primarily based on interview and may be subject to recall bias.
2. Validation of information on exposure is difficult, or incomplete, or even impossible.
3. By definition, concerned with one disease only.
4. Cannot usually provide information on incidence rates of disease.
5. Generally incomplete control of extraneous variables.
6. Choice of appropriate control group may be difficult.

7. Methodology may be hard to comprehend for nonepidemiologists, and correct interpretation of results may be difficult.

Cohort studies:
Advantages:

1. Allow complete information on the subject's exposure, including quality control of data, and experience thereafter.
2. Provide a clear temporal sequence of exposure and disease.
3. Give an opportunity to study multiple outcomes related to a specific exposure.
4. Permit calculation of incidence rates (absolute risk) as well as relative risk.
5. Methodology and results are easily understood by nonepidemiologists.
6. Enable the study of relatively rare exposures.

Disadvantages:

1. Not suited for the study of rare diseases because a large number of subjects are required.
2. Not suited when the time between exposure and disease manifestation is very long, although this can be overcome in historical cohort studies.
3. Exposure patterns, for example, the composition of oral contraceptives, may change during the course of the study and make the results irrelevant.
4. Maintaining high rates of follow-up can be difficult.
5. Expensive to carry out because a large number of subjects are usually required.
6. Baseline data may be sparse because the large number of subjects does not allow for long interviews.

[From Metric O. Cohort and Case–Control Studies, WHO.]

34. (A) Nonparametric tests are used when the data are not normally distributed. These tests include (1) the Wilcoxon signed-rank test (for comparing the difference between paired groups, as in t-test for parametric data); (2) the Mann–Whitney U-test or the Wilcoxon ranks sum test (for comparing two sets of data that are derived from two different sets of subjects); and (3) the Kruskal–Wallis test (for comparing two or more independent groups, as in ANOVA for parametric data).

35. (B) See Table 14.6.

36. (A) Categorical data include (1) nominal data that describe data that can be in categories but have no particular order or magnitude differences (such as single ventricle and biventricular surgical strategies or antiarrhythmic agent for supraventricular tachycardia) and (2) ordinal data that are data that can be allocated to an ordered set of categories (such as severity of AV valve regurgitation from mild to severe).

Numerical data include (1) discrete data that can only be certain whole numbers (such as number of reinterventions after Norwood procedure) and (2) continuous data that can be any numerical value (such as blood pressure measurements before and after ACE inhibitors).

37. (B) A case–control study is a retrospective study that studies the relationship between risk factor and outcome and

TABLE 14.6 Summary of Statistical Methods

	Numerical Data	Categorical Data
Single group	One-sample t-test or sign test[a]	Test of single proportion or sign test[a]
Two groups, paired	Paired t-test or Wilcoxon signed-rank test[a]	McNemar test
Two groups, unpaired	Unpaired t-test or Wilcoxon rank sum test[a] (Mann–Whitney U-test)	χ^2 test or Fisher exact test[a] (<5)
Multiple (>2) groups	ANOVA (one way) or Kruskal–Wallis test[a]	χ^2 test

[a]Nonparametric tests (relevant for populations that do not have a normal distribution).
[b]Used when expected frequencies are small.

uses relevant exposure or condition information from a sample of individuals with the disease or condition (cases) rather than examining the entire population.

A case series refers to the qualitative study of a single patient or small group of patients with a similar disease.

A cohort study (also termed follow-up, longitudinal, or prospective study) is a prospective observational study with study subjects (cohort) assigned to an exposure or condition category and then all followed for a defined observation period to see whether they develop disease. A historical cohort study, as the name implies, is a group of patients from the past and would not involve active enrollment of new study subjects.

38. (C) This study fits phase III criteria. Phase 0—administration of a single subtherapeutic doses of the drug to a small group (10 to 15 subjects) to gather preliminary data on pharmacokinetics and pharmacodynamics; phase I—a small group (20 to 80 subjects) of volunteers to assess the safety and pharmacokinetic profile of the medication; phase II—a large group (20 to 300 of subjects) to assess safety in a larger group of patients as well as effectiveness of the drug; phase III—randomized controlled multicenter trial on a relatively large group (300 to 3,000 or more subjects) depending on the medical condition and to assess the effectiveness of the drug in comparison with an accepted therapy; and phase IV—involves safety surveillance and ongoing technical support of a drug after permission for it to be distributed.

39. (E) The Fisher's exact test is used when the numbers in the contingency table of categorical variables are relatively small while the χ^2 test is a measure of the difference between actual and expected frequencies with categorical variables with larger (>5) populations. Both are tests used for categorical data. The other tests are all used for numerical data.

Parametric tests are used to compare samples of normally (or Gaussian) distributed data. These tests include (1) the Student t-test (used to compare two samples to test the probability that the samples come from a population with the same mean value) and (2) the ANOVA (used to compare the means of two or more

samples to see whether they are derived from the same population). The Kolmogorov–Smirnov test is used to test the hypothesis that the collected data are from a normal distribution, so that the parametric statistics can be used. Nonparametric tests are used when the data are not normally distributed, so that the above tests are not appropriate. These tests include the Wilcoxon signed-rank test (for comparing the difference between paired groups, as in t-test for parametric data).

40. (C) Incidence describes the frequency of occurrence of new cases during a time period, whereas prevalence describes what proportion of the population has the disease at a specific point in time. The prevalence P depends on both the incidence I and duration D of the disease ($P = I \times D$) (see explanation under Question 6).

Prevalence (P) (also prevalence rate, point prevalence rate, or prevalence proportion) (0–1 or %):

$$P = \frac{\text{Existing number of individuals having the disease at a specific time}}{\text{Number of individuals in the population at that point in time}}$$

41. (D) A CEA is an economic assessment method in which the costs and consequences of alternative interventions are expressed in costs per unit of health outcome. Another economic tool is the CUA, which uses quality-of-life measurements expressed as utilities (such as QALY) in the value equation. A third economic assessment methodology is the CBA, which seeks to translate all relevant healthcare considerations into monetary terms by analyzing economic and social costs of medical care and benefits of reduced loss of net earnings due to preventing premature death or disability (see Answer 14).

42. (C) A designation from level A to I as described by the US Preventive Services Task Force can be made for each review: (1) level A—good scientific evidence (benefits substantially outweigh risk); (2) level B—at least fair scientific evidence (benefits outweigh the risk); (3) level C—at least fair scientific evidence (benefit and risk too close); (4) level D—at least fair scientific evidence that risks outweigh the benefit; and (5) level I—scientific evidence is lacking, or poor quality, or conflicting.

43. (C)

44. (B)

45. (A)

46. (A)

47. (B) See Table 14.7.

TABLE 14.7 Disease and Test Result

	Disease		
Test Result	Present	Absent	Total
Positive	A	B	A + B
Negative	C	D	C + D
Total	A + C	B + D	A + B + C + D

Sensitivity: A/A + C (how often the test is positive if the patient has the disease)

Specificity: D/D + B (how often the test is negative if the patient is healthy)

PPV: A/A + B (likelihood that patient has disease if test is positive)

NPV: D/D + C (likelihood that patient is healthy if test is negative)

An LR is the likelihood that a test result would be expected in a patient with the condition compared to the likelihood that the same result would be in a patient without the condition. To calculate this: LR = sensitivity/(1 − specificity).

The higher the calculated value, the more valuable the test as the perfect test will have a calculated value of 1. The ECG as a screening tool in this case had a relatively low sensitivity and PPVs (hence one of the criticisms of ECG as a screening tool) but acceptable NPV.

48. (A) Risk ratio (also relative risk), used in prospective cohort studies, is calculated by dividing the risk in the treated or exposed group by the risk in the control or unexposed group (as in odds ratio, risk ratio can be <1,1, or >1 and given with their 95% CI—if the CI includes 1, it is not statistically significant). In this case, the risk ratio is 2.5/10 = 0.25 or 25%.

The RRR is the proportion by which the intervention reduces the event rate while the ARR is the difference between the event rates in the intervention versus control groups. The RRR in this study is 10 − 2.5/10 = 0.75 or 75%.

The NNT is the number of patients who need to be treated for one to get benefit and is the reciprocal of ARR (NNT = 100/AAR). The ARR in this case is 10 − 2.5 = 7.5%, so the NNT = 100/ARR = 100/7.5 = 13.3.

49. (B) Risk ratio (also relative risk), used in prospective cohort studies, is calculated by dividing the risk in the treated or exposed group by the risk in the control or unexposed group (as in odds ratio, risk ratio can be <1,1, or >1 and given with their 95% CI—if the CI includes 1, it is not statistically significant). In this case, the risk ratio is 2.5/10 = 0.25 or 25%.

The RRR is the proportion by which the intervention reduces the event rate while the ARR is the difference between the event rates in the intervention versus control groups. The RRR in this study is 10 − 2.5/10 = 0.75 or 75%.

The NNT is the number of patients who need to be treated for one to get benefit and is the reciprocal of ARR (NNT = 100/AAR). The ARR in this case is 10 − 2.5 = 7.5%, so the NNT = 100/ARR = 100/7.5 = 13.3.

50. (A) Risk ratio (also relative risk), used in prospective cohort studies, is calculated by dividing the risk in the treated or exposed group by the risk in the control or unexposed group (as in odds ratio, risk ratio can be <1,1, or >1 and given with their 95% CI—if the CI includes 1, it is not statistically significant). In this case, the risk ratio is 2.5/10 = 0.25 or 25%.

The RRR is the proportion by which the intervention reduces the event rate while the ARR is the difference between the event rates in the intervention versus control groups. The RRR in this study is 10 − 2.5/10 = 0.75 or 75%.

The NNT is the number of patients who need to be treated for one to get benefit and is the reciprocal of ARR (NNT = 100/AAR). The ARR in this case is 10 − 2.5 = 7.5%, so the NNT = 100/ARR = 100/7.5 = 13.3.

51. (B) Reliability is the degree to which a study produces stable and consistent results. One way to improve reliability is to minimize bias within the study. Randomization refers to the practice of randomly assigning enrolled patients in one of the treatment or control groups. Double blinding involves designing the study in such a way that providers administering the intervention, those measuring the outcomes, and patients receiving the therapy are not aware of which patients are in the treatment group and which patients are in the control group. Both randomization and double blinding can minimize the susceptibility bias which occurs when differences in the subjects at baseline between the compared groups cause differences in outcomes beyond what the difference in interventions would cause otherwise. Use of a placebo control group is also important to assure changes would not be seen in the study groups regardless of the intervention.

52. (E) Case–control studies involve reviewing risk factors for those patients who have the disease of interest and comparable control patients who do not. This type of study is used to determine the likelihood that various risk factors are more (or less) associated with the cases versus the controls. Cohort studies entail prospectively following those patients with a given exposure and those without. Some of the advantages of case–control study include the ability to study multiple risk factors and rare conditions making it appropriate for the use of evaluating congenital heart disease in children of diabetic mothers.

53. (D) A cross-sectional study involves the collection and analysis of data collected from a population at one specific point in time. In the study described in this question a representative cohort of families were surveyed to help determine the prevalence of chest pain in the pediatric population. A census would not be a type of study design and therefore is not the correct answer. A retrospective cohort study would involve the review of records from a cohort of patients described, but that was not done in this case. A prospective cohort study would involve following a group of patients forward in time to determine which of them developed disease rather than a point in time analysis as described in this study. A cross-sectional study is very useful for determining prevalence of a disease making it an appropriate study design choice for the clinical question of interest.

54. (A) The more participants that enroll in a study, the higher the sensitivity is for detecting adverse events. Type II error refers to the inability to reject the null hypothesis when a difference between study groups truly exists. In other terms, this can be thought of as a false-negative finding. One way to decrease this risk is to increase the sample size studied thereby increasing the power and the ability to find a difference if one truly exists. Type I error refers to the rejection of the null hypothesis when a true difference does not exist (i.e., false-positive study results). This is changed by adjusting the significance rate which is typically set at 0.05 where statistical analysis of results must show a less than 5% chance that the results are related to chance rather than a true difference to be termed "significant".

55. (C) A prospective cohort study is a type of study design in which patients with exposure to the intervention of interest (angiotensin II receptor blocker therapy) and those without are followed forward in time for the development of the measured outcome (aortic root dilation). This is not a retrospective study because patients were followed forward in time rather than review of previous records. This study would not be useful to determine the natural epidemiology of aortic root dilation in Marfan syndrome because there is an intervention. The healthy entrant effect refers to a lower morbidity/mortality in patients entering a study than the general population due to the design of the study. The healthy entrant effect is not a factor in this study.

56. (D) Specificity refers to the ability of a test to correctly identify those without the disease. In this case, transient QT prolongation can be seen in patients following syncope [Van Dorn CS, Johnson JN, Taggart NW, et al. QTc values among children and adolescents presenting to the emergency department. *Pediatrics.* 2011;128(6):e1395–e1401.]; so an ECG showing QT prolongation in a patient following syncope is not specific for the diagnosis of long QT syndrome. A negative predictive value refers to the ability of a negative test to truly predict patients without the disease. Reliability refers to the ability of a test (ECG) to demonstrate the same (QTc) value on repeat checks and validity refers to a test's ability to demonstrate an accurate (QTc) value. Neither reliability nor validity are in question for the ECG obtained in the emergency department.

57. (D) Studies are comprised of a representative sample of the population of interest which in this case is older adolescents with hyperlipidemia. Data are collected on these patients and a mean value is determined based on the measured outcome (cholesterol level). A 95% confidence interval is calculated around the mean value for each group. The 95% confidence interval is the range of values that are 95% certain to contain the true mean for a population based on data from the representative cohort. It does NOT represent the values between which 95% of the sample or population values fall. In this case the 95% confidence values for cholesterol level in adolescents with the intervention (food intake recording, weekly weigh-ins, and weekly group education) was 149 to 173.

58. (C) Recall bias is a type of systematic error which occurs as a result of inaccurate recollection of events by study participants when asked to describe events from the past. This is particularly challenging and prone to bias for events with a significant emotional component such as the death of a child. Lead-time (aka length) bias refers to the inaccurate perception that a given test improves survival time for an illness when in reality survival is not prolonged, but rather a patient is recognized as having the disease at an early point in the disease course. Selection bias is another type of systematic error which results from the nonrandom collection of participants in a study such that certain traits are selected for. Referral bias is the bias created when only a subset of the population is included in the study. This typically happens when the center performing the study is a tertiary referral center and the patients who are referred to the center represent the most complicated subset of patients and not the disease pattern seen in the general community. This creates a study cohort which is not truly representative of the population of interest.

59. (B) The odds ratio statistically describes the association between an exposure and the risk of the outcome of interest. In this case, the odds ratio describes the association between having an AV canal defect and the risk of anemia. Since the odds ratio is <1, this indicates a decreased risk for anemia in

patients with AV canal defect. An odds ratio >1 indicates an increased association. This odds ratio is likely to be statistically significant ($P < 0.05$) because the 95% confidence interval does not include 1.

60. (A) This study describes the use of a continuous variable (number of rejection episodes) both pre- and postintervention (initiation of sirolimus) in the same patient. Because this is a continuous variable with sample size >25, you can use a parametric test which in this case would be Student *t*-test. The correct answer is to use the paired Student *t*-test because each patient is studied both before and after the intervention thereby providing two matched cohorts. The Wilcoxon signed-rank test is a nonparametric test used to compare cohort means in samples that are nonnormally distributed or with low number of participants. Chi-squared is an analysis used to compare categorical outcomes rather than continuous variables. An odds ratio demonstrates the odds of developing a given outcome in those patients with a particular exposure and those without. A Kaplan–Meier curve is a method to display survival results graphically and not a form of statistical analysis.

61. (A) The odds ratio describes the odds of the outcome of interest (endocarditis) in those patients with the exposure (valve replacement). It is calculated by the equation $(A \times D)/(B \times C)$; see Table 14.8. Odds ratio can be calculated from multiple different study designs including case–control studies.

TABLE 14.8 A Case–Control Study in Cardiology: Determination of the Odds Ratio

	Endocarditis Present	No Endocarditis Present
Prosthetic valve replacement	A = 10	B = 40
No prosthetic valve replacement	C = 2	D = 48

62. (A) Chi-squared analysis is used to statistically evaluate nominal data but is not the appropriate test for continuous data. To use chi-squared analysis several assumptions must be fulfilled including random and completely independent study groups, all cells of the table must have an expected value of >5, and data must be able to be arranged in a table form (i.e., nominal data). We generally define a statistically significant *P*-value as <0.05 which means that there is less than a 5% chance that the data distribution seen in the study could have occurred by random chance.

63. (A) The normal distribution of data in a study refers to the fact that random data will demonstrate a bell-shaped curve when graphed. However, data can often be skewed or nonnormally distributed particularly if there are a small number of participants in the study. The Fischer exact test is a nonparametric test used to statically analyze the association between two groups which are not normally distributed and therefore would have been the appropriate test to use in the study described. In order to use chi-squared analysis, you must have normally distributed data with at least five participants in each cell of the table. The study described does not satisfy these criteria and therefore chi-squared analysis would not be appropriate to use and may provide a falsely low *P*-value. The Wilcoxon signed-rank test and *t*-test are both used for the analysis of continuous data rather than categorical data.

64. (A) In a survival curve, patients are defined as being censored or noncensored. Those patients who are censored dropped out of the study for reasons other than the event of interest, which in this case is death. That can be due to withdrawal from the study, being lost to follow-up, or being alive at the end of the study period. Those patients who had the event of interest (death) are defined as being noncensored.

65. (A) A number needed to treat (NNT) cannot be calculated with continuous data. Data must be categorical and binary to appropriately calculate the NNT. Remember that the NNT = 1/ absolute risk reduction (ARR).

66. (B) The kappa statistic demonstrates agreement between two groups when there is no clear gold standard. The kappa statistic can range from −1 (negative association) to 1 (positive association) with 0 demonstrating no association between the two groups. Sensitivity calculations and a receiver operating curve can be used to evaluate a test when there is a clear gold standard, but this type of analysis would not be appropriate in this study. Regression analysis can demonstrate the relationship between a dependent variable and one or more independent variables; however, in this study the two scores cannot be defined as dependent and independent, so this would not be the appropriate statistical analysis.

67. (A) The Fischer exact test is a nonparametric test used to analyze categorical data with sample sizes that are too small to allow for the use of the χ^2 analysis. For χ^2 analysis to be used there must be more than five patients in each cell and this would not be the case for the study described, hence it would not be appropriate to utilize this test for the data presented. The Student

t-test is for continuous data which were not reported in this study. ANOVA analysis is used to compare the mean values from three or more groups and the Kruskal–Wallis test is the nonparametric equivalent of the ANOVA analysis.

68. (A) ANOVA analysis is a parametric test used to compare group means when there are three or more independent groups in a study. If the *P*-value calculated using ANOVA analysis is statistically significant (typically defined as $P < 0.05$) this indicates that there is a difference in the group means among the multiple study groups, but not specifically where the difference lies or how great a difference there is. Additional analysis comparing each group to the other is required to tease out the exact difference.

69. (A) The graph shown in the question demonstrates a skewed distribution of the data. Although the distribution for the other two groups is not shown, you can assume that these may be non-normally distributed as well due to the small number of patients in each group. The Kruskal–Wallis test is used to compare the mean values among multiple groups when ANOVA testing is not appropriate, such as this case in which the data are not normally distributed. χ^2 analysis is used to evaluate categorical data rather than group means and therefore would not be appropriate to use. Student *t*-test is for analyzing two mean values, but in this case there are three groups again making this an incorrect test to choose.

70. (C) If *P* is <0.05, then the null hypothesis has been disproven and there is a difference between the study groups. The null hypothesis when comparing multiple independent variables (genetic markers) to one dependent outcome (presence of DiGeorge syndrome) is that none of the independent variables is associated with the outcome of interest. The null hypothesis is accepted if *P* is >0.05. Type I error occurs if the null hypothesis is rejected but is really true (false positive). A type II error occurs when the null hypothesis is not rejected but there is really a difference between the groups (false negative).

SUGGESTED READINGS

Ahlbom A, Norell S. *Introduction to Modern Epidemiology.* Chestnut Hill, MA: Epidemiology Resources Inc.; 1990.

Harris M, Taylor G. *Medical Statistics Made Easy.* London: Taylor and Francis; 2004.

Last JM. *A Dictionary of Epidemiology.* Oxford: Oxford University Press; 2001.

Petrie A, Sabin C. *Medical Statistics at a Glance.* Oxford: Blackwell Publishing; 2005.

Index

Note: Page number followed by f and t indicates figure and table respectively.

C

Percutaneous balloon angioplasty, of peripheral pulmonary artery stenosis, 31, 51
Pericardial calcification, noncontrast CT for, 107, 120
Pericardial defect, magnetic resonance imaging for, 43, 57–58
Pericardial effusion, 63, 71, 186, 194–195
   with cardiac tamponade, 100, 115
Pericardial tamponade, 201, 211
Pericardial volume and pericardial pressure, relationship between, 203, 212
Pericardiocentesis
   indication for, 62, 70
   sudden circulatory collapse and, 76, 90
Pericardium, calcified, 86, 86f, 94
Pericytes, 16
Permanent junctional reciprocating tachycardia (PJRT), 129, 159
Persistent left superior vena cava (LSVC), 29, 50
Persistent pulmonary hypertension, 214
Phase-contrast (velocity-encoded) cine imaging, 107, 119
Phenoxybenzamine, 233, 243
Phenylephrine, 61, 70
Phenylketonuria, maternal, 23, 46
Phenytoin, in LQTS type 1, 234, 243
Platypnea-orthodeoxia syndrome, 270, 285
Poiseuille–Hagen relationship, 2, 13
Polycythemia, 85, 94
Polysplenia, 1, 13, 101, 116
Pompe disease, 134, 134f, 162
Postcoarctectomy hypertension, 200, 209
Postpericardiotomy syndrome, fever and, 256, 263
Poststenotic pulmonary artery dilation, 80, 80f, 92
Posttransplant lymphoproliferative disorder (PTLD), 222, 227
Potassium abnormality, on ECG, 142, 143f, 165
Potts shunt, 120, 249, 258
Power of study, 295, 305
Pregnancy
   absolute contraindication to, 268, 284
   ACE inhibitors in, 268, 284
   risk of cardiac complication during, 268, 270, 284, 285
Prehypertension, 182, 190
Premature atrial beats, in fetus, 129, 159
Premature atrial contractions (PAC), 105, 118, 123, 157
Prevalence, 294, 298, 304, 309
Primum atrial septal defect, 130, 160
PR interval, 105, 118
Procainamide, 238, 247
Propranolol, for SVT in Wolff–Parkinson–White syndrome, 129, 159
Prospective cohort study, 300, 310–311
Prostacyclin, 200, 210, 235, 244
Prostaglandin, 13, 34, 53
Prostaglandin E1 (PGE1), side effects of, 235, 244
Protamine, 82, 92
Proton pump inhibitor, discontinuation of, 237, 246
PTPN11 mutations, 46
Pulmonary arterial hypertension (PAH), 184, 192
Pulmonary arteries, 2, 13
Pulmonary arteriolar resistance, 77, 80, 91, 92
Pulmonary arteriovenous fistulae, 29, 50, 259
Pulmonary arteriovenous malformations, 86, 94, 250, 258
Pulmonary artery banding, 42, 57
Pulmonary artery pressure, in children living at altitude, 9, 18
Pulmonary artery sling, 27, 49
Pulmonary artery thrombus, 199, 209

Pulmonary atresia
   and intact ventricular septum, 31, 51, 52, 88, 95, 105, 118, 136, 137f, 162–163, 252, 260
   with VSD, 32, 33, 35, 52, 53, 253, 260
Pulmonary blood flow, 77, 91, 267, 283–284
Pulmonary hypertension, 150, 150f, 166, 200, 209, 210
   atrial septal defect and, 24, 46
   irreversible, risk factors for, 202, 212
   mitral valve stenosis and, 37, 54
   after repair for total anomalous pulmonary venous drainage, 203, 212
Pulmonary overcirculation, in infant, 183, 191
Pulmonary sequestration, 93
Pulmonary situs, 117
Pulmonary stenosis, 252, 260
   classification of severity of, 31, 50
   congenital rubella syndrome and, 68, 74
   and left ventricular hypertrophy, 62, 70
   in neonate, 100, 115
   and valvuloplasty, 31, 50
   worsening of, 65, 72
Pulmonary to systemic blood flow ratio, in single ventricle physiology patients, 202, 211
Pulmonary valve ejection click, 70
Pulmonary valve regurgitation, 193
Pulmonary valvuloplasty, recommendations for, 88, 95, 95t
Pulmonary vascular resistance (PVR), 81, 83, 92, 93, 235, 244, 293, 303
Pulmonary vasoconstrictors, 204, 211, 213
Pulmonary vasodilators, 201, 211
Pulmonary veins, cardiac myocytes in, 9, 19
Pulmonary venous desaturation, 86, 94
Pulmonary venous plexus, 11, 20
Pulsatility index, 106, 119
Pulsed-wave (PW) Doppler, 97, 112
Pulsus paradoxus, 185, 193
   and pericardiocentesis, 62, 70
PVR. *See* Pulmonary vascular resistance (PVR)
PW Doppler, 99, 114

R
Randomized controlled trial (RCT), 296, 307
Rastelli operation, 56
RA waveform, components of, 84, 93
RCM. *See* Restrictive cardiomyopathy (RCM)
Recall bias, 300, 311
Receiver operating characteristic (ROC) curve, 295, 306, 306f
Reentrant supraventricular tachycardia, 125, 158
Referral bias, 311
Regression analysis, 304, 312
Relative risk reduction (RRR), 295, 299, 306, 310
Reliability, 297, 299, 308, 310
Renin, 2, 13
Respiratory acidosis, acute, 12, 21
Restrictive cardiomyopathy (RCM), 45, 59, 67, 73, 204, 213, 220, 221, 225, 226
   and elevated right atrial pressure, 203, 212
   glycogen-storage disease and, 186, 194
Restrictive LV physiology, echocardiographic hallmarks of, 98, 113
Restrictive physiology, 85, 94
REV procedure, 56
RF. *See* Rheumatic fever (RF)